Alcoholic Liver Disease: An Issue of Clinics in Liver Disease

Alcoholic Liver Disease: An Issue of Clinics in Liver Disease

Editor: Seth Norton

AMERICAN
MEDICAL PUBLISHERS
www.americanmedicalpublishers.com

AMERICAN
MEDICAL PUBLISHERS
www.americanmedicalpublishers.com

Cataloging-in-Publication Data

Alcoholic liver disease : an issue of clinics in liver disease / edited by Seth Norton.
p. cm.
Includes bibliographical references and index.
ISBN 978-1-63927-864-0
1. Alcoholic liver diseases. 2. Alcoholic liver diseases--Diagnosis.
3. Alcoholic liver diseases--Treatment. 4. Liver--Diseases. 5. Alcoholism--Complications.
I. Norton, Seth.
RC848.A42 A43 2023
616.362--dc23

American Medical Publishers,
41 Flatbush Avenue,
1st Floor, New York,
NY 11217, USA

ISBN 978-1-63927-864-0 (Hardback)

Contents

Preface

Every book is initially just a concept; it takes months of research and hard work to give it the final shape in which the readers receive it. In its early stages, this book also went through rigorous reviewing. The notable contributions made by experts from across the globe were first molded into patterned chapters and then arranged in a sensibly sequential manner to bring out the best results.

The chronic liver disease which is caused by excessive consumption of alcohol is known as alcoholic liver disease. It has various stages, and can progress from alcoholic fatty liver to alcoholic steatohepatitis. It can also lead to more severe medical conditions such as cirrhosis and hepatocellular cancer. The severity to which this disease affects different people can be influenced by epigenetic, genetic and non-genetic factors. A few of its major symptoms are fluid buildup in legs, abnormal bleeding, poor appetite and redness of palms. Alcoholic liver disease can be diagnosed through physical tests, imaging tests and blood tests. The degree of the progression of this disease can be determined by tests such as transient elastography, ultrasonography, MRI and liver biopsy. This book contains some path-breaking studies on alcoholic liver disease. It strives to provide a fair idea about this liver disease and to help develop a better understanding of the latest advances towards its treatment. Researchers and students actively engaged in the field of hepatology will find this book full of crucial and unexplored concepts.

It has been my immense pleasure to be a part of this project and to contribute my years of learning in such a meaningful form. I would like to take this opportunity to thank all the people who have been associated with the completion of this book at any step.

Editor

1

Fenretinide Improves Intestinal Barrier Function and Mitigates Alcohol Liver Disease

Xiao-Han Tang[1†], *Marta Melis*[1†], *Karen Mai*[2], *Lorraine J. Gudas*[1] *and Steven E. Trasino*[1,2*]

[1]Department of Pharmacology, Weill Cornell Medical College of Cornell University, New York, NY, United States, [2]Nutrition Program, Hunter College, City University of New York, New York, NY, United States

***Correspondence:**
Steven E. Trasino
steven.trasino@hunter.cuny.edu

†These authors have contributed equally to this work and share first authorship

Alcohol liver disease (ALD) is a major cause of liver-related mortality globally, yet there remains an unmet demand for approved ALD drugs. The pathogenesis of ALD involves perturbations to the intestinal barrier and subsequent translocation of bacterial endotoxin that, acting through toll-like receptor 4 (TLR4), promotes hepatic inflammation and progression of ALD. In the present study we investigated the ability of fenretinide (Fen) [N-(4-hydroxyphenyl) retinamide], a synthetic retinoid with known anti-cancer and anti-inflammatory properties, to modulate intestinal permeability and clinical hallmarks of ALD in a mouse model of chronic ethanol (EtOH) exposure. Our results show that EtOH-treated mice had reductions in mRNA and protein expression of intestinal tight junction proteins, including claudin one and occludin, and increases in intestinal permeability and endotoxemia compared to pair-fed mice. Also, EtOH-treated mice had marked increases in hepatic steatosis, liver injury, and expression of pro-inflammatory mediators, including TNF-α, and TLR4-positive macrophages, Kupffer cells, and hepatocytes in the intestines and liver, respectively. In contrast, EtOH + Fen-treated mice were resistant to the effects of EtOH on promoting intestinal permeability and had higher intestinal protein levels of claudin one and occludin. Also, EtOH + Fen-treated mice had significantly lower plasma levels of endotoxin, and reductions in expression of TNF-α and TLR4 positive macrophages, Kupffer cells, and hepatocytes in the intestine and liver. Lastly, we found that EtOH + Fen-treated mice exhibited major reductions in hepatic triglycerides, steatosis, and liver injury compared to EtOH-treated mice. Our findings are the first to demonstrate that Fen possesses anti-ALD properties, potentially through modulation of the intestinal barrier function, endotoxemia, and TLR4-mediated inflammation. These data warrant further pre-clinical investigations of Fen as a potential anti-ALD drug.

Keywords: alcohol, fenretinide, gut barrier, endotoxemia, toll-like receptor 4, steatosis, inflammation, tumor necrosis factor-α

INTRODUCTION

Alcohol liver disease (ALD) is responsible for almost half of all liver-related deaths around the world and is the second most common cause of all liver transplants (Rehm et al., 2013). There are currently no FDA-approved drugs for the treatment of ALD, and therapeutic drugs that aid in alcohol abstinence are generally ineffective (Osna et al., 2017). The pathogenesis of ALD is complex and multifactorial, but multiple lines of evidence support that chronic alcohol intake disrupts gastrointestinal tight junction proteins (TJPs), increasing the gut translocation of bacterial lipopolysaccharide (LPS) into the systemic blood, where it stimulates the release of pro-inflammatory mediators including tumor necrosis factor-α (TNF-α) from liver Kupffer cells through toll-like receptor 4 (TLR4) (Bode et al., 1987; Rao, 2009; Samuelson et al., 2019). Moreover alcohol sensitizes Kupffer cells and hepatocytes to the pro-inflammatory effects of LPS and TNF-α, creating a vicious gut-liver inflammation cycle (Petrasek et al., 2010).

Conversely, mice harboring inactivating mutations in TLR4 or TNF- α receptor I (TNFRI) are protected against alcohol-mediated gut barrier disruption, hepatic steatosis, and progression ALD (Uesugi et al., 2001; Chen et al., 2015). Moreover, a convincing body of evidence shows that anti-inflammatory dietary medium chain fatty acids and ω-3 polyunsaturated fatty acids (PUFAs) preserve gut barrier and inhibit TLR4 mediated inflammation and ALD in alcohol-fed rodents (Kirpich et al., 2012; Zhong et al., 2013). Despite the known role that dysregulation of the gut barrier has in the development of ALD (Bode et al., 1987; Rao, 2009; Samuelson et al., 2019), to date no drugs have been examined for their potential to protect barrier function and mitigate the progression of hallmarks of ALD, including hepatic steatosis, steatohepatitis, and fibrosis.

Fenretinide (Fen) [N-4-hydroxyphenyl-retinamide, 4-HPR] is a synthetic derivative of all-trans retinoic acid that has been primarily studied for its promising anti-cancer properties in numerous clinical trials of adult and pediatric cancers (Veronesi et al., 2006; Cooper et al., 2017). Fen inhibits cancer cell proliferation through the induction of reactive oxygen species (ROS) and apoptosis through mechanisms that are incompletely understood [reviewed in (Hail et al., 2006)]. Recently, studies have demonstrated that Fen possesses anti-inflammatory properties (López-Vales et al., 2010; Lachance et al., 2013; Kanagaratham et al., 2014; Lin et al., 2016), marked by inhibition of LPS-induced expression of inflammatory mediators such as IL-1β and TNF-α in mouse models of allergic asthma (Kanagaratham et al., 2014), and LPS-disruption of the blood brain barrier TJP occludin (Li et al., 2020). Moreover, evidence shows that Fen also possesses anti-diabetic properties (Preitner et al., 2009) and can mitigate hepatic fatty steatosis in genetic and dietary models of non-alcoholic fatty liver disease (NAFLD) (Preitner et al., 2009; Koh et al., 2012), which shares pathological features of ALD (Sanyal et al., 2016). Therefore, in light of these data, and its history of safety and low toxicity in humans (Veronesi et al., 2006; Cooper et al., 2017), we sought to examine for the first time the effects of Fen on intestinal barrier function and progression of ALD in a model of chronic ethanol exposure in mice.

MATERIALS AND METHODS

Animals

All animal experiments were conducted in accordance with the Guide for the Care and Use of Laboratory Animals as adopted and promulgated by the U.S. National Institutes of Health and the Institutional Animal Care and Use Committee (IACUC) guidelines at Hunter College.

Liquid Ethanol Diet

Male Wild type (Wt) C57BL/6J mice (8–9-week-old) (n = 20) were purchased from Jackson Laboratory and were housed in standard cages with 2-mice per cage and fed standard laboratory chow (rodent diet #2014, Harlan-Teklad, Madison, WI, United States) prior to initiation of liquid diet feeding. After 7 days, mice were switched from chow diet to a nutritionally sufficient, control liquid diet (Lieber-DeCarli-shake and pour control liquid diet, Bio-Serve, Inc. diet #F1259SP) for 5 days. After 5 days, mice were randomly assigned to either remain on a liquid control diet (n = 8) or switched to an ethanol liquid diet (n = 12) (Lieber-DeCarli-shake and pour ethanol liquid diet, Bio-Serve, #F1258SP) for acclimatization as follows: 1% ethanol (v/v) for 2 days, 2% (v/v) for 3 days. After 5 days, ethanol-fed mice were switched to either 5% ethanol v/v (approximately 27.6% kcal from ethanol) plus vehicle [0.1% DMSO] in their liquid diet (EtOH-treated, n = 6), or 5% ethanol plus fenretinide (Apexbio, Inc) [10 mg/kg/day] (EtOH + Fen). A group of liquid control-fed mice (n = 4) were switched to Fen at a dose of 10 mg/kg/day. All control diet-fed mice were pair-fed (no EtOH) to the mean 24 h intake of 5% EtOH-treated mice. Control and ethanol diets were prepared fresh daily. All groups remained on their diets for 25 days. Changes to food intake and body weight were similar across all experimental groups throughout the study period (**Supplementary Figures S1A,B**).

In vivo Intestinal Permeability Assay

Determination of intestinal permeability was performed as previously described (Volynets et al., 2016). Mice were fasted for 4 h and then administered fluorescein isothiocyanate (FITC)-dextran D4000 (4-kDa, dissolved in sterile PBS 100 mg/ml) (Sigma-Aldrich, #FD4) at a dose of 600 mg/kg body weight by oral gavage. Two hours after gavage, blood was collected from the tail vein in heparinized tubes, protected from light, and immediately centrifuged (2,000 ×g) to collect plasma fractions. Plasma FITC-dextran was measured at an excitation wavelength of 490 nm and an emission wavelength of 520 nm on a fluorescence spectrophotometer. Standard curves were generated with serial dilutions of FITC-dextran in nontreated mouse plasma to determine plasma concentrations.

Plasma Biochemical Assays

Blood samples for the following biochemical assays were collected from the tail vein 2 h after lights off when blood alcohol content (BAC) levels peak in rodents (Freund, 1970). BAC levels were measured in plasma samples using a commercially available ethanol assay kit (Sigma-Aldrich, Inc.). Plasma alanine aminotransferase (ALT) and aspartate aminotransferase (AST) activity were measured using commercially available enzymatic assay kits (BioAssay Systems, Inc.) following the manufacturer's protocol. Plasma endotoxin (LPS) was measured under pyrogen-free conditions using a Limulus amebocyte lysate (LAL) chromogenic LPS kit following the manufacturer's protocol (Thermo, Inc).

Immunohistochemistry

Immunohistochemistry (IHC) was performed as previously described (Trasino et al., 2016). Briefly, after deparaffinization and re-hydration with graded alcohol concentrations, deparaffinized ileum and liver tissue sections were incubated with the following primary antibodies overnight at 4°C: Occludin 1 (Rabbit polyclonal, #13409, Proteintech, Inc.), claudin 1 (Rabbit polyclonal, #13050, Proteintech, Inc.), TNF-α (Rabbit polyclonal, #A0277, Abclonal, Inc.), TLR4 (Mouse monoclonal, clone 76B357.1, Novus, Inc.), F4/80 (Rat monoclonal, #ab6640, Abcam, Inc.), α-Smooth Muscle Actin (Rabbit monoclonal #19245, Cell Signaling Inc.), and 4 Hydroxynonenal (4-HNE) (Rabbit polyclonal, #ab46545, Abcam, Inc.). After overnight incubation, samples were treated with the appropriate HRP- or fluorescent-conjugated secondary antibodies (SuperBoost Goat anti-Rabbit Poly HRP, Thermo, Inc.), or goat anti-rabbit IgG, Alexa Fluor 488 and 594 (Thermo, Inc.). HRP-conjugated antibodies were visualized with 3,3-diaminobenzidine (DAB).

Liver Fibrosis and Collagen Deposition

To determine liver collagen deposition and fibrosis, paraffin embedded liver sections were stained with Masson's Trichrome Kit (Poly Scientific, Bayshore, NY, United States), according to the manufacturers' protocol. Liver collagen was then analyzed by color densitometry analysis using Fiji ImageJ software as described (Schindelin et al., 2012).

Quantitation of Immunofluorescence and Immunohistochemistry

For quantitation of intestinal and liver antibody staining, slide images were photographed using a Nikon Ts2-inverted fluorescent microscope. Approximately 10-15 FITC-488, TRITC-594, and DAB tissue positive fields per slide, with one slide per mouse, and four to six mice per dietary group, for a total of 40–90 antibody positive fields per experimental group, were analyzed by color densitometry analysis using Fiji ImageJ software as described (Schindelin et al., 2012).

RNA Isolation and Quantitative RT-PCR

Total RNA was extracted and purified from 2 cm portions of ileum (approximately 10–15 mg) and liver samples (approximately 10–15 mg) using the RNeasy Mini Kit (Qiagen, Inc.). RNA concentration and purity were measured on a Nanodrop One (Thermo, Inc.). Total RNA (1 μg) was used to synthesize cDNA using the RevertAid First Strand cDNA Synthesis Kit (Thermo, Inc.). Quantitative RT-PCR (q-PCR) was performed as previously described (Trasino et al., 2016) using SYBR Green PCR master mix on an Agilent Mx3000P Real Time PCR system (Agilent, Inc.). Gene specific primers (**Supplementary Table S1**) were used to amplify target mRNAs that were normalized to the internal control mRNA, *36B4*. Relative gene expression fold changes were calculated using the delta, delta Ct method (Livak and Schmittgen, 2001).

Quantification of Intestinal Bacterial

Total DNA was extracted and purified from the intestinal cecum using QIAamp DNA Mini Kit (Qiagen, Inc). Cecum DNA (1 μg) was amplified for total bacterial species using universal bacterial primers (Horz et al., 2005) (**Supplementary Table S1**) on an Agilent Mx3000P Real Time PCR system (Agilent, Inc.). The relative levels of total bacterial species are expressed as relative fold change compared to pair-fed mice.

Statistical Analysis

Group means differences are reported as means +/− SD and were analyzed using repeated measures ANOVA and Dunnett's multiple comparison test. Group means were treated as independent variables and computed using ANOVA and Dunnett's multiple comparison test when sample numbers were not equal. Significant differences were defined as *p*-values of less than 0.05, and all usage of the term "significant" throughout the text refers to means differences with a $p < 0.05$. All statistical analyses were performed using GraphPad Prism version 8.0 statistical software (GraphPad Software, Inc.).

RESULTS

Fenretininde Reduces Ethanol-Induced Intestinal Permeability and Endotoxemia

Alcohol-induced intestinal hyper-permeability and endotoxemia are key contributors to the pathogenesis of ALD (Bode et al., 1987; Rao, 2009); therefore, we measured intestinal permeability *in vivo* with an oral dose FITC-dextran into the systemic blood as previously described (Volynets et al., 2016). We found that chronic alcohol exposure markedly altered intestinal permeability, as we detected over a 110% increase in blood FITC-dextran concentrations in EtOH-treated compared to pair-fed mice (**Figure 1A**), whereas blood concentrations of FITC-dextran levels were reduced by 36% in EtOH + Fen-treated compared to EtOH-treated mice (**Figure 1A**). No differences in FITC-dextran blood levels were detected between pair-fed and pair-fed + Fen-treated mice (**Figure 1A**). Given that the intestine is the source of bacterial LPS in the pathogenesis of ALD (Keshavarzian et al., 2009), we next sought to determine the effect of Fen treatments on LPS translocations into the systemic blood in both EtOH cohorts of mice. We found that systemic LPS levels in EtOH-treated mice were increased ~2.2-fold compared to pair-fed mice and, consistent with the reductions in gut permeability (**Figure 1A**), EtOH + Fen-treated mice showed reductions in systemic LPS and endotoxemia of over 30% compared to EtOH-treated mice (**Figure 1B**).

Human and experimental animal models have demonstrated that chronic alcohol exposure is associated with intestinal microbiota dysbiosis, which is marked by bacterial overgrowth that can contribute to increased intestinal hyper-permeability (Rao, 2009; Yan et al., 2011). Therefore, we next measured intestinal bacterial load in the cecum by qPCR using universal 16s rRNA bacterial primers (**Supplementary Table S1**). Consistent with previous rodent studies (Keshavarzian et al., 2009; Yan et al., 2011), we found that the cecal total bacteria contents in EtOH-treated were

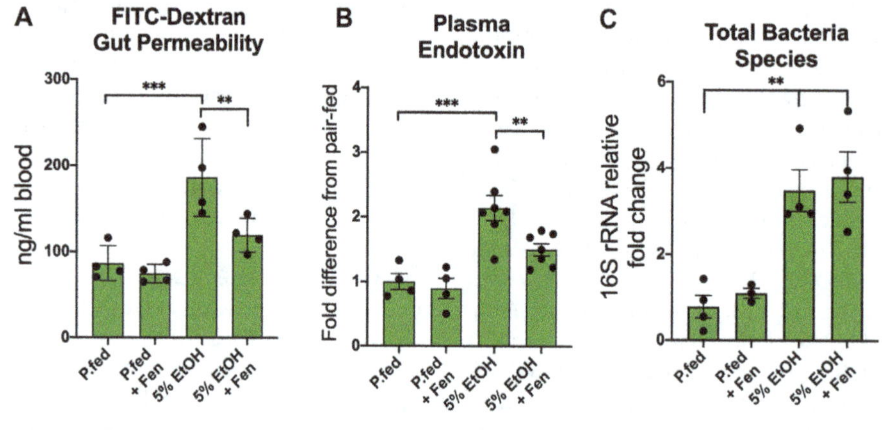

FIGURE 1 | Fenretininde prevents intestinal hyper-permeability and endotoxemia. **(A)** Blood levels of 4-kDa fluorescein isothiocyanate (FITC) dextran 2 h after oral gavage. **(B)** Plasma endotoxin (LPS) fold change 2 h after peak blood alcohol content relative to pair-fed mice. **(C)** Intestinal total bacterial species measured as cecum 16S rDNA fold change relative to pair-fed mice. All data error bars represent ±SD, with $^{**}p < 0.01$, $^{***}p < 0.001$.

approximately 4.5-fold higher compared to pair-fed mice (**Figure 1C**). We did not detect mean differences in cecal total bacterial content between EtOH-treated and EtOH + Fen-treated mice (**Figure 1C**). Given that food intake and peak blood alcohol levels were unchanged between EtOH-treated and EtOH + Fen-treated mice (**Supplementary Figures S1A,C**), the Fen-associated improvements to the intestinal barrier and systemic endotoxemia were likely not a result of alterations in gut bacterial overgrowth or alcohol exposure.

Fenretininde Increases Expression of Intestinal Tight Junction Proteins

Intestinal barrier function is mediated by tight-junction proteins (TJPs), such as occludin, claudins, zona occludins 1 (ZO-1), and other adaptor proteins such as cingulin and fordrin (Groschwitz and Hogan, 2009). Numerous lines of evidence demonstrate that alcohol-mediated increases in intestinal permeability are associated with perturbations and reductions in the expression and function of TJPs, such as occludin and claudins, permitting paracellular translocation and translocation of bacterial products and further exacerbating local and systemic endotoxemia and inflammation (Wang et al., 2014; Samuelson et al., 2019). Therefore, given that we detected increases in gut permeability and endotoxemia in EtOH-treated mice, we assessed mRNA and protein levels of TJPs in the intestinal ileum using qPCR and immunofluorescence (IF). By qPCR analysis EtOH-treated mice showed approximately 2.5-fold reductions in ileum mRNA levels of TJPs claudin 1, occludin, and ZO-1 (**Figures 2A–C**). We also found that, compared to pair-fed mice, ileum mRNA levels of the TJP adaptor proteins fordin and symplekin were reduced in EtOH-treated mice by 1.8 and 1.7-fold, respectively (**Figures 2D,E**). Ileum mRNA levels of the adaptor protein cingulin were reduced in EtOH-treated mice by approximately 1.4-fold, but these reductions did not reach statistical significance (**Figure 2F**). In contrast, ileum mRNA transcripts of the TJPs claudin 1, occludin, fordin, and symplekin were significantly higher in EtOH + Fen-treated compared to EtOH-treated mice (**Figures 2A,B,D,E**). We did not detect statistically significant differences in ileum mRNA levels of ZO-1 (**Figure 2C**) and cingulin (**Figure 2F**) between EtOH-treated and EtOH + Fen-treated mice. Ileum mRNA levels of all of the TJPs measured were unchanged between pair-fed and pair-fed + Fen-treated mice (**Figures 2A–F**). Using IF, we found that ileum immunoreactivity for the TJPs occludin (**Figures 2M *vs.* 2K, white arrows, 2S**) and claudin 1 (**Figure 2Q *vs.* 2O, white arrows, 2T**), was reduced in EtOH-treated mice by 72 and 68%, respectively, compared to pair-fed mice. In contrast and consistent with our qPCR findings, ileum immunoreactivity of occludin (**Figure 2N *vs.* 2M, white arrows, 2S**) and claudin 1 (**Figure 2R *vs.* 2Q, white arrows, 2T**) was increased by 93 and 80%, respectively, in EtOH + Fen-treated mice compared to EtOH-treated mice. Despite the reductions in ileum TJPs, ileum histological analysis did not show any gross morphological differences in intestinal villi across all experimental groups (**Figures 2G–J**).

Fenretininde Reduces Intestinal Toll-like Receptor 4-Positive Macrophages and Inflammatory Mediators

Toll-like receptor 4 (TLR4) is a key component of the innate immune response that binds to bacterial LPS, triggering an anti-microbial response that includes secretion of inflammatory cytokines, including TNF-α (Uematsu and Akera, 2006). TLR4 is expressed in cells of the innate immune response, including macrophages (Uematsu and Akira, 2006), and a convincing body of evidence shows that TLR4 and LPS mediate reductions in intestinal barrier function and expression of TJPs (Guo et al., 2015; Li et al., 2013; Uesugi et al., 2001). Given our findings of increased intestine hyperpermeability and LPS translocation in EtOH-treated cohorts (**Figures 1A,B**), we next examined ileum expression of TLR4 using qPCR and immunofluorescence (IF). Our qPCR data show that compared to pair-fed, EtOH-treated mice exhibited an approximately 3-fold increase in ileum TLR4

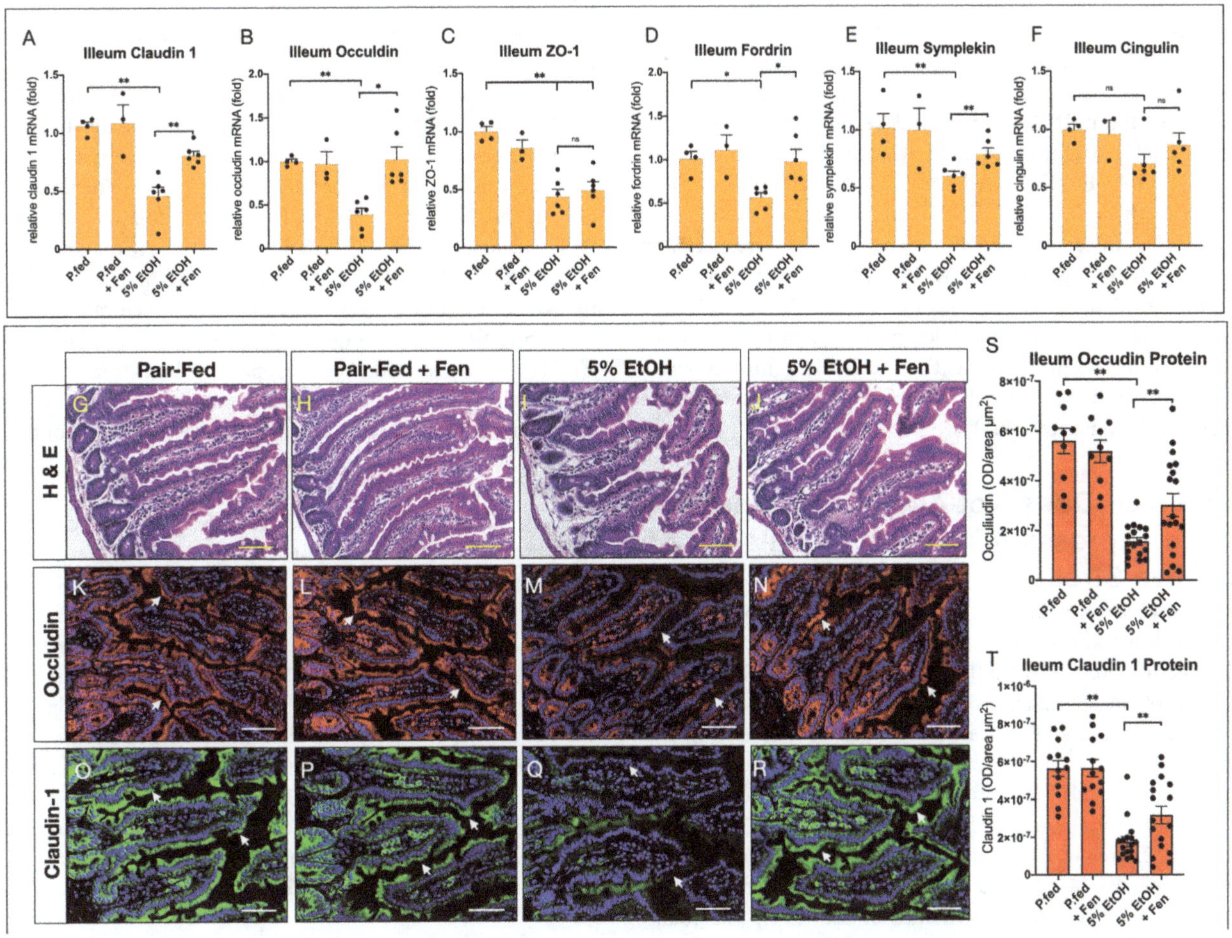

FIGURE 2 | Fenretininde increases intestinal expression of tight junction proteins. Ileum mRNA levels of tight junction proteins **(A)** *Claudin 1*, **(B)**, *Occludin*, **(C)** *ZO-1*, **(D)** *Fordrin*, **(E)** *Symplekin*, **(F)** *Cingulin* were measured using qPCR as described in materials and methods. **(G–J)** Representative images of hematoxylin and eosin stain ileum sections. Magnification: ×100; Scale Bar = 50 μm. Representative immunofluorescence (IF) images of ileum sections stained with antibodies against: occludin K-N), or claudin one O-R). Magnification: ×100; Scale Bar = 50 μm. Quantification of ileum IF optical intensity of occludin S), and claudin 1 T). All data errors bars represent ±SD, with $^{**}p < 0.01$, ns = not significant.

transcripts (**Supplementary Figure S2A**). EtOH + Fen-treated mice displayed approximately 37% reductions in ileum TLR4 mRNA levels compared to the EtOH-treated mice (**Supplementary Figure S2A**). Compared to pair-fed, we did not detect changes to TLR4 mRNA in pair-fed + Fen-treated mice (**Supplementary Figure S2A**).

We next sought to determine ileum TLR4 protein levels, and more specifically, the percentage of TLR4 positive macrophages in the ileum lamina in pair-fed and EtOH-treated groups. Using double IF and antibodies against the macrophage glycoprotein F4/80 and TLR4, we detected, compared to pair-fed mice, 3-fold and 2-fold increases in villi lamina F4/80 positive macrophages in EtOH-treated and EtOH + Fen-treated mice, respectively (**Supplementary Figures 2B,G *vs.* 2F, and 2I *vs.* 2F**). The differences in the percentages of villi lamina F4/80 positive macrophages between EtOH-treated and EtOH + Fen-treated mice did not meet statistical significance (**Supplementary Figure S2B**). However, we found that, compared to pair-fed mice, the percentages of F4/80:TLR4 double positive macrophages increased by 13-fold in EtOH-treated mice (**Supplementary Figures S2B,G *vs.* S2F**, [white arrows]), and were reduced by 46% in EtOH-Fen mice (**Supplementary Figures S2B,I *vs.* S2G** [white arrows]). Pair-fed-Fen mice, compared to paid-fed mice, showed no differences in the percentages of villi lamina F4/80 positive and F4/80:TLR4 double positive macrophages (**Supplementary Figures S2B,H *vs.* S2F**).

We next measured ileum mRNA levels of TNF-α, a major downstream cytokine of TLR4 (Petrasek et al., 2010; Uematsu and Akira, 2006), and of the TNF-α receptor (TNFR1), both of which play key roles in alcohol-mediated disruption of the intestinal barrier function and liver injury in ALD (Chen et al., 2015; Yin et al., 1999). Our qPCR data show that ileum TNF-α mRNA levels were increased by ~2.3-fold in EtOH-treated compared to pair-fed mice (**Supplementary Figure S2C**), whereas ileum TNFR1 transcripts were increased by approximately 1.5-fold in EtOH-treated *vs.* pair-fed mice, but these changes were not statistically significant (**Supplementary Figure S2D**). Using IHC, we sought to confirm our qPCR findings and found, similarly, that ileum

TNF-α immunoreactivity was increased by 2.2-fold in EtOH-treated compared to pair-fed mice (**Supplementary Figures S2E,K *vs.* S2J**). These data are consistent with a previous study showing that chronic alcohol intakes markedly increase intestinal TNF-α mRNA and protein levels in mice and humans (Chen et al., 2015). Our qPCR and IHC analysis also showed that, compared to EtOH-treated mice, ileum mRNA and immunoreactivity levels of TNF-α were reduced in EtOH + Fen-treated mice by 44% and 39%, respectively (**Supplementary Figures S2C,M *vs.* S2K,E**). We found no differences in ileum mRNA levels of TLR4, TNF-α, and TNF-α protein between pair-fed and pair-fed-Fen-treated mice (**Supplementary Figures S2A,C,E**), and TNFR1 mRNA levels between EtOH-treated and EtOH + Fen-treated mice (**Supplementary Figure S2D**).

Fenretinide Does Not Alter Tight Junction Protein Expression Through Modulation of Oxidative Stress

Previous studies have demonstrated that Fen can inhibit LPS and TNF-α mediated inflammation (López-Vales et al., 2010), and LPS mediated disruption of TJPs at the blood brain barrier (BBB) though activation of the Nrf2-antioxidant response element signaling pathway and reductions in reactive oxygen species (ROS) and oxidative stress (Li et al., 2020). Moreover, data show that modulation of cellular ROS is involved in the chemopreventive actions of Fen in a number of cancers (Hail et al., 2006; Sheikh et al., 1995). Therefore, using IHC, we next measured ileum levels of 4-hydroxynonenal (4-HNE), a lipid peroxidation product and a marker of oxidative stress (Esterbauer et al., 1991). We found that, compared to paid-fed mice, EtOH-treated and EtOH + Fen-treated mice showed an almost 10-fold increase in ileum levels of 4-HNE (**Supplemental Figures S3B,D *vs.* S3A,E**), suggesting a large increase intestinal ROS and oxidative stress. We found no differences in the ileum levels of 4-HNE between EtOH-treated and EtOH + Fen-treated mice, however (**Supplementary Figures S3D *vs.* S3B,E**). Using qPCR we next measured the mRNA transcripts of Gsta1 and Gstm1, two Nrf-regulated genes involved in the cellular antioxidant defense response (Ma, 2013), and found, consistent with our 4-HNE IHC data showing increased levels of ileum oxidative stress, that EtOH-treated mice had 2.4 and 3.2-fold increases in ileum transcripts of the Nrf-target genes Gsta1 and Gstm1, respectively (**Supplemental Figures S3F,G**). Also consistent with our 4-HNE-IHC data, we did not detect differences in ileum mRNA levels of Gsta1 and Gstm1 between EtOH-treated and EtOH + Fen-treated mice (**Supplemental Figures S3F,G**).

Fenretininde Reduces Hepatic Steatosis and Liver Injury

We next evaluated the effects of ethanol feeding on liver steatosis and injury in EtOH-treated and EtOH + Fen-treated mice. Histological evaluations of livers showed that compared to pair-fed mice, EtOH-treated mice developed hepatic steatosis (**Figures 3C *vs.* 3A** [yellow arrows]) marked by 4-fold and 3-fold increases in Oil-red O lipid staining (**Figures 3G *vs.* 3E,M**) and hepatic triglyceride levels (**Figure 3N**), respectively. In contrast, we found that livers of EtOH + Fen-treated mice showed marked reductions in hepatic steatosis compared to EtOH-treated mice (**Figures 3D *vs.* 3C**[yellow arrows]), with reductions in Oil-red O lipid staining (**Figures 3H *vs.* 3G,M**) and hepatic triglyceride levels (**Figure 3N**) of 34% and 39%, respectively. Given these modulations of liver triglycerides and steatosis, we next measured hepatic mRNA levels of key lipogenic mediators involved in ALD-steatosis, including FASN, SREBP1-c, ACC1 and PPARγ, by qPCR. Our data show that, compared to pair-fed mice, hepatic mRNA levels of both *FASN* and *PPARγ* were elevated by 2–2.5-fold (**Supplementary Figures S4A,B**), in EtOH-treated and ETOH + Fen-treated mice. Hepatic *FASN* transcripts were 20% lower in EtOH + Fen-compared EtOH-treated mice (**Supplementary Figure S4A**); however, we found no significant differences in hepatic mRNA levels of *FASN* or *PPARγ* between the EtOH-treated and EtOH + Fen-treated groups (**Supplementary Figures S4A,B**). Also, hepatic transcripts of *SREBP1c* and *ACC1* were not significantly different among all groups (**Supplementary Figures S4C,D**).

Alcohol-mediated liver injury can be assessed by plasma levels of the hepatic transaminases alanine aminotransferase (ALT) and aspartate aminotransferase (AST) (Reichling and Kaplan, 1988). We found that, compared to pair-fed mice, plasma ALT and AST enzyme activity levels were elevated in EtOH-treated mice by 50% and 27%, respectively (**Figure 3O,P**). In contrast, plasma levels of ALT and AST were reduced by 30% and 17% in EtOH-Fen-treated compared to EtOH-treated mice (**Figures 3O,P**). Compared to pair-fed mice, hepatic steatosis and plasma levels of ALT and AST in pair-fed-Fen treated mice were not different (**Figures 3M–P**).

Fenretininde Reduces Hepatic Expression of Toll-like Receptor 4 and Inflammatory Mediators

In chronic alcohol exposure and endotoxemia, LPS promotes an inflammatory response through TLR4 (Petrasek et al., 2010), which in the liver is expressed in both hepatocytes (Liu et al., 2002; Jia et al., 2018) and Kupffer cells (Petrasek et al., 2010). Therefore, we next measured hepatic mRNA levels of TLR4 and some of its downstream inflammatory mediators shown to be involved in alcohol and LPS-induced liver inflammation (Petrasek et al., 2010; Neuman et al., 2015). Our qPCR analysis showed that, compared to pair-fed mice, hepatic transcripts of *TLR4*, *IL-6*, *IL-1β* and *TNF-α* were all significantly increased in EtOH-treated mice (**Figures 3Q–T**) and, with the exception of *IL-6*, our analysis also showed that hepatic mRNA levels of these inflammatory mediators were significantly lower in EtOH + Fen-treated compared to EtOH-treated mice (**Figures 3Q–T**). We next used IHC to measure hepatic TNF-α protein levels, given our *TNF-α* qPCR data (**Figure 3T**) and the key role of TNF-α in the pathogenesis of ALD (Yin et al., 1999; Neuman et al., 2015). We found, compared to pair-fed mice, that hepatic TNF-α protein immunoreactivity and levels increased by more than 120% in EtOH-treated mice (**Figures 3K *vs.* 3I,U**), and consistent with our qPCR data, that hepatic TNF-α protein levels were reduced by approximately 40% in EtOH + Fen-treated compared to EtOH-treated mice (**Figures 3L *vs.*3K,U**). Using IF, we next measured

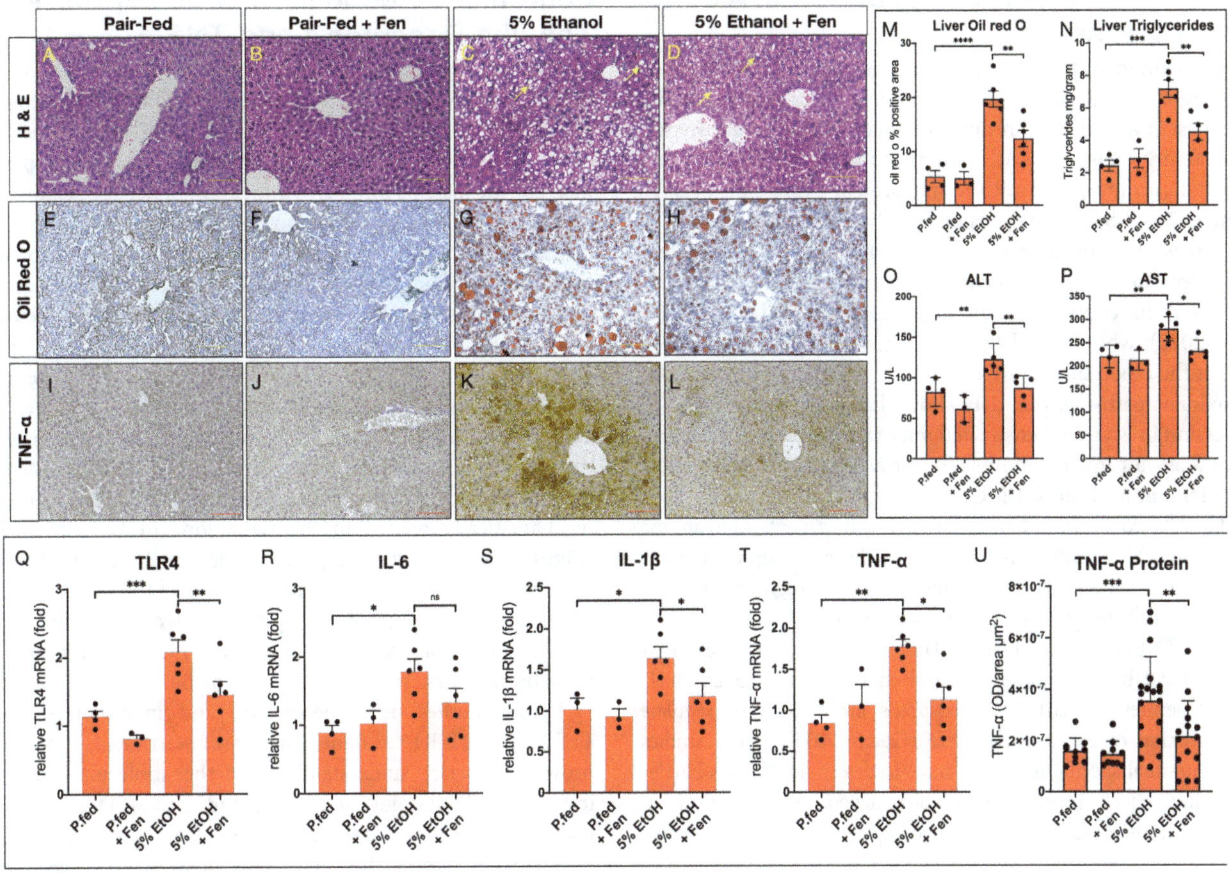

FIGURE 3 | Fenretininde reduces alcohol liver disease (ALD) and liver inflammation. **(A–D)** Representative images of hematoxylin and eosin; **(E–H)** Oil-Red O-stained liver sections Magnification: ×100; Scale Bar = 50 μm; **(I–L)** Representative immunohistochemistry (IHC) images of liver sections stained with an antibody against tumor necrosis factor α (TNF-α) Magnification: ×100; Scale Bar = 50 μm. **(M)** Quantification of liver Oil-red-O stained liver sections. **(N)** Liver triglyceride concentrations (mg/Gram tissue weight). Plasma activity levels (U/L) of **(O)** alanine amino transferase (ALT) and **(P)** aspartate amino transferase (AST). Hepatic mRNA levels of inflammatory mediators **(Q)** *TLR4*, **(R)** *IL-6*, **(S)** *IL-1β*, **(T)** *TNF-α*. **(U)** Quantification of hepatic IHC for TNF-α protein levels. All data errors bars represent ±SD, with *$p < 0.05$, **$p < 0.01$. ***$p < 0.001$, ns = not significant.

hepatic TLR4 protein expression in hepatocytes and Kupffer cells, and found, compared to pair-fed mice, that the percentages of F4/80: TLR4 double positive Kupffer cells (**Supplementary Figures S5B *vs.* S5A[white arrows], S5E**), and TLR4 positive hepatocytes (**Supplementary Figures S5B *vs.* 5A,E**) increased by 15.6-fold and 13.7-fold respectively, in EtOH-treated mice. In contrast, compared to EtOH-treated mice, the percentages of F4/80:TLR4 double positive hepatic Kupffer cells (**Supplementary Figures 5D *vs.* 5B [white arrows], 5E**), and TLR4 positive hepatocytes (**Supplementary Figures 5D *vs.* 5B,E**), were reduced by 55% and by 60% in EtOH + Fen-treated mice, respectively.

Hepatic steatosis and inflammation can lead to excessive liver collagen deposition, fibrotic scarring, and injury (Osna et al., 2017). Therefore, given that we detected increases in hepatic steatosis (**Figures 3M,N**) and expression of inflammatory cytokines, including TNF-α (**Figures 3Q–U**), in the EtOH-cohorts, we next assessed liver fibrosis by using both IHC for the fibrogenic marker α-smooth muscle actin (α-SMA) and Masson's trichrome staining for collagen. Compared to pair-fed mice, we detected no increases in hepatic levels of α-SMA (**Supplementary Figures 4I,J *vs.* 4G,O**), or evidence of excessive liver collagen deposition or fibrosis in the EtOH-treated and EtOH + Fen-treated mice (**Supplementary Figure 4M,N *vs.* 4K,P**).

DISCUSSION

Multiple lines of evidence indicate that chronic alcohol intake promotes disruption of intestinal barrier integrity (Rao, 2009; Samuelson et al., 2019). The mechanisms through which this occurs are incompletely understood, but modulation of gut bacterial growth (Bode et al., 1987; Rao, 2009; Samuelson et al., 2019), mucosal immunity, and intestinal inflammation have been proposed (Bishehsari et al., 2017). Still, experimental and human data consistently show that in the early stages of ALD, ethanol negatively affects expression of intestinal TJPs (Bode et al., 1987; Rao, 2009; Samuelson et al., 2019), leading to endotoxemia and a pro-inflammatory cascade that damages both the gut and liver (Bode et al., 1987; Rao, 2009; Samuelson et al., 2019).

Fenretinide Preserves Gut Barrier in Alcohol Liver Disease

Here we demonstrate for the first time that Fen, a synthetic analog of all-trans retinol widely studied for its anti-cancer properties (Veronesi et al., 2006), can mitigate ethanol-induced gut hyper-permeability (**Figure 1A**), endotoxemia (**Figure 1B**), and reductions to intestinal mRNA and protein expression of TJPs (**Figures 2A–E,S,T**). Fen does not directly modulate expression of TJPs, as we did not detect changes in TJP mRNA and protein expression in pair-fed Fen-treated mice (**Figures 2A–F,S,T**). Moreover, in contrast to findings reported by Li et al. (Li et al., 2020), who showed that Fen mitigates LPS disruption of TJPs at the blood brain barrier through stimulation of the Nrf2-antioxidant pathway, our data show that perseveration of TJP expression in EtOH + Fen-treated mice (**Supplementary Figures 2S,T**) does not involve modulation of Nrf2 and oxidative stress (**Supplemental Figures 3E–G**).

Our data do show, in contrast, that Fen treatments mitigate the TLR4 and TNF-α inflammatory axis in the gut (**Supplementary Figures S2**). These findings could provide insight into Fen's preservation of the gut barrier with alcohol intake, as mice lacking TLR4 or TNF-α receptor I (TNFRI) are protected against alcohol-mediated gut barrier dysfunction and endotoxemia (Uesugi et al., 2001; Chen et al., 2015). As retinoids are known to regulate differentiation of gut epithelial cells (Gudas, 2011), future studies using intestinal specific RAR null-mice to determine if Fen's barrier preserving effect involves retinoid-mediated differentiation of intestinal epithelial cells are warranted.

Fenretinide Inhibits Hepatic Steatosis and Liver Injury

Our data also show positive effects of Fen treatments on mitigating clinical hallmarks of ALD, including hepatic steatosis (**Figures 2M,N**) and liver injury (**Figures 2O,P**). The reductions in liver triglyceride content in EtOH + Fen-treated mice (**Figure 3N**) did not correlate with changes in hepatic expression of lipogenic genes such as FASN and SREBP1-c (**Supplementary Figures 4A–D**). As food intake and alcohol-exposure was unchanged between both EtOH experimental groups (**Supplementary Figure 1B**), it remains unclear how Fen reduces alcohol-mediated hepatic steatosis and liver injury. Moreover, we have evidence that the anti-ALD effects of Fen do not involve activation of RARs, as hepatic mRNA expression of the well-established retinoid-mediated target genes, RARβ2 and Cyp26A1 (Gudas, 2011), were unchanged in EtOH + Fen and pair-fed + Fen-treated mice compared to pair-fed and EtOH-treated mice respectively (**Supplementary Figures 4E,F**). This is consistent with the data showing that the anti-cancer actions of Fen are largely through non-RAR mediated pathways (Sheikh et al., 1995; Hail et al., 2006). Still, it is likely that Fen has unappreciated effects on the complex regulation of alcohol-mediated lipogenesis and lipid metabolism. Therefore, in future studies next-generation RNA sequencing could be performed to explore the hepatic gene networks impacted by Fen in chronic alcohol exposure.

Fenretinide Reduces Hepatic Expression of Toll-like Receptor 4 and TNF-α

The concomitant reductions in endotoxemia (**Figure 1B**) and hepatic and Kupffer cell expression of TLR4 (**Supplemental Figure S5**) and TLR4 targets, including TNF-α (**Figures 3I–L, 3U**), in the livers of EtOH + Fen-treated mice could provide mechanistic insights into Fen's mitigation of hepatic steatosis and liver injury, as LPS is a potent stimulator of the TLR4 inflammatory axis (Uematsu and Akira, 2006). Moreover, there is a convincing body of evidence of a nexus between the innate immune inflammatory axis and nutrient and metabolic pathways (Hotamisligil, 2006), including studies showing that TNF-α and LPS:TLR4 signaling promote lipogenesis in hepatocytes *in vivo* (Feingold and Grunfeld, 1987; Feingold et al., 1992; Jia et al., 2018). Nevertheless, we recognize that the preservation of gut barrier function (**Figure 1A**) and reductions in endotoxemia (**Figure 1B**) may not be mechanistically related to the reductions in hepatic steatosis (**Figure 3M,N**) and liver injury (**Figures 3O,P**), in EtOH + Fen-treated mice. Moreover, it is unclear if the modulations of TLR4 and TNF-α in both the guts and livers of EtOH + Fen-treated mice are a direct effect of Fen on TLR4 signaling, are from reductions in systemic endotoxemia, or both.

Future studies using hepatocyte and macrophage-specific TLR4 or TNFR1 mutant mice are warranted, and could provide a better understanding of the molecular pathways involved in Fen's gut preserving and anti-ALD effects. Still, taken together, our data are consistent with a number of recent studies reporting that Fen possess anti-TLR4, anti-inflammatory, and TJP-preserving actions (López-Vales et al., 2010; Lachance et al., 2013; Kanagaratham et al., 2014; Lin et al., 2016).

CONCLUSION

Given that few therapeutics for ALD have been developed which can preserve both gut integrity and liver functions, the data presented here suggest that Fen may possess properties that target both gut barrier function and clinical hallmarks of ALD. Also, given the decades of safety data for Fen from numerous human clinical trials (Veronesi et al., 2006), our findings warrant further pre-clinical testing of Fen as an anti-ALD drug.

AUTHOR CONTRIBUTIONS

X-HT, MM, KM, LG, and ST conducted research, data collection and provided data interpretation, manuscript writing and critical review.

ACKNOWLEDGMENTS

We would like to thank the Hunter College Animal Care Facility with all their help in animal handling and care.

REFERENCES

Bishehsari, F., Magno, E., Swanson, G., Desai, V., Voigt, R. M., Forsyth, C. B., et al. (2017). Alcohol and gut-derived inflammation. *Alcohol. Res.* 38 (2), 163–171.

Bode, C., Kugler, V., and Bode, J. C. (1987). Endotoxemia in patients with alcoholic and non-alcoholic cirrhosis and in subjects with no evidence of chronic liver disease following acute alcohol excess. *J. Hepatol.* 4 (1), 8–14. doi:10.1016/s0168-8278(87)80003-x

Chen, P., Stärkel, P., Turner, J. R., Ho, S. B., and Schnabl, B. (2015). Dysbiosis-induced intestinal inflammation activates tumor necrosis factor receptor I and mediates alcoholic liver disease in mice. *Hepatology* 61 (3), 883–894. doi:10.1002/hep.27489

Cooper, J. P., Reynolds, C. P., Cho, H., and Kang, M. H. (2017). Clinical development of fenretinide as an antineoplastic drug: Pharmacology perspectives. *Exp. Biol. Med. (Maywood)* 242 (11), 1178–1184. doi:10.1177/1535370217706952

Esterbauer, H., Schaur, R. J., and Zollner, H. (1991). Chemistry and biochemistry of 4-hydroxynonenal, malonaldehyde and related aldehydes. *Free Radic. Biol. Med.* 11 (1), 81–128. doi:10.1016/0891-5849(91)90192-6

Feingold, K. R., and Grunfeld, C. (1987). Tumor necrosis factor-alpha stimulates hepatic lipogenesis in the rat *in vivo*. *J. Clin. Invest.* 80 (1), 184–190. doi:10.1172/JCI113046

Feingold, K. R., Staprans, I., Memon, R. A., Moser, A. H., Shigenaga, J. K., Doerrler, W., et al. (1992). Endotoxin rapidly induces changes in lipid metabolism that produce hypertriglyceridemia: low doses stimulate hepatic triglyceride production while high doses inhibit clearance. *J. Lipid Res.* 33 (12), 1765–1776. doi:10.1016/s0022-2275(20)41334-3

Freund, G. (1970). Alcohol consumption and its circadian distribution in mice. *J. Nutr.* 100 (1), 30–36. doi:10.1093/jn/100.1.30

Groschwitz, K. R., and Hogan, S. P. (2009). Intestinal barrier function: molecular regulation and disease pathogenesis. *J. Allergy Clin. Immunol.* 124 (1), 3–2. doi:10.1016/j.jaci.2009.05.038

Gudas, L. J. (2011). Emerging roles for retinoids in regeneration and differentiation in normal and disease states. *Biochim. Biophys. Acta (Bba)— Mol. Cel Biol. Lipids*, 1821 (11), 213. doi:10.1016/j.bbalip.2011.08.002

Guo, S., Nighot, M., Al-Sadi, R., Alhmoud, T., Nighot, P., and Ma, T. Y. (2015). Lipopolysaccharide regulation of intestinal tight junction permeability is mediated by TLR4 signal transduction pathway activation of FAK and MyD88. *J. Immunol.* 195 (10), 4999–5010. doi:10.4049/jimmunol.1402598

Hail, N., Kim, H. J., and Lotan, R. (2006). Mechanisms of fenretinide-induced apoptosis. *Apoptosis* 11 (10), 1677–1694. doi:10.1007/s10495-006-9289-3

Horz, H. P., Vianna, M. E., Gomes, B. P., and Conrads, G. (2005). Evaluation of universal probes and primer sets for assessing total bacterial load in clinical samples: general implications and practical use in endodontic antimicrobial therapy. *J. Clin. Microbiol.* 43 (10), 5332–5337. doi:10.1128/JCM.43.10.5332-5337.2005

Hotamisligil, G. S. (2006). Inflammation and metabolic disorders. *Nature* 444 (7121), 860–867. doi:10.1038/nature05485

Jia, L., Chang, X., Qian, S., Liu, C., Lord, C. C., Ahmed, N., et al. (2018). Hepatocyte toll-like receptor 4 deficiency protects against alcohol-induced fatty liver disease. *Mol. Metab.* 14, 121–129. doi:10.1016/j.molmet.2018.05.015

Kanagaratham, C., Kalivodová, A., Najdekr, L., Friedecký, D., Adam, T., Hajduch, M., et al. (2014). Fenretinide prevents inflammation and airway hyperresponsiveness in a mouse model of allergic asthma. *Am. J. Respir. Cel Mol Biol.* 51 (6), 783–792. doi:10.1165/rcmb.2014-0121OC

Keshavarzian, A., Farhadi, A., Forsyth, C. B., Rangan, J., Jakate, S., Shaikh, M., et al. (2009). Evidence that chronic alcohol exposure promotes intestinal oxidative stress, intestinal hyperpermeability and endotoxemia prior to development of alcoholic steatohepatitis in rats. *J. Hepatol.* 50 (3), 538–547. doi:10.1016/j.jhep.2008.10.028

Kirpich, I. A., Feng, W., Wang, Y., Liu, Y., Barker, D. F., Barve, S. S., et al. (2012). The type of dietary fat modulates intestinal tight junction integrity, gut permeability, and hepatic toll-like receptor expression in a mouse model of alcoholic liver disease. *Alcohol. Clin. Exp. Res.* 36 (5), 835–846. doi:10.1111/j.1530-0277.2011.01673.x

Koh, I. U., Jun, H. S., Choi, J. S., Lim, J. H., Kim, W. H., Yoon, J. B., et al. (2012). Fenretinide ameliorates insulin resistance and fatty liver in obese mice. *Biol. Pharm. Bull.* 35 (3), 369–375. doi:10.1248/bpb.35.369

Lachance, C., Wojewodka, G., Skinner, T. A., Guilbault, C., De Sanctis, J. B., and Radzioch, D. (2013). Fenretinide corrects the imbalance between omega-6 to omega-3 polyunsaturated fatty acids and inhibits macrophage inflammatory mediators *via* the ERK pathway. *PLoS One* 8 (9), e74875. doi:10.1371/journal.pone.0074875

Li, T., Zheng, L.-N., and Han, X.-H. (2020). Fenretinide attenuates lipopolysaccharide (LPS)-induced blood-brain barrier (BBB) and depressive-like behavior in mice by targeting Nrf-2 signaling. *Biomed. Pharmacother.* 125, 109680. doi:10.1016/j.biopha.2019.109680

Li, X., Wang, C., Nie, J., Lv, D., Wang, T., and Xu, Y. (2013). Toll-like receptor 4 increases intestinal permeability through up-regulation of membrane PKC activity in alcoholic steatohepatitis. *Alcohol* 47 (6), 459–465. doi:10.1016/j.alcohol.2013.05.004

Lin, C. H., Lee, S. Y., Zhang, C. C., Du, Y. F., Hung, H. C., Wu, H. T., et al. (2016). Fenretinide inhibits macrophage inflammatory mediators and controls hypertension in spontaneously hypertensive rats *via* the peroxisome proliferator-activated receptor gamma pathway. *Drug Des. Devel Ther.* 10, 3591–3597. doi:10.2147/DDDT.S114879

Liu, S., Gallo, D. J., Green, A. M., Williams, D. L., Gong, X., Shapiro, R. A., et al. (2002). Role of toll-like receptors in changes in gene expression and NF-kappa B activation in mouse hepatocytes stimulated with lipopolysaccharide. *Infect. Immun.* 70 (7), 3433–3442. doi:10.1128/iai.70.7.3433-3442.2002

Livak, K. J., and Schmittgen, T. D. (2001). Analysis of relative gene expression data using real-time quantitative PCR and the 2(-Delta Delta C(T)) Method. *Methods* 25 (4), 402–408. doi:10.1006/meth.2001.1262

López-Vales, R., Redensek, A., Skinner, T. A., Rathore, K. I., Ghasemlou, N., Wojewodka, G., et al. (2010). Fenretinide promotes functional recovery and tissue protection after spinal cord contusion injury in mice. *J. Neurosci.* 30 (9), 3220–3226. doi:10.1523/JNEUROSCI.5770-09.2010

Ma, Q. (2013). Role of nrf2 in oxidative stress and toxicity. *Annu. Rev. Pharmacol. Toxicol.* 53, 401–426. doi:10.1146/annurev-pharmtox-011112-140320

Neuman, M. G., Maor, Y., Nanau, R. M., Melzer, E., Mell, H., Opris, M., et al. (2015). Alcoholic liver disease: role of cytokines. *Biomolecules* 5 (3), 2023–2034. doi:10.3390/biom5032023

Osna, N. A., Donohue, T. M., and Kharbanda, K. K. (2017). Alcoholic liver disease: pathogenesis and current management. *Alcohol. Res.* 38 (2), 147–161.

Petrasek, J., Mandrekar, P., and Szabo, G. (2010). Toll-like receptors in the pathogenesis of alcoholic liver disease. *Gastroenterol. Res. Pract.*, 2010, 1–12. doi:10.1155/2010/710381

Preitner, F., Mody, N., Graham, T. E., Peroni, O. D., and Kahn, B. B. (2009). Long-term Fenretinide treatment prevents high-fat diet-induced obesity, insulin resistance, and hepatic steatosis. *Am. J. Physiol. Endocrinol. Metab.* 297 (6), E1420–E1429. doi:10.1152/ajpendo.00362.2009

Rao, R. (2009). Endotoxemia and gut barrier dysfunction in alcoholic liver disease. *Hepatology* 50 (2), 638–644. doi:10.1002/hep.23009

Rehm, J., Samokhvalov, A. V., and Shield, K. D. (2013). Global burden of alcoholic liver diseases. *J. Hepatol.* 59 (1), 160–168. doi:10.1016/j.jhep.2013.03.007

Reichling, J. J., and Kaplan, M. M. (1988). Clinical use of serum enzymes in liver disease. *Dig. Dis. Sci.* 33 (12), 1601–1614. doi:10.1007/BF01535953

Samuelson, D. R., Gu, M., Shellito, J. E., Molina, P. E., Taylor, C. M., Luo, M., et al. (2019). Intestinal microbial products from alcohol-fed mice contribute to intestinal permeability and peripheral immune activation. *Alcohol. Clin. Exp. Res.* 43 (10), 2122–2133. doi:10.1111/acer.14176

Sanyal, A. J., Mathurin, P., and Nagy, L. A. (2016). Commonalities and distinctions between alcoholic and nonalcoholic fatty liver disease. *Gastroenterology* 150 (8), 1695–1697. doi:10.1053/j.gastro.2016.04.038

Schindelin, J., Arganda-Carreras, I., Frise, E., Kaynig, V., Longair, M., Pietzsch, T., et al. (2012). Fiji: an open-source platform for biological-image analysis. *Nat. Methods* 9 (7), 676–682. doi:10.1038/nmeth.2019

Sheikh, M. S., Shao, Z. M., Li, X. S., Ordonez, J. V., Conley, B. A., Wu, S., et al. (1995). N-(4-hydroxyphenyl)retinamide (4-HPR)-mediated biological actions involve retinoid receptor-independent pathways in human breast carcinoma. *Carcinogenesis* 16 (10), 2477–2486. doi:10.1093/carcin/16.10.2477

Trasino, S. E., Tang, X. H., Jessurun, J., and Gudas, L. J. (2016). A retinoic acid receptor β2 agonist reduces hepatic stellate cell activation in nonalcoholic fatty liver disease. *J. Mol. Med.* 94 (10), 1143–1151. doi:10.1007/s00109-016-1434-z

Uematsu, S., and Akira, S. (2006). Toll-like receptors and innate immunity. *J. Mol. Med.* 84 (9), 712–725. doi:10.1007/s00109-006-0084-y

Uesugi, T., Froh, M., Arteel, G. E., Bradford, B. U., and Thurman, R. G. (2001). Toll-like receptor 4 is involved in the mechanism of early alcohol-induced liver injury in mice. *Hepatology* 34 (1), 101–108. doi:10.1053/jhep.2001.25350

Veronesi, U., Mariani, L., Decensi, A., Formelli, F., Camerini, T., Miceli, R., et al. (2006). Fifteen-year results of a randomized phase III trial of fenretinide to prevent second breast cancer. *Ann. Oncol.* 17 (7), 1065–1071. doi:10.1093/annonc/mdl047

Volynets, V., Reichold, A., Bárdos, G., Rings, A., Bleich, A., and Bischoff, S. C. (2016). Assessment of the intestinal barrier with five different permeability tests in healthy C57bl/6J and BALB/cJ mice. *Dig. Dis. Sci.* 61 (3), 737–746. doi:10.1007/s10620-015-3935-y

Wang, Y., Tong, J., Chang, B., Wang, B., and Zhang, D. (2014). Effects of alcohol on intestinal epithelial barrier permeability and expression of tight junction-associated proteins. *Mol. Med. Rep.* 9 (6), 2352–2356. doi:10.3892/mmr.2014.2126

Yan, A. W., Fouts, D. E., Brandl, J., Stärkel, P., Torralba, M., Schott, E., et al. (2011). Enteric dysbiosis associated with a mouse model of alcoholic liver disease. *Hepatology* 53 (1), 96–105. doi:10.1002/hep.24018

Yin, M., Wheeler, M. D., Kono, H., Bradford, B. U., Gallucci, R. M., Luster, M. I., et al. (1999). Essential role of tumor necrosis factor alpha in alcohol-induced liver injury in mice. *Gastroenterology* 117 (4), 942–952. doi:10.1016/s0016-5085(99)70354-9

Zhong, W., Li, Q., Xie, G., Sun, X., Tan, X., Sun, X., et al. (2013). Dietary fat sources differentially modulate intestinal barrier and hepatic inflammation in alcohol-induced liver injury in rats. *Am. J. Physiol. Gastrointest. Liver Physiol.* 305 (12), G919–G932. doi:10.1152/ajpgi.00226.2013

2

Non-Invasive Biomarkers of Liver Inflammation and Cell Death in Response to Alcohol Detoxification

***Manuela G. Neuman*[1]*, *Johannes Mueller*[2] *and Sebastian Mueller*[2,3]**

[1] *In Vitro Drug Safety and Biotechnology, Department of Pharmacology and Toxicology, Temerity Faculty of Medicine, University of Toronto, Toronto, ON, Canada,* [2] *Center for Alcohol Research, University of Heidelberg, Heidelberg, Germany,* [3] *Department of Internal Medicine, Salem Medical Center, Heidelberg, Germany*

Correspondence:
Manuela G. Neuman
m_neuman@rogers.com

Introduction: Alcohol-related liver disease (ALD) represents the most common liver disease worldwide, however, the underlying molecular mechanisms are still poorly understood. Namely centrilobular inflammation and programmed cell death are characteristic to ALD and it remains to be elucidated why they persist despite the absence of alcohol.

Aims: To study the effects of alcohol withdrawal in a cohort of heavy drinkers and the role of cirrhosis by using non-invasive biomarkers such as cytokines, apoptotic and angiogenic markers.

Methods: Caspase 3-cleaved M30, M65, cytokines (IL-6, IL-8), tumor necrosis factor alpha (TNF-α), transforming growth factor (TGF-β) and vascular endothelial growth factor (VEGF) were measured in 114 heavy drinkers. The role of alcohol detoxification was investigated in 45 patients. The liver histology was available in 23 patients. Fibrosis stage and steatosis were assessed by measuring liver stiffness (LS) and controlled attenuation parameter (CAP) in all patients using transient elastography (FibroScan, Echosens, Paris). Mean observation interval between the measurements was 5.7 ± 1.4 days (mean + –SD).

Results: Patients consumed a mean of 204 ± 148 g/day alcohol with a heavy drinking duration of 15.3 ± 11.0 years. Mean LS was 20.7 ± 24.4 kPa and mean CAP was 303 ± 51 dB/m. Fibrosis distribution was F0–38.1%, F1-2–31%, F3–7.1 and F4–23.9%. Apoptotic markers M30 and M65 were almost five times above normal. In contrast, TNF-α a, IL-8 and VEGF were only slightly elevated. Patients with manifest liver cirrhosis (F4) had significantly higher levels of M30, M65, IL-6 and IL-8. Histology features such as hepatocyte ballooning, Mallory-Denk bodies, inflammation and fibrosis were all significantly associated with elevated LS, and serum levels of TNF-alpha, M30 and M65 but not with CAP and other cytokines. During alcohol detoxification, LS, transaminases, TGF- β, IL-6, IL-8 and VEGF decreased significantly. In contrast, no significant changes were observed for M30, M65 and TNF- α and M30 even increased during detoxification in non-cirrhotic patients. Profibrogenic cytokine TGF-beta and pro-angiogenic cytokine VEGF showed a delayed decrease in patients with manifest cirrhosis.

Conclusion: Patients with alcohol-related cirrhosis have a pronounced apoptotic activity and a distinct inflammatory response that only partly improves after 1 week of alcohol detoxification. Alcohol withdrawal may represent an important approach to better dissect the underlying mechanisms in the setting of alcohol metabolism.

Keywords: cytokines, liver stiffness, alcoholic liver disease, apoptosis, inflammation/hepatitis

INTRODUCTION

Alcohol-related liver disease (ALD) is the most common liver disease worldwide ranging from steatosis to liver cirrhosis (Seitz et al., 2018). ALD both depends on various genetic and non-genetic factors including ethnicity (Roerecke et al., 2016) or co-morbidities such as obesity and HCV infection (Mueller et al., 2009; Neuman et al., 2012). In addition, cirrhosis is considered an important pre-cancerogenic lesion ultimately leading to hepatocellular carcinoma (HCC) (Morgan et al., 2004). Most patients with ALD typically present for medical care after developing jaundice or complications of cirrhosis (Zimmerman et al., 1998; Wiesner et al., 2003; Louvet et al., 2017). Given its high prevalence and economic burden, ALD is receiving increasing attention by health authorities and the liver medical and academic communities (Neuman et al., 2001; Yoon and Chen, 2016).

The recent development of non-invasive tools to diagnose various disease stages of ALD by elastography (Mueller et al., 2014), CAP (Thiele et al., 2018), or room temperature susceptometry (Mueller J. et al., 2017) has significantly improved the screening of ALD patients (Moreno et al., 2019). However, optimized non-invasive approaches and refined diagnostic algorithms are still needed to explore promising pharmacological approaches for alcoholic steatohepatitis (ASH), or the rare cases of fatal acute alcoholic hepatitis (AH). Moreover, the therapeutic armamentarium is still limited, and abstinence remains the most effective treatment option in patients with ALD. While studies suggest that early liver transplantation can be successfully performed in highly selected patients with AH its application is limited in most countries due to organ shortage and compliance (Forster et al., 1993; Molina et al., 2002; Neuman et al., 2014a).

The underlying molecular mechanisms of ALD are still incompletely understood. Liver damage due to high alcohol consumption produces a cytokine storm syndrome characterized by the release of pro-inflammatory cytokines. The activation of the immune system is a host defense mechanism (Neuman et al., 2002, 2014b; Neuman, 2007). In response to chronic, heavy alcohol exposure, hepatocytes express and secrete chemokines (Neuman et al., 2017; Le Daré et al., 2019). The role of inflammation in chronic liver disease has also recently lead to a new terminology called acute-on-chronic liver failure (ACLF). Although systemic inflammation is a hallmark of ACLF, its role in the development of this syndrome is poorly understood (Moreau, 2016). Important exogenous inducers further include bacterial products such as pathogen-associated molecular patterns (PAMPs) and virulence factors. Pathogen-associated molecular patterns elicit inflammation *via* innate pattern-recognition receptors (PRRs), whereas virulence factors generally trigger inflammation *via* functional feature identification. Endogenous inducers are called danger-associated molecular patterns (DAMPs) and include molecules released by necrotic cells and products of extracellular matrix breakdown (Neuman et al., 2017; Gao et al., 2019; Gaul et al., 2021).

Increasing evidence suggests an important role for hepatocyte apoptosis in the progression of ALD (Malhi and Gores, 2008; Lavallard et al., 2011), although several other forms of cell death have been described including necrosis, necroptosis, autophagic cell death, and others (Vandenabeele et al., 2010). Both apoptosis and necrosis have also been proposed to be responsible for the development and progression of liver fibrosis (Mehal and Imaeda, 2010). Early during apoptosis, caspases are activated and cleave various substrates including cytokeratin 18 (K18) (Leers et al., 1999; Bantel et al., 2000). K18 is a member of the intermediate filament family of cytoskeletal proteins (Romano et al., 1986). Cytokeratine-generated cleavage fragments of K18 can be detected in serum by the M30 antibody, which specifically labels early apoptotic fragments of cells (Bantel et al., 2000). An increase of apoptotic activity has been demonstrated in heavy drinkers undergoing alcohol detoxification (Mueller S. et al., 2017). This study indicated a link between apoptotic activity and incidence of hepatocellular carcinoma (HCC). The data from detoxification patients suggested that alcohol may inhibit apoptosis and therefore diminishing an important clearance pathway of tumor cells.

Recent studies confirmed the strong association of M30 with steatohepatitis on biopsy in a cohort of patients with severe alcoholic hepatitis (Atkinson et al., 2020). Moreover, in this study, M30 and M65 were associated with 90-day mortality, independent of age and Model for End-stage Liver Disease (MELD). Also, Schlossberger et al. (2019) showed also measured M30 levels in sera of 184 patients with ALD and they did not find significant differences in M30 levels among fibrosis stages and cirrhosis was predicted with a sensitivity of 84.5% and a negative predictive value of 73.5%.

Abbreviations: ALD, alcohol-related liver disease; ACLF, acute-on-chronic liver failure; AH, Alcoholic hepatitis; ALD, Alcohol-related liver disease; ALT, alanine aminotransferase (glutamic-pyruvic transaminase; GPT); ALP, alkaline phosphatase; AMA, anti-mitochondrial antibody; ANA, antinuclear antibody; AST-aspartate aminotransferase (glutamic-oxalic- transaminase; GOT); ASH alcoholic steatohepatitis; BMI, body mass index; CAP, controlled attenuation parameter; CCK, caspase cleaved cytokeratin (8 and 18)- M30-M 65; DAMPs, danger-associated molecular patterns; EGF, epithelial growth factor; FDA- Food and Drug Administration; GGT-γ-glutamyl-transferase; HBV, hepatitis virus B; HCV, hepatitis virus C; HGF, hepatocyte growth factor; IL, Interleukin: IL-6; IL-8, INR, International Normalized Ratio; Mean ± SD, mean ± standard deviation; PAMPs, pathogen-associated molecular patterns; PRRs, pattern-recognition receptors; TGF-beta, transforming growth factor beta; TNF- α, Tumor necrosis factor.

In a cohort of Caucasian heavy drinkers with well characterized disease stages we study the role of alcohol withdrawal and we correlate the clinical information with serum markers of apoptosis and inflammation. In addition, we analyze their association with histological features of ALD in a smaller subcohort. Moreover, we specifically explore the role of cirrhosis in modulating these markers during alcohol withdrawal. Based on proposed role of hepatic arterialization for sustained fibrosis progression (Mueller S., 2016; Piecha et al., 2016), we analyze VEGF to obtain insights on the pro-angiogenic status in the context of inflammation and fibrosis stage.

MATERIALS AND METHODS

Patient Cohorts and Clinical Data

The study design is shown in **Figure 1**.

A total of 114 Caucasian heavy drinkers were prospectively enrolled at Salem Medical Center. All patients with ALD were heavy drinkers (> 80 g per day in males and > 60 g per day in females) with a mean alcohol consumption of 204 ± 148 g/day.

Patient's characteristics are given in **Table 1**. All patients were Caucasians with no viral hepatitis B or C (HBV, HCV) infection or human immunodeficiency (HIV) viral infection.

Liver histology data were available in n = 23 patients. The study protocol was reviewed and approved by the local Ethics Committee and all patients gave written informed consent prior to inclusion. Other causes of liver diseases were ruled out in all patients serologically by screening for AMA (anti-mitochondrial antibody) and ANA (antinuclear antibody).

Data before and after alcohol detoxification could be obtained in a cohort of 45 individuals. According to the study protocol, blood tests, ultrasound and transient elastography were performed within 24 h after admission and after completion of alcohol detoxification therapy on the day of release from the hospital. Liver biopsies were performed within 48 h after admission.

A cohort of 80 Caucasian healthy individuals served as control group. None of the controls were drinkers or social drinkers. Values for demographic and routine laboratory data are also given in **Table 1**. All the controls were part of the *In Vitro* Drug Safety and Biotechnology cohort.

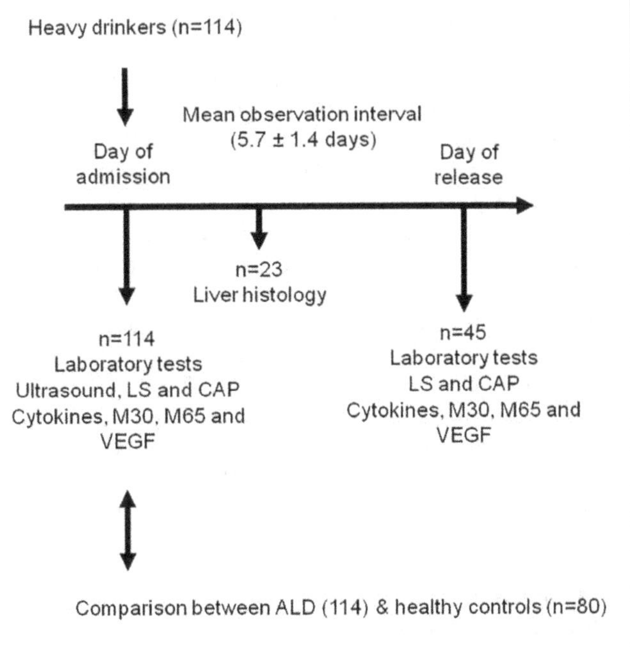

FIGURE 1 | Study design.

Ultrasound, Transient Elastography (TE) and CAP

Liver size, signs of cirrhosis, spleen size, ascites formation and semi-quantitative liver steatosis (0–3) were assessed by abdominal ultrasound. Liver stiffness was measured (in kPa)

TABLE 1 | Patient characteristics.

Parameters	ALD	Control	*P*-value
General data			
Number of patients	114	80	
Sex (male)	68%	55%	0.0759
Age (years)	49.9 ± 12.4	34 ± 16	<0.0001
BMI (kg/m^2)	26.2 ± 5.3	24.0 ± 2.1	0.0005
Alcohol consumption (g/day)	204 ± 148	12 ± 5	<0.0001
Duration of heavy alcohol drinking (years)	15.3 ± 11.0	0	<0.0001
Ultrasound data			
Liver size (cm)	16.4 ± 3.7	15.4 ± 2.1	0.0303
Hepatic steatosis (US) (0-3)	1.82 ± 0.86	0.52 ± 0.36	<0.0001
Spleen size (cm)	10.5 ± 2.8	9.9 ± 1.2	0.0730
Presence of Ascites (%)	10%	0%	<0.0001
Signs of cirrhosis (US) (%)	21%	0%	<0.0001
Elastography data			
Liver stiffness (kPa)	20.7 ± 24.4	NA	
CAP (dB/m)	303 ± 51	NA	
Laboratory parameters			
AST (U/L)	115 ± 101	22 ± 10	<0.0001
ALT (U/L)	74 ± 67	24 ± 15	<0.0001
GGT (U/L)	502 ± 688	33 ± 12	<0.0001
AP(U/L)	115 ± 71	73 ± 21	<0.0001
Bilirubin total (mg/dL)	1.76 ± 3.23	0.3 ± 0.4	<0.0001
INR	1.00 ± 0.27	1.00 ± 0.15	1.0000
Crea (mg/dL)	0.70 ± 0.27	0.72 ± 0.21	0.5795
Hb (g/dL)	13.8 ± 1.9	14.2 ± 1.1	0.0920
Platelets (/nL)	194 ± 81	221 ± 92	0.0320
Apoptosome and Inflammamosome data			
M30 (U/L)	566 ± 617	80.0 ± 25.0	<0.0001
M65 (U/L)	1,106 ± 1,040	120.0 ± 60.0	<0.0001
TNF-alpha (pg/mL)	45.6 ± 40.0	90 ± 10.0	<0.0001
TGF-beta (ng/mL)	26.1 ± 23.4	25.0 ± 5.0	0.6796
IL-6 (pg/mL)	47.2 ± 32.9	40.0 ± 15.0	0.0692
IL-8 (pg/mL)	65.9 ± 72.9	40.0 ± 10.0	0.0019
VEGF (pg/mL)	78.0 ± 50.2	60.0 ± 25.0	0.0035

using the FibroScan 502 platform (Echosens SA, Paris, France) using both the M and XL probe (Mueller, 2020). Hepatic fat content was also assessed with the Fibroscan device by measuring the controlled attenuation parameter (CAP) (Thiele et al., 2018). CAP values are expressed in dB/m and range from 100 to 400 dB/m. TE was performed by physicians with at least 12 months of experience in abdominal ultrasound and transient elastography on the right lobe of the liver in intercostal position according to established protocols (Mueller, 2020). Fibrosis stages were determined based on the aspartate amino-transferase (AST)-adapted cut-off values as described recently (Mueller et al., 2015).

Liver Histology

Liver biopsy was available in 23 patients with a mean biopsy lengths of 16.1 ± 12.5 mm). The tissue was fixed in formalin and embedded in paraffin. The histological analysis was performed in 4 μm sections. The tissue was further dewaxed and stained with hematoxylin and eosin (H&E), using standard procedures. Histological scoring was performed as described by Kleiner et al. (2005). The histological diagnosis of steatohepatitis was based on the minimal criteria of steatosis (micro and macro), ballooned hepatocytes, lobular inflammation and Mallory–Denk bodies. In addition, we correlated histological confounders with LS. We also looked at the small nodules (micro-nodular cirrhosis) that surrounded by connective tissue.

Cytokine Measurements and Apoptosis Markers

Cytokine levels and apoptosis markers were measured at *In Vitro* Drug Safety and Biotechnology, in Toronto, Canada using enzyme-linked immunosorbent-assay (ELISA) with in-house validated controls. Cytokine Kits were as follows: TGF- β (R&D Systems, Inc.; Minneapolis, MN, United States), VEGF, TNF- α levels, IL-6 and IL-8 (pg/mL), (PeproTech Asia, Rehovot, Israel).

The tests were performed according to the manufacturer specifications. For cytokine and apoptosis determination, each specimen was analyzed in duplicate with 95% sensitivity and 92% specificity.

Levels of M30 and M65 were assessed by ELISA using the M30 Apoptosense® ELISA Kit from Bender MedSystems (Vienna, Austria). The procedure is routine in *In Vitro* Drug Safety laboratory. The standards and reference reagents were from the National Institute for Biological Standards and Controls (NIBSC, Herts, United Kingdom).

Statistical Analysis

For a statistical description of the groups we used mean and standard deviation. Between-group differences were tested for statistical significance using the independent samples *T*-test for continuous variables and the chi-square test for binary data. Change of paired data was tested using the paired samples *T*-test. Correlation analysis was performed using the Spearman's rank correlation coefficient. *P*-values < 0.05 were considered significant.

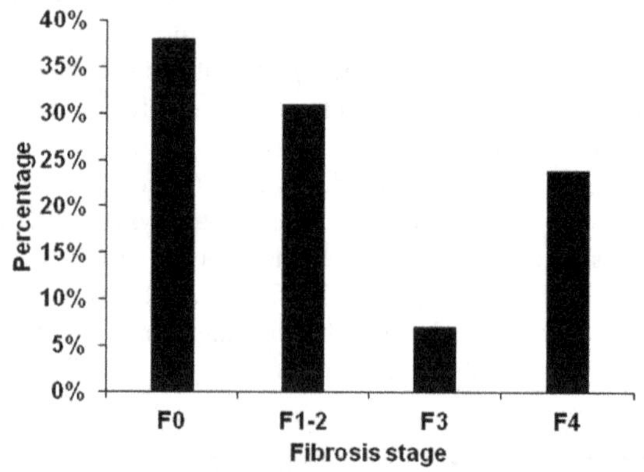

FIGURE 2 | Fibrosis distribution in all 114 patients. Fibrosis stage was non-invasively assessed by transient elastography using AST-adapted cutoff values for liver stiffness (Mueller et al., 2015).

RESULTS

Patients Characteristics

Patient characteristics are given in **Table 1**. The heavy drinkers consumed 204 ± 148 g/day alcohol for a duration of 15.3 ± 11.0 years. The liver stiffness (kPa) was 20.7 ± 24.4 (mean ± standard deviation) and CAP was 303 ± 51 dB/m. Mean spleen size was only slightly elevated and ascites was present in 11%.

Fibrosis distribution was F0–38.1%, F1–2–31%, F3–7.1% and F4–23.9% (**Figure 2**).

All laboratory parameters showed a typical profile for a heavy drinker cohort presenting fibrosis and steatosis (Mueller et al., 2014). Consequently, AST, alanine amino-transferase (ALT) and gamma-gluthamyl transpeptidase (GGT) levels were elevated and showed an AST/ALT ratio > 1. Mean total bilirubin was slightly elevated with 1.76 mg/dL. International Normalized Ratio (INR) was normal (1.00). In contrast, apoptotic marker M30 and necrotic marker M65 were five times above normal. Levels of cytokines and chemokines: TNF-α, IL-6, IL-8 and VEGF were only slightly elevated. Correlation analysis is shown in **Supplementary Table 1**.

LS was significantly correlated with M30 and M65 levels. Serum TNF- α was highly correlated with hemoglobin (r = -0.299, $P < 0.01$) and the presence of ascites (r = 0.288, $P < 0.01$), TGF-b and IL-8 with bilirubin (r = 0.232, $P < 0.05$ and r = 0.241, $P < 0.05$), while VEGF correlated highly with hepatic steatosis (r = -0.271, $P < 0.01$), platelets (r = 0.382, $P < 0.001$) and AST (r = -0.307, $P < 0.001$).

In summary, the fibrosis distribution and laboratory parameters of our cohort are representative for a heavy drinker cohort with drastically increased apoptosis markers and slightly elevated cytokines.

Liver Histology and Inflammation/Apoptosis

The available liver histology from the 23 patients showed the following: Steatosis distribution was: S0 (4.4%), S1 (26%), S2

(17.4%), and S3 (52.2%). Fibrosis distribution was F0 (8.7%) F1 (13.0%), F2 (8.7%), F3 (26.1%), and F4 (43.5%). 82.6% showed ballooning and 87% were classified as steatohepatitis. As shown in **Table 2**, LS was significantly associated with signs of ballooning, Mallory hyaline bodies, inflammation and fibrosis while no correlation was seen with the degree of steatosis.

Correlation analysis of histology with serum markers are shown in **Supplementary Table 2**.

M30 and M65 correlated with ballooning ($r = 0.419$ and 0.449, $P < 0.05$), lobular inflammation ($r = 0.506$ and 0.489, $P < 0.05$) and Mallory hyaline ($r = 0.575$ and 0.661, $P < 0.001$). TNF-α correlated significantly with hepatic steatosis ($r = 0.415$, $P < 0.05$), lobular inflammation ($r = 0.441$, $P < 0.05$), ballooning ($r = 0.557$, $P < 0.01$), steatohepatitis ($r = 0.466$, $P < 0.05$) and fibrosis septa around the central vein ($r = 0.487$, $P < 0.05$).

IL-6 correlated negatively with steatosis grade ($r = -0.544$, $P < 0.01$), ballooning ($r = -0.432$, $P < 0.05$), acidophil bodies ($r = -0.440$, $P < 0.05$), classification of steatohepatitis ($r = -0.415$, $P < 0.05$) and fibrosis septa around the central vein ($r = -0.580$, $P < 0.01$). No significant correlations were seen for TGF-β, IL-8 and VEGF. Typical ALD-related features of histology correlated highly with LS and apoptosis markers.

Role of Alcohol Detoxification

In the 45 individuals that underwent detoxification, both LS and CAP decreased significantly over a mean observation interval of 5.7 days in confirmation of earlier reports (Mueller et al., 2010; Thiele et al., 2018). Thus, LS decreased from 32.9 ± 29.7 to 24.8 ± 27.1 ($p < 0.05$) while CAP values declined from 310 ± 50 to 264 ± 77 ($p < 0.05$). In **Table 3** we present the changes of laboratory and elastography parameters before and after detoxification.

Levels of alanine and aspartate aminotransferases (ALT, AST), alkaline phosphatase (AP) and gamma glutamyl transpeptidase (GGT) also decreased during alcohol withdrawal as described earlier (Mueller et al., 2010). A significant decrease, however, was only observed for AST, GGT and AP but not for ALT and bilirubin. No significant changes were observed for M30, M65 and TNF-α while levels of TGF-beta decreased slightly ($P < 0.05$) or drastically in case of IL-6, IL-8 and VEGF ($P < 0.001$).

We calculated the Spearman correlations of the changes of cytokines during detoxification with other laboratory parameters (**Supplementary Tables 3A,B**).

The change of M30 was significantly associated with the change in GGT ($r = 0.367$, $P < 0.05$) and absolute hemoglobin levels ($r = 0.408$, $P < 0.05$). The change of M65 was significantly associated with changes in AST ($r = 0.581$, $P < 0.001$), ALT ($r = 0.529$, $P < 0.01$) and GGT ($r = 0.350$, $P < 0.05$) but also absolute GGT levels ($r = -0.356$, $P < 0.05$). The change in IL-8 was significant associated with initial levels of bilirubin ($r = -0.376$, $P < 0.05$) and white blood cells ($r = -0.333$, $P < 0.05$). The change in IL-6 was associated with white blood cells ($r = 0.329$, $P < 0.05$). No relevant associations were seen for VEGF and TGF-β. In conclusion, a significant improvement was observed after 1 week of detoxification for LS, CAP, TGF-β and VEGF but not the other cytokines.

Role of Cirrhosis Status on Biomarkers During Alcohol Withdrawal

We next studied the role of cirrhosis status on apoptotic markers and cytokines, since cirrhosis itself impairs the immune response, affects programmed cell death and is considered a pre-cancerogenic lesion. **Supplementary Table 4** shows comparison between cirrhotic (F4) vs. non-cirrhotic patients (F0-F3) in all 114 patients before detoxification. Cirrhosis was classified

TABLE 2 | Spearman correlations of LS with histological parameters ($n = 23$).

Histological parameter	Correlation with LS	
	R	*p*
Ballooning 0–2	0.741	0.0001
Lobular inflammation 0–3	0.733	0.0001
Classification steatohepatitis 0–2	0.648	0.0011
Fibrosis stage 0–4	0.611	0.0025
Large lipo-granulomas 0–1	0.467	0.0284
Mallory hyaline 0–1	0.451	0.0352
Micro-granulomas 0–1	0.387	0.0756
Microvesicular 0–1	0.362	0.0983
Glycogenated nuclei 0–1	0.346	0.1142
Portal inflammation 0–1	0.303	0.1704
Steatosis grade 0–3	0.298	0.1781
Location 0–3	0.195	0.3845
Pigmented macrophages 0–1	0.131	0.5615
Acidophil bodies 0–1	0.130	0.5653
Megamitochondria 0–1	0.009	0.9698

TABLE 3 | Laboratory and elastography parameters before and after alcohol detoxification ($n = 45$).

Parameter	Before detox	After detox	*P*-value
Laboratory parameter			
AST (U/L)	134 ± 96	99 ± 107	0.0144
ALT (U/L)	79 ± 74	76 ± 118	0.7748
GGT (U/L)	764 ± 861	453 ± 503	0.0005
AP (U/L)	149 ± 94	117 ± 71	0.0016
Bilirubin total (mg/dL)	2.6 ± 3.89	2.65 ± 4.45	0.8394
INR	1.06 ± 0.27	1.04 ± 0.30	0.8977
Urea (mg/dL)	20.62 ± 12.6	23.1 ± 12.7	0.2230
Creatinine (mg/dL)	0.69 ± 0.29	0.76 ± 0.29	0.0291
Hb (g/dL)	13.1 ± 2.0	13.1 ± 1.9	0.8490
Serum markers of inflammation and apoptosis			
M30 (U/L)	811 ± 795	771 ± 626	0.7417
M65 (U/L)	1391 ± 1173	1327 ± 1096	0.5237
TNF-alpha (pg/mL)	56.1 ± 34.9	56.7 ± 95.9	0.9662
TGF-beta (ng/mL)	27.1 ± 31.5	16.7 ± 6.2	0.0280
IL-6 (pg/mL)	43.5 ± 29.6	28.9 ± 13.6	0.0002
IL-8 (pg/mL)	92.6 ± 93.1	60.7 ± 43.3	0.0004
VEGF (pg/mL)	90.8 ± 62.4	61.0 ± 36.0	<0.0001
Transient elastography			
Liver stiffness (kPa)	32.9 ± 29.7	24.8 ± 27.1	0.0421
CAP (dB/m)	310.3 ± 50.03	264 ± 76.7	0.0277

according to AST-adapted cutoff-values for LS (Mueller et al., 2015). Cirrhotics were significantly older (54.4 ± 9.1 vs. 48.6 ± 12.9 years, $P < 0.05$), had a significantly longer duration of heavy alcohol drinking (20.1 ± 12.6 vs. 14.3 ± 10.3 years, $P < 0.05$) and had a significantly elevated LS (60.1 ± 14.6 vs. 8.3 ± 8.2 kPa, $P < 0.001$).

Alcohol consumption was slightly decreased in patients with cirrhosis (189 ± 193 vs. 208 134 g/day). They also had significantly higher levels of alcaline phosphatase (AP) (173 ± 94 vs. 95 ± 43, $P < 0.001$), GGT (793 ± 834 vs. 403 ± 613 U/L, $P < 0.05$), bilirubin (3.6 ± 4.3 g/dL, $P < 0.001$) and INR (1.21 ± 0.23 vs. 0.93 ± 0.24, $P < 0.001$) but lowered hemoglobin (12.7 ± 2.2 vs. 14.1 ± 1.7 g/dL, $P < 0.001$) and platelets (161 ± 83 vs. 206 ± 77/nL, $P < 0.01$).

No significant differences were observed with regard to gender distribution, steatosis degree, BMI and levels of ALT and leukocytes. Both M30 and M65 levels were significantly increased in cirrhotics (949 ± 821 vs. 434 ± 473 U/L, $P < 0.001$ for M30 and 1852 ± 1157 vs. 851 ± 864 U/L, $P < 0.001$ for M65). Among the cytokines, only IL-8 was significantly elevated in cirrhotics (97 ± 111 vs. 55 ± 51 pg/mL, $P < 0.01$).

TGF-β and VEGF levels were slightly reduced in patients with established cirrhosis, however, they did not reach levels of significance. The kinetics of cytokine levels, and M30/65 during alcohol withdrawal depends on the cirrhosis status (**Table 4**).

Cirrhosis was classified using AST-adapted cutoff-values for LS (Mueller et al., 2015).

Pro-fibrogenic cytokine TGF-β decreased significantly in patients with cirrhosis during alcohol detoxification. The levels of TGF-β were identical in cirrhotic and non-cirrhotic individuals after the detoxification period. No significant changes of M30/65 were observed (**Table 4**).

M30 tended to increase during detox in non-cirrhotics while a decrease was seen in cirrhotic individuals. Despite a smaller cohort size in the cirrhosis subgroup, all changes were slightly significant in response to alcohol withdrawal except VEGF. VEGF remained higher in the cirrhosis group despite the absence of alcohol. Among the biomarkers, only M65 was significantly higher in the cirrhosis group after detoxification.

In conclusion, despite impaired synthesis capacity in patients with cirrhosis, both markers of inflammation and apoptosis were significantly elevated in these patients. Significant reduction of cytokine levels were seen in the cirrhosis group after detoxification.

TABLE 4 | Biomarkers in cirrhosis (N = 18) vs. non-cirrhosis (N = 18) before and after alcohol withdrawal.

Parameter	Before	After	P
Non-cirrhotics F0-3 *N* = 26			
M30 (U/L)	622 ± 654	658 ± 649	0.6581
M65 (U/L)	979 ± 1,019	953 ± 1,101	0.5580
TNF-alpha (pg/mL)	50.4 ± 33.3	40.5 ± 21.4	0.0052
TGF-beta (ng/mL)	30.3 ± 40.4	16.8 ± 6.7	0.0977
IL-6 (pg/mL)	40.5 ± 29.2	25.2 ± 13.6	0.0024
IL-8 (pg/mL)	72.4 ± 65.9	52.1 ± 31.1	0.0197
VEGF (pg/mL)	96.8 ± 69.7	59.4 ± 36.6	0.0002
Cirrhotics F4 *N* = 18			
M30 (U/L)	1,046 ± 931	873 ± 583	0.3846
M65 (U/L)	19,02 ± 1,168	1721 ± 898	0.7379
TNF-alpha (pg/mL)	60.4 ± 33.9	46.0 ± 24.6	0.0040
TGF-beta (ng/mL)	23.2 ± 11.2	16.6 ± 5.8	0.0037
IL-6 (pg/mL)	49.7 ± 30.0	34.8 ± 11.9	0.0327
IL-8 (pg/mL)	114.9 ± 118.4	69.5 ± 54.6	0.0124
VEGF (pg/mL)	86.2 ± 50.6	65.3 ± 35.5	0.0023

DISCUSSION

In a cohort of well characterized heavy drinkers apoptosis. inflammation and vascular activities are mechanistic factors. Apoptosis, as measured by levels of M30, is drastically increased in cirrhotics. Alcohol detoxification for less than 1 week rapidly improved various parameters such as liver stiffness and transaminase levels but not the apoptosis rate. Both markers of inflammation and apoptosis were significantly elevated in these patients.

LS declines significantly in heavy drinkers after only 1 week of alcohol abstinence. This confirms earlier reports (Mueller et al., 2010). This decrease was statistically significant in 45.3% of the patients and resulted in a decrease of the estimated stage of fibrosis in 23.3% of them. LS was also significantly associated with histological features of fibrosis, ballooning and inflammation but not steatosis. The findings that LS was even higher correlated with inflammation than fibrosis is due to smaller sample size in comparison to an earlier report (Mueller and Lackner, 2020). Apoptosis rate was highly associated with histological features of ballooning, lobular inflammation and fibrosis (Stärkel et al., 2019). These data suggested that alcohol has a strong inhibiting effect on cell regeneration and apoptosis while withdrawal will enhance cell regeneration.

In the present study we provide further evidence that M30 levels are generally higher in cirrhotic patients. The increase of M30 in response to withdrawal is only seen in non-cirrhotic patients. These novel findings suggest that patients with cirrhosis have a liver micro- environment that, independent of amount of alcohol consumption, causes continued cell death by apoptosis. Significantly elevated M65 levels in cirrhotic patients after detoxification confirms the continue hepatocyte death by necrosis. Due to the smaller sample size in this study, no levels of significance were reached with regard to M30 differences after detoxification. In contrast to apoptosis markers, TNF-α, IL-6, IL-8 and VEGF were only slightly elevated while no difference was seen with TGF-β in comparison to controls.

In our small sub-cohort with liver histology, only TNF-a correlated significantly with hepatic steatosis, lobular inflammation, ballooning, and fibrosis septa around the central vein while no significant correlations were seen for TGF-b, IL-8 and VEGF. IL-6, IL-8 and VEGF decreased drastically during alcohol withdrawal while TNF- a and TGF- b showed only a moderate decrease. However, when looking at the cirrhotic subcohort, the pro-fibrogenic TGF- b decreased highly significantly reaching almost identical levels in both subgroups. This is in line with other reports where statistically significant reductions in TGF b after the detoxification period show a positive correlation with the reduction of fibrosis (Neuman et al., 2015a,b, 2020).

In the cirrhosis subgroup, cytokine changes were significant in response to alcohol withdrawal. Only VEGF levels remained higher in the cirrhosis group. This could be a first support for the recently introduced sinusoidal pressure hypothesis (SPH) to explain fibrosis progression (Mueller S., 2016). SPH identifies as an elevation of sinusoidal pressure (SP) as cause of fibrosis/cirrhosis. This postulates that elevated SP is the major upstream event that initiates fibrosis progression *via* biomechanical signaling by stretching of perisinusoidal cells. SPH further postulates that arterialization of the stiff cirrhotic liver causes the final self-perpetuating key event exposing the low-pressure-organ to pathologically high pressures. This arterialization, however, is strongly driven by angiogenetic signaling pathways including hypoxia signaling. Since VEGF is one of the major target genes of hypoxia inducible factor 1 alpha, sustained levels of VEGF in cirrhotics during alcohol detoxification could be a first hint that angiogenesis and revascularization is an important process in manifest cirrhosis in support of SPH.

In summary, we here demonstrate important findings on biomarkers of apoptosis, inflammation and angiogenesis in patients with ALD undergoing detoxification. While apoptosis seems to be a hallmark primarily in patients with manifest cirrhosis, it further increases especially in non-cirrhotic patients after alcohol withdrawal. Moreover, both pro-fibrogenic TGF-beta and pro-angiogenic VEGF responded especially effectively in cirrhotics to alcohol withdrawal. These findings seem to be in line with clinical observations and may pave the way to novel targeted therapeutic approaches. Finally, in our opinion, studies on heavy drinkers undergoing alcohol withdrawal represents a valid approach to better understand molecular mechanisms of liver damage and resolution in patients with ALD.

AUTHOR CONTRIBUTIONS

This work resulted from a collaboration between an academic clinician (SM) and an academic clinical biochemist and toxicologist (MN). MN and SM: substantial contributions to the conception or design of the work acquisition, analysis, and interpretation of data for the work. MN, SM, and JM: writing—original draft preparation, and review and editing. All authors have read and agreed to the published version of the manuscript and are accountable for all aspects of the work in ensuring the accuracy of any part of the work.

REFERENCES

Atkinson, S. R., Grove, J. I., Liebig, S., Astbury, S., Vergis, N., Goldin, R., et al. (2020). In severe alcoholic hepatitis, serum Keratin-18 fragments are diagnostic, prognostic, and theragnostic biomarkers. *Am. J. Gastroenterol.* 115, 1857–1868. doi: 10.14309/ajg.0000000000000912

Bantel, H., Ruck, P., and Schulze-Osthoff, K. (2000). In situ monitoring of caspase activation in hepatobiliary diseases. *Cell Death Differ.* 7, 504–505. doi: 10.1038/sj.cdd.4400669

Forster, L. E., Pollow, R., and Stoller, E. P. (1993). Alcohol use and potential risk for alcohol-related adverse drug reactions among community-based elderly. *J. Community Health* 18, 225–239. doi: 10.1007/bf01324433

Gao, B., Ahmad, M. F., Nagy, L. E., and Tsukamoto, H. (2019). Inflammatory pathways in alcoholic steatohepatitis. *J. Hepatol.* 70, 249–259. doi: 10.1016/j.jhep.2018.10.023

Gaul, S., Leszczynska, A., Alegre, F., Kaufmann, B., Johnson, C. D., Adams, L. A., et al. (2021). Hepatocyte pyroptosis and release of inflammasome particles induce stellate cell activation and liver fibrosis. *J. Hepatol.* 74, 156–167. doi: 10.1016/j.jhep.2020.07.041

Kleiner, D. E., Brunt, E. M., Van Natta, M., Behling, C., Contos, M. J., Cummings, O. W., et al. (2005). Design and validation of a histological scoring system for nonalcoholic fatty liver disease. *Hepatology* 41, 1313–1321. doi: 10.1002/hep.20701

Lavallard, V. J., Bonnafous, S., Patouraux, S., Saint-Paul, M. C., Rousseau, D., Anty, R., et al. (2011). Serum markers of hepatocyte death and apoptosis are non invasive biomarkers of severe fibrosis in patients with alcoholic liver disease. *PLoS One* 6:e17599. doi: 10.1371/journal.pone.0017599

Le Daré, B., Lagente, V., and Gicquel, T. (2019). Ethanol and its metabolites: update on toxicity, benefits, and focus on immunomodulatory effects. *Drug Metab. Rev.* 51, 545–561. doi: 10.1080/03602532.2019.1679169

Leers, M. P., Kolgen, W., Bjorklund, V., Bergman, T., Tribbick, G., Persson, B., et al. (1999). Immunocytochemical detection and mapping of a cytokeratin 18 neo-epitope exposed during early apoptosis. *J. Pathol.* 187, 567–572. doi: 10.1002/(sici)1096-9896(199904)187:5<567::aid-path288>3.0.co;2-j

Louvet, A., Labreuche, J., Artru, F., Bouthors, A., Rolland, B., Saffers, P., et al. (2017). Main drivers of outcome differ between short term and long term in severe alcoholic hepatitis: a prospective study. *Hepatology* 66, 1464–1473. doi: 10.1002/hep.29240

Malhi, H., and Gores, G. J. (2008). Cellular and molecular mechanisms of liver injury. *Gastroenterology* 134, 1641–1654. doi: 10.1053/j.gastro.2008.03.002

Mehal, W., and Imaeda, A. (2010). Cell death and fibrogenesis. *Semin. Liver Dis.* 30, 226–231. doi: 10.1055/s-0030-1255352

Molina, P. E., McClain, C., Valla, D., Guidot, D., Diehl, A. M., Lang, C. H., et al. (2002). Molecular pathology and clinical aspects of alcohol-induced tissue injury. *Alcohol. Clin. Exp. Res.* 26, 120–128. doi: 10.1097/00000374-200201000-00017

Moreau, R. (2016). The pathogenesis of ACLF: the inflammatory response and immune function. *Semin. Liver Dis.* 36, 133–140. doi: 10.1055/s-0036-1583199

Moreno, C., Mueller, S., and Szabo, G. (2019). Non-invasive diagnosis and biomarkers in alcohol-related liver disease. *J. Hepatol.* 70, 273–283. doi: 10.1016/j.jhep.2018.11.025

Morgan, T. R., Mandayam, S., and Jamal, M. M. (2004). Alcohol and hepatocellular carcinoma. *Gastroenterology* 127, S87–S96.

Mueller, J., Raisi, H., Rausch, V., Peccerella, T., Simons, D., Ziener, C. H., et al. (2017). Sensitive and non-invasive assessment of hepatocellular iron using a novel room-temperature susceptometer. *J. Hepatol.* 67, 535–542. doi: 10.1016/j.jhep.2017.04.019

Mueller, S. (2016). Does pressure cause liver cirrhosis? The sinusoidal pressure hypothesis. *World J. Gastroenterol.* 22, 10482–10501. doi: 10.3748/wjg.v22.i48.10482

Mueller, S. (2020). *Liver Elastography: Clinical Use and Interpretation.* Berlin: Springer.

Mueller, S. (ed.), and Lackner, C. (2020). "Histological confounders of liver stiffness," in *Liver Elastography*. Berlin: Springer.

Mueller, S., Englert, S., Seitz, H. K., Badea, R. I., Erhardt, A., Bozaari, B., et al. (2015). Inflammation-adapted liver stiffness values for improved fibrosis staging in patients with hepatitis C virus and alcoholic liver disease. *Liver Int.* 35, 2514–2521. doi: 10.1111/liv.12904

Mueller, S., Millonig, G., and Seitz, H. K. (2009). Alcoholic liver disease and hepatitis C: a frequently underestimated combination. *World J. Gastroenterol.* 15, 3462–3471.

Mueller, S., Millonig, G., Sarovska, L., Friedrich, S., Reimann, F. M., Pritsch, M., et al. (2010). Increased liver stiffness in alcoholic liver disease: differentiating fibrosis from steatohepatitis. *World J. Gastroenterol.* 16, 966–972. doi: 10.3748/

wjg.v16.i8.966

Mueller, S., Nahon, P., Rausch, V., Peccerella, T., Silva, I., Yagmur, E., et al. (2017). Caspase-cleaved keratin-18 fragments increase during alcohol withdrawal and predict liver-related death in patients with alcoholic liver disease. *Hepatology* 66, 96–107. doi: 10.1002/hep.29099

Mueller, S., Seitz, H. K., and Rausch, V. (2014). Non-invasive diagnosis of alcoholic liver disease. *World J. Gastroenterol.* 20, 14626–14641. doi: 10.3748/wjg.v20.i40.14626

Neuman, M. G. (2007). Cytokine – chemokines modulate fibrosis in alcoholic hepatitis. *Rom J. Hepatol.* 3, 19–34.

Neuman, M. G., Brenner, D. A., Rehermann, B., Taieb, J., Chollet-Martin, S., Cohard, M., et al. (2001). Mechanisms of alcoholic liver disease: cytokines. *Alcohol. Clin. Exp. Res.* 25, 251s–253s.

Neuman, M. G., Cohen, L., Zakhari, S., Nanau, R. M., Mueller, S., Schneider, M., et al. (2014a). Alcoholic liver disease: a synopsis of the Charles Lieber's memorial Symposia 2009-2012. *Alcohol Alcohol.* 49, 373–380. doi: 10.1093/alcalc/agu021

Neuman, M. G., French, S. W., French, B. A., Seitz, H. K., Cohen, L. B., Mueller, S., et al. (2014b). Alcoholic and non-alcoholic steatohepatitis. *Exp. Mol. Pathol.* 97, 492–510.

Neuman, M. G., French, S. W., Zakhari, S., Malnick, S., Seitz, H. K., Cohen, L. B., et al. (2017). Alcohol, microbiome, life style influence alcohol and non-alcoholic organ damage. *Exp. Mol. Pathol.* 102, 162–180. doi: 10.1016/j.yexmp.2017.01.003

Neuman, M. G., Katz, G. G., Malkiewicz, I. M., Mathurin, P., Tsukamoto, H., Adachi, M., et al. (2002). Alcoholic liver injury and apoptosis - synopsis of the symposium held at ESBRA 2001. 8th congress of the European Society for Biomedical Research on Alcoholism, Paris, September 16, 2001. *Alcohol* 28, 117–128.

Neuman, M. G., Malnick, S., Maor, Y., Nanau, R. M., Melzer, E., Ferenci, P., et al. (2015a). Alcoholic liver disease: clinical and translational research. *Exp. Mol. Pathol.* 99, 596–610.

Neuman, M. G., Maor, Y., Nanau, R. M., Melzer, E., Mell, H., Opris, M., et al. (2015b). Alcoholic liver disease: role of cytokines. *Arch. Toxicol.* 5, 2023–2034.

Neuman, M. G., Schmilovitz-Weiss, H., Hilzenrat, N., Bourliere, M., Marcellin, P., Trepo, C., et al. (2012). Markers of inflammation and fibrosis in alcoholic hepatitis and viral hepatitis C. *Int. J. Hepatol.* 2012:231210.

Neuman, M. G., Seitz, H. K., French, S. W., Malnick, S., Tsukamoto, H., Cohen, L. B., et al. (2020). Alcoholic-hepatitis, links to brain and microbiome: mechanisms. clinical and experimental research. *Biomedicines* 8:63. doi: 10.3390/biomedicines8030063

Piecha, F., Peccerella, T., Bruckner, T., Seitz, H. K., Rausch, V., and Mueller, S. (2016). Arterial pressure suffices to increase liver stiffness. *Am. J. Physiol. Gastrointest. Liver Physiol.* 311, G945–G953.

Roerecke, M., Nanau, R., Rehm, J., and Neuman, M. (2016). Ethnicity matters: a systematic review and meta-analysis of the non-linear relationship between alcohol consumption and prevalence and incidence of hepatic steatosis. *EBioMedicine* 8, 317–330. doi: 10.1016/j.ebiom.2016.04.023

Romano, V., Hatzfeld, M., Magin, T. M., Zimbelmann, R., Franke, W. W., Maier, G., et al. (1986). Cytokeratin expression in simple epithelia. i. Identification of mRNA coding for human cytokeratin no. 18 by a cDNA clone. *Differentiation* 30, 244–253. doi: 10.1111/j.1432-0436.1986.tb00787.x

Schlossberger, V., Worni, M., Kihm, C., Montani, M., Datz, C., Hampe, J., et al. (2019). Plasma levels of K18 fragments do not correlate with alcoholic liver fibrosis. *Gut Liver* 13, 77–82. doi: 10.5009/gnl18037

Seitz, H. K., Bataller, R., Cortez-Pinto, H., Gao, B., Gual, A., Lackner, C., et al. (2018). Alcoholic liver disease. *Nat. Rev. Dis. Primers* 4:16.

Stärkel, P., Schnabl, B., Leclercq, S., Komuta, M., Bataller, R., Argemi, J., et al. (2019). Deficient IL-6/Stat3 signaling, High TLR7, and Type i interferons in early human alcoholic liver disease: a triad for liver damage and fibrosis. *Hepatol. Commun.* 3, 867–882. doi: 10.1002/hep4.1364

Thiele, M., Rausch, V., Fluhr, G., Kjaergaard, M., Piecha, F., Mueller, J., et al. (2018). Controlled attenuation parameter and alcoholic hepatic steatosis: diagnostic accuracy and role of alcohol detoxification. *J. Hepatol.* 68, 1025–1032. doi: 10.1016/j.jhep.2017.12.029

Vandenabeele, P., Galluzzi, L., Vanden Berghe, T., and Kroemer, G. (2010). Molecular mechanisms of necroptosis: an ordered cellular explosion. *Nat. Rev. Mol. Cell Biol.* 11, 700–714. doi: 10.1038/nrm2970

Wiesner, R., Edwards, E., Freeman, R., Harper, A., Kim, R., Kamath, P., et al. (2003). Model for end-stage liver disease (MELD) and allocation of donor livers. *Gastroenterology* 124, 91–96. doi: 10.1053/gast.2003.50016

Yoon, Y.-H., and Chen, C. M. (2016). *Liver Cirrhosis Mortality in the United States: National, State, and Regional Trends, 2000–2013*. Bethesda, MD: NIAAA.

Zimmerman, J. E., Wagner, D. P., Draper, E. A., Wright, L., Alzola, C., and Knaus, W. A. (1998). Evaluation of acute physiology and chronic health evaluation III predictions of hospital mortality in an independent database. *Crit. Care Med.* 26, 1317–1326. doi: 10.1097/00003246-199808000-00012

3

Insomnia Promotes Hepatic Steatosis in Rats Possibly by Mediating Sympathetic Overactivation

Zongding Wang[1,2†], Xiaoyan Liang[3,4†], Yanmei Lu[3,4], Tiemin Jiang[1,2], Tuerganaili Aji[1,2], Kalibixiati Aimulajiang[1], Huaxin Sun[3,4], Ling Zhang[3,4], Xianhui Zhou[3,4], Baopeng Tang[3,4] and Hao Wen[1,2*]*

[1]State Key Laboratory of Pathogenesis, Prevention, and Treatment of High Incidence Diseases in Central Asia, The First Affiliated Hospital of Xinjiang Medical University, Urumqi, China, [2]Hepatobiliary and Hydatid Disease Department, First Affiliated Hospital of Xinjiang Medical University, Urumqi, China, [3]Department of Pacing and Electrophysiology, The First Affiliated Hospital of Xinjiang Medical University, Xinjiang, China, [4]Xinjiang Key Laboratory of Cardiac Electrophysiology and Cardiac Remodeling, The First Affiliated Hospital of Xinjiang Medical University, Xinjiang, China

***Correspondence:**
Hao Wen
dr.wenhao@163.com
Baopeng Tang
tangbaopeng1111@163.com

†These authors have contributed equally to this work*

Background: Insomnia is a widespread problem that can lead to the occurrence of other diseases and correlates closely with sympathetic nerve hyperactivation. Obesity-induced hepatic steatosis is mediated by sympathetic overactivation. However, it remains unclear whether insomnia may cause hepatic steatosis. The goal of this study was to preliminarily investigate whether insomnia caused hepatic steatosis in rats *via* sympathetic hyperactivation.

Methods: A total of 32 Sprague-Dawley male rats were divided randomly into four groups: model, sympathetic denervation (Sd), estazolam, and control (eight rats/group). Model group received sustained sleep deprivation using the modified multiple platform method. In the Sd group, rats underwent sleep deprivation after receiving Sd by 6-hydroxydopamine (6-OHDA). Estazolam group: the rats concurrently received sleep deprivation and treatment with estazolam. The other eight rats housed in cages and kept in a comfortable environment were used as control. Blood samples were obtained for analysis of plasma lipids and hepatic function. Sympathetic hyperactivation-related indexes and hepatic steatosis in liver tissues were tested.

Results: Liver enzymes, plasma lipid levels, and hepatic steatosis were elevated in insomnia rats, and sympathetic hyperactivation was found. Insomnia-induced hepatic steatosis was effectively lowered with pharmacological ablation of the hepatic sympathetic nerves. Furthermore, the treatment of insomnia with estazolam inhibited sympathetic activation and reduced hepatic steatosis.

Conclusion: Sustained sleep deprivation-induced insomnia promotes hepatic steatosis in rats possibly by mediating sympathetic overactivation.

Keywords: insomnia, sleep deprivation, sympathetic nerve, hepatic steatosis, lipid droplets

INTRODUCTION

Insomnia is a common problem that warrants increased attention from clinicians (Buysse, 2013). Previous studies indicated a high incidence of sleep disturbance in the general population, including insomnia (Kalmbach et al., 2019), hypersomnia (Belenky et al., 2003), circadian rhythm sleep disorders, and other sleep dysfunction (Kammerer et al., 2021), especially chronic insomnia, which is highly correlated with increased morbidity and mortality (Lu et al., 2018). People with long-term insomnia are prone to nonrestorative or poor-quality sleep and even suffering from depression, anxiety (Okun et al., 2018), cognitive impairment (Fortier-Brochu and Morin, 2014), mental disorder (Medrano-Martinez and Ramos-Platon, 2016), concomitant cardiovascular, and other diseases if left untreated (Jarrin et al., 2018). Some studies have suggested an association of insomnia with increased sympathetic activity (Carter et al., 2018). The possible mechanism might be correlated with dysregulation of the hypothalamic-pituitary-adrenal axis (van Liempt et al., 2013). In addition, chronic insomnia is often accompanied by impairment of the sympathetic baroreflex (Carter et al., 2018). Therefore, sympathetic hyperactivation may be closely related to the development of insomnia.

The liver is the major organ responsible for lipid metabolism, modulating hepatic lipid metabolism and homeostasis (Jensen-Cody and Potthoff, 2021). Its main functions include lipid synthesis, metabolism, and transportation. Lipids mainly include triglycerides (TGs), phospholipids, and cholesterol (Schulze and McNiven, 2019). Dysregulation of hepatic lipid metabolism leads to abnormal accumulation of lipids and the formation of lipid droplets in liver tissues, ultimately predisposing patients to fatty liver. Furthermore, patients with fatty liver are increasingly susceptible to steatohepatitis and cirrhosis compared with those nonfatty liver (Gluchowski et al., 2017). Thus, fatty liver is gaining increasing attention.

The liver receives innervation from the autonomic nervous system, including the sympathetic and parasympathetic nervous systems (Furness et al., 2014). Sympathetic nerves, as regulators, are involved in hepatic lipid metabolism (Amir et al., 2020). Sympathetic hyperactivation promoted hepatic steatosis. In contrast, sympathetic denervation could ameliorate high-fat diet-induced fatty liver in obese mice (Hurr et al., 2019). These results provide clues for sympathetic nerves to regulate hepatic lipid metabolism.

However, the hepatic sympathetic nerve activity of chronic insomnia is involved in lipid metabolism is unknown. Here, a chronic insomnia model was established. The present study aimed to validate the hypothesis that hepatic sympathetic nerve activity mediates hepatic steatosis in rats with chronic insomnia.

MATERIALS AND METHODS

Animals and Welfare

Sprague-Dawley (SD) male rats (180–220g; 6–8weeks) were purchased from our institution and randomly divided into four groups (eight rats per group). The four groups were the control, model group, sympathetic denervation group (Sd), and treatment group (estazolam). The present study protocol was reviewed and approved by the Institutional Animal Ethics Committee of Xinjiang Medical University (IACUC-20210301-01), in accordance with the 588th regulation of animal experiments issued by the Chinese Government in 2011. Rats were euthanized by anesthetic overdose. Blood samples and liver specimens were obtained for analysis.

Intraperitoneal Administration of 6-Hydroxydopamine

The sympathetic denervation group received 6-hydroxydopamine (6-HODA; #28094-15-7, Nanjing Chemical Co., Ltd.). Rats were injected intraperitoneally once daily for 3 consecutive days (50mg/kg/day; Chen et al., 2016; Hurr et al., 2019). Subsequently, these rats received sleep deprivation.

Animal Model Establishment

Multiple modified platforms were used to establish the sleep deprivation model (Alkadhi and Alhaider, 2016). Except for eight rats in the normal control group, the remaining rats were prepared to establish the chronic insomnia model. In brief, rats were placed on a small fixed platform surrounded by water for 8weeks to sustainably maintain sleep deprivation and had access to water and food only. The normal control rats were housed in cages and kept in a comfortable environment under a 12-h light/dark cycle with water and food available *ad libitum*. All rats were fed with common pellet diets, and each group were given the same total amount of food every day. The treated rats received combined sleep deprivation and 5mg/kg/day disulfiram by estazolam (Hirase et al., 2008). The schematic of the experimental timeline was delineated in the **Supplementary Figure 1**.

Hepatic Function and Lipid Level Assay

Blood samples were centrifuged, and the supernatant was collected for hepatic function tests. The levels of aspartate transaminase (ALT) and alanine aminotransferase (AST) were determined by an automatic biochemical analyzer (Mindray-120, Guangzhou, China) in accordance with the instructions. Free fatty acids (FFAs) and TGs were measured by kits with a colorimetric method (Nanjing Jianchen Biotech Inc., Nanjing, China).

Histological Analysis and Immunohistochemistry

Paraffin-embedded liver sections were deparaffinized, baked, dewaxed and hydrated. Hematoxylin-eosin (HE) staining was performed according to routine protocols. For oil red O staining, the cardiac tissue was sliced using a freezing microtome, rinsed, kept in 60% isopropanol, and finally stained with 0.5% oil red O solution (Sigma, St. Louis, United States) for 20min or maintained in 60% isopropanol for differentiation.

The process of immunohistochemical staining was performed following the manual instructions. In brief, endogenous peroxidase activity was quenched using 3% hydrogen peroxidase, samples were subjected to heat-mediated antigen retrieval (citrate buffer, pH6), and samples were then blocked with goat serum for 30 min. Primary antibody incubation was performed overnight at 4°C using different dilutions, including Perilipin-2 (1:500, OriGene, Rockville, United States) and growth-associated protein-43 (GAP43; 1:1,000, Abcam, Cambridge, United States), and the secondary antibody was incubated for 1 h at room temperature. The sections were washed three times (5 min/wash) after each step. Substitution of PBS for the primary antibody served as the negative control. Diaminobenzidin (DAB; ZSGB-BIO, Beijing, China) was used to stain the sections. Then, sections were counterstained with hematoxylin. The stained sections were examined by a Leica DMI 3000R microscope (Leica Microsystems, Germany) and images were captured under an Olympus microscope (Olympus, DP26, Japan). Immunostaining was quantified using ImageJ software.

Immunofluorescence Assay

Liver tissues were fixed in 4% formaldehyde over 24 h, dehydrated, and embedded in paraffin. Sections (5 μm) were deparaffinized and sequentially incubated overnight at 4°C with primary antibodies against GAP43 (1:100, Abcam, Cambridge, United States) and TH (1:50, Bioss, Beijing, China), washed and incubated for 1 h with appropriate conjugated secondary antibodies (Alexa Fluor 488-conjugated donkey anti-mouse IgG and CoraLite 594-conjugated goat anti-rabbit IgG, Proteintech, United States). Nuclei were stained with 4', 6-diamidino-2-phenylindole (DAPI). Confocal microscopy imaging and colocalization analysis were carried out on a confocal laser scanning microscope (Leica, Germany).

ELISA

After weighing and mashing, fresh liver tissues were lysed in PBS buffer supplemented with protease inhibitors (Mini EDTA-free Protease Inhibitor, Roche, Switzerland) and broken by sonication. After centrifugation (5,000 × *g*, 10 min), the supernatant was used for nerve growth factor (NGF) assays according to the manufacturer's protocol (Jianglai Biotechnology Co., Shanghai, China). Absorbance at 450 nm was measured using a microplate reader (Bio-Rad, Hercules, United States). Each measurement was performed in triplicate.

Transmission Electron Microscopy

The subcellular organelles in liver tissues were observed by Transmission Electron Microscopy (TEM, JEM-1220, JEOL Ltd., Japan) and images were captured under an Olympus microscope (Olympus Soft Imaging Solutions, Morada G3, Japan). The method for liver preprocessing was in line with those from previous studies (Du et al., 2017). Briefly, the liver tissue was fixed with 4% glutaraldehyde for 24 h, dehydrated by an ethanol gradient series, postfixed in 0.5% osmium tetroxide, 2% uranyl acetate, and 0.1% tannic acid, followed by epoxy resin fixation.

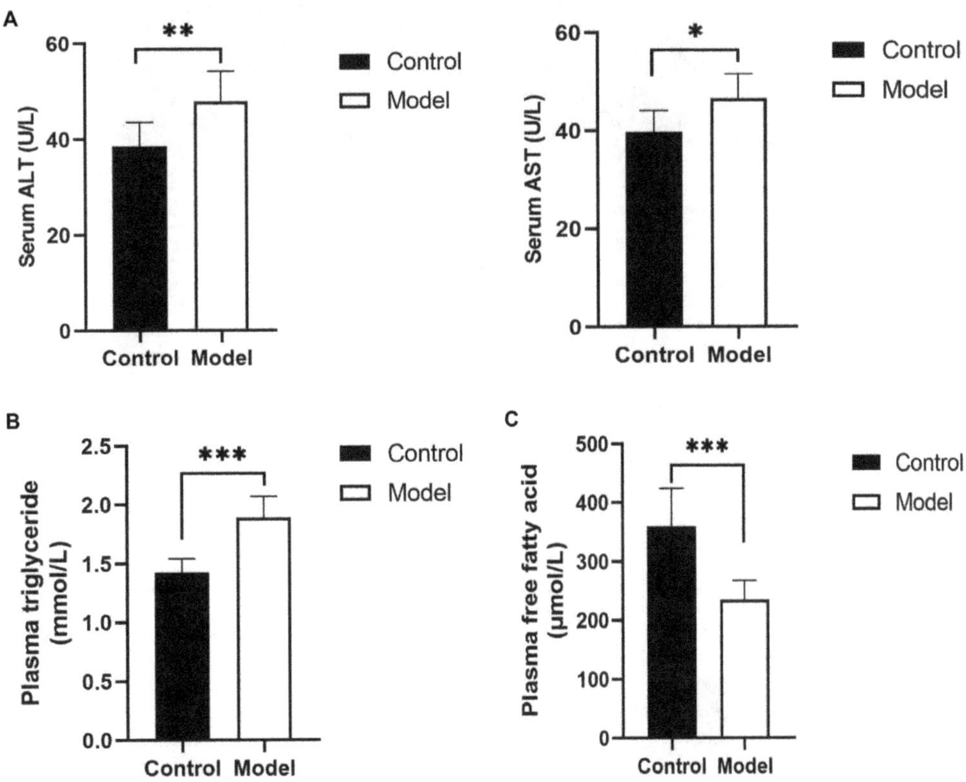

FIGURE 1 | Changes in hepatic function and blood lipids. **(A)** Serum was analyzed for liver enzyme [aspartate transaminase (ALT) and alanine aminotransferase (AST)] levels; **(B)** plasma triglyceride levels in insomnia rats were clearly higher than those in controls; and **(C)** Plasma free fatty acid (FFA) levels in insomnia rats were significantly lower than those in controls. The results were obtained from two independent experiments and are expressed as the mean ± SD, $n = 8$ per group, *$p < 0.05$; **$p < 0.01$; and ***$p < 0.001$.

High-Performance Liquid Chromatography-Tandem Mass Spectrometry

In this study, high-performance liquid chromatography-tandem mass spectrometry (HP-LC-MS/MS) was used to test the norepinephrine (NE) content in the liver. First, 10.0 mg of NE (Zhongshan Golden Bridge, Beijing, China) was added to 0.1% ascorbic acid solution (1 mg ascorbic acid dissolved in 1 ml of methanol). The pretreatment of samples was conducted according to a previous study (Tsunoda et al., 2002). Then, the 250-μl sample was dried with a nitrogen gun and reconstituted with 50 μl of acetonitrile: water (85:15) solution (containing 2% formic acid), and 20 μl of sample and NE standard were added to the LC/MS vial. High-performance liquid chromatography (ACQUITY UPLC, Waters, United States) and mass spectrometry (ACQUITY TQD, Waters, United States) were used for analysis. The MS conditions were as follows: cone gas flow rate of 150 L/h, desolvation gas flow rate of 900 L/h, source temperature of 150°C, desolvation temperature of 550°C, and ionization mode ESI+. Finally, the samples were subjected to gradient elution as follows: mobile phase A (5:95 acetonitrile containing 30 mM formic acid: Milli-Q water) and mobile phase B (85:15 acetonitrile containing 30 mM formic acid: Milli-Q water).

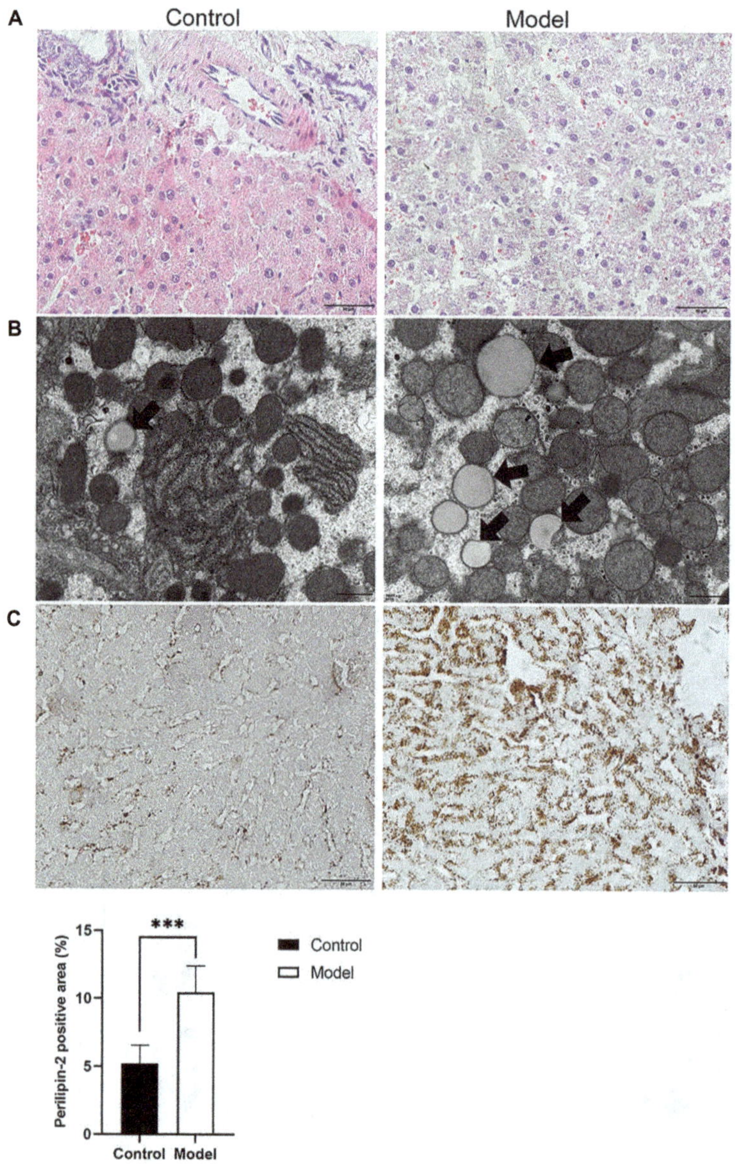

FIGURE 2 | Histopathology, immunohistochemistry, and transmission electron microscopy (TEM) were performed to determine the degree of hepatic steatosis. **(A)** Hematoxylin-eosin (HE) staining of the liver showed steatosis of most hepatocytes in the model group (scale bar: 50 μm). **(B)** Lipid droplets in hepatocytes were examined by TEM (scale bar: 1 μm). **(C)** Immunohistochemical staining for Perilipin-2 was observed predominantly in hepatocytes, where positive staining was brown-yellow (scale bar: 50 μm). The results were obtained from two independent experiments and are expressed as the mean ± SD, $n = 8$ per group, $^{***}p < 0.001$.

Statistical Analysis

The data are presented as the mean ± SD, comparisons between two groups were carried out using the independent T test and among multiple groups using single factor ANOVA. About $p < 0.05$ was considered statistically significant. All statistical calculations were performed using the statistical software program (GraphPad Prism 8.0 software, United States).

RESULTS

Sustained Sleep-Deprivation Occurred in the Model Group

After receiving 8 weeks of sleep deprivation, the mental state, activity, and hair luster of the rats were selected as the main observation indexes in the present experiment. The rats in the model group showed obvious retarded reactions, reduced activity, and dull hair. The rats in the treatment group and the sympathetic denervation group exhibited shiny fur and improvements in the previously mentioned symptoms. However, no abnormal findings were observed in the control group.

Liver Enzymes and Lipid Metabolism Tests Were Abnormal in Insomnia Rats

To determine the change in hepatic function of the insomnia rats, serum ALT, and AST were detected. Compared with the control group, the rats in the model group displayed a higher level of liver enzymes (ALT, 47.8 ± 6.3 vs. 38.5 ± 4.9 U/L, $p = 0.0058$; AST, 46.4 ± 5.0 vs. 39.7 ± 4.3 U/L,

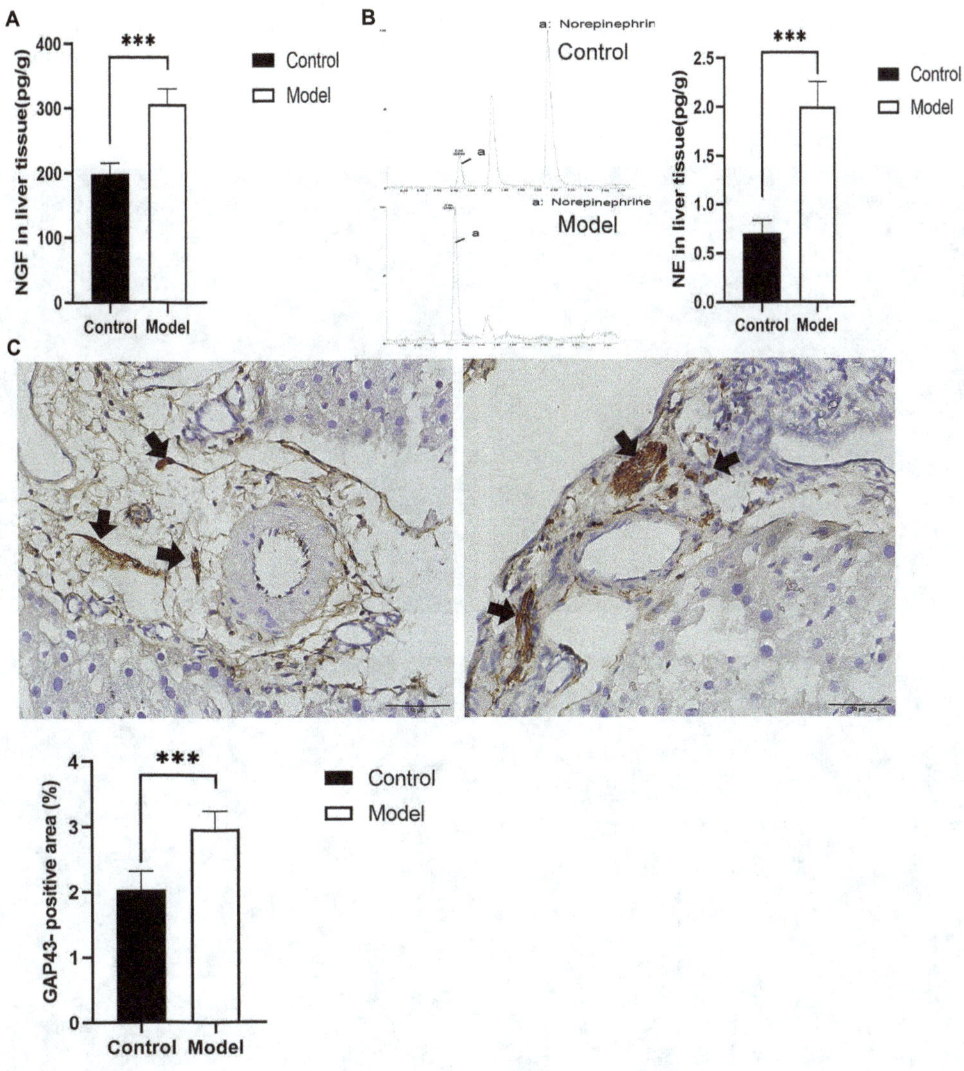

FIGURE 3 | Determination of nerve growth-related indexes in liver tissue. **(A)** Nerve growth factor (NGF) was determined by ELISA in liver tissues. **(B)** Norepinephrine (NE) in liver tissues was quantified by high-performance liquid chromatography-tandem mass spectrometry (HP-LC-MS/MS), presenting an increase in the model group. **(C)** Immunohistochemical staining of growth-associated protein-43 (GAP43) was used to assess nerve growth (scale bar: 50 μm). The results were obtained from two independent experiments and are expressed as the mean ± SD, $n = 8$ per group, $^{***}p < 0.001$. NE, norepinephrine.

$p = 0.0124$ U/L; **Figure 1A**). Moreover, to evaluate insomnia-induced plasma lipid changes, we analyzed the plasma lipids of the control and model groups. The level of triglycerides in the model group was significantly higher than that in the control group (1.88 ± 0.18 vs. 1.42 ± 0.11 mmol/L, $p < 0.0001$; **Figure 1B**). Conversely, a greater reduction in the free fatty acid content was observed in the model group (233.95 ± 33.92 vs. 359.51 ± 63.90 μmol/L, $p = 0.0002$; **Figure 1C**).

To further investigate the effects of insomnia on fatty liver, we inspected the pathology and microstructure of the liver. HE staining of the liver in the model group indicated that more lipid droplets accumulated in the hepatocytes of the model group than in the hepatocytes of the control rats (**Figure 2A**). Additionally, the subsequent results from electron microscopy also supported this conclusion (**Figure 2B**). Perilipin-2, which is expressed around lipid droplets, was assessed to determine the extent of fat accumulation in the liver. The immunohistochemistry results revealed that compared to the control group, the expression of Perilipin-2 was significantly increased in the model group (10.45 ± 1.95 vs. 5.21 ± 1.34%, $p < 0.0001$; **Figure 2C**).

Sympathetic Activation and Hyperplasia in the Livers of the Model Group

To explore the effect of insomnia on the growth of the sympathetic innervation status in the liver. We first examined the levels of NGF and NE in hepatic tissue. Our results showed that the levels were significantly elevated in the model group compared with the control group (NGF, 306.24 ± 23.64 vs. 197.98 ± 17.13 pg/g, $p < 0.0001$; NE, 2.00 ± 0.29 vs. 0.70 ± 0.12 pg/g, $p < 0.0001$; **Figures 3A,B**). Immunohistochemistry for GAP43, an indicator of neuronal growth, was performed to investigate axonal regeneration in liver tissue, which suggested more active nerve sprouting in the model group (0.54 ± 0.08 vs. 2.02 ± 0.25%, $p < 0.0001$; **Figure 3C**). To identify these nerves, immunofluorescence was used to colocalize GAP43 with TH in the liver tissue. These observations suggested active

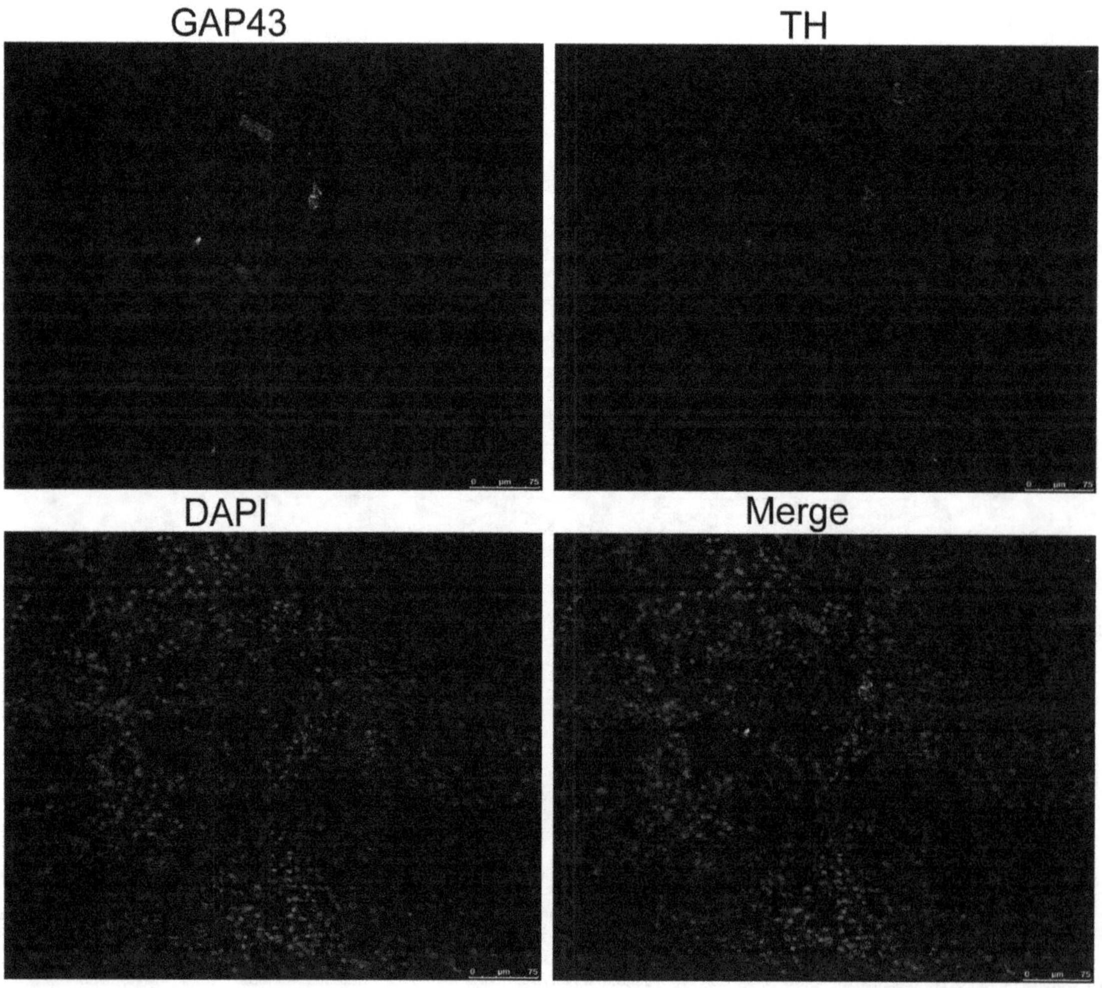

FIGURE 4 | Identification of sympathetic nerves in the liver by confocal laser scanning microscopy. GAP43/TH colocalization indicated hyperplastic sympathetic nerves in the livers of insomnia rats (scale bar: 75 μm).

and hyperplastic sympathetic nerves in the livers of the model group (**Figure 4**).

Sympathetic Denervation Improved Hepatic Steatosis

Injection of 6-OHDA is commonly used as a model of sympathetic denervation. To determine the effects of denervation, NE was measured in hepatic tissue after administration. In comparison with the model group, the NE content in the sympathetic denervation group evidently decreased (2.00 ± 0.25 vs. 0.70 ± 0.12 pg/g, $p < 0.0001$; **Figure 5A**).

In addition, the plasma levels of FFAs and TGs were analyzed, as well as the protein levels of Perilipin-2 in the liver tissues. Compared with the model group, TGs and Perilipin-2 levels decreased significantly in the 6-OHDA administration group, while FFAs showed the opposite trend (FFAs, 298.01 ± 24.44 vs. 233.95 ± 33.92 μmol/L, $p = 0.0007$; TGs, 1.56 ± 0.13 vs. 1.88 ± 0.18 mmol/L, $p = 0.001$; Perilipin-2: 7.61 ± 1.23 vs. 10.45 ± 1.95%, $p = 0.0038$; **Figures 5B,C,F**). Similar results were obtained by HE staining and TEM images (**Figures 5D,E**). These results suggested that the sympathetic nerve was involved in insomnia-induced liver steatosis, exerting a promotion function.

Estazolam Alleviated Fatty Liver in Insomnia Rats

Estazolam is the first-line therapy for insomnia. To evaluate the effect of estazolam on fatty liver in insomnia rats, the plasma FFAs and TGs levels were determined, as well as histopathological examinations. Compared with the model group, the plasma FFAs level was markedly elevated (335.65 ± 29.41 vs. 233.95 ± 33.92 μmol/L, $p < 0.0001$), while the TGs level was decreased in the treatment group (1.50 ± 0.10 vs. 1.88 ± 0.18 mmol/L, $p = 0.0038$; **Figures 6A,B**).

Subsequently, we investigated the change in Perilipin-2 in the liver after treatment. Immunohistochemical staining showed that hepatic steatosis was significantly decreased in the treatment group (7.03 ± 1.06 vs. 10.45 ± 1.95%, $p = 0.0007$; **Figure 6E**). Moreover, the HE and microscopic tests were similar to the above immunohistochemical results (**Figures 6C,D**). It appears that supplementation with estazolam ameliorates fatty liver in insomnia rats.

Estazolam Administration Inhibited Sympathetic Activation

To further explore whether estazolam prevents sympathetic activation in fatty liver in insomnia rats, the growth of sympathetic innervation in the liver was evaluated. NGF and NE in liver

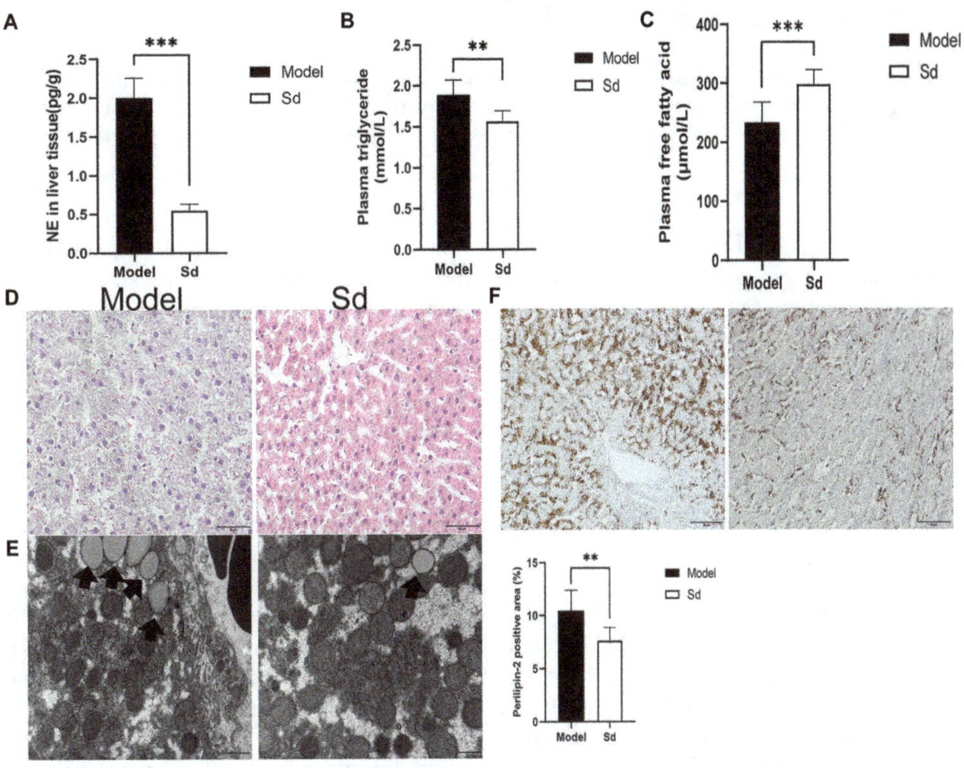

FIGURE 5 | The effect of sympathetic denervation on hepatic steatosis. **(A)** NE of sympathetic neuromediators in liver was detected. **(B)** The plasma triglyceride levels in the liver tissues were analyzed. **(C)** The plasma free fatty acid levels were detected. **(D)** HE staining (scale bar: 50 μm). **(E)** TEM was performed to observe lipid droplets (scale bar: 1 μm). **(F)** Quantitative analysis of lipid droplets was measured by Perilipin-2 immunohistochemistry (scale bar: 50 μm). The results were obtained from two independent experiments and are expressed as the mean ± SD, $n = 8$ per group, $^{**}p < 0.01$; and $^{***}p < 0.001$. Sd, sympathetic denervation group; NE, norepinephrine.

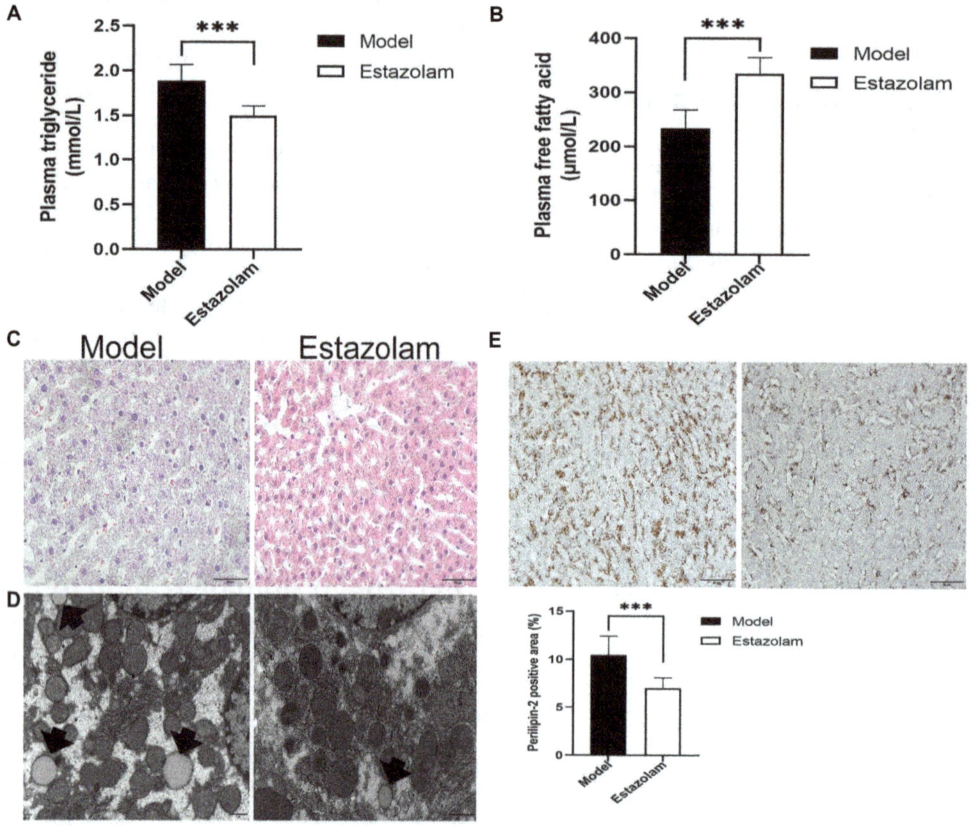

FIGURE 6 | Blood lipids and hepatic steatosis were detected to evaluate the effect of estazolam on fatty liver in insomnia rats. **(A)** The plasma triglyceride levels. **(B)** The plasma free fatty acid levels. **(C)** HE staining (scale bar: 50μm). **(D)** Detection of lipid droplets by TEM (scale bar: 1 μm). **(E)** Expression of Perilipin-2 was determined by immunohistochemistry (scale bar: 50μm). The results were obtained from two independent experiments and are expressed as the mean ± SD, $n=8$ per group, $^{***}p<0.001$.

tissues showed that estazolam administration could suppress the growth of sympathetic nerves in the treatment group compared to the model group (NGF, 248.26 ± 49.23 vs. 306.24 ± 23.64 pg/g, $p=0.0095$; NE, 0.42 ± 0.13 vs. 2.00 ± 0.29 pg/g, $p<0.0001$; **Figures 7A,B**). The immunohistochemistry results also suggested that GAP43 expression in the treatment group was significantly attenuated (2.16 ± 0.30 vs. 2.96 ± 0.27%, $p<0.0001$; **Figure 7C**).

DISCUSSION

Persistent insomnia can lead to an impairment in the quality of life and mental health (Fadeuilhe et al., 2021). Recently, insomnia has been gaining attention. In the present study, we first observed that sustained sleep deprivation contributed to fatty liver. To determine whether the sympathetic nerve was involved in insomnia-mediated hepatic steatosis, we performed sympathetic denervation experiments with 6-OHDA. We found that fatty liver can be alleviated by the use of 6-OHDA prior to suffering from sustained sleep deprivation. These initial results suggested that the sympathetic nerve has a facilitatory role in fatty liver associated with insomnia. This result is consistent with the results of previous studies (Hurr et al., 2019). We then assessed whether this phenomenon would also be seen in the heart muscle. No myocardial steatosis in insomnia rats was found in the results of Oil Red O staining. This result might correlate with the fact that the liver was the major tissue site for fat deposition and metabolism (**Supplementary Figure 2**).

Estazolam is an effective agent for insomnia control (Cohn et al., 1991). Based on the experimental data, there was an alleviation in the severity of fatty liver in the rats that received estazolam treatment. Furthermore, to understand the mechanisms underlying these experimental phenomena, we examined sympathetic activation, NGF and its neurotransmitter. Thus, these results offer preliminary evidence that estazolam inhibits sympathetic activation and relieves hepatic steatosis in insomnia rats. Besides, serum aminotransferase activity was measured in insomnia group and control group. The main purpose of this data was to evaluate the effects of sustained sleep deprivation on hepatic function only. Since both Sd group and estazolam group underwent pharmacological intervention, these drugs might produce liver enzyme abnormalities that would likely complicate the results shown in our study.

The modified multiple platform method was used to establish the sleep deprivation model, which is currently a widely used

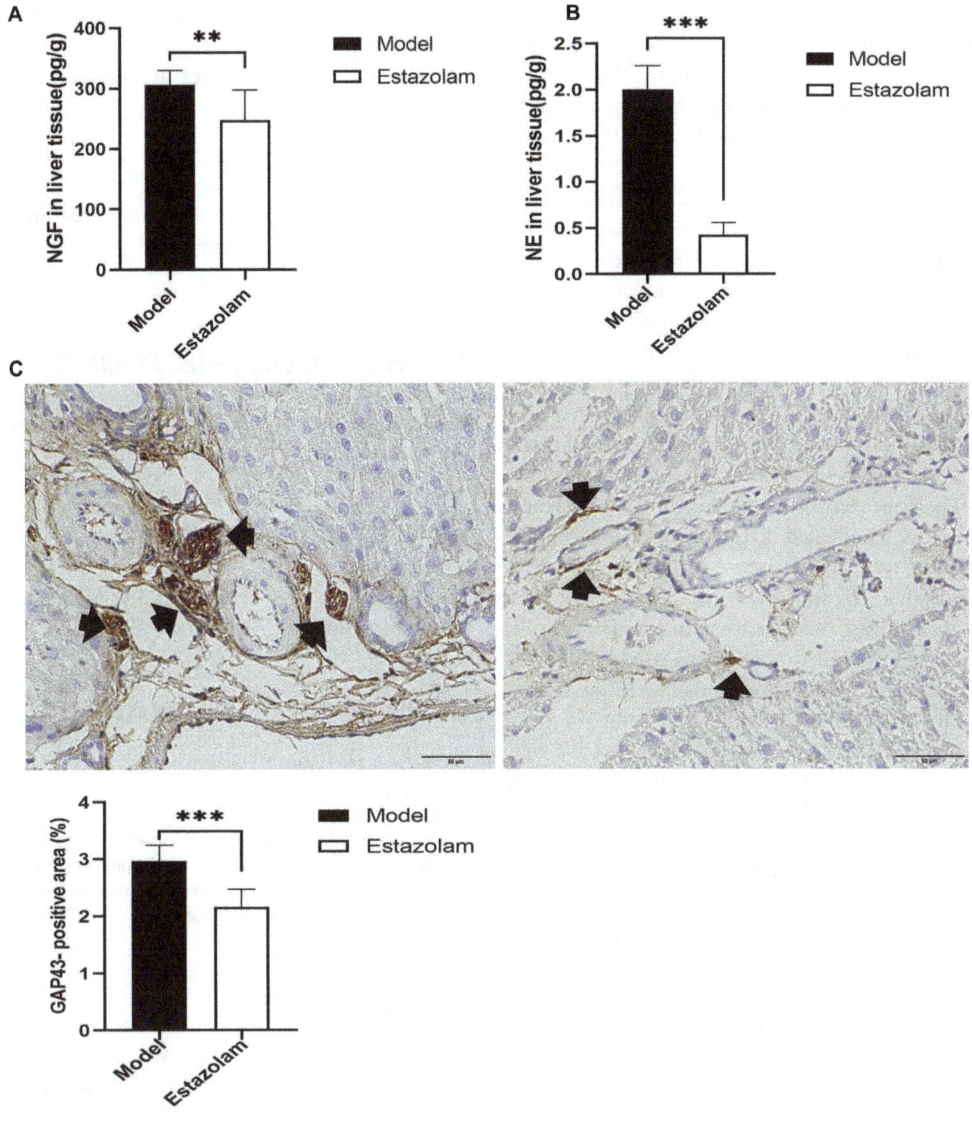

FIGURE 7 | Sympathetic innervation in liver was evaluated. **(A)** The NGF level was tested in liver tissues. **(B)** NE in liver tissues was detected by HP-LC-MS/MS. **(C)** GAP43 staining was observed in the liver as a qualitative metric of neural growth by immunohistochemistry (scale bar: 50 μm). The results were obtained from two independent experiments and are expressed as the mean ± SD, $n = 8$ per group, $^{**}p < 0.01$ and $^{***}p < 0.001$. NE, norepinephrine.

sleep deprivation rat model. The primary advantage of this method is its simplicity. When rats reached the sleep phase, muscle atonia caused them to lose balance on a platform and fall into the water and awaken (Machado et al., 2004). In our experiments, rats underwent sustained sleep deprivation for 8 weeks, with the main aim of achieving complete insomnia. These rats subsequently developed unusual presentations, including retarded reactions, reduced activity, and dull hair. However, these results are not completely consistent with previous studies showing that rats increased their activity after suffering from short-term sleep deprivation.

In addition, the relationship between the sympathetic nerve and insomnia is complex and tightly linked. Sympathetic overactivation would cause insomnia, and insomnia in turn would exacerbate a range of physical and mental health problems (Taylor et al., 2016). The insomnia rat model was established by long-term sleep deprivation in our study, which was associated with sympathetic hyperactivity. Estazolam for insomnia has been widely employed. In one group of animals, eight rats received both estazolam therapy and sleep deprivation. The results indicated that estazolam was an efficacious pharmacological treatment for insomnia and suppressed sympathetic activation in the liver. These results also suggested that this agent is effective in reversing sympathetic hyperactivity in insomnia rats.

The liver plays a crucial regulatory role in fat metabolism (Alves-Bezerra and Cohen, 2017). Sympathetic overactivation in the insomnia model contributed to fatty liver. However, after treatment with 6-OHDA to destroy sympathetic nerves, hepatic steatosis significantly improved. These data suggested that sympathetic nerves are involved in the regulation of hepatic lipid metabolism. Furthermore, some studies have shown that obesity-induced hepatic steatosis is associated with hepatic sympathetic hyperactivity. Hepatic sympathetic denervation by 6-OHDA reduced obesity-induced hepatic steatosis (Hurr et al., 2019). This phenomenon coincided with our experimental conclusions.

From the clinical point of view, insomnia is a risk factor for nonalcoholic fatty liver disease (NAFLD; Kim et al., 2013). Recent studies have shown that insomnia is associated with metabolic disorders, including glucose metabolism and lipid metabolism (Mir et al., 2013; Seelig et al., 2013). Therefore, that is one reason short sleep duration is associated with diabetes, obesity, and fatty liver. Consistent results have also been found in a population-based observational study, showing that good sleep is associated with lower presence of NAFLD (Deng et al., 2021). However, the mechanisms for this result remain unclear. So, we conducted a preliminary exploration of this issue from the sympathetic nerve activity perspective.

In our research results, HE and microscopic tests were used to evaluate the degree of liver steatosis. In addition, Perilipin-2, which is expressed around lipid droplets, was used to directly assess lipid droplets by immunohistochemistry. These results could provide useful information for the evaluation of fatty liver. Hepatic steatosis is closely related to blood lipid levels. FFAs are a major secretory product of lipid droplets or adipocytes as a result of lipolysis of stored TGs. The major process of lipolysis involves the hydrolysis of TGs to FFAs and glycerol (Quiroga and Lehner, 2018). Therefore, TGs and FFAs levels were measured in the present study. These results indicated that TGs level were elevated as a result of insomnia and that FFAs levels were lower. In contrast, the opposite results were found in rats suffering insomnia treated with estazolam. These data implied that pharmacotherapy altered the metabolic states of synthesis or breakdown in insomnia rats. However, this requires further validation.

Regarding sympathetic nerve assessment, we first analyzed the expression of the nerve growth marker GAP43. The results suggested that hepatic autonomic nerves were in an active growth state in insomnia rats. Therefore, it was necessary to identify the sympathetic nerves using colocalization by fluorescence confocal microscopy. Further analysis was conducted on NGF and neurotransmitters in liver tissues. These results also provided preliminary evidence to support sympathetic overactivation.

However, our research still has some shortcomings and limitations. Firstly, pharmacological intervention for hepatic sympathetic denervation by 6-OHDA included intraperitoneal injection, which disrupted all sympathetic neurons in the abdominal cavity, thus lacking specificity. Secondly, the sample size in our initial exploratory study is small. In the future, we will expand the sample size to confirm these results. Thirdly, the relationship between insomnia, psychological stress, and sympathetic overactivation is intricate. To date, there have been few animal models of insomnia that can avoid the effects of psychological stress. Similarly, other mechanisms of benzodiazepines may also contribute to facilitation of falling asleep. Moreover, the detailed mechanisms that are involved in sympathetic nerve regulation of hepatic steatosis remain unclear, and further studies are warranted.

CONCLUSION

In conclusion, sustained sleep deprivation-induced insomnia promotes hepatic steatosis in rats possibly by mediating sympathetic overactivation.

AUTHOR CONTRIBUTIONS

ZW and XL wrote the manuscript. All authors contributed to the article and approved the submitted version.

ACKNOWLEDGMENTS

We thank Boer Liao from Xinjiang Medical University Central Laboratory for excellent technical assistance about HP-LC-MS.

SUPPLEMENTARY MATERIAL

Supplementary Figure 1 | Schematic presentation of experimental timeline and design. Experimental grouping rats were randomly divided into four groups, as indicated in the figure.

Supplementary Figure 2 | Oil red O staining was performed to visualize myocardial steatosis in both control and insomnia rats (scale bar: 50 μm). The results showed that the gross observations of myocardial steatosis from the two groups were no significant difference.

REFERENCES

Alkadhi, K. A., and Alhaider, I. A. (2016). Caffeine and REM sleep deprivation: effect on basal levels of signaling molecules in area CA1. *Mol. Cell. Neurosci.* 71, 125–131. doi: 10.1016/j.mcn.2015.12.015

Alves-Bezerra, M., and Cohen, D. E. (2017). Triglyceride metabolism in the liver. *Compr. Physiol.* 8, 1–8. doi: 10.1002/cphy.c170012

Amir, M., Yu, M., He, P., and Srinivasan, S. (2020). Hepatic autonomic nervous system and neurotrophic factors regulate the pathogenesis and progression of non-alcoholic fatty liver disease. *Front. Med.* 7:62. doi: 10.3389/fmed.2020.00062

Belenky, G., Wesensten, N. J., Thorne, D. R., Thomas, M. L., Sing, H. C., Redmond, D. P., et al. (2003). Patterns of performance degradation and restoration during sleep restriction and subsequent recovery: a sleep dose-response study. *J. Sleep Res.* 12, 1–12. doi: 10.1046/j.1365-2869.2003.00337.x

Buysse, D. J. (2013). Insomnia. *JAMA* 309, 706–716. doi: 10.1001/jama.2013.193

Carter, J. R., Grimaldi, D., Fonkoue, I. T., Medalie, L., Mokhlesi, B., and Cauter, E. V. (2018). Assessment of sympathetic neural activity in chronic insomnia: evidence for elevated cardiovascular risk. *Sleep* 41:zsy048. doi: 10.1093/sleep/zsy048

Chen, W., Chang, Y., He, L., Jian, X., Li, L., Gao, L., et al. (2016). Effect of renal sympathetic denervation on hepatic glucose metabolism and blood pressure in a rat model of insulin resistance. *J. Hypertens.* 34, 2465–2474. doi: 10.1097/HJH.0000000000001087

Cohn, J. B., Wilcox, C. S., Bremner, J., and Ettinger, M. (1991). Hypnotic efficacy of estazolam compared with flurazepam in outpatients with insomnia. *J. Clin. Pharmacol.* 31, 747–750. doi: 10.1002/j.1552-4604.1991.tb03771.x

Deng, Y. Y., Zhong, Q. W., Zhong, H. L., Xiong, F., Ke, Y. B., and Chen, Y. M. (2021). Higher healthy lifestyle score is associated with lower presence of non-alcoholic fatty liver disease in middle-aged and older Chinese adults: a community-based cross-sectional study. *Public Health Nutr.* 1–9. doi: 10.1017/S1368980021000902 [Epub ahead of print]

Du, J., Zhang, X., Han, J., Man, K., Zhang, Y., Chu, E. S., et al. (2017). Pro-inflammatory CXCR3impairs mitochondrial function in experimental non-alcoholic steatohepatitis. *Theranostics* 7, 4192–4203. doi: 10.7150/thno.21400

Fadeuilhe, C., Daigre, C., Richarte, V., Grau-Lopez, L., Palma-Alvarez, R. F., Corrales, M., et al. (2021). Insomnia disorder in adult attention-deficit/hyperactivity disorder patients: clinical, comorbidity, and treatment correlates. *Front. Psychol.* 12:663889. doi: 10.3389/fpsyt.2021.663889

Fortier-Brochu, E., and Morin, C. M. (2014). Cognitive impairment in individuals with insomnia: clinical significance and correlates. *Sleep* 37, 1787–1798. doi: 10.5665/sleep.4172

Furness, J. B., Callaghan, B. P., Rivera, L. R., and Cho, H. J. (2014). The enteric nervous system and gastrointestinal innervation: integrated local and central control. *Adv. Exp. Med. Biol.* 817, 39–71. doi: 10.1007/978-1-4939-0897-4_3

Gluchowski, N. L., Becuwe, M., Walther, T. C., and Farese, R. V. (2017). Lipid droplets and liver disease: from basic biology to clinical implications. *Nat. Rev. Gastroenterol. Hepatol.* 14, 343–355. doi: 10.1038/nrgastro.2017.32

Hirase, M., Ishida, T., and Kamei, C. (2008). Rebound insomnia induced by abrupt withdrawal of hypnotics in sleep-disturbed rats. *Eur. J. Pharmacol.* 597, 46–50. doi: 10.1016/j.ejphar.2008.08.024

Hurr, C., Simonyan, H., Morgan, D. A., Rahmouni, K., and Young, C. N. (2019). Liver sympathetic denervation reverses obesity-induced hepatic steatosis. *J. Physiol.* 597, 4565–4580. doi: 10.1113/JP277994

Jarrin, D. C., Ivers, H., Lamy, M., Chen, I. Y., Harvey, A. G., and Morin, C. M. (2018). Cardiovascular autonomic dysfunction in insomnia patients with objective short sleep duration. *J. Sleep Res.* 27:e12663. doi: 10.1111/jsr.12663

Jensen-Cody, S. O., and Potthoff, M. J. (2021). Hepatokines and metabolism: deciphering communication from the liver. *Mol. Metab.* 44:101138. doi: 10.1016/j.molmet.2020.101138

Kalmbach, D. A., Cheng, P., Arnedt, J. T., Anderson, J. R., Roth, T., Fellman-Couture, C., et al. (2019). Treating insomnia improves depression, maladaptive thinking, and hyperarousal in postmenopausal women: comparing cognitive-behavioral therapy for insomnia (CBTI), sleep restriction therapy, and sleep hygiene education. *Sleep Med.* 55, 124–134. doi: 10.1016/j.sleep.2018.11.019

Kammerer, M. K., Mehl, S., Ludwig, L., and Lincoln, T. M. (2021). Sleep and circadian rhythm disruption predict persecutory symptom severity in day-to-day life: a combined actigraphy and experience sampling study. *J. Abnorm. Psychol.* 130, 78–88. doi: 10.1037/abn0000645

Kim, C. W., Yun, K. E., Jung, H. S., Chang, Y., Choi, E. S., Kwon, M. J., et al. (2013). Sleep duration and quality in relation to non-alcoholic fatty liver disease in middle-aged workers and their spouses. *J. Hepatol.* 59, 351–357. doi: 10.1016/j.jhep.2013.03.035

Lu, J. L., Freire, A. X., Molnar, M. Z., Kalantar-Zadeh, K., and Kovesdy, C. P. (2018). Association of chronic insomnia with mortality and adverse renal outcomes. *Mayo Clin. Proc.* 93, 1563–1570. doi: 10.1016/j.mayocp.2018.05.032

Machado, R. B., Hipolide, D. C., Benedito-Silva, A. A., and Tufik, S. (2004). Sleep deprivation induced by the modified multiple platform technique: quantification of sleep loss and recovery. *Brain Res.* 1004, 45–51. doi: 10.1016/j.brainres.2004.01.019

Medrano-Martinez, P., and Ramos-Platon, M. J. (2016). Cognitive and emotional alterations in chronic insomnia. *Rev. Neurol.* 62, 170–178.

Mir, H. M., Stepanova, M., Afendy, H., Cable, R., and Younossi, Z. M. (2013). Association of sleep disorders with nonalcoholic fatty liver disease (NAFLD): a population-based study. *J. Clin. Exp. Hepatol.* 3, 181–185. doi: 10.1016/j.jceh.2013.06.004

Okun, M. L., Mancuso, R. A., Hobel, C. J., Schetter, C. D., and Coussons-Read, M. (2018). Poor sleep quality increases symptoms of depression and anxiety in postpartum women. *J. Behav. Med.* 41, 703–710. doi: 10.1007/s10865-018-9950-7

Quiroga, A. D., and Lehner, R. (2018). Pharmacological intervention of liver triacylglycerol lipolysis: the good, the bad and the ugly. *Biochem. Pharmacol.* 155, 233–241. doi: 10.1016/j.bcp.2018.07.005

Schulze, R. J., and McNiven, M. A. (2019). Lipid droplet formation and lipophagy in fatty liver disease. *Semin. Liver Dis.* 39, 283–290. doi: 10.1055/s-0039-1685524

Seelig, E., Keller, U., Klarhofer, M., Scheffler, K., Brand, S., Holsboer-Trachsler, E., et al. (2013). Neuroendocrine regulation and metabolism of glucose and lipids in primary chronic insomnia: a prospective case-control study. *PLoS One* 8:e61780. doi: 10.1371/journal.pone.0061780

Taylor, K. S., Murai, H., Millar, P. J., Haruki, N., Kimmerly, D. S., Morris, B. L., et al. (2016). Arousal from sleep and sympathetic excitation during wakefulness. *Hypertension* 68, 1467–1474. doi: 10.1161/HYPERTENSIONAHA.116.08212

Tsunoda, M., Takezawa, K., Masuda, M., and Imai, K. (2002). Rat liver and kidney catechol-O-methyltransferase activity measured by high-performance liquid chromatography with fluorescence detection. *Biomed. Chromatogr.* 16, 536–541. doi: 10.1002/bmc.202

van Liempt, S., Arends, J., Cluitmans, P. J., Westenberg, H. G., Kahn, R. S., and Vermetten, E. (2013). Sympathetic activity and hypothalamo-pituitary-adrenal axis activity during sleep in post-traumatic stress disorder: a study assessing polysomnography with simultaneous blood sampling. *Psychoneuroendocrinology* 38, 155–165. doi: 10.1016/j.psyneuen.2012.05.015

4

Soluble TIM3 and its Ligands Galectin-9 and CEACAM1 are in Disequilibrium During Alcohol-Related Liver Disease and Promote Impairment of Anti-Bacterial Immunity

Antonio Riva[1,2], Elena Palma[1,2], Dhruti Devshi[1,2], Douglas Corrigall[1,2,3], Huyen Adams[1,2,4], Nigel Heaton[5], Krishna Menon[5], Melissa Preziosi[5], Ane Zamalloa[5], Rosa Miquel[6], Jennifer M. Ryan[7], Gavin Wright[3], Sarah Fairclough[3], Alexander Evans[4], Debbie Shawcross[2], Robert Schierwagen[8], Sabine Klein[8], Frank E. Uschner[8], Michael Praktiknjo[9], Krum Katzarov[10], Tanya Hadzhiolova[10], Slava Pavlova[10], Marieta Simonova[10], Jonel Trebicka[8,11], Roger Williams[1,2] and Shilpa Chokshi[1,2]**

[1] Institute of Hepatology, Foundation for Liver Research, London, United Kingdom, [2] Faculty of Life Sciences & Medicine, King's College London, London, United Kingdom, [3] Department of Gastroenterology, Basildon University Hospital, Basildon, United Kingdom, [4] Department of Gastroenterology, Royal Berkshire Hospital, Reading, United Kingdom, [5] Institute of Liver Studies, King's College London, London, United Kingdom, [6] Liver Histopathology Laboratory, Institute of Liver Studies, King's College Hospital, London, United Kingdom, [7] Gastrointestinal and Liver Services, Royal Free Hospital, London, United Kingdom, [8] Translational Hepatology, Department of Internal Medicine I, University Hospital Frankfurt, Frankfurt, Germany, [9] Department of Internal Medicine I, University of Bonn, Bonn, Germany, [10] Department of Gastroenterology, Hepatobiliary Surgery and Transplantology, Military Medical Academy, Sofia, Bulgaria, [11] European Foundation for the Study of Chronic Liver Failure (EF-CLIF), Barcelona, Spain

***Correspondence:**
Shilpa Chokshi
s.chokshi@researchinliver.org.uk
Antonio Riva
a.riva@researchinliver.org.uk

Background and Aims: Immunoregulatory checkpoint receptors (CR) contribute to the profound immunoparesis observed in alcohol-related liver disease (ALD) and *in vitro* neutralization of inhibitory-CRs TIM3/PD1 on anti-bacterial T-cells can rescue innate and adaptive anti-bacterial immunity. Recently described soluble-CR forms can modulate immunity in inflammatory conditions, but the contributions of soluble-TIM3 and soluble-PD1 and other soluble-CRs to immune derangements in ALD remain unclear.

Methods: In Alcoholic Hepatitis (AH; n = 19), alcohol-related cirrhosis (ARC; n = 53) and healthy control (HC; n = 27) subjects, we measured by Luminex technology (i) plasma levels of 16 soluble-CRs, 12 pro/anti-inflammatory cytokines and markers of gut bacterial translocation; (ii) pre-hepatic, post-hepatic and non-hepatic soluble-CR plasma levels in ARC patients undergoing TIPS; (iii) soluble-CRs production from ethanol-treated immunocompetent precision cut human liver slices (PCLS); (iv) whole-blood soluble-CR expression upon bacterial challenge. By FACS, we assessed the relationship between soluble-TIM3 and membrane-TIM3 and rescue of immunity in bacterial-challenged PBMCs.

Results: Soluble-TIM3 was the dominant plasma soluble-CR in ALD vs. HC (p = 0.00002) and multivariate analysis identified it as the main driver of differences between groups. Soluble-CRs were strongly correlated with pro-inflammatory cytokines, gut bacterial translocation markers and clinical indices of disease severity. Ethanol exposure or bacterial challenge did not induce soluble-TIM3 production from PCLS nor from whole-blood. Bacterial challenge prompted membrane-TIM3 hyperexpression on PBMCs from ALD patient's vs. HC ($p < 0.002$) and was inversely correlated with plasma soluble-TIM3 levels in matched patients. TIM3 ligands soluble-Galectin-9 and soluble-CEACAM1 were elevated in ALD plasma (AH > ARC; $p < 0.002$). *In vitro* neutralization of Galectin-9 and soluble-CEACAM1 improved the defective anti-bacterial and anti-inflammatory cytokine production from *E. coli*-challenged PBMCs in ALD patients.

Conclusions: Alcohol-related liver disease patients exhibit supra-physiological plasma levels of soluble-TIM3, particularly those with greater disease severity. This is also associated with increased levels of soluble TIM3-ligands and membrane-TIM3 expression on immune cells. Soluble-TIM3 can block the TIM3-ligand synapse and improve anti-bacterial immunity; however, the increased levels of soluble TIM3-binding ligands in patients with ALD negate any potential immunostimulatory effects. We believe that anti-TIM3 neutralizing antibodies currently in Phase I clinical trials or soluble-TIM3 should be investigated further for their ability to enhance anti-bacterial immunity. These agents could potentially represent an innovative immune-based supportive approach to rescue anti-bacterial defenses in ALD patients.

Keywords: TIM3, immune checkpoint, alcohol, biomarker, alcohol-related liver disease

INTRODUCTION

Alcohol-related liver disease (ALD) represents a significant public health burden, and according to the World Health Organization alcohol is "the third highest risk factor for premature mortality, disability and loss of health worldwide" (Soria Saucedo, 2013). Whilst ALD encompasses a spectrum of clinical manifestations, it is well recognized that advanced disease is associated with multiple derangements in host immunity and one of the major and most common complications that patients face is an increased vulnerability to bacterial infection, which can lead to worsening of disease and multi-organ failure (Louvet and Mathurin, 2015; Albillos et al., 2014; EASL, 2018).

Patients with alcohol-related cirrhosis (ARC) are highly susceptible to overwhelming bacterial infections, which increases their probability of death by 3.75-fold, reaching 30% at 1-month and 63% at 1-year (Albillos et al., 2014; Gustot et al., 2014; Jalan et al., 2014; Louvet and Mathurin, 2015). In patients with alcoholic hepatitis (AH), the most florid form of ALD, the susceptibility to infection is further heightened and is the leading cause of death, with infection observed in up to 65% of cases (Louvet et al., 2009, 2015). It is also the commonest precipitating event for acute-on-chronic liver failure (ACLF) (Arroyo et al., 2015; Trebicka et al., 2020).

The disease state in advanced ALD represents an immunological paradox. Patients exhibit a multi-systemic hyperactivated immunity at the clinical and molecular level, which can co-exist with immune inactivation. This landscape, which is progressively established during ARC and is a hallmark of AH (Mathurin and Lucey, 2012; Albillos et al., 2014; Louvet and Mathurin, 2015; Markwick et al., 2015; EASL, 2018), underlies the rampant inflammation and profound predisposition to bacterial infection (Mathurin and Lucey, 2012; Louvet and Mathurin, 2015; EASL, 2018). To date, therapeutics have primarily focussed on (i) curtailing the infection with use of widespread antibiotics, concerningly this has promoted development of multi-drug resistant microbes (Merli et al., 2015; Fernandez et al., 2016; EASL, 2018), or (ii) bridling the rampant inflammation with immunosuppressive agents. However, this latter strategy can potentiate the immunocompromised state and increase the risk of secondary infections (Louvet et al., 2009; Thursz et al., 2015; Vergis et al., 2017; Chokshi, 2018). Targeted immunomodulatory approaches to restore the disrupted balance

Abbreviations: ALD, alcohol-related liver disease; ARC, alcohol-related cirrhosis; BH FDR, Benjamini–Hochberg False Discovery Rate; BHq, BH FDR adjusted *p*-value (i.e., *q*-value); BTLA, B- and T-lymphocyte attenuator; C.I., confidence interval; CD, cluster of differentiation; CEACAM1, carcinoembryonic antigen-related cell adhesion molecule 1; DMSO, dimethyl sulfoxide; Gal9, galectin-9; GITR, glucocorticoid-induced TNFR-related protein; HC, healthy controls; HVEM, herpesvirus entry mediator; IDO, indoleamine 2,3-dioxygenase; IFN, interferon; IL, interleukin; IQR, interquartile range; KWp, Kruskal–Wallis *p*-value; LAG3, lymphocyte-activation gene 3; MELD, model end-stage liver disease; membrane-CR(s), membrane checkpoint receptor(s); mfi, median fluorescence intensity; MWp, Mann–Whitney *p*-value; PBMC(s), peripheral blood mononuclear cell(s); PBS, phosphate-buffered saline; PD1, programmed death 1; PDL1/PDL2, programmed death ligand 1/2; rcf, relative centrifugal force; (S)AH, (severe) alcoholic hepatitis; soluble-CR(s), soluble checkpoint receptor(s); TIM3, T-cell immunoglobulin and mucin domain 3 (also known as Hepatitis A virus cellular receptor 2, HAVCR2); TNF, tumor necrosis factor.

between protective anti-pathogen immunity and host-induced immunopathology are lacking.

Preservation of this homeostatic equilibrium physiologically is achieved through multi-faceted immunoregulatory networks and a major 'tenet' are checkpoint receptors (CRs), which activate or inhibit immune cells in a temporal and anatomically coordinated manner (Riva and Chokshi, 2018). Best known for their involvement in suppressing anti-tumor immunity, blockade with neutralizing antibodies to PD1 has obtained FDA approval in multiple cancers including hepatocellular carcinoma. Pre-clinical and clinical studies have also described a role for checkpoint receptors including PD1 and TIM3 in sepsis (Patil et al., 2017) and septic shock, where increased membrane-bound immune cell expression has been associated with a higher rate of nosocomial infections and mortality (Guignant et al., 2011). Of note, a recent phase-1b randomized controlled trial of checkpoint inhibitor therapy in 31 immunocompromised patients with sepsis (Hotchkiss et al., 2019b) found it well tolerated with no evidence of treatment-related hypercytokinemia. Further to this, a second study assessing the utility of anti-PDL1 in sepsis was also well tolerated and at higher doses there was evidence of immune restoration (Hotchkiss et al., 2019a).

We were the first to demonstrate that membrane-bound PD1 and membrane-bound TIM3 on T-cells impair their anti-bacterial functionality in AH (Markwick et al., 2015). Moreover, we showed that *ex vivo* blockade using neutralizing antibodies led to reconstitution of both innate and adaptive arms of the anti-bacterial immunity without exacerbating the production of cytokines associated with systemic inflammation. However, the individual contributions of these two membrane-bound checkpoints remained unclear. Furthermore, while CRs were initially discovered as membrane-bound molecules (membrane-CRs), we now know that many can exist in soluble form (soluble-CRs), generated by alternative mRNA splicing or metalloprotease-mediated ectodomain shedding (Gu et al., 2018; Riva and Chokshi, 2018). These soluble-CRs can act as agonists or antagonistic molecular decoys and can orchestrate host immunity distally, performing paracrine tasks similar to stimulatory or inhibitory cytokines. Systemic concentrations of several soluble-CRs rise during inflammation, autoimmunity (Jung et al., 2003; Lahat et al., 2003; Ip et al., 2005, 2006; Cao et al., 2012; Delmastro et al., 2012; Chiba et al., 2017; Zhao D. et al., 2017; Lin et al., 2018), infectious diseases (Cao et al., 2011; Clayton et al., 2015; Ren et al., 2015; Zilber et al., 2019), and cancer (Prigent et al., 1999; Triebel et al., 2006; Hock et al., 2009; Heo et al., 2012; Ge et al., 2017; Silva et al., 2017; Zhao Q. et al., 2017; He et al., 2018; Li N. et al., 2018) often mirroring immune dysfunction, disease progression and increased mortality. Measurements of systemic soluble-CRs are useful both as potential diagnostic/prognostic biomarkers (Chen et al., 2017; Li Y. M. et al., 2018) but also to expose mechanisms underlying immunopathogenesis of disease. The contribution of soluble-CRs in ALD, particularly soluble-PD1 and soluble-TIM3, remains unclear and defining it was the aim of this investigation.

We report that the soluble-TIM3/ligand axis is significantly dysregulated in ALD, whereas the soluble-PD1 pathway does not seem to be involved. We show that soluble-TIM3 and both its soluble ligands Galectin-9 and CEACAM-1 were significantly elevated in the plasma of ALD patients. Interestingly, we show that unlike the membrane-bound form, the soluble-TIM3 pathway is immunostimulatory. However, we suggest that in the context of ALD, the immune potentiating properties of this pathway may be hampered by the high levels of ligand-receptor neutralisation in the systemic circulation.

MATERIALS/PATIENTS AND METHODS

Subjects and Samples

The study was performed conforming to the declaration of Helsinki, with full informed patient consent and ethical approval from all recruiting centers (United Kingdom Research Ethics Committee reference numbers 13/SW/0219, 08/H0702/52 and 12/SC/0359; Bulgarian Ethics Protocol 1/27.02.18). We included: AH, $n = 19$, with Maddrey's discriminant function ≥ 32 (Maddrey et al., 1978), excluding patients receiving immunosuppressants prior-to/at-time-of sampling; Compensated/decompensated ARC, $n = 33$, excess active alcohol drinkers (>60g/>80g female/male per day) seen as out-patients, excluding patients with cancer, gastrointestinal bleeding, untreated sepsis, or immunomodulatory treatments; Healthy volunteers as healthy controls (HC, $n = 27$).

In sub-groups of patients we assessed: (i) soluble-CRs in plasma and in whole-blood or peripheral blood mononuclear cell (PBMC) cultures challenged with *Escherichia coli*; (ii) membrane-CRs on PBMCs, challenged with *E. coli* as previously described (Riva et al., 2018); (iii) *in vitro* biological activity of soluble-TIM3 in PBMCs challenged with *E. coli* and treated with/without recombinant soluble-TIM3. Soluble-CR levels were also measured (iv) in whole-blood plasma obtained from four anatomical sites (portal/hepatic/cubital vein, right cardiac atrium) from 20 decompensated ARC patients during Transjugular Intrahepatic Portosystemic Shunt (TIPS) procedure (ascites = 17; varices = 3) (Bonn University Ethics Committee reference number 029/13) and (v) in a novel human organotypic liver culture model of acute ethanol exposure (precision-cut liver slices, PCLS). PCLS were prepared from the healthy (tumor-free) portion of liver resections from 3 patients undergoing partial hepatectomy for colorectal liver metastases (fibrosis score F1–F2, $n = 2$; F2–F3, $n = 1$) and 1 patient undergoing partial hepatectomy for adrenocortical carcinoma liver metastases (United Kingdom Research Ethics Committee reference number 17/NE/0340, IRAS ID222302) as previously described (Palma et al., 2020). **Table 1** summarizes the clinical characteristics of patients.

Preparation of Fixed *Escherichia coli*

Escherichia coli (*E. coli*) DH5-alpha was prepared as previously described (Riva et al., 2018). Briefly, *E. coli*

TABLE 1 | Baseline patient characteristics.

	p-value	HC	ARC	SAH	PCLS	TIPS
Gender (M/F/na)*		10/15/2	23/10/0	13/6/0	1/3/0	12/8/0
Age (years)	7.3E-10	32.00	56.00	47.00	60.00	61.00
		(26, 41)	(49, 64)	(41, 52.5)	(46.5–73.5)	(53.75–66.00)
Child-Pugh category (A/B/C)*		–	8/12/12	–	–	1/15/4
Child-pugh score	4.1E-3	–	9.0	11.0	–	8
			(6.75, 10)	(10, 12)		(7–9)
MELD score	3.0E-4	–	13.67	21.41	–	15.00
			(8, 20.33)	(19.87, 26.98)		(10.50–18.25)
Maddrey's discriminant function		–	–	44.19	–	–
				(37.96, 58.1)		
Creatinine (μmol/L)		–	70.00	71.00	81.00	119.34
			(56.5, 101)	(60.5, 87.5)	(62.5–103.5)	(91.94–145.86)
Total bilirubin (μmol/L)	1.6E-7	–	34.00	251.00	6.00	24.62
			(19, 62)	(146, 369)	(3–10.5)	(15.9–45.14)
AST (IU/L)	7.1E-4	–	54.50	115.00	26.50	51.00
			(43.5, 65.75)	(92, 234)	(24.25–78.25)	(26.05–72.50)
GGT (IU/L)		–	127.50	341.00	–	166.50
			(93, 208)	(116, 679)		(96.00–265.25)
ALP (IU/L)	8.3E-3	–	140.50	248.00	97.50	135.00
			(95.25, 177.5)	(149, 312.5)	(94.75–99)	(104.75–149.75)
Albumin (g/dL)	6.1E-3	–	33.00	28.00	4.00	31.30
			(27, 38)	(24.5, 32)	(3.4–4.15)	(25.90–35.80)
INR		–	1.50	1.60	1.02	1.20
			(1.2, 1.7)	(1.5, 1.85)	(0.99–1.06)	(1.10–1.43)
Sodium (mmol/L)	4.2E-2	–	135.50	133.00	139.50	138.00
			(133.75, 140)	(132.5, 135)	(138.5–140.25)	(136.00–139.75)
Platelets (billion/L)		–	114.00	117.00	241.50	165.00
			(73, 173)	(83, 182.5)	(237.25–259)	(114.50–221.50)
Total leukocytes (billion/L)	2.2E-5	–	5.90	11.10	6.26	7.96
			(4.21, 7.87)	(8.1, 16.95)	(5.75–6.95)	(6.51–10.51)
Neutrophils (billion/L)	2.8E-5	–	3.46	9.71	3.79	5.65
			(2.21, 4.9)	(5.77, 12.21)	(3.63–4.18)	(3.90–7.46)
Lymphocytes (billion/L)		–	1.29	1.59	1.60	1.60
			(0.86, 1.65)	(1.11, 2.18)	(1.49–1.96)	(1.10–2.04)
Monocytes (billion/L)	7.7E-5	–	0.42	1.00	0.35	0.92
			(0.3, 0.6)	(0.84, 1.3)	(0.29–0.43)	(0.66–1.40)
Neutrophil-to-lymphocyte ratio (NLR)	3.5E-3	–	2.64	6.48	2.24	3.66
			(1.65, 3.8)	(3.12, 7.99)	(1.96–2.82)	(2.2–4.93)
Monocyte-to-lymphocyte ratio (MLR)	5.0E-3	–	0.34	0.57	0.18	0.63
			(0.24, 0.48)	(0.42, 0.76)	(0.12–0.3)	(0.35–0.77)

**Absolute counts.*

All other parameters = median (IQR).

ALP, alkaline phosphatase; ARC, alcohol-related cirrhosis; AST, aspartate transaminase; GGT, gamma-glutamyl transpeptidase; HC, healthy control; INR, international normalized ratio; MELD, model for end-stage liver disease; SAH, severe alcoholic hepatitis; TOT, total number.

batches were grown in RPMI 1640 medium, fixed in BD Cytofix buffer (formaldehyde 4% in PBS, BD-Biosciences, United Kingdom) for 10 min at room temperature, extensively washed in PBS (Gibco/Thermo Fisher Scientific, United Kingdom) and stored at 4–8°C (or −80°C for long-term storage). Bacterial concentrations were determined by visual counting with a Neubauer-Petroff 0.02 mm chamber.

Soluble-CR and Cytokine Production From Whole-Blood Cultures Challenged With *E. coli*

Fresh whole-blood cultures were established within 2 h of collection. Briefly, whole blood was cultured at 37°C, 5% CO_2 in round-bottom cell-culture tubes for 2 h, with or without stimulation with *E. coli* at 10 bacteria-per-cell (BpC);

supernatants were cryopreserved at −80°C for Luminex analysis of soluble-CR and cytokine production.

Soluble-CR Production From a Human Organotypic Liver Culture Model of Acute Ethanol Exposure

An immunocompetent human precision-cut liver slice (PCLS) model of acute ethanol exposure was utilized to assess soluble-CR production in response to ethanol. Slices were prepared according to established protocols (Palma et al., 2019, 2020). After 2 h of recovery, slices were treated with ethanol 250 mmol/L for 24 h. At the end of culture, slices were harvested for haematoxylin/eosin staining. PCLS culture supernatants were cryopreserved at −80°C for Luminex analysis. To assess ethanol treatment toxicity, cytokeratin (CK) 18 fragments, surrogate markers of cell toxicity and apoptotic cell death, were measured in PCLS supernatants by ELISA according to manufacturer's guidelines (Peviva, M65 EPIDEATH® ELISA and M30 CYTODEATH™ ELISA).

Temporal Relationship Between Membrane- and Soluble-CR Production From PBMCs Challenged With *E. coli*

PBMCs were isolated and cryopreserved according to well established protocols (Riva et al., 2014). PBMCs were defrosted, counted and cultured at 37°C, 5% CO_2, in round-bottom 96-well plates (300,000/200 μL/well) in complete supplemented (s)RPMI medium [RPMI 1640, 100 IU/mL Penicillin/Streptomycin, 2.2 mmol/L L-glutamine, 23mmol/L HEPES (Gibco/Thermo Fisher Scientific, United Kingdom)] with 10% human AB serum (Sigma-Aldrich/Merck, United Kingdom). Cell viability was determined with an automated ADAM cell counter. For membrane-CR/soluble-CR kinetics, PBMCs from HC, ARC and SAH (n = 10/10/10) were unstimulated/stimulated with *E. coli* (10 BpC) in replicates for 7 days. Daily supernatants were collected and cryopreserved at −80°C for soluble-CR Luminex analysis. On days 1, 4, and 7 PBMCs were collected for flow cytometric evaluation of membrane-CR expression. Briefly, cells were pelleted, resuspended in PBS and stained with Ghost Dye™ Red 710 (Tonbo Biosciences/Cambridge Bioscience, Cambridge, United Kingdom) for live/dead discrimination. Cells were then washed, resuspended in FACS buffer (PBS without Ca^{2+}/Mg^{2+}, 1% FBS) and stained with antibodies (20 min, 4°C) to: CD3, CD4, CD8, CD14, CD19, CD56, CD16, and TIM3, then washed and fixed with BD Cytofix buffer for analysis.

Functional assessments were conducted by blocking the interaction between TIM3 and its ligands using alpha-lactose 30 mmol/L (L2643, Sigma-Aldrich/Merck, United Kingdom) and/or recombinant soluble TIM3-Ig fusion protein at 5 μg/mL (rhsTIM3-Ig, 2365-TM, Bio-Techne, United Kingdom) cultured with PBMCs from HC and SAH (n = 5/5) for 1 h. When in combination, alpha-lactose was administered for 1 h, followed by soluble-TIM3 for another hour. Subsequently, *E. coli* was added for 1 h and intracellular transports were blocked with Brefeldin-A 10 μg/mL (B7651, Sigma-Aldrich/Merck, United Kingdom) during the last overnight incubation. Cells were incubated overnight, resuspended in FACS buffer and stained for intracellular flow cytometry as previously described (Riva et al., 2018) for CD3, CD4 and CD8 and with intracellular antibodies for IFNγ, IL-17A and IL-10.

Specific Galectin-9 neutralization was subsequently assessed in PBMC cultures from SAH patients (n = 4) blocked with a monoclonal neutralizing anti-Galectin-9 antibody at 10 μg/mL (MABT834, clone 9S2-1, Sigma-Aldrich/Merck, United Kingdom) for 1 h. *E. coli* was added for 1 h and intracellular transports were blocked with Brefeldin-A 10 μg/mL (B7651, Sigma-Aldrich/Merck, United Kingdom). Cells were incubated for up to 48 h, resuspended in FACS buffer and stained for intracellular flow cytometry as previously described (Riva et al., 2018) for CD3, CD4, CD8, and CD14 and with intracellular antibodies for IFNγ, IL-17A and IL-10.

For antibody clones and fluorochromes see **Supplementary Table 1**.

Multiplex Quantification of Soluble-CRs, Cytokines and Bacterial Translocation Markers

Soluble-CRs were quantified by Luminex following manufacturer's instructions, using a MAGPix instrument with xPonent v4.2 software (LuminexCorp, 's-Hertogenbosch, Netherlands). Soluble-CRs included TIM3, CD80, LAG3, HVEM, BTLA, CD27, CD28, CD137, CD152, GITR, IDO, PDL1, PDL2, and PD1) (Thermo Fisher Scientific, United Kingdom). Using the same platform, we also measured TIM3 soluble ligands Galectin-9 and soluble-CEACAM1, 10 pro-/anti-inflammatory cytokines (IL-1a, IL-1b, IL-1Ra, IL-6, IL-8, IL-10, IL-18, IL-33, IFNg, and TNFa), and the gut bacterial translocation marker soluble-CD163 (R&D-Systems/Bio-Techne, Abingdon-Oxford, United Kingdom). Another gut bacterial translocation marker, D-lactate, was measured by colorimetric assay (AbCam, Cambridge, United Kingdom).

Statistical Analyses

We used: Mann–Whitney (MW) test or Kruskal–Wallis (KW) test with Dunn's *post hoc* correction for independent samples; Wilcoxon Signed Rank test or Repeated-Measures Two-way ANOVA with Holm–Sidak's *post hoc* correction for paired samples; Mixed Model analysis for time-dependent cell-culture kinetics; Chi-square test for categorical variables; Pearson's R or Spearman's r correlation coefficients as appropriate. Multiple hypothesis testing adjustments were: Benjamini–Hochberg false discovery rate (BH, FDR) for group comparisons; Bonferroni family-wise error (FWER) for correlations. Group differences for multiplex assays were considered 'significant' with $p \leq$ BH-threshold or 'trends' with BH-threshold $< p \leq 0.05$. Multicollinearity was investigated by correlation matrix analysis (bivariate) and Variance Inflation Factor (VIF) regression diagnostics (multivariate). Basic statistics were calculated with IBM SPSS 25 (Armonk, NY, United States), GraphPad Prism 8 (San Diego, CA, United States) and Microsoft Excel 2016 (Redmond, WA, United States). Correlation heatmaps were produced with RStudio 1.3.959, R 5.3.2 and the package 'corrplot' (Wei and Simko, 2017; R_Core_Team, 2020; RStudio_Team, 2020).

Multivariate analysis (MVA) was performed by Principal Component Analysis (PCA, unsupervised) and Partial Least Squares (Projection-to-Latent-Structures) discriminant analysis (PLS-DA, supervised). Data for MVA were Log10-transformed, mean-centered and unit-variance scaled. Goodness-of-fit and internal predictive performance were assessed by cumulative R2X/R2Y and Q2, respectively. Model validation and significance were measured by cross-validated residuals ANOVA (CV-ANOVA) and misclassification tables. MVA was performed with Umetrics SIMCA 15 (Umeå/Malmö, Sweden).

Statistical significance, FWER and FDR were all set at two-tailed alpha = 5.0E-2.

RESULTS

Patients Characteristics

As summarized in **Table 1**, AH patients were significantly sicker than ARC, having higher Child-Pugh score, MELD score and INR, increased concentrations of bilirubin, AST, ALP and GGT and lower albumin levels. AH patients also had higher leukocyte count (particularly neutrophils and monocytes), neutrophil-to-lymphocyte ratio (NLR) and monocyte-to-lymphocyte ratio (MLR) compared to ARC patients. ALD patients were older than HC and among ARC patients, those with Child-Pugh A were younger.

Soluble-TIM3 Is Severely Dysregulated in ALD

Systemic levels of soluble-TIM3 were highly elevated in ALD patients and the most significantly different between groups amongst all the soluble-CRs (**Supplementary Table 2** and **Figures 1A,B**). Increased levels of soluble-CD80 were also observed (ALD > HC, **Figures 1A,C**). Compared to HC, soluble-LAG3 was also greater in patients (ALD > HC), while soluble-HVEM was lower in patients (ALD < HC); however, differences for soluble-LAG3 and soluble-HVEM between groups were only borderline significant (**Figures 1A,D**). All other soluble-CRs were comparable between patients and controls (**Figures 1A,E**), and interestingly soluble-PD1 was the least different amongst all (**Figures 1A,F**).

To investigate the combined effect of multiple soluble-CRs on the performance of soluble-TIM3 as a disease marker, multivariate analysis of plasma soluble-CRs was performed in the three study groups. Principal component analysis (PCA) highlighted a degree of unsupervised internal clustering linked to differential soluble-CR plasma levels (**Figure 1G**). Superimposition of clinical categories (HC, ARC, and SAH) by partial least squares discriminant analysis (PLS-DA) indicated soluble-TIM3 as the strongest driver of these differences (**Figure 1H**).

Soluble-TIM3 and Its Ligands Correlate With ALD Severity and Inflammation

The relationship between plasma soluble-TIM3, other soluble-CRs and indices of inflammation and disease severity was then assessed by correlation analysis.

Soluble-CRs were strongly positively intercorrelated with each other in ALD patients (**Figure 2A** and **Supplementary Table 3**) and in controls (**Figure 2B** and **Supplementary Table 4**). However, soluble-TIM3 and soluble-CD80 correlations were peculiar: the majority of soluble-TIM3 intercorrelations were only present in patients, while most soluble-CD80 intercorrelations were only present in controls. Some multivariate collinearity was also detected by Variance Inflation Factor (VIF) regression diagnostics (**Supplementary Table 5**). Of note, plasma levels for both TIM3 soluble ligands Galectin-9 and soluble-CEACAM1 were higher in ALD patients (SAH > ARC) compared to HC (**Figure 2C**). To estimate receptor-ligand binding, the normalized molar ratios for each soluble ligand and soluble-TIM3 were calculated, and for both Galectin-9 and soluble-CEACAM1 these values were comparable across groups (**Figure 2D**), suggesting a disease-independent molar (quantitative) equilibrium. In ALD patients, the top-three hyper-expressed soluble-CRs displayed several positive correlations with Child-Pugh score (soluble-TIM3, soluble-CD80, and soluble-LAG3), MELD score (soluble-TIM3 and soluble-CD80), INR (soluble-CD80 and soluble-LAG3) and negative correlations with albumin (soluble-TIM3, soluble-CD80, and soluble-LAG3), GGT (soluble-LAG3), sodium (soluble-TIM3) and lymphocyte count (soluble-LAG3) (**Figure 3C** and **Supplementary Table 6**). Soluble-TIM3 was also the only soluble-CR positively correlated with the monocyte-to-lymphocyte ratio (MLR), a surrogate index of inflammation (**Figure 3C** and **Supplementary Table 6**).

As expected, elevated plasma levels of pro-inflammatory IL-1a, IL-1b, IL-1ra, IL-6, IL-8, IL-18, TNFa, and IFNg were observed in ALD compared to HC (**Figure 3A** and **Supplementary Figure 1**). By contrast, IL-10 and IL-33 were comparable between groups. Soluble-TIM3 was the only soluble-CR correlated with the archetypal pro-inflammatory cytokine IL-6 in ALD patients (**Figure 3C** and **Supplementary Table 6**). Other cytokine correlations were observed for soluble-CD80 (IL-1b, IL-18, and IFNg) and soluble-IDO (IL-1a, IL-1b, IL-1ra, and IL-18) (**Figure 3C** and **Supplementary Table 6**). Of note, no correlations were found in HC between soluble-CRs and cytokines (**Supplementary Table 7**).

As expected, plasma concentrations of both D-lactate and soluble-CD163, two surrogate markers of gut permeability and bacterial translocation, (i) were significantly higher in ALD patients (SAH > ARC) compared to HC (**Figure 3B**) reconfirming our previous findings (Markwick et al., 2015; Riva et al., 2018, 2020), and (ii) were strongly correlated with clinical indices of disease severity (Child-Pugh score, MELD score,

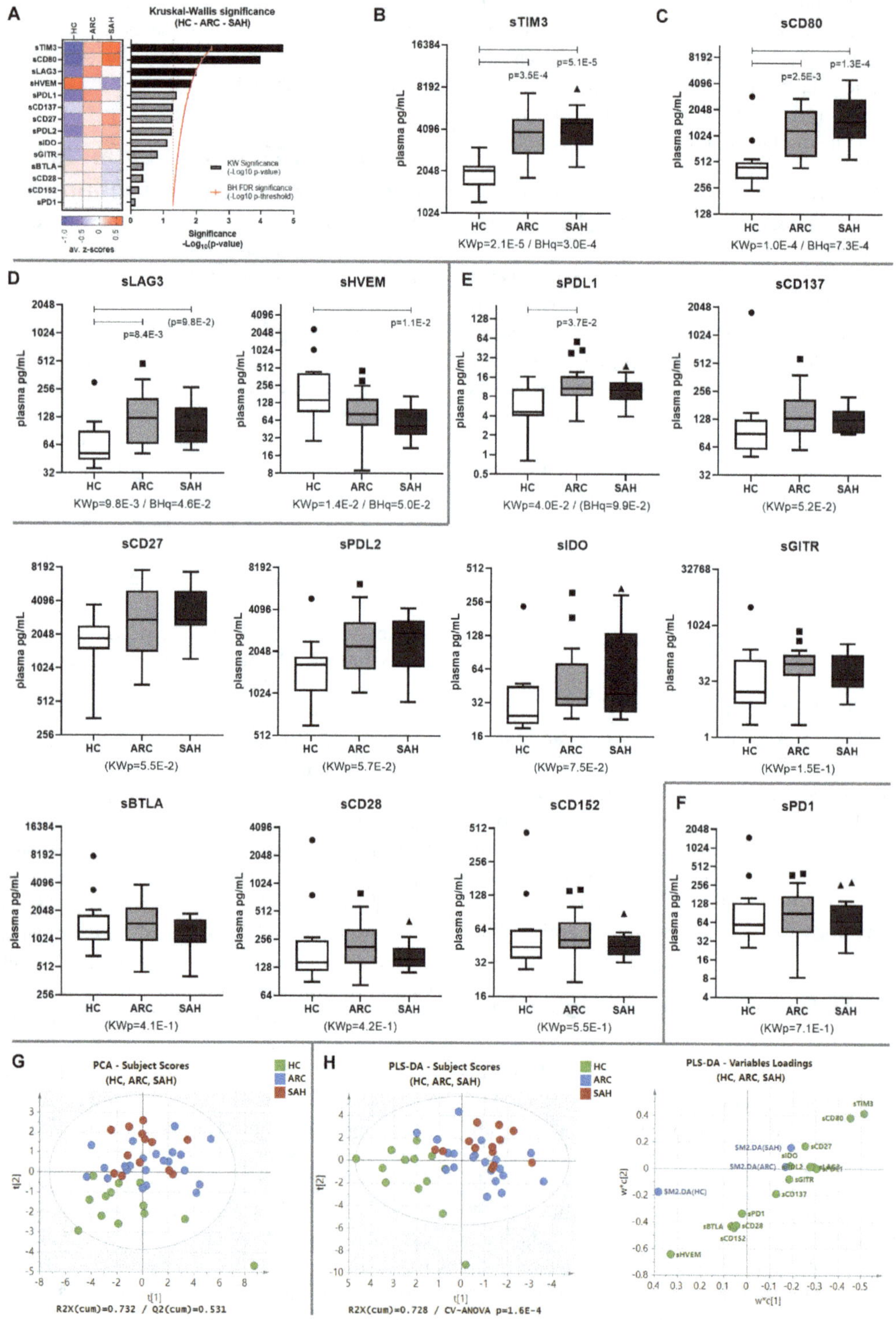

FIGURE 1 | Soluble-CR networks in ALD patients. **(A)** Significance plot summarizing the soluble-CR differential expression in HC, ARC and SAH; soluble-CR measurements: standardized *z*-scores; significance: $-\text{Log}_{10}$(*p*-value); red continuous line: BH significance threshold; red dotted line: $p = 0.05$; black bars: significantly different soluble-CRs; gray bars: non-significant soluble-CRs. **(B)** Soluble-TIM3 is the most different and highly upregulated soluble-CR in patients vs. HC, followed by **(C)** soluble-CD80, **(D)** soluble-LAG3 and soluble-HVEM. **(E)** Soluble-CRs comparable between groups. **(F)** Soluble-PD1 is the most similar in patients and controls. KWp, raw Kruskal–Wallis *p*-value; BHq, FDR-adjusted *q*-value; p, significant multiple comparisons with Dunn's correction. Boxplots (median, IQR, ± Tukey's whiskers/outliers) ordered by decreasing statistical significance. **(G)** Subject clustering by unsupervised PCA. **(H)** 3-way supervised clustering by PLS-DA, with superimposition of HC, ARC, and SAH categories; soluble-TIM3 is the main driver of supervised clustering, as shown in the 'Variables Loadings' plot; subject re-classification based on this model: 70.8% accuracy (HC-ARC-SAH = 100%–86.4%–15.4%, Fisher's $p = 8.7\text{E-}9$). 'Subject Scores' plots: each dot represents a subject; 'Variables Loadings' plots: each dot represents a soluble-CR.

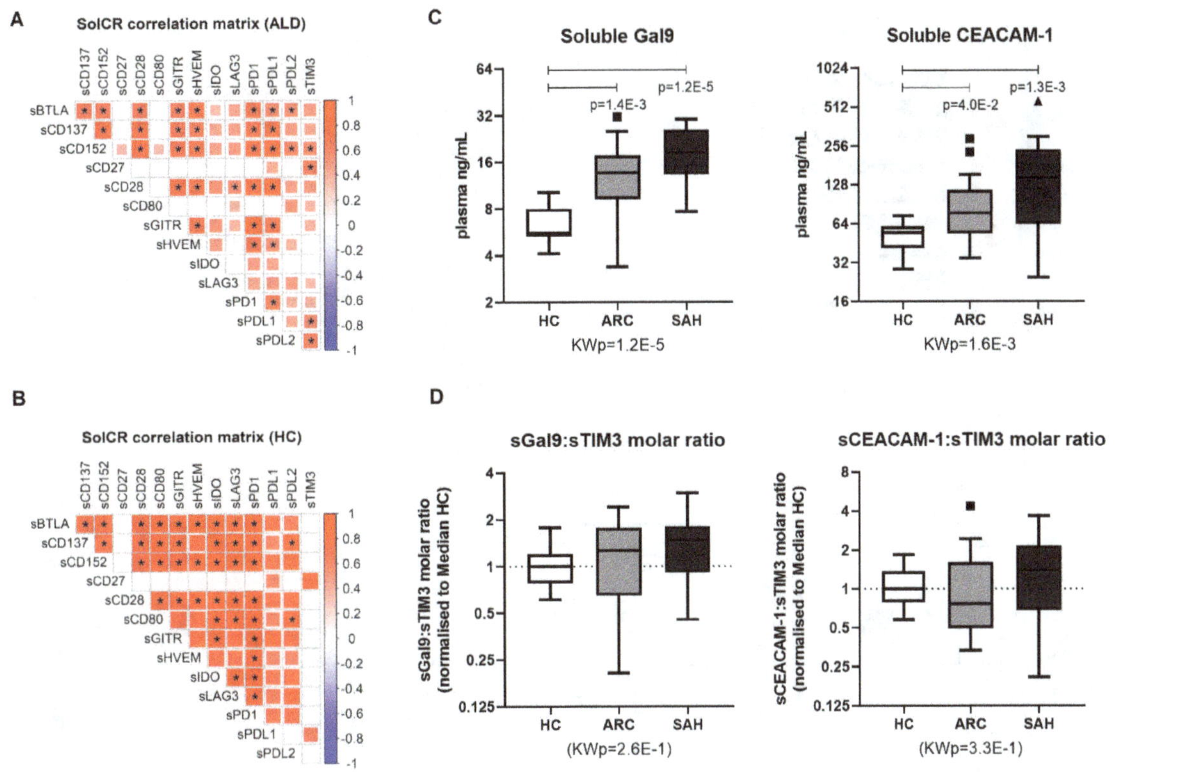

FIGURE 2 | Soluble-TIM3 intercorrelations and soluble-TIM3 ligands. **(A)** Intercorrelation matrix of individual soluble-CRs in ALD patients and **(B)** controls; the color scale and the size of individual matrix squares represent the value of significant Pearson correlation coefficients ($p \leq 0.05$); blank squares indicate lack of significant correlation; starred squares indicate significant correlations by Bonferroni correction. **(C)** Plasma levels of TIM3 soluble ligands Galectin-9 and soluble-CEACAM1 in HC, ARC and SAH. **(D)** Molar ratios between plasma Galectin-9 or soluble-CEACAM1 and soluble-TIM3 in HC, ARC and SAH, normalized vs. median (HC) (Kruskal–Wallis test with Dunn's multiple comparison correction).

bilirubin) (**Figure 3C** and **Supplementary Table 6**). D-lactate was also positively correlated with total leukocyte, neutrophil and monocyte counts, and with all the cytokine measurements (**Figure 3C** and **Supplementary Table 6**). D-lactate and soluble-CD163 were also positively correlated to soluble-TIM3 and soluble-CD80 (**Figure 3C** and **Supplementary Table 6**) reinforcing the association between bacterial translocation, hyper-inflammation, soluble-CRs and disease severity in ALD patients.

Investigating the Source of Soluble-TIM3 in ALD Patients and the Relationship Between Soluble-TIM3 and Membrane-TIM3 in Response to Bacterial Challenge

To investigate the source of soluble-TIM3, soluble-CR concentrations were measured in plasma samples obtained from pre-hepatic (portal vein), post-hepatic (hepatic vein), and systemic (cubital vein and right cardiac atrium) blood beds in ARC patients during TIPS procedure. As shown in **Figure 4A**, intestinal/splanchnic or hepatic alterations during established ALD did not affect systemic levels of soluble-TIM3, and similar results were also obtained for all the soluble-CRs measured (**Supplementary Figure 2**).

To assess whether an acute alcohol 'hit' would trigger hepatic soluble-TIM3 production, human precision cut liver slices (PCLS) were treated with ethanol 250 mmol/L for 24 h but no release of soluble-TIM3 was observed upon this treatment, as shown in **Figure 4B**. This was also true for all the other soluble-CRs (**Supplementary Figure 3A**). Liver slices retained the immune infiltrate, viability (**Supplementary Figure 3B**) and tissue architecture during the culture period (**Supplementary Figure 3C**).

To investigate whether an acute bacterial challenge could provoke release of soluble-TIM3 in the whole blood, we measured soluble-CR concentrations in whole blood cultured with *E. coli* from ALD or HC subjects. As shown in **Figure 4C**, bacterial stimulation did not induce release of soluble-TIM3 or all the other soluble-CRs measured (**Supplementary Figure 4**). Of note, whole-blood soluble-TIM3 levels (in the absence of bacterial stimulation) were only different between groups (**Figure 4C**), in line with the plasma findings.

To assess whether soluble-TIM3 production from peripheral blood immune cells changes over time and to assess its relationship with membrane-TIM3 expression during anti-bacterial responses, membrane-TIM3 and soluble-TIM3

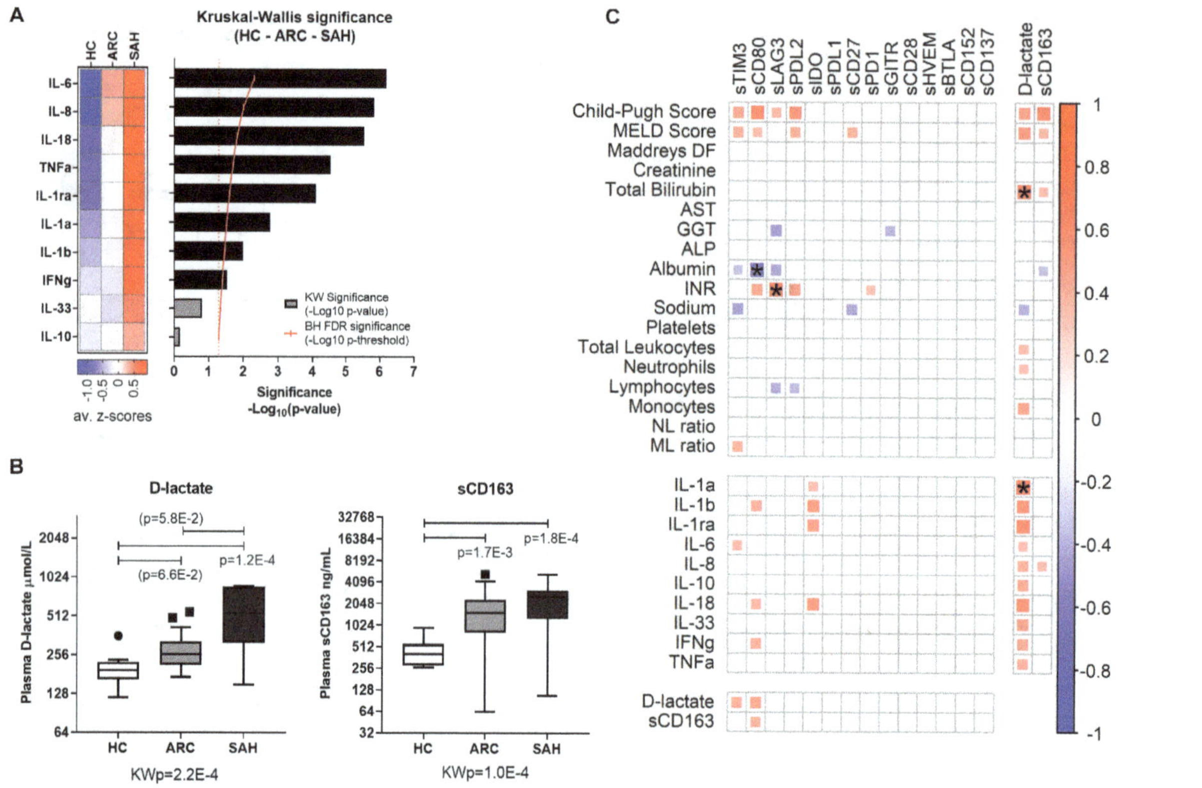

FIGURE 3 | Inflammatory cytokines, bacterial translocation and overall association with the hyper-inflamed state in ALD patients. **(A)** Significance plot summarizing cytokine differential expression in HC, ARC, and SAH; cytokine measurements: standardized *z*-scores; significance: $-\text{Log}_{10}(p\text{-value})$; red continuous line: BH significance threshold; red dotted line: $p = 0.05$; black bars: significantly different cytokines; gray bars: non-significant cytokines. **(B)** Boxplot representation of D-lactate and soluble-CD163 as surrogate markers of bacterial translocation, indicating higher levels in ALD patients compared to HC. KWp, Kruskal–Wallis *p*-value; p, significant multiple comparisons with Dunn's correction. Boxplots (median, IQR, ± Tukey's whiskers/outliers). **(C)** Correlation matrix of individual soluble-CRs with clinical parameters, cytokine measurements and markers of bacterial translocation in ALD patients; the color scale and the size of the individual matrix squares represent the value of significant Pearson correlation coefficients ($p \leq 0.05$); blank squares indicate lack of significant correlation; starred squares indicate significant correlations by Bonferroni correction.

were measured daily by flow cytometry and Luminex assays, respectively, in *E. coli*-challenged PBMC cultures from ALD patients and HC (representative FACS gating shown in **Supplementary Figure 5**). Baseline unstimulated (basal) membrane-TIM3 expression was significantly higher in ALD compared to HC (SAH > ARC) on T, B, and NK-cells but not on monocytes (mfi, **Figure 5A**; %, **Supplementary Figure 6A**), confirming our previously published results (Markwick et al., 2015). Bacterial stimulation caused progressive changes of membrane-TIM3 expression. In particular, membrane-TIM3 increased on T, B, and NK-cells (mfi, **Figure 5B**; %, **Supplementary Figure 6B**) and decreased on monocytes (mfi, **Figure 5B**). These changes were comparable between ARC and HC but were less pronounced in SAH (**Figure 5B** and **Supplementary Figure 6B**). Measurements of soluble-TIM3 in cell-culture supernatants revealed lack of bacteria-stimulated soluble-TIM3 production by PBMCs in all groups (**Figure 5C**).

In correlation analyses (**Supplementary Figure** 7), plasma soluble-TIM3 was strongly positively correlated with basal membrane-TIM3% in CD4 T-cells and both NK-cell subsets ($r \geq 0.529$, $p \leq 3.1\text{E-}2$); with basal membrane-TIM3mfi in CD8 T-cells and both NK-cell subsets ($r \geq 0.529$, $p \leq 1.8\text{E-}2$); and with unstimulated membrane-TIM3mfi in day-4 CD56dim NK-cells and day-7 CD8 T-cells ($r \geq 0.474$, $p \leq 4.0\text{E-}2$). Regarding the changes of membrane-TIM3 expression induced by bacterial stimulation, plasma soluble-TIM3 was strongly negatively correlated with the early (day-1) membrane-TIM3 response in CD56dim NK-cells (% and mfi; $r \leq -0.475, p \leq 4.0\text{E-}2$); and with the membrane-TIM3 mfi response in both day-4 CD56dim NK-cells and day-7 CD8 T-cells ($r \leq -0.544$, $p \leq 2.0\text{E-}2$). Overall, subjects with high baseline plasma levels of soluble-TIM3 had higher basal membrane-TIM3 expression on NK-/T-cell subsets but also significantly weaker/null membrane-TIM3 upregulation on CD56dim NK-cells and CD8 T-cells upon bacterial challenge.

Soluble-TIM3 Competitively Activates Anti-bacterial Immunity in ALD Patients

To investigate the biological function of soluble-TIM3 in ALD patients, in the context of anti-bacterial responses, the TIM3 receptor-ligand equilibrium was assessed with *in vitro* PBMC

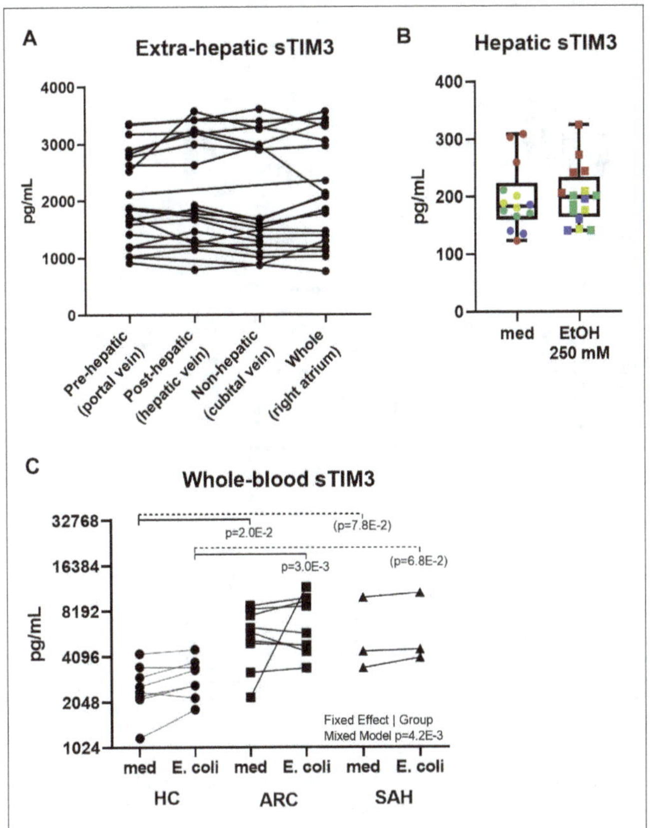

FIGURE 4 | Anatomical distribution and peripheral origin of soluble-TIM3. **(A)** No differences in soluble-TIM3 measured in plasma obtained from four anatomical compartments in 20 ARC patients undergoing TIPS; measurements are matched by subject (Friedman's paired test). **(B)** Lack of soluble-TIM3 production in PCLS treated with ethanol 250 mM for 24 h (Mann–Whitney test. Each dot represents one slice; each color represents one subject). Boxplots (median, IQR, ±full range). **(C)** Unchanged soluble-TIM3 levels in *E. coli*-pulsed whole blood (Mixed Model analysis, with significant fixed effect by subject group but not by stimulation).

cultures by neutralizing Galectin-9 with alpha-lactose and by competitive saturation using an excess of recombinant human soluble-TIM3-Ig fusion protein (rhsTIM3-Ig). As illustrated in **Figure 6A**, PBMC stimulation with *E. coli* induced T-cell IFNγ only in HC but not SAH, confirming our previously published observations (Markwick et al., 2015; Riva et al., 2018). T-cell production of anti-bacterial IL-17A and anti-inflammatory IL-10 were unchanged (**Figures 6B,C**) and monocyte IL-10 was induced in both groups (**Figure 6D**). Pre-treatment with rhsTIM3-Ig alone had no effect on *E. coli*-stimulated cytokines (**Figures 6A–D**). However, following Galectin-9 neutralization with alpha-lactose, rhsTIM3-Ig unlocked anti-bacterial T-cell IFNγ (**Figure 6A**) and IL-17A (**Figure 6B**) production in SAH patients, and strongly stimulated their T-cell/monocyte IL-10 production (**Figures 6C,D**, respectively). Of note, this immune reactivation was selective for ALD patients (SAH), as neither treatments elicited any effects in HC.

Control experiments on Galectin-9 neutralization in PBMCs from SAH patients stimulated with *E. coli* in the presence or absence of a blocking anti-Galectin-9 monoclonal antibody (**Supplementary Figure 8**) indicated that Galectin-9 blockade alone was not sufficient to recapitulate all the changes observed when Galectin-9 neutralization was achieved with alpha-lactose and excess rhsTIM3-Ig. In particular, Galectin-9 blockade could not rescue the production of *E. coli*-stimulated anti-bacterial IFNγ (**Supplementary Figure 8A**), while its effects on the production of pro-inflammatory IL-17A by CD8 T-cells (**Supplementary Figure 8B**) and anti-inflammatory IL-10 by monocytes (**Supplementary Figure 8D**) were only marginal.

DISCUSSION

We have previously shown that the compromised innate and adaptive anti-bacterial immunity in SAH could be maneuvered to a more favorable state through *ex vivo* neutralization of membrane-bound checkpoint receptors TIM3 and PD1 on lymphocytes, without inducing the production of cytokines associated with systemic inflammatory response syndrome (Markwick et al., 2015). However, the role of the recently discovered functional soluble (cell-free) CRs in the immune dysregulation associated with ALD is not well understood and this was the aim of the current study.

The main finding from our analysis is that soluble-TIM3 and its soluble ligands Galectin-9 and soluble-CEACAM1 are closely associated with the severity of ALD. Multivariate assessments (PCA and PLS-DA) of soluble-CRs highlighted disease-based differences among subjects and indicated soluble-TIM3 as the strongest driver of these differences in ALD. Soluble-TIM3 was also strongly correlated with a highly inflammatory state, increased bacterial translocation and clinical indices of disease severity in ALD patients, highlighting a novel potential immune-related pathogenetic mechanism associated with disease progression. These findings led us to focus our subsequent work on the characterisation of the soluble-TIM3 pathway and its role in ALD.

The immunosuppressive activity of membrane-TIM3 has been characterized in detail; the engagement of membrane-TIM3 by its ligands Galectin-9 and CEACAM1 activates downstream intracellular signaling pathways leading to functional inactivation of the immune cell (Davidson et al., 2007; Lee et al., 2011; Rangachari et al., 2012; Clayton et al., 2014; Das et al., 2017). Blocking membrane-TIM3 with neutralizing antibodies prevents T-cell 'shutdown' and reactivates immune function (Sabatos-Peyton et al., 2018), underpinning pre-clinical and clinical studies for TIM3-based immunotherapy (Riva and Chokshi, 2018; Friedlaender et al., 2019). In the present study, we found that during ALD, and predominantly in SAH patients, membrane-TIM3 is hyper-expressed on immune cells, reconfirming previously published results (Markwick et al., 2015), and plasma levels of Galectin-9 and CEACAM1 are also highly increased. In these circumstances, over-expression of both ligands and their membrane receptor may drive widespread immune impairment. However, the soluble cell-free form of

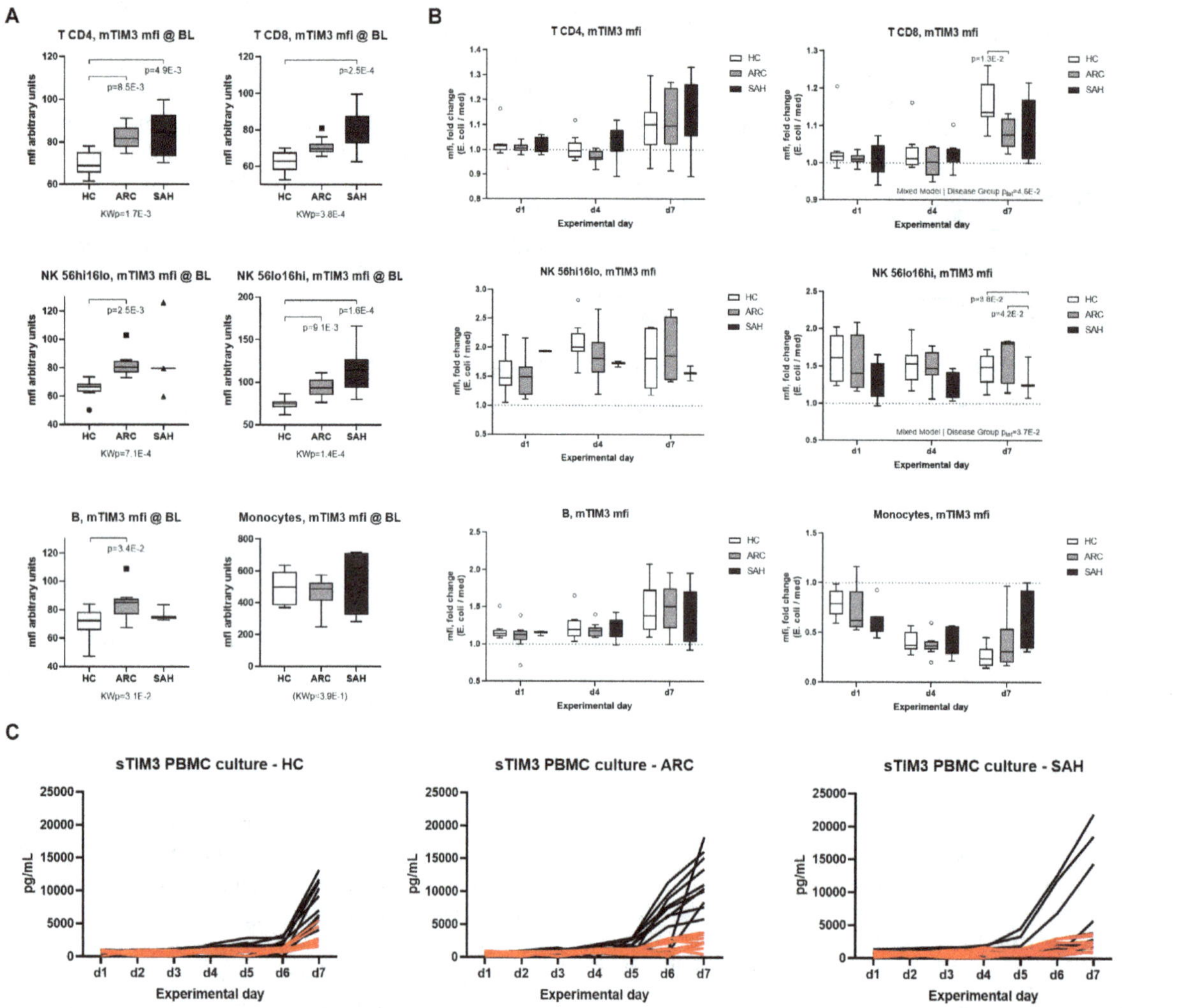

FIGURE 5 | Expression of membrane-TIM3 on immune subsets and modulation by *E. coli*. **(A)** membrane-TIM3 mfi at baseline (day 1, unstimulated) on T-cells (CD4/CD8), NK-cells (CD56hi/CD56lo), B-cells and monocytes (Kruskal–Wallis test with Dunn's multiple comparison correction). **(B)** Modulation of membrane-TIM3 mfi during a 7-day *E. coli*-stimulated culture; assessments performed at days 1–4–7; data expressed as *E. coli* fold ratio vs. unstimulated medium (Mixed Model analysis, with fixed effect comparisons by group). Boxplots: median, IQR, ±Tukey's whiskers/outliers. **(C)** Soluble-TIM3 in daily PBMC culture supernatants; black lines indicate soluble-TIM3 levels in unstimulated medium; red lines represent soluble-TIM3 in *E. coli*-stimulated cultures. $N = 10$ for each HC, ARC, and SAH.

TIM3 is known to act as a 'decoy antagonist' and when plasma levels are supra-physiological, like those found in ALD patients in the present study, sequestration of Galectin-9 and CEACAM1 may prevent immune suppression mediated via membrane-TIM3 (Jones et al., 2008; Muthukumarana et al., 2008; Vega-Carrascal et al., 2011; Nebbia et al., 2012; Wu et al., 2012; de Kivit et al., 2013, 2017; Xiao et al., 2013; Kojima et al., 2014). In fact, detectable complexes of soluble-TIM3 and Galectin-9 have been described in the literature (Silva et al., 2017) and we would suggest that the heightened production of soluble-TIM3 in ALD could be an attempt to counter the immunosuppressive properties of Galectin-9 and CEACAM1.

However, the binding between TIM3, Galectin-9 and CEACAM1 does not occur in a 1-to-1 ratio. Whilst TIM3 is monomeric, Galectin-9 is homodimeric and both Galectin-9 and CEACAM1 are molecular mixtures of several isoforms (Zhu et al., 2005; Nagaishi et al., 2008; Huang et al., 2015; Horst et al., 2018; Kim et al., 2019). Thus, even when quantitative molar ratios are comparable, the number of binding sites for TIM3 may be in excess. As such, Galectin-9 and CEACAM1 could act as 'molecular sponges' for soluble-TIM3 while still retaining enough unsaturated binding sites to ligate membrane-TIM3 on immune cells, thereby suppressing immune responses and inhibiting anti-bacterial immunity.

To explore this, we saturated bacteria-stimulated PBMC cultures with recombinant human soluble-TIM3 (rhsTIM3-Ig fusion protein) and biochemically neutralized Galectin-9 with alpha-lactose; we found that this cocktail was able to unlock anti-bacterial immunity (IFNγ and IL-17) and restore anti-inflammatory IL-10 production in AH patients. As expected,

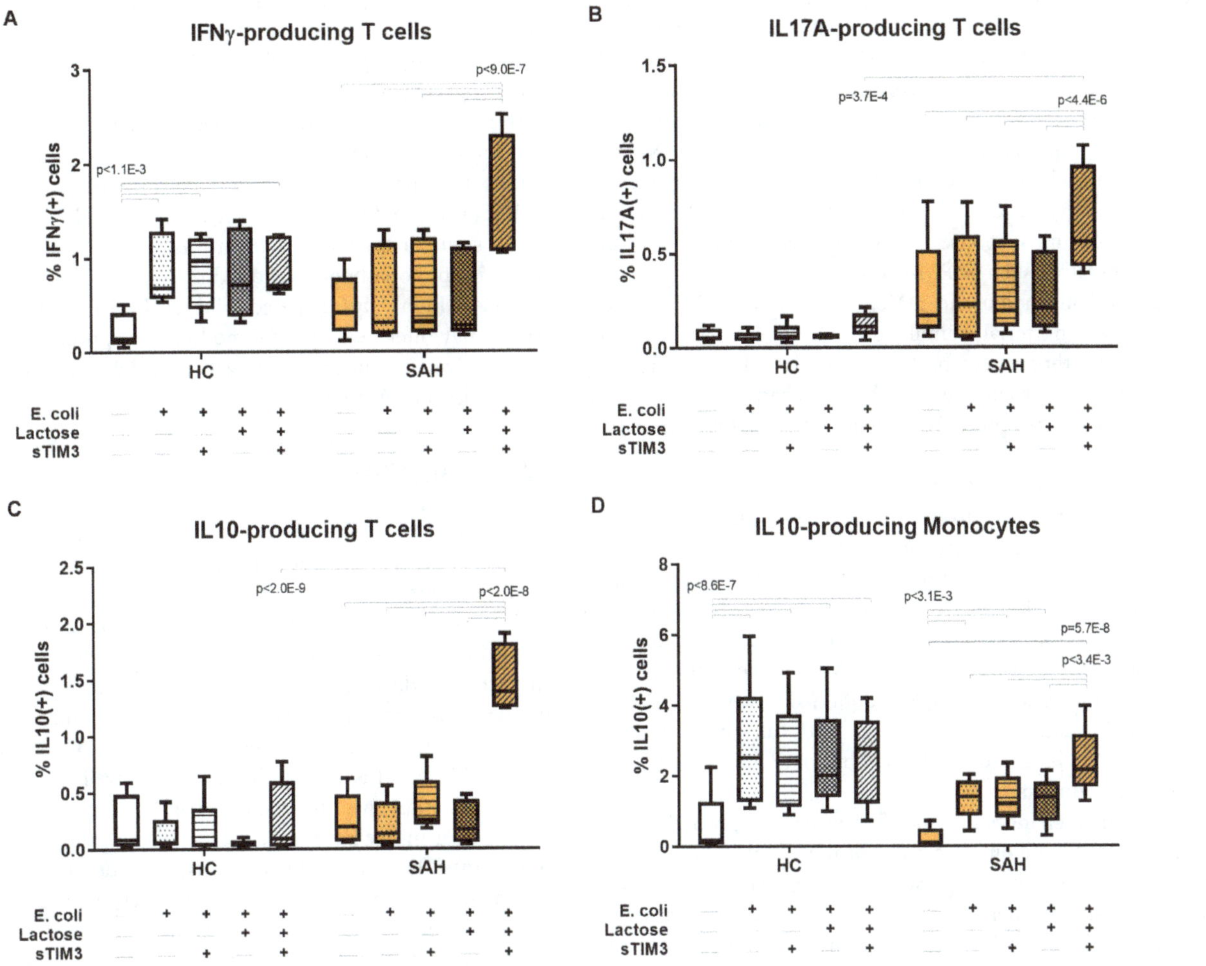

FIGURE 6 | Soluble-TIM3 pathway and soluble-TIM3 functional characterisation. **(A)** Recombinant human soluble-TIM3 (rhsTIM3-Ig fusion protein) shows a stimulatory effect on *E. coli*-stimulated T-cell production of IFNγ, **(B)** T-cell IL-17A, **(C)** T-cell IL-10, and **(D)** monocyte IL-10 in PBMC cultures from SAH, after Galectin-9 binding neutralization with alpha-lactose; no effects observed in HC PBMC cultures (2-way ANOVA with Holm–Sidak's *post hoc* correction for paired samples); orange bars represent SAH PBMCs; white bars represent HC PBMCs; shading identifies different culture conditions as specified along each graph's *x*-axis. Boxplots: median, IQR, ±Tukey's whiskers/outliers.

immune rescue was not observed in controls, where the TIM3 pathway was not dysregulated. Notably, Galectin-9 blockade alone with a neutralizing anti-Gal9 monoclonal antibody was not sufficient to recapitulate the immune rescue effects observed when soluble-TIM3 was used in combination with alpha-lactose. It is important to mention that several publications confirm that the type of recombinant human soluble-TIM3 used in the present study can selectively bind TIM3 ligands, is biologically active and has comparable blocking activity to anti-TIM3 antibodies (Vega-Carrascal et al., 2011; Nebbia et al., 2012; Wu et al., 2012; de Kivit et al., 2013, 2017; Kojima et al., 2014). The *in vitro* immune rescue activity of this rhsTIM3-Ig has been shown to be highly antigen-specific, with no effects upon generalized stimuli such as PMA/Ionomycin or anti-CD3/CD28 (Nebbia et al., 2012; Wu et al., 2012), which may be relevant in the context of bacteria-specific responses. Furthermore, rhsTIM3-Ig has also demonstrated the ability to enhance compensatory type-2 responses (Wang et al., 2015) potentially dampening type 1 inflammation, which may be highly relevant in ALD and specifically SAH patients where chronic inflammation underlies immunopathology. Taken together our study would suggest that TIM3 ligands Galectin-9 and soluble-CEACAM1 may be central to the immune impairment in AH and that therapeutic administration of soluble-TIM3 may be a novel option to improve anti-bacterial effector functions in AH.

We next turned our attention to investigate the possible sources of soluble-TIM3 in ALD. Firstly we aimed to understand if there was a direct and temporal relationship between the expression of membrane-TIM3 on immune cells and the production of the soluble form, and whether the latter was upregulated during bacterial challenge. During *E. coli* challenge of PBMCs, we observed progressive loss of membrane-TIM3 expression in monocytes from both ALD patients and controls, and dampened membrane-TIM3 upregulation on Natural Killer cells and CD8 T-cells from ALD patients, the latter being in strong negative correlation with higher plasma soluble-TIM3 in the same patients. However, these membrane-TIM3 changes were not accompanied by increased soluble-TIM3 in our culture supernatants upon *E. coli* stimulation. Notably, it has been shown that monocytes (Moller-Hackbarth et al., 2013) and activated CD8 T-cells (Clayton et al., 2015) release soluble-TIM3 in response to lipopolysaccharide and other broad stimulators such as PMA/Ionomycin, but no information is available on membrane-TIM3 and soluble-TIM3 kinetics during direct bacterial stimulation. More research is needed to clarify whether direct bacterial stimulation acts differently on soluble-TIM3 shedding or other mechanisms are at play, such as recapture, proteolytic degradation, sequestration or epitope masking.

Next, we assessed whether systemic soluble-TIM3 originated from the liver during ALD. Using a novel human immunocompetent precision cut liver slice model of ALD, we found that upon treatment with high ethanol concentrations, soluble-TIM3 levels were not prompted. This finding was confirmed in plasma from patients undergoing TIPS procedure, where soluble-TIM3 concentrations were measured in plasma samples obtained from pre-hepatic, post-hepatic, and systemic blood beds in ARC patients: soluble-TIM3 levels were high but not different between these compartments.

Rather than changes in a specific source, the elevated soluble-TIM3 levels may be due to activity of metalloproteases involved in soluble-TIM3 shedding, such as ADAM10 or ADAM17, which warrants further investigation. In fact, it is well described that inflammatory responses lead to increased metalloprotease activity and in these conditions production of soluble-TIM3 by proteolytic cleavage may be facilitated (Moller-Hackbarth et al., 2013; Clayton et al., 2015; Ren et al., 2015). However, their ubiquitous expression, relative lack of specificity and broadly diverse biological roles *in vivo* (Weber and Saftig, 2012; Giebeler and Zigrino, 2016; Wetzel et al., 2017; Zunke and Rose-John, 2017; Saha et al., 2019) would make them difficult therapeutic targets.

Interestingly, the soluble form of PD1 and its ligands were not different between groups, despite our previous finding of membrane-PD1 being upregulated on immune cells in ALD patients (Markwick et al., 2015). There are several soluble isoforms of PD1, one of which retains ligand binding capacity and is therefore putatively biologically active (Nielsen et al., 2005), but whether our quantification measured total soluble-PD1 or any of its isoforms is unclear, as currently no commercially available reagents allow the measurement of distinct isoforms. The existence of different soluble isoforms may affect other soluble-CRs as well, including soluble-CD80 (Lahat et al., 2003; Kakoulidou et al., 2007), soluble-LAG3 (Li et al., 2007), soluble-HVEM (Heo et al., 2012; Li et al., 2020), and the already discussed soluble-TIM3 (Moller-Hackbarth et al., 2013; Clayton et al., 2015; Ren et al., 2015), Galectin-9 and CEACAM1 (Zhu et al., 2005; Nagaishi et al., 2008; Huang et al., 2015; Horst et al., 2018; Kim et al., 2019), and we believe this also to be the reason for the discrepancy between our findings and a recent publication by Li et al. (2020) where soluble-HVEM was found to be the most significantly dysregulated soluble-CR in AH patients (Wang et al., 2001; Heo et al., 2012; Zhao Q. et al., 2017; Li et al., 2020). There is currently no information on the relative balance between soluble-CR isoforms in health and disease, but since changes in this equilibrium may have pathophysiological consequences, this may be important to discern for future advances in the field.

To summarize, the data from this study reveal new insights in the immunopathogenesis of ALD. In particular, we describe a novel and highly dysregulated soluble-TIM3/ligand axis in ALD, which may offer new immunomodulatory approaches to restore an effective state of anti-pathogen host defense in these highly immunocompromised patients.

LAY SUMMARY

Alcohol-related liver disease (ALD) is an escalating global problem and is responsible for >2.5 million deaths/year. One of the major and most common complications that ALD patients face is an increased susceptibility to infection, which can lead to worsening of liver disease and multi-organ failure. In fact, the development of bacterial infection often signals the terminal phase in ALD, increasing the probability of death to 30% at 1 month and >60% by 1 year. The mechanisms responsible for this susceptibility are not well understood and it is vital that we understand why patients with alcohol-related liver injury have impaired defenses against infection and the factors that may influence this, in order to develop new treatments beyond the use of antibiotics, which are driving the selection of multi-drug resistant bacteria in this patient group. In this study, we present novel findings describing the central role of the immunoregulatory molecule TIM3 and its binding partners Galectin-9 and CEACAM1 in the impaired immunity in ALD patients. We also show that the soluble form of TIM3 may be a promising therapeutic target to facilitate rescue of anti-microbial immunity without exacerbating damaging inflammatory responses.

AUTHOR CONTRIBUTIONS

AR: study design and supervision, experimental work, data acquisition, analysis, presentation, manuscript preparation, and revision. SC: study design and supervision, funding, manuscript revision, and final approval. EP, DD, and DC: additional laboratory work. DC, HA, NH, KM, MeP, AZ, RM, JR, GW, SF, AE, DS, RS, SK, FU, MiP, KK, TH, SP, MS, and JT: provision of samples. RW: critical evaluation of the manuscript for important intellectual content and study funding. All authors reviewed and approved the final version of the manuscript.

REFERENCES

Albillos, A., Lario, M., and Alvarez-Mon, M. (2014). Cirrhosis-associated immune dysfunction: distinctive features and clinical relevance. *J. Hepatol.* 61, 1385–1396. doi: 10.1016/j.jhep.2014.08.010

Arroyo, V., Moreau, R., Jalan, R., Gines, P., Easl-Clif Consortium, C. A. N. O. N. I. C., and Study. (2015). Acute-on-chronic liver failure:

a new syndrome that will re-classify cirrhosis. *J. Hepatol.* 62 (1 Suppl.), S131–S143. doi: 10.1016/j.jhep.2014.11.045

Cao, J., Zhang, L., Huang, S., Chen, P., Zou, L., Chen, H., et al. (2011). Aberrant production of soluble co-stimulatory molecules CTLA-4 and CD28 in patients with chronic hepatitis B. *Microbial Pathogenesis* 51, 262–267. doi: 10.1016/j.micpath.2011.06.003

Cao, J., Zou, L., Luo, P., Chen, P., and Zhang, L. (2012). Increased production of circulating soluble co-stimulatory molecules CTLA-4, CD28 and CD80 in patients with rheumatoid arthritis. *Int. Immunopharmacol.* 14, 585–592. doi: 10.1016/j.intimp.2012.08.004

Chen, D., Peng, W., Jiang, H., Yang, H., Wu, J., Wang, H., et al. (2017). Noninvasive detection of acute renal allograft rejection by measurement of soluble Tim-3 in urine. *Mol. Med. Rep.* 16, 915–921. doi: 10.3892/mmr.2017.6670

Chiba, M., Yanaba, K., Hayashi, M., Yoshihara, Y., and Nakagawa, H. (2017). Clinical significance of serum soluble T-cell immunoglobulin and mucin domain 3 levels in systemic sclerosis: association with disease severity. *J. Dermatol.* 44, 194–197. doi: 10.1111/1346-8138.13610

Chokshi, S. (2018). Can we reliably predict response to corticosteroid treatment in severe alcoholic hepatitis? *Hepatol. Commun.* 2, 625–627. doi: 10.1002/hep4.1191

Clayton, K. L., Douglas-Vail, M. B., Rahman, N.-U. A. K. M., Medcalf, K. E., Xie, I. Y., Chew, G. M., et al. (2015). Soluble T cell immunoglobulin mucin domain 3 is shed from CD8+ T cells by the sheddase ADAM10, is increased in plasma during untreated HIV infection, and correlates with HIV disease progression. *J. Virol.* 89, 3723–3736. doi: 10.1128/jvi.00006-15

Clayton, K. L., Haaland, M. S., Douglas-Vail, M. B., Mujib, S., Chew, G. M., Ndhlovu, L. C., et al. (2014). T cell Ig and mucin domain-containing protein 3 is recruited to the immune synapse, disrupts stable synapse formation, and associates with receptor phosphatases. *J. Immunol.* 192, 782–791. doi: 10.4049/jimmunol.1302663

Das, M., Zhu, C., and Kuchroo, V. K. (2017). Tim-3 and its role in regulating anti-tumor immunity. *Immunol. Rev.* 276, 97–111. doi: 10.1111/imr.12520

Davidson, D., Schraven, B., and Veillette, A. (2007). PAG-associated FynT regulates calcium signaling and promotes anergy in T lymphocytes. *Mol. Cell Biol.* 27, 1960–1973. doi: 10.1128/MCB.01983-06

de Kivit, S., Kostadinova, A. I., Kerperien, J., Morgan, M. E., Muruzabal, V. A., Hofman, G. A., et al. (2017). Dietary, nondigestible oligosaccharides and *Bifidobacterium breve* M-16V suppress allergic inflammation in intestine via targeting dendritic cell maturation. *J. Leukoc. Biol.* 102, 105–115. doi: 10.1189/jlb.3A0516-236R

de Kivit, S., Kraneveld, A. D., Knippels, L. M., van Kooyk, Y., Garssen, J., and Willemsen, L. E. (2013). Intestinal epithelium-derived galectin-9 is involved in the immunomodulating effects of nondigestible oligosaccharides. *J. Innate Immun.* 5, 625–638. doi: 10.1159/000350515

Delmastro, M. M., Styche, A. J., Trucco, M. M., Workman, C. J., Vignali, D. A. A., and Piganelli, J. D. (2012). Modulation of redox balance leaves murine diabetogenic TH1 T Cells "LAG-3-ing" behind. *Diabetes* 61, 1760–1768. doi: 10.2337/db11-1591

EASL (2018). EASL clinical practice guidelines: management of alcohol-related liver disease. *J Hepatol* 69, 154–181. doi: 10.1016/j.jhep.2018.03.018

Fernandez, J., Bert, F., and Nicolas-Chanoine, M. H. (2016). The challenges of multi-drug-resistance in hepatology. *J. Hepatol.* 65, 1043–1054. doi: 10.1016/j.jhep.2016.08.006

Friedlaender, A., Addeo, A., and Banna, G. (2019). New emerging targets in cancer immunotherapy: the role of TIM3. *ESMO Open* 4(Suppl. 3):e000497. doi: 10.1136/esmoopen-2019-000497

Ge, W., Li, J., Fan, W., Xu, D., and Sun, S. (2017). Tim-3 as a diagnostic and prognostic biomarker of osteosarcoma. *Tumor Biol.* 39:1010428317715643. doi: 10.1177/1010428317715643

Giebeler, N., and Zigrino, P. (2016). A Disintegrin and Metalloprotease (ADAM): historical overview of their functions. *Toxins* 8:122. doi: 10.3390/toxins8040122

Gu, D., Ao, X., Yang, Y., Chen, Z., and Xu, X. (2018). Soluble immune checkpoints in cancer: production, function and biological significance. *J. Immunother. Cancer* 6:132. doi: 10.1186/s40425-018-0449-0

Guignant, C., Lepape, A., Huang, X., Kherouf, H., Denis, L., Poitevin, F., et al. (2011). Programmed death-1 levels correlate with increased mortality, nosocomial infection and immune dysfunctions in septic shock patients. *Critic. Care* 15:R99. doi: 10.1186/cc10112

Gustot, T., Felleiter, P., Pickkers, P., Sakr, Y., Rello, J., Velissaris, D., et al. (2014). Impact of infection on the prognosis of critically ill cirrhotic patients: results from a large worldwide study. *Liver Int.* 34, 1496–1503. doi: 10.1111/liv.12520

He, Y., Wang, Y., Zhao, S., Zhao, C., Zhou, C., and Hirsch, F. R. (2018). sLAG-3 in non-small-cell lung cancer patients' serum. *OncoTargets Ther.* 11, 4781–4784. doi: 10.2147/ott.s164178

Heo, S. K., Ju, S. A., Kim, G. Y., Park, S. M., Back, S. H., Park, N. H., et al. (2012). The presence of high level soluble herpes virus entry mediator in sera of gastric cancer patients. *Exp. Mol. Med.* 44, 149–158. doi: 10.3858/emm.2012.44.2.010

Hock, B. D., Starling, G. C., Patton, W. N., Salm, N., Bond, K., McArthur, L. T., et al. (2009). Identification of a circulating soluble form of CD80: levels in patients with hematological malignancies. *Leukem. Lymphoma* 45, 2111–2118. doi: 10.1080/10428190410001712199

Horst, A. K., Najjar, S. M., Wagener, C., and Tiegs, G. (2018). CEACAM1 in liver injury, metabolic and immune regulation. *Int. J. Mol. Sci.* 19:3110. doi: 10.3390/ijms19103110

Hotchkiss, R. S., Colston, E., Yende, S., Angus, D. C., Moldawer, L. L., and Crouser. (2019a). Immune checkpoint inhibition in sepsis: a phase 1b randomized, placebo-controlled, single ascending dose study of antiprogrammed cell death-ligand 1 Antibody (BMS-936559). *Crit. Care Med.* 47, 632–642. doi: 10.1097/ccm.0000000000003685

Hotchkiss, R. S., Colston, E., Yende, S., Crouser, Martin, G. S., Albertson, T., et al. (2019b). Immune checkpoint inhibition in sepsis: a Phase 1b randomized study to evaluate the safety, tolerability, pharmacokinetics, and pharmacodynamics of nivolumab. *Intens. Care Med.* 45, 1360–1371. doi: 10.1007/s00134-019-05704-z

Huang, Y. H., Zhu, C., Kondo, Y., Anderson, A. C., Gandhi, A., Russell, A., et al. (2015). CEACAM1 regulates TIM-3-mediated tolerance and exhaustion. *Nature* 517, 386–390. doi: 10.1038/nature13848

Ip, W. K., Wong, C. K., Leung, T. F., and Lam, C. W. (2005). Elevation of plasma soluble T cell costimulatory molecules CTLA-4, CD28 and CD80 in children with allergic asthma. *Int. Arch. Allergy Immunol.* 137, 45–52. doi: 10.1159/000084612

Ip, W. K., Wong, C. K., Leung, T. F., and Lam, C. W. (2006). Plasma concentrations of soluble CTLA-4, CD28, CD80 and CD86 costimulatory molecules reflect disease severity of acute asthma in children. *Pediatr. Pulmonol.* 41, 674–682. doi: 10.1002/ppul.20432

Jalan, R., Fernandez, J., Wiest, R., Schnabl, B., Moreau, R., Angeli, P., et al. (2014). Bacterial infections in cirrhosis: a position statement based on the EASL Special Conference 2013. *J. Hepatol.* 60, 1310–1324. doi: 10.1016/j.jhep.2014.01.024

Jones, R. B., Ndhlovu, L. C., Barbour, J. D., Sheth, P. M., Jha, A. R., Long, B. R., et al. (2008). Tim-3 expression defines a novel population of dysfunctional T cells with highly elevated frequencies in progressive HIV-1 infection. *J. Exp. Med.* 205, 2763–2779. doi: 10.1084/jem.20081398

Jung, H. W., La, S. J., Kim, J. Y., Heo, S. K., Kim, J. Y., Wang, S., et al. (2003). High levels of soluble herpes virus entry mediator in sera of patients with allergic and autoimmune diseases. *Exp. Mol. Med.* 35, 501–508. doi: 10.1038/emm.2003.65

Kakoulidou, M., Giscombe, R., Zhao, X., Lefvert, A. K., and Wang, X. (2007). Human soluble CD80 is generated by alternative splicing, and recombinant soluble CD80 binds to CD28 and CD152 influencing T-cell activation. *Scand. J. Immunol.* 66, 529–537. doi: 10.1111/j.1365-3083.2007.02009.x

Kim, W. M., Huang, Y. H., Gandhi, A., and Blumberg, R. S. (2019). CEACAM1 structure and function in immunity and its therapeutic implications. *Semin. Immunol.* 42:101296. doi: 10.1016/j.smim.2019.101296

Kojima, R., Ohno, T., Iikura, M., Niki, T., Hirashima, M., Iwaya, K., et al. (2014). Galectin-9 enhances cytokine secretion, but suppresses survival and degranulation, in human mast cell line. *PLoS One* 9:e86106. doi: 10.1371/journal.pone.0086106

Lahat, N., Rahat, M. A., Ballan, M., Weiss-Cerem, L., Engelmayer, M., and Bitterman, H. (2003). Hypoxia reduces CD80 expression on monocytes but enhances their LPS-stimulated TNF-alpha secretion. *J. Leukoc. Biol.* 74, 197–205. doi: 10.1189/jlb.0303105

Lee, J., Su, E. W., Zhu, C., Hainline, S., Phuah, J., Moroco, J. A., et al. (2011). Phosphotyrosine-dependent coupling of Tim-3 to T-cell receptor signaling pathways. *Mol. Cell Biol.* 31, 3963–3974. doi: 10.1128/MCB.05297-11

Li, N., Jilisihan, B., Wang, W., Tang, Y., and Keyoumu, S. (2018). Soluble LAG3 acts as a potential prognostic marker of gastric cancer and its positive correlation with CD8+T cell frequency and secretion of IL-12 and INF-γ in peripheral blood. *Cancer Biomark.* 23, 341–351. doi: 10.3233/cbm-181278

Li, N., Wang, Y., Forbes, K., Vignali, K. M., Heale, B. S., Saftig, P., et al. (2007). Metalloproteases regulate T-cell proliferation and effector function via LAG-3. *EMBO J.* 26, 494–504. doi: 10.1038/sj.emboj.7601520

Li, W., Xia, Y., Yang, J., Guo, H., Sun, G., Sanyal, A. J., et al. (2020). Immune checkpoint axes are dysregulated in patients with alcoholic hepatitis. *Hepatol. Commun.* 4, 588–605. doi: 10.1002/hep4.1475

Li, Y. M., Shi, Y. Y., Li, Y., Yan, L., Tang, J. T., Bai, Y. J., et al. (2018). Soluble Tim-3 and Gal-9 are associated with renal allograft dysfunction in kidney transplant recipients: a cross-sectional study. *Int. Immunopharmacol.* 55, 330–335. doi: 10.1016/j.intimp.2018.01.008

Lin, M., Huang, J., Huang, J., Liu S-l, and Chen, W.-C. (2018). Level of serum soluble Tim-3 expression in early-phase acute pancreatitis. *Turkish J. Gastroenterol.* 30, 188–191. doi: 10.5152/tjg.2018.18137

Louvet, A., Labreuche, J., Artru, F., Boursier, J., Kim, D. J., O'Grady, J., et al. (2015). Combining data from liver disease scoring systems better predicts outcomes of patients with alcoholic hepatitis. *Gastroenterology* 149, e16–e17. doi: 10.1053/j.gastro.2015.04.044

Louvet, A., and Mathurin, P. (2015). Alcoholic liver disease: mechanisms of injury and targeted treatment. *Nat. Rev. Gastroenterol. Hepatol.* 12, 231–242. doi: 10.1038/nrgastro.2015.35

Louvet, A., Wartel, F., Castel, H., Dharancy, S., Hollebecque, A., Canva-Delcambre, V., et al. (2009). Infection in patients with severe alcoholic hepatitis treated with steroids: early response to therapy is the key factor. *Gastroenterology* 137, 541–548. doi: 10.1053/j.gastro.2009.04.062

Maddrey, W. C., Boitnott, J. K., Bedine, M. S., Weber, F. L. Jr., Mezey, E., and White, R. I. Jr. (1978). Corticosteroid therapy of alcoholic hepatitis. *Gastroenterology* 75, 193–199. doi: 10.1016/0016-5085(78)90401-8

Markwick, L. J., Riva, A., Ryan, J. M., Cooksley, H., Palma, E., Tranah, T. H., et al. (2015). Blockade of PD1 and TIM3 restores innate and adaptive immunity in patients with acute alcoholic hepatitis. *Gastroenterology* 148, 590.e10–602.e10. doi: 10.1053/j.gastro.2014.11.041

Mathurin, P., and Lucey, M. R. (2012). Management of alcoholic hepatitis. *J. Hepatol.* 56(Suppl. 1), S39–S45. doi: 10.1016/S0168-8278(12)60005-1

Merli, M., Lucidi, C., Di Gregorio, V., Falcone, M., Giannelli, V., Lattanzi, B., et al. (2015). The spread of multi drug resistant infections is leading to an increase in the empirical antibiotic treatment failure in cirrhosis: a prospective survey. *PLoS One* 10:e0127448. doi: 10.1371/journal.pone.0127448

Moller-Hackbarth, K., Dewitz, C., Schweigert, O., Trad, A., Garbers, C., Rose-John, S., et al. (2013). A disintegrin and metalloprotease (ADAM) 10 and ADAM17 are major sheddases of T cell immunoglobulin and mucin domain 3 (Tim-3). *J. Biol. Chem.* 288, 34529–34544. doi: 10.1074/jbc.M113.488478

Muthukumarana, P. A. D. S., Zheng, X. X., Rosengard, B. R., Strom, T. B., and Metcalfe, S. M. (2008). In primed allo-tolerance, TIM-3-Ig rapidly suppresses TGFβ, but has no immediate effect on Foxp3. *Transplant. Int.* 21, 593–597. doi: 10.1111/j.1432-2277.2008.00654.x

Nagaishi, T., Chen, Z., Chen, L., Iijima, H., Nakajima, A., and Blumberg, R. S. (2008). CEACAM1 and the regulation of mucosal inflammation. *Mucosal Immunol.* 1(Suppl. 1), S39–S42. doi: 10.1038/mi.2008.50

Nebbia, G., Peppa, D., Schurich, A., Khanna, P., Singh, H. D., Cheng, Y., et al. (2012). Upregulation of the Tim-3/galectin-9 pathway of T cell exhaustion in chronic hepatitis B virus infection. *PLoS One* 7:e47648. doi: 10.1371/journal.pone.0047648

Nielsen, C., Ohm-Laursen, L., Barington, T., Husby, S., and Lillevang, S. T. (2005). Alternative splice variants of the human PD-1 gene. *Cell Immunol.* 235, 109–116. doi: 10.1016/j.cellimm.2005.07.007

Palma, E., Doornebal, E. J., and Chokshi, S. (2019). Precision-cut liver slices: a versatile tool to advance liver research. *Hepatol. Int.* 13, 51–57. doi: 10.1007/s12072-018-9913-7

Palma, E., Riva, A., Moreno, C., Odena, G., Mudan, S., Manyakin, N., et al. (2020). Perturbations in mitochondrial dynamics are closely involved in the progression of Alcoholic Liver Disease. *Alcohol Clin. Exp. Res.* 44, 856–865. doi: 10.1111/acer.14299

Patil, N. K., Guo, Y., Luan, L., and Sherwood, E. R. (2017). Targeting immune cell checkpoints during sepsis. *Int. J. Mol. Sci.* 18:2413. doi: 10.3390/ijms18112413

Prigent, P., Mir, S. E., Dréano, M., and Triebel, F. (1999). Lymphocyte activation gene-3 induces tumor regression and antitumor immune responses. *Eur. J. Immunol.* 29, 3867–3876. doi: 10.1002/(sici)1521-4141(199912)29:12<3867::aid-immu3867<3.0.co;2-e

Rangachari, M., Zhu, C., Sakuishi, K., Xiao, S., Karman, J., Chen, A., et al. (2012). Bat3 promotes T cell responses and autoimmunity by repressing Tim-3-mediated cell death and exhaustion. *Nat. Med.* 18, 1394–1400. doi: 10.1038/nm.2871

Ren, F., Li, J., Jiang, X., Xiao, K., Zhang, D., Zhao, Z., et al. (2015). Plasma soluble Tim-3 emerges as an inhibitor in sepsis: sepsis contrary to membrane Tim-3 on monocytes. *Tissue Anti.* 86, 325–332. doi: 10.1111/tan.12653

Riva, A., and Chokshi, S. (2018). Immune checkpoint receptors: homeostatic regulators of immunity. *Hepatol. Int.* 12, 223–236. doi: 10.1007/s12072-018-9867-9

Riva, A., Gray, E. H., Azarian, S., Zamalloa, A., McPhail, M. J., Vincent, R. P., et al. (2020). Faecal cytokine profiling as a marker of intestinal inflammation in acutely decompensated cirrhosis. *JHEP Rep.* 2:100151. doi: 10.1016/j.jhepr.2020.100151

Riva, A., Laird, M., Casrouge, A., Ambrozaitis, A., Williams, R., Naoumov, N. V., et al. (2014). Truncated CXCL10 is associated with failure to achieve spontaneous clearance of acute hepatitis C infection. *Hepatology* 60, 487–496. doi: 10.1002/hep.27139

Riva, A., Patel, V., Kurioka, A., Jeffery, H. C., Wright, G., Tarff, S., et al. (2018). Mucosa-associated invariant T cells link intestinal immunity with antibacterial immune defects in alcoholic liver disease. *Gut* 67, 918–930. doi: 10.1136/gutjnl-2017-314458

RStudio_Team (2020). *RStudio: Integrated Development Environment for R.* Boston, MA: RStudio_Team.

R_Core_Team (2020). *R: A Language and Environment for Statistical Computing.* Vienna: R Foundation for Statistical Computing.

Sabatos-Peyton, C. A., Nevin, J., Brock, A., Venable, J. D., Tan, D. J., Kassam, N., et al. (2018). Blockade of Tim-3 binding to phosphatidylserine and CEACAM1 is a shared feature of anti-Tim-3 antibodies that have functional efficacy. *Oncoimmunology* 7:e1385690. doi: 10.1080/2162402X.2017.1385690

Saha, N., Robev, D., Himanen, J. P., and Nikolov, D. B. (2019). ADAM proteases: emerging role and targeting of the non-catalytic domains. *Cancer Lett.* 467, 50–57. doi: 10.1016/j.canlet.2019.10.003

Silva, I. G., Yasinska, I. M., Sakhnevych, S. S., Fiedler, W., Wellbrock, J., Bardelli, M., et al. (2017). The Tim-3-galectin-9 secretory pathway is involved in the immune escape of human acute myeloid leukemia cells. *EBioMedicine* 22, 44–57. doi: 10.1016/j.ebiom.2017.07.018

Soria Saucedo, R. (2013). *Harmful Use of Alcohol, Alcohol Use Disorders and Alcoholic Liver Diseases.* Geneva: World Health Organization.

Thursz, M. R., Richardson, P., Allison, M., Austin, A., Bowers, M., Day, C. P., et al. (2015). Prednisolone or pentoxifylline for alcoholic hepatitis. *N. Engl. J. Med.* 372, 1619–1628. doi: 10.1056/NEJMoa1412278

Trebicka, J., Fernandez, J., Papp, M., Caraceni, P., Laleman, W., Gambino, C., et al. (2020). PREDICT identifies precipitating events associated with the clinical course of acutely decompensated cirrhosis. *J. Hepatol.* doi: 10.1016/j.jhep.2020.11.019 [Epub ahead of print].

Triebel, F., Hacene, K., and Pichon, M.-F. (2006). A soluble lymphocyte activation gene-3 (sLAG-3) protein as a prognostic factor in human breast cancer expressing estrogen or progesterone receptors. *Cancer Lett.* 235, 147–153. doi: 10.1016/j.canlet.2005.04.015

Vega-Carrascal, I., Reeves, E. P., Niki, T., Arikawa, T., McNally, P., O'Neill, S. J., et al. (2011). Dysregulation of TIM-3-galectin-9 pathway in the cystic fibrosis airways. *J. Immunol.* 186, 2897–2909. doi: 10.4049/jimmunol.1003187

Vergis, N., Atkinson, S. R., Knapp, S., Maurice, J., Allison, M., Austin, A., et al. (2017). In patients with severe alcoholic hepatitis, prednisolone increases susceptibility to infection and infection-related mortality, and is associated with high circulating levels of bacterial DNA. *Gastroenterology* 152, 1068–77e4. doi: 10.1053/j.gastro.2016.12.019

Wang, J., Lo, J. C., Foster, A., Yu, P., Chen, H. M., Wang, Y., et al. (2001). The regulation of T cell homeostasis and autoimmunity by T cell-derived LIGHT. *J. Clin. Invest.* 108, 1771–1780. doi: 10.1172/JCI13827

Wang, S., Cao, C., Piao, H., Li, Y., Tao, Y., Zhang, X., et al. (2015). Tim-3 protects decidual stromal cells from toll-like receptor-mediated apoptosis and inflammatory reactions and promotes Th2 bias at the maternal-fetal interface. *Sci. Rep.* 5:9013. doi: 10.1038/srep09013

Weber, S., and Saftig, P. (2012). Ectodomain shedding and ADAMs in development. *Development* 139, 3693–3709. doi: 10.1242/dev.076398

Wei, T., and Simko, V. (2017). *R Package "corrplot": Visualization of a Correlation Matrix, v0.84.*

Wetzel, S., Seipold, L., and Saftig, P. (2017). The metalloproteinase ADAM10: A useful therapeutic target? *Biochim. Biophys. Acta Mol. Cell Res.* 1864(11 Pt B)), 2071–2081. doi: 10.1016/j.bbamcr.2017.06.005

Wu, W., Shi, Y., Li, S., Zhang, Y., Liu, Y., Wu, Y., et al. (2012). Blockade of Tim-3 signaling restores the virus-specific CD8(+) T-cell response in patients with chronic hepatitis B. *Eur. J. Immunol.* 42, 1180–1191. doi: 10.1002/eji.201141852

Xiao, L., Wang, D., Sun, C., Li, P., Jin, Y., Feng, L., et al. (2013). Enhancement of SIV-specific cell mediated immune responses by co-administration of soluble PD-1 and Tim-3 as molecular adjuvants in mice. *Hum. Vac. Immunotherap.* 10, 724–733. doi: 10.4161/hv.27340

Zhao, D., Guo, M., Liu, B., Lin, Q., Xie, T., Zhang, Q., et al. (2017). Frontline Science: tim-3-mediated dysfunctional engulfment of apoptotic cells in SLE. *J. Leukocyte Biol.* 102, 1313–1322. doi: 10.1189/jlb.3hi0117-005rr

Zhao, Q., Zhang, G. L., Zhu, X., Su, D., Huang, Z. L., Hu, Z. X., et al. (2017). The paradoxical changes of membrane and soluble herpes virus entry mediator in hepatocellular carcinoma patients. *J. Gastroenterol. Hepatol.* 32, 1520–1524. doi: 10.1111/jgh.13678

Zhu, C., Anderson, A. C., Schubart, A., Xiong, H., Imitola, J., Khoury, S. J., et al. (2005). The Tim-3 ligand galectin-9 negatively regulates T helper type 1 immunity. *Nat. Immunol.* 6, 1245–1252. doi: 10.1038/ni1271

Zilber, E., Martin, G. E., Willberg, C. B., Fox, J., Nwokolo, N., Fidler, S., et al. (2019). Soluble plasma PD-1 and Tim-3 in primary HIV infection. *AIDS* 33, 1253–1256. doi: 10.1097/qad.0000000000002165

Zunke, F., and Rose-John, S. (2017). The shedding protease ADAM17: physiology and pathophysiology. *Biochim. Biophys. Acta Mol. Cell Res.* 1864(11 Pt B), 2059–2070. doi: 10.1016/j.bbamcr.2017.07.001

5

Functional Microbial Responses to Alcohol Abstinence in Patients with Alcohol use Disorder

Bei Gao[1], Atoosa Emami[1], Rongrong Zhou[1], Sonja Lang[1], Yi Duan[1,2], Yanhan Wang[1,2], Lu Jiang[1,2], Rohit Loomba[1], David A. Brenner[1], Peter Stärkel[3] and Bernd Schnabl[1,2]**

[1] Department of Medicine, University of California, San Diego, San Diego, CA, United States, [2] Department of Medicine, VA San Diego Healthcare System, San Diego, CA, United States, [3] St. Luc University Hospital, Université catholique de Louvain, Brussels, Belgium

***Correspondence:**
Bei Gao
begao@ucsd.edu
Bernd Schnabl
beschnabl@ucsd.edu

Excessive alcohol consumption is associated with hepatic steatosis and dysregulation of the gut microbiota in patients with alcohol use disorder (AUD). However, how gut microbiota responds when patients stop drinking has not been well studied. In this study, we use shotgun metagenomic sequencing to elucidate the alterations in the functional capacity of gut microbiota in patients with AUD when they stop drinking for 2-weeks. Sensitive microbial pathways to alcohol abstinence were identified in AUD patients. Further, we found the functional microbial responses to alcohol abstinence were different in AUD patients with different degree of hepatic steatosis. Our results provide insights into the link between functional alterations of the gut microbiota and steatosis associated with alcohol consumption.

Keywords: microbiome, metagenomics, steatosis, AUD, CAP

INTRODUCTION

Alcohol-related health problems are a major medical burden worldwide. In response to moderate to large amounts of alcohol consumption, steatosis develops in 90–95% of patients with alcohol-use disorder (EASL, 2012). Controlled attenuation parameter (CAP) is a non-invasive method to detect hepatic steatosis using transient elastography (Myers et al., 2012). CAP values range from 100 to 400 dB/m, where higher values indicate more severe steatosis (Mikolasevic et al., 2016). In addition to steatosis, chronic and excessive alcohol consumption contributes to gut barrier dysfunction, increased intestinal permeability, and dysregulation of the gut microbiota (Szabo, 2015). The gut metagenome, encoding 100-fold more unique genes than human genome, has a vast metabolic capacity. Metagenomic analysis of the gut microbiota reveals the functional capacity of the gut community and allows for further understanding of their potential metabolic functions (Qin et al., 2010).

The impact of alcohol on the composition of the gut microbiota has been reported previously (Qin et al., 2010; Mutlu et al., 2012; Bull-Otterson et al., 2013; Dubinkina et al., 2017; Wang et al., 2018). However, how the gut metagenome responds when alcohol use disorder (AUD) patients stop drinking has not been investigated. In this study, we use shotgun metagenomic sequencing to elucidate the alterations in the functional capacity of gut microbiota in AUD patients when they stop drinking for 2 weeks. Our aim is to identify sensitive microbial pathways to alcohol abstinence in AUD patients.

MATERIALS AND METHODS

Patients

Patient cohorts have been described (Brandl et al., 2018; Duan et al., 2019; Gao et al., 2019; Lang et al., 2019). Eight (8) non-alcoholic controls and 30 patients with AUD were included in this study. AUD patients were recruited from an alcohol withdrawal unit where they followed a highly standardized and controlled 3-weeks detoxification and rehabilitation program consisting of 1 week inpatient detoxification (day 1–7) followed by 1 week outpatient care (day 8–14) and 1 week hospital readmission for consolidation (day 15–21). The diagnosis of AUD was based on the DSM IV criteria (Ball et al., 1997). Patients reported long-term (>1 year) alcohol consumption >60 g/day and were actively drinking until the day of admission for elective alcohol withdrawal. Complete physical examination, medication and medical history are taken at admission. Serum samples were collected, and patients underwent FibroScan® (Echosens, Paris, France) with determination of liver stiffness and continued attenuation parameter (CAP) measurements on the day of admission. Stool samples were collected from the first bowel movement after each hospital admission. These samples and procedures were labeled "WEEK 1" for the initial hospitalization and "WEEK 3" after hospital readmission. We collected fecal samples from spontaneous bowel movements of patients, and timing of these evacuations varies depending on the patient. Because of this, the collection time was not precisely controlled, and diurnal variations in fecal microbiota may contribute to the variations in the metagenomics data, which was one limitation of this study. Non-alcoholic controls were social drinkers consuming less than 20 g of alcohol per day, which was one inclusion criteria. Non-alcoholic controls and AUD patients did not take antibiotics or immunosuppressive medication during the 2 months preceding enrollment. Other exclusion criteria were diabetes, inflammatory bowel disease, known liver disease of any other etiology, and clinically significant cardio-vascular, pulmonary or renal co-morbidities. Written informed consent was signed by each participant after the nature and possible consequences of the studies were explained. The study protocol was approved by the Institutional Review Board from each institution involved.

Continued Attenuation Parameter (CAP) Measurements

Liver steatosis was assessed non-invasively by CAP (Nguyen-Khac et al., 2018). The measurements were performed with the Fibroscan® device (Echosens, Paris, France) by an experienced examiner blinded to patient's data. CAP was deemed valid if at least ten validated measurements were obtained with an interquartile range ≤40 dB/m. Final results were the median of all obtained valid measurements. The patients were divided into CAP High group (≥300 dB/m, severe steatosis, n = 13) and CAP Low group (<300 dB/m, n = 17). This cutoff was derived from recent studies performed in NAFLD patients (Buzzetti et al., 2015; Karlas et al., 2017; Caussy et al., 2018; Eddowes et al., 2019).

Shotgun Metagenomic Analysis

DNA was extracted from fecal samples using FastDNA Spin Kit (MP-Biomedicals). Shotgun metagenomic sequencing was performed on Illumina HiSeq 4000 generating 150 bp paired-end reads. KneadData version 0.7.2 was used for the quality control of shotgun metagenomic raw sequencing reads. MetaPhlAn2 version 2.7.7 and HUMAnN2 version 0.11.1 was used for the profiling of composition of the microbial communities and microbial pathways, respectively (Truong et al., 2015; Franzosa et al., 2018). Each of the HUMAnN2 abundance output was normalized into relative abundance.

Short-Chain Fatty Acids Measurement

Short-chain fatty acids extraction and quantification was performed as described in our previous study (Nusbaum et al., 2018). Briefly, short-chain fatty acids were extracted from 10 mg feces with 700 µL of 5:1:1 water, hydrochloric acid and methyl tert-butyl ether. Samples were homogenized and centrifuged. Supernatant underwent dehydration and tert-butyldimethylsilylation with tert-Butyldimethylsilyl-N-methyltrifluoroacetamide (MTBSTFA, Sigma-Aldrich). Samples were shaken at 80°C for 30 min and injected into an Agilent 5977A GC-quadrupole mass spectrometer with selected ion monitoring mode. Agilent Mass Hunter Quantitative Analysis software (B.07.00) was used for data processing. Data were quantified against authentic standards.

Statistical Analysis

Linear discriminant analysis effect size (LEfSe) was used for the biomarker discovery (Segata et al., 2011). For LEfSe analysis, all-against-all strategy was used. Alpha value for the factorial Kruskal–Wallis test among classes was set to 0.05. Threshold on the logarithmic linear discriminant analysis (LDA) score for discriminative features was set to 2.0. For the statistical analysis of butyrate concentration, wilcoxon rank-sum test was used. Spearman correlation was used to test the correlation between two variables.

RESULTS

Patient Characteristics

Serum and fecal samples were collected from 8 non-alcoholic controls and 30 patients with AUD. The AUD patients were divided into CAP Low (n = 17) and CAP High (n = 13) groups as defined by a CAP cutoff of 300 dB/m (Buzzetti et al., 2015; Karlas et al., 2017; Caussy et al., 2018; Eddowes et al., 2019). The baseline characteristics of patients with AUD and control subjects are shown in **Supplementary Table S1**. Subjects were predominantly males, and there was no difference in gender and age when compared between controls and AUD patients. The BMI was not different between control and patients with AUD (CAP Low and High), but patients in CAP Low group had a higher BMI than CAP High group (p-value = 0.02). Even though, BMI is still within normal range. There was no difference between CAP Low and High groups for the comparison of laboratory parameters including albumin, aspartate aminotransferase (AST), alanine aminotransferase (ALT), gamma-glutamyl transferase (GGT), total bilirubin, platelet counts, creatinine, and international normalized ratio (INR).

Sensitive Microbial Pathways to Alcohol

To identify the sensitive microbial pathways, we compared the gut microbial pathway in AUD patients at WEEK 1 and WEEK 3. A total of seven microbial pathways were sensitive to alcohol abstinence with LDA score > 2.0, all of which were enriched at WEEK 3 (**Figure 1A**), including isoprene biosynthesis I, phytol degradation, L-isoleucine biosynthesis II, superpathway of geranylgeranyl diphosphate biosynthesis II (via MEP), NAD salvage pathway II, glutaryl-CoA degradation and superpathway of geranylgeranyldiphosphate biosynthesis I (via mevalonate).

Furthermore, to investigate whether these seven sensitive microbial pathways were also different between AUD patients and control subjects, we compared all detected microbial pathways between control subjects and AUD patients at WEEK 1 and WEEK 3, respectively. At WEEK 1, a total of 34 and 22 microbial pathways were enriched in AUD patients and control subjects, respectively (**Supplementary Figure S1**). Notably, glutaryl-CoA degradation was enriched in control subjects, which was one of the sensitive microbial pathways enriched in AUD patients at WEEK 3 (**Figure 1B**). Next, we compared microbial pathways between control subjects and AUD patients at WEEK 3 and found 46 and 17 microbial pathways were enriched in AUD patients and control subjects, respectively (**Supplementary Figure S2**). Four sensitive microbial pathways were found, among which three were enriched in AUD patients at WEEK 3, including isoprene biosynthesis I, phytol degradation, and superpathway of geranylgeranyldiphosphate biosynthesis I (via mevalonate). Meanwhile, glutaryl-CoA degradation was enriched in control subjects, which was also enriched in control subjects when comparing controls with AUD patients at WEEK 1 (**Figure 1B**). The remaining three microbial pathways were not significantly different between control subjects and AUD patients either at WEEK 1 or WEEK 3, including L-isoleucine biosynthesis II, superpathway of geranylgeranyl diphosphate biosynthesis II (via MEP) and NAD salvage pathway II (**Figure 1B**).

Different Microbial Functional Responses in CAP High and Low Patients

The functional microbial responses to alcohol abstinence were different in CAP High (≥300 dB/m) and CAP Low (<300 dB/m) patients. Five microbial pathways were significantly increased at WEEK 3 in CAP High patients with LDA score > 2.0, including L-isoleucine biosynthesis II, superpathway of β-D-glucuronosides degradation, superpathway of hexuronide and hexuronate degradation, superpathway of geranylgeranyl diphosphate biosynthesis II (via MEP), and glutaryl-CoA degradation (**Figure 2A**). In contrast, heterolactic fermentation was decreased at WEEK 3 in CAP High patients (LDA score > 2.0, **Figure 2A**). When comparing WEEK 1 and WEEK 3 microbial pathways in CAP Low patients, we found five microbial pathways were enriched at WEEK 1 (LDA score > 2.0, **Figure 2B**), including adenosine nucleotides degradation II, guanosine nucleotides degradation III, superpathway of pyrimidine ribonucleosides degradation, purine nucleotides degradation II aerobic, and ppGpp biosynthesis.

DISCUSSION

By comparing the WEEK 3 metagenomic sequencing data with WEEK 1 in AUD patients, we found seven sensitive pathways, among which four pathways were different when comparing control subjects with AUD patients at WEEK 1 or WEEK 3. Especially, the relative abundance of glutaryl-CoA degradation was lower in AUD patients at WEEK 1 when compared with controls and it was increased in AUD patients at WEEK 3 compared with AUD patients at WEEK 1. However, its relative abundance was still lower at WEEK 3 when comparing with controls (**Figure 1B**). During glutaryl-CoA degradation process, glutaryl-CoA is turned into acetyl-CoA through β-oxidation, which functions as an intermediate in many metabolic pathways. *F. prausnitzii* is a major contributor to glutaryl-CoA degradation (**Supplementary Figure S3A**). *F. prausnitzii* is one of the most abundant species in the human microbiome (Martín et al., 2017). In the present study, AUD patients showed a lower relative abundance of *F. prausnitzii* compared with control group (**Supplementary Figure S3B**), which is consistent with previous findings in alcohol-dependent subjects (Leclercq et al., 2014). A high-fat diet feeding mouse model shows that *F. prausnitzii* supplementation improves hepatic health and reduces adipose tissue inflammation (Munukka et al., 2017). *F. prausnitzii* is known as a butyrate producer. Therefore, we measured the level of short-chain fatty acids in patients with AUD and then performed spearman correlation between short-chain fatty acids and *F. prausnitzii*. We found increased *F. prausnitzii* was associated with elevated butyrate level in fecal samples (**Supplementary Figure S3C**). We further checked the fecal level of butyrate in non-alcoholic controls and AUD patients, however, no significant difference was found (**Supplementary Figure S3D**).

The microbial functional responses to alcohol abstinence were different in CAP High (≥300 dB/m) and CAP Low (<300 dB/m) patients. Among the six significantly different microbial pathways in CAP High patients, β-glucuronidase was involved in two processes, including superpathway of β-D-glucuronosides degradation and superpathway of hexuronide and hexuronate degradation. During the superpathway of β-D-glucuronosides degradation process, β-glucuronosides undergo hydrolysis by β-glucuronidase to yield D-glucuronate. Similarly to the superpathway of β-D-glucuronosides degradation, β-glucuronidase is also the first enzyme utilized in the degradation of hexuronide and hexuronate (Mandrand-Berthelot et al., 2004). Besides,

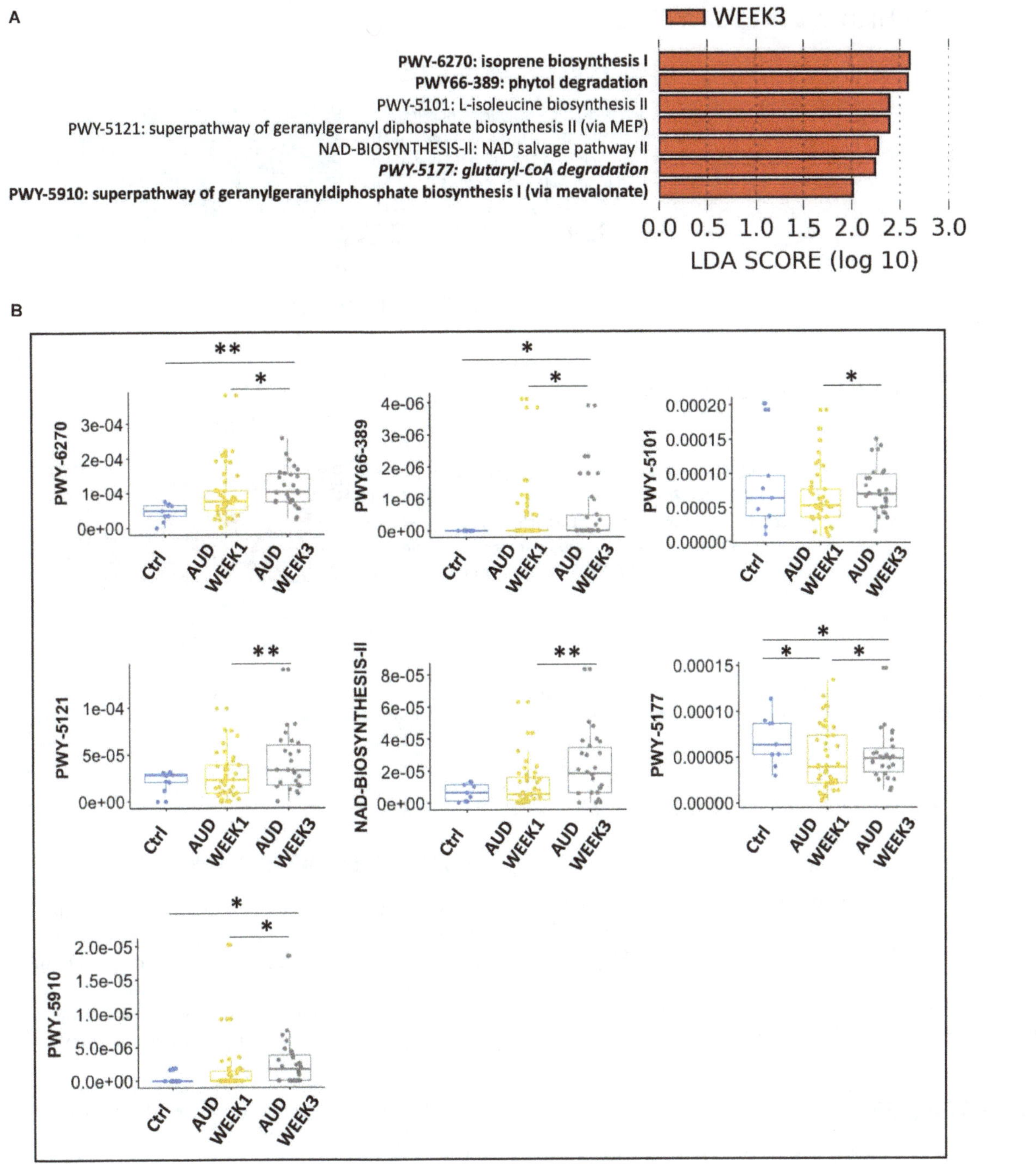

FIGURE 1 | Seven sensitive microbial pathways to alcohol abstinence in alcohol use disorder patients. **(A)** Seven microbial pathways were enriched at WEEK 3 compared with WEEK 1. Italic: significantly altered pathway comparing control subjects and alcohol use disorder patients at WEEK 1. Bold: significantly altered pathways comparing control subjects and alcohol use disorder patients at WEEK 3. **(B)** Pairwise comparison of control subjects, alcohol use disorder patients at WEEK 1 and alcohol use disorder patients at WEEK 3. *: *p*-value < 0.05; **: *p*-value < 0.01.

L- isoleucine biosynthesis II was increased in the CAP High patients at WEEK 3 compared with WEEK 1. Branched chain amino acids including isoleucine have been found to alleviate steatosis by suppressing gene and protein expression level of fatty acid synthase (Honda et al., 2017). Rats deficient in isoleucine had higher levels of triglyceride in the liver compared with rats with normal levels (Lyman et al., 1964). While in CAP Low patients, the microbial processes involved in nucleotides and nucleosides degradation was lower at WEEK 3. Different microbial functional responses to alcohol abstinence in CAP

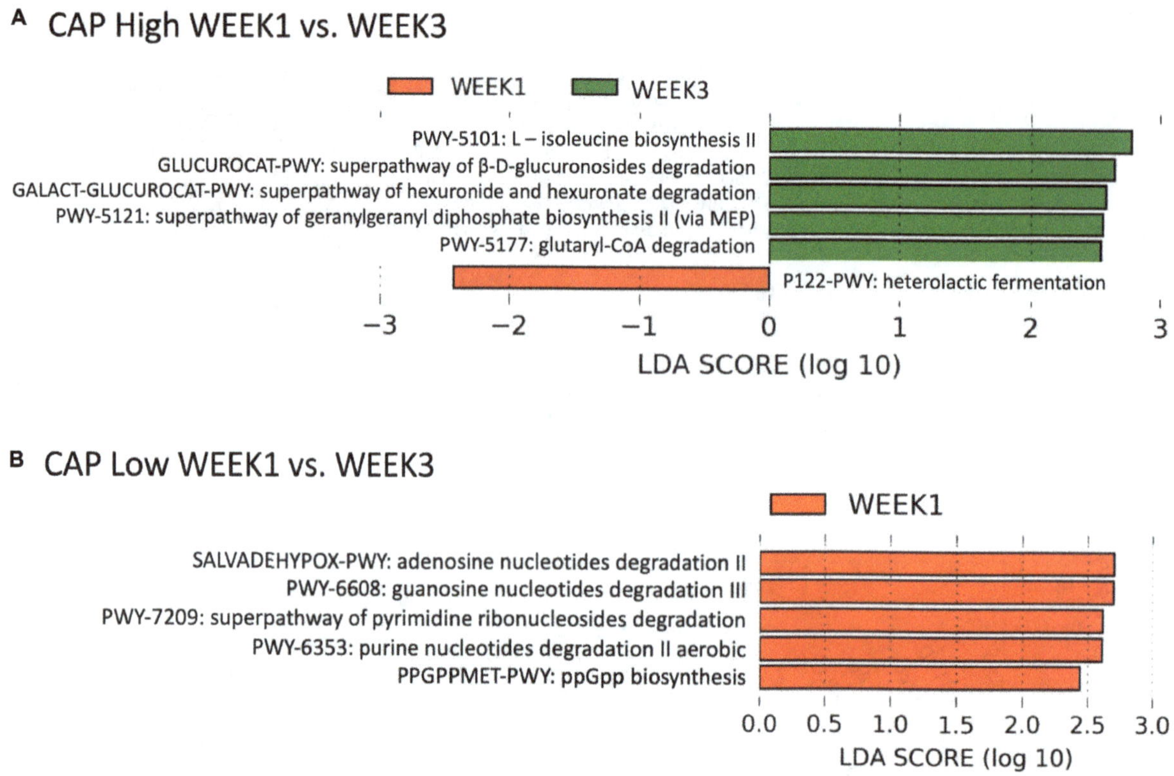

FIGURE 2 | Functional microbial response to alcohol abstinence were different in CAP High and CAP Low patients. **(A)** In CAP High patients, five microbial pathways were enriched at WEEK 3 (Green) and one microbial pathways were enriched at WEEK 1 (Red). **(B)** In CAP Low patients, five microbial pathways were enriched at WEEK 1 (Red).

High and Low patients suggested the complex interplay between alcohol, microbiota and the hepatic steatosis.

In summary, we identified sensitive microbial pathways to alcohol abstinence and found different microbial functional responses to alcohol abstinence in CAP High and Low patients. Our study provides insights into the link between functional alterations of the gut microbiota and steatosis induced by alcohol consumption. One limitation of our study is that the sample size is small and these findings need to be validated in a larger patient cohort.

AUTHOR CONTRIBUTIONS

BG was responsible for data analysis and manuscript editing. AE was responsible for manuscript writing. RZ, SL, and LJ were responsible for the analysis of clinical data. YD and YW were responsible for sample preparation. RL and DB were responsible for manuscript editing. PS and BS were responsible for the study concept and design, manuscript editing, and study supervision.

REFERENCES

Ball, S. A., Tennen, H., Poling, J. C., Kranzler, H. R., and Rounsaville, B. J. (1997). Personality, temperament, and character dimensions and the DSM-IV personality disorders in substance abusers. *J. Abnorm. Psychol.* 106, 545–553. doi: 10.1037/0021-843x.106.4.545

Brandl, K., Hartmann, P., Jih, L. J., Pizzo, D. P., Argemi, J., Ventura-Cots, M., et al. (2018). Dysregulation of serum bile acids and FGF19 in alcoholic hepatitis. *J. Hepatol.* 69, 396–405. doi: 10.1016/j.jhep.2018.03.031

Bull-Otterson, L., Feng, W., Kirpich, I., Wang, Y., Qin, X., Liu, Y., et al. (2013). Metagenomic analyses of alcohol induced pathogenic alterations in the intestinal microbiome and the effect of *Lactobacillus rhamnosus* GG treatment. *PLoS One* 8:e53028. doi: 10.1371/journal.pone.0053028

Buzzetti, E., Lombardi, R., De Luca, L., and Tsochatzis, E. A. (2015). Noninvasive assessment of fibrosis in patients with nonalcoholic fatty liver disease. *Int. J. Endocrinol.* 2015:343828.

Caussy, C., Alquiraish, M. H., Nguyen, P., Hernandez, C., Cepin, S., Fortney, L. E., et al. (2018). Optimal threshold of controlled attenuation parameter with MRI-PDFF as the gold standard for the detection of hepatic steatosis. *Hepatology* 67, 1348–1359. doi: 10.1002/hep.29639

Duan, Y., Llorente, C., Lang, S., Brandl, K., Chu, H., Jiang, L., et al. (2019). Bacteriophage targeting of gut bacterium attenuates alcoholic liver disease. *Nature* 575, 505–511. doi: 10.1038/s41586-019-1742-x

Dubinkina, V. B., Tyakht, A. V., Odintsova, V. Y., Yarygin, K. S., Kovarsky, B. A., Pavlenko, A. V., et al. (2017). Links of gut microbiota composition with alcohol dependence syndrome and alcoholic liver disease. *Microbiome* 5, 141–141. doi: 10.1186/s40168-017-0359-2

EASL, (2012). EASL clinical practical guidelines: management of alcoholic liver disease. *J. Hepatol.* 57, 399–420. doi: 10.1016/j.jhep.2012.04.004

Eddowes, P. J., Sasso, M., Allison, M., Tsochatzis, E., Anstee, Q. M., Sheridan, D., et al. (2019). Accuracy of fibroscan controlled attenuation parameter and liver stiffness measurement in assessing steatosis and fibrosis in patients with nonalcoholic fatty liver disease. *Gastroenterology* 156, 1717–1730. doi: 10.1053/j.gastro.2019.01.042

Franzosa, E. A., Mciver, L. J., Rahnavard, G., Thompson, L. R., Schirmer, M., Weingart, G., et al. (2018). Species-level functional profiling of metagenomes and metatranscriptomes. *Nat. Methods* 15, 962–968. doi: 10.1038/s41592-018-0176-y

Gao, B., Lang, S., Duan, Y., Wang, Y., Shawcross, D. L., Louvet, A., et al. (2019). Serum and fecal oxylipins in patients with alcohol-related liver disease. *Dig. Dis. Sci.* 64, 1878–1892. doi: 10.1007/s10620-019-05638-y

Honda, T., Ishigami, M., Luo, F., Lingyun, M., Ishizu, Y., Kuzuya, T., et al. (2017). Branched-chain amino acids alleviate hepatic steatosis and liver injury in choline-deficient high-fat diet induced NASH mice. *Metab. Clin. Exp.* 69, 177–187. doi: 10.1016/j.metabol.2016.12.013

Karlas, T., Petroff, D., Sasso, M., Fan, J.-G., Mi, Y.-Q., De Lédinghen, V., et al. (2017). Individual patient data meta-analysis of controlled attenuation parameter (CAP) technology for assessing steatosis. *J. Hepatol.* 66, 1022–1030. doi: 10.1016/j.jhep.2016.12.022

Lang, S., Duan, Y., Liu, J., Torralba, M. G., Kuelbs, C., Ventura-Cots, M., et al. (2019). Intestinal fungal dysbiosis and systemic immune response to fungi in patients with alcoholic hepatitis. *Hepatology* 71, 522–538. doi: 10.1002/hep.30832

Leclercq, S., Matamoros, S., Cani, P. D., Neyrinck, A. M., Jamar, F., Stärkel, P., et al. (2014). Intestinal permeability, gut-bacterial dysbiosis, and behavioral markers of alcohol-dependence severity. *Proc. Natl. Acad. Sci. U.S.A.* 111, E4485–E4493. doi: 10.1073/pnas.1415174111

Lyman, R. L., Cook, C. R., and Williams, M. A. (1964). Liver lipid accumulation in isoleucine-deficient rats. *J. Nutr.* 82, 432–438. doi: 10.1093/jn/82.4.432

Mandrand-Berthelot, M., Condemine, G., and Hugouvieux-Cotte-Pattat, N. (2004). Catabolism of hexuronides, hexuronates, aldonates, and aldarates. *EcoSal Plus* 1. doi: 10.1128/ecosalplus.3.4.2

Martín, R., Miquel, S., Benevides, L., Bridonneau, C., Robert, V., Hudault, S., et al. (2017). Functional characterization of novel *Faecalibacterium prausnitzii* strains isolated from healthy volunteers: a step forward in the use of *F. prausnitzii* as a next-generation probiotic. *Front. Microbiol.* 8:1226. doi: 10.3389/fmicb.2017.01226

Mikolasevic, I., Orlic, L., Franjic, N., Hauser, G., Stimac, D., and Milic, S. (2016). Transient elastography (FibroScan(®)) with controlled attenuation parameter in the assessment of liver steatosis and fibrosis in patients with nonalcoholic fatty liver disease - Where do we stand? *World J. Gastroenterol.* 22, 7236–7251. doi: 10.3748/wjg.v22.i32.7236

Munukka, E., Rintala, A., Toivonen, R., Nylund, M., Yang, B., Takanen, A., et al. (2017). Faecalibacterium prausnitzii treatment improves hepatic health and reduces adipose tissue inflammation in high-fat fed mice. *ISME J.* 11, 1667–1679. doi: 10.1038/ismej.2017.24

Mutlu, E. A., Gillevet, P. M., Rangwala, H., Sikaroodi, M., Naqvi, A., Engen, P. A., et al. (2012). Colonic microbiome is altered in alcoholism. *Am. J. Physiol. Gastrointest. Liver Physiol.* 302, G966–G978. doi: 10.1152/ajpgi.00380.2011

Myers, R. P., Pollett, A., Kirsch, R., Pomier-Layrargues, G., Beaton, M., Levstik, M., et al. (2012). Controlled attenuation parameter (CAP): a noninvasive method for the detection of hepatic steatosis based on transient elastography. *Liver Int.* 32, 902–910. doi: 10.1111/j.1478-3231.2012.02781.x

Nguyen-Khac, E., Thiele, M., Voican, C., Nahon, P., Moreno, C., Boursier, J., et al. (2018). Non-invasive diagnosis of liver fibrosis in patients with alcohol-related liver disease by transient elastography: an individual patient data meta-analysis. *Lancet Gastroenterol. Hepatol.* 3, 614–625. doi: 10.1016/S2468-1253(18)30124-9

Nusbaum, D. J., Sun, F., Ren, J., Zhu, Z., Ramsy, N., Pervolarakis, N., et al. (2018). Gut microbial and metabolomic profiles after fecal microbiota transplantation in pediatric ulcerative colitis patients. *FEMS Microbiol. Ecol.* 94:fiy133. doi: 10.1093/femsec/fiy133

Qin, J., Li, R., Raes, J., Arumugam, M., Burgdorf, K. S., Manichanh, C., et al. (2010). A human gut microbial gene catalogue established by metagenomic sequencing. *Nature* 464, 59–65. doi: 10.1038/nature08821

Segata, N., Izard, J., Waldron, L., Gevers, D., Miropolsky, L., Garrett, W. S., et al. (2011). Metagenomic biomarker discovery and explanation. *Genome Biol.* 12:R60.

Szabo, G. (2015). Gut-liver axis in alcoholic liver disease. *Gastroenterology* 148, 30–36. doi: 10.1053/j.gastro.2014.10.042

Truong, D. T., Franzosa, E. A., Tickle, T. L., Scholz, M., Weingart, G., Pasolli, E., et al. (2015). MetaPhlAn2 for enhanced metagenomic taxonomic profiling. *Nat. Methods* 12:902. doi: 10.1038/nmeth.3589

Wang, G., Liu, Q., Guo, L., Zeng, H., Ding, C., Zhang, W., et al. (2018). Gut Microbiota and Relevant Metabolites Analysis in Alcohol Dependent Mice. *Front. Microbiol.* 9:1874. doi: 10.3389/fmicb.2018.01874

6

Contrasting Effects of Fasting on Liver-Adipose Axis in Alcohol-Associated and Non-Alcoholic Fatty Liver

Karuna Rasineni[1,2†], Clayton W. Jordan[1†], Paul G. Thomes[1,2], Jacy L. Kubik[1,2], Elizabeth M. Staab[1], Sarah A. Sweeney[1], Geoffrey A. Talmon[3], Terrence M. Donohue[1,2,4], Mark A. McNiven[5], Kusum K. Kharbanda[1,2,4‡] and Carol A. Casey[1,2,4‡]*

[1] Department of Internal Medicine, University of Nebraska Medical Center, Omaha, NE, United States, [2] Research Service, Veterans Affairs Nebraska-Western Iowa Health Care System, Omaha, NE, United States, [3] Department of Pathology and Microbiology, University of Nebraska Medical Center, Omaha, NE, United States, [4] Department of Biochemistry and Molecular Biology, University of Nebraska Medical Center, Omaha, NE, United States, [5] Department of Biochemistry and Molecular Biology and the Center for Digestive Diseases, Mayo Clinic, Rochester, MN, United States

***Correspondence:**
Carol A. Casey
ccasey@unmc.edu

† These authors have contributed equally to this work and share first authorship

‡ These authors have contributed equally to this work and share last authorship

Background: Fatty liver, a major health problem worldwide, is the earliest pathological change in the progression of alcohol-associated (AFL) and non-alcoholic fatty liver disease (NAFL). Though the causes of AFL and NAFL differ, both share similar histological and some common pathophysiological characteristics. In this study, we sought to examine mechanisms responsible for lipid dynamics in liver and adipose tissue in the setting of AFL and NAFL in response to 48 h of fasting.

Methods: Male rats were fed Lieber-DeCarli liquid control or alcohol-containing diet (AFL model), chow or high-fat pellet diet (NAFL model). After 6–8 weeks of feeding, half of the rats from each group were fasted for 48 h while the other half remained on their respective diets. Following sacrifice, blood, adipose, and the liver were collected for analysis.

Results: Though rats fed AFL and NAFL diets both showed fatty liver, the physiological mechanisms involved in the development of each was different. Here, we show that increased hepatic *de novo* fatty acid synthesis, increased uptake of adipose-derived free fatty acids, and impaired triglyceride breakdown contribute to the development of AFL. In the case of NAFL, however, increased dietary fatty acid uptake is the major contributor to hepatic steatosis. Likewise, the response to starvation in the two fatty liver disease models also varied. While there was a decrease in hepatic steatosis after fasting in ethanol-fed rats, the control, chow and high-fat diet-fed rats showed higher levels of hepatic steatosis than pair-fed counterparts. This diverse response was a result of increased adipose lipolysis in all experimental groups except fasted ethanol-fed rats.

Conclusion: Even though AFL and NAFL are nearly histologically indistinguishable, the physiological mechanisms that cause hepatic fat accumulation are different as are their responses to starvation.

Keywords: alcohol-associated fatty liver disease, non-alcoholic fatty liver disease, starvation, hepatic lipid metabolism, adipose lipolysis, liver-adipose crosstalk

INTRODUCTION

Fatty liver is a major health problem both in the United States and around the globe. It is the earliest and most common response to excessive ethanol consumption or over-consumption of a high-fat/high-sugar diet (Singal and Anand, 2013; Li et al., 2019; Wong et al., 2019; Mitra et al., 2020). It is characterized by the accumulation of fats, chiefly as triglycerides (TG), in the liver (Kharbanda et al., 2007a, 2012; Rasineni et al., 2016). Upon excessive lipid accumulation, the liver is susceptible to inflammatory mediators and toxic agents which cause progressive liver injury (Lieber, 2004; Gao et al., 2019). About 100 million individuals in the United States are estimated to have non-alcoholic fatty liver disease as a result of consumption of a high-fat/high-sugar diet, known as a Western diet (Cotter and Rinella, 2020; Cotter et al., 2020). It is estimated that 90–100% of alcohol consumers develop fatty liver (Singal et al., 2013; Tapper and Parikh, 2018). Fatty liver development after heavy alcohol consumption (AFL, alcohol-associated fatty liver) or that after high caloric-intake (NAFL, non-alcoholic fatty liver) have similar phenotypes, showing excessive hepatocellular lipid accumulation in the form of larger lipid droplets (Rasineni et al., 2016).

In the body, liver and adipose tissue play prominent roles in maintaining energy homeostasis in both fed and fasting states. Specifically, hepatocytes play an important role in glucose homeostasis by storing or producing glucose in response to a fed or fasted state (Klover and Mooney, 2004). Adipose tissue serves as a storage site for fat derived from excess food consumption. Fat is utilized to fulfill subsequent metabolic requirements to other tissues, including the liver. During times of little or no food consumption, adipose tissue releases non-esterified fatty acids (NEFA) into circulation (Tang et al., 2017). In the liver, NEFA can be oxidized by mitochondria or re-esterified to form TG within the endoplasmic reticulum to be stored in lipid droplets or secreted/exported into the blood as a component of very-low-density lipoprotein (VLDL) (Kawano and Cohen, 2013). Unlike adipose tissue, the liver is not intended as a storage site for excess lipids. However, ethanol misuse or the over-consumption of a high-fat/high-sugar diet increases hepatocyte TG accumulation, which leads to the development of fatty liver disease. Many mechanisms have been reported to play a role in the development of AFL, including increased flow of fatty acids to the liver from enhanced adipose tissue lipolysis (Wei et al., 2013), impaired fat transport out of the liver via reduced VLDL secretion (Kharbanda et al., 2009), increased lipogenesis and decreased fatty acid oxidation (Rasineni and Casey, 2012; Osna et al., 2017; You and Arteel, 2019). Similarly, several mechanisms have been proposed to contribute to the development of high-fat/high-sugar diet induced non-alcoholic hepatic steatosis, including carbohydrate and fatty acid substrate overload and/or impairment of fatty acid disposal pathways (Chao et al., 2019). Although the causes of AFL and NAFL are different, both share some common pathophysiological mechanism(s) for fat accumulation and are histologically similar (Rasineni et al., 2016).

Extensive studies conducted in our laboratory as well as others have shown that multiple pathways in adipose-liver crosstalk contribute to the development and progression of liver disease in both AFL and NAFL (Lomonaco et al., 2012; Rasineni et al., 2019b). It is also known that nutrient deprivation or fasting activates many tissue-specific metabolic pathways to provide energy to the body by coordination of organ-organ interactions. It is mainly liver and adipose tissue that act as a metabolic buffering system for adipose-released NEFA and its utilization by the liver to produce glucose for survival (Klover and Mooney, 2004; Tang et al., 2017). But how this liver-adipose axis is affected by fasting against a backdrop of hepatic fat accumulation remains unknown. Here, we sought to examine mechanisms involved in both AFL and NAFL to reveal similarities and differences between shared physiological pathways. Specifically, our study was aimed at deciphering the mechanism(s) responsible for lipid dynamics in liver and adipose tissue in the settings of AFL and NAFL and the response of each to a 48 h fast.

MATERIALS AND METHODS

Reagents

Antibodies and reagents were purchased from the following companies: Ethanol was purchased from Pharmaco-AAPER (Brookfield, CT, United States). IRDye infrared secondary antibodies (Abs) and blocking buffer were from LI-COR Biosciences (Lincoln, NE, United States). Antibodies for adipose triacylglycerol lipase (ATGL), hormone sensitive lipase (HSL), and phosphorylated HSL (pHSL) were purchased from Cell Signaling (Danvers, MA, United States), phosphorylated pATGL was obtained from Abcam (Cambridge, MA, United States), and perilipin 2 (PLIN2) antibody was from Fitzgerald (Acton, MA, United States). All other chemicals were obtained from Sigma Chemical Co. (St. Louis, MO, United States) unless stated otherwise.

Animal Maintenance and Tissue Collection

Male Wistar rats (175–200 g) were purchased from Charles River Laboratories (Portage, MI, United States). For the AFL model, rats were weight-matched and pair-fed Lieber-DeCarli ethanol liquid diet (Dyets Inc., Bethlehem, PA, United States; Cat# 710260; 18% of total energy as protein, 35% as fat, 11% as carbohydrates, and 36% as ethanol) or control diet (Cat# 710027; ethanol replaced isocalorically with maltodextrin) for 6–8 weeks as described previously (Rasineni et al., 2016). Rats were housed singly for the ethanol feeding experiments, as it is necessary to pair their feeding with control rats for proper experimental protocol. In addition, the rats in the AFL group were housed in wire-bottom cages so that the rats don't eat their feces, a necessary component to control nutritional equivalence. This type of single caging has been utilized at the Omaha VAMC for alcohol feeding protocols and does not appear to add significant stress to the animals. For the NAFL model, rats were fed *ad libitum* either high-fat pellet diet (Research Diets #D08060104; 60% of calories derived from fat, 20% from carbohydrates, and 20% from protein) or maintained on standard chow pellet diet (Research Diets #D12450K; 10% of total calories from fat, 20% from protein, and 70% from carbohydrates as mainly corn starch, maltodextrin). NAFL and chow groups were allowed *ad libitum* access to their pellet diets and water (Rasineni et al., 2016). Rats in the NAFL model groups were housed in standard cages with bedding and a PVC pipe for enrichment. Forty-eight hours prior to termination of feeding, half of the rats in each of the four groups had their liquid or pellet diets removed. These rats were considered to be in fasting condition at the end of the 48 h time period (Cuervo et al., 1995; Schneider et al., 2014; Kaushik and Cuervo, 2015). These rats had *ad libitum* access to water during the fasting period. Note that chronic ethanol-fed rats did not exhibit any sudden alcohol withdrawal effects such as delirium tremens, hyperreactivity, psychological discomfort or death following the removal of alcohol diet during fasting. At the termination of the experimental period, all rats were anesthetized with isoflurane and blood was collected from the vena cava. Livers and epididymal adipose tissue were collected, rinsed in TE buffer (10 mM Tris–HCL, 1 mM EDTA) and weighed. Tissue sections were placed in 10% formalin for sectioning and remaining tissue was frozen in liquid nitrogen and stored at −80°C until further use. All animals received humane care in accordance with the guidelines established by the American Association for the Accreditation of Laboratory Animal Care. All protocols were approved by the Institutional Animal Care and Use Committee at the VA NWIHCS Research Service.

Histology by H&E Staining

Paraffin-embedded liver and epididymal white adipose tissue was deparaffinized and stained with hematoxylin followed by counter-staining with eosin.

Serum Analysis

Serum levels of alanine aminotransferase (ALT), alkaline phosphatase (ALP), and cholesterol were measured by a Vetscan chemistry analyzer (Abaxis, Union City, CA, United States) using a Mammalian Liver Profile reagent rotor (#89126-004). Serum non-esterified fatty acids (NEFA) were measured in an enzymatic colorimetric assay using a HR Series NEFA-HR2 kit (Wako Chemicals, Richmond, VA, United States). Serum triglycerides (TG) were quantified using a colorimetric diagnostic kit (#TR22421) from Thermo Fisher Scientific (Middletown, VA, United States).

Hepatic TG

Measurement of liver TG were performed by lipid extraction of frozen liver pieces by the Folch procedure (Folch et al., 1957). Aliquots of the lipid extract were saponified to quantify the triglyceride mass using the triglyceride diagnostics kit (#TR22421) from Thermo Fisher Scientific (Middletown, VA, United States). Triglyceride levels were normalized to grams of liver tissue.

Immunohistochemistry

Immunohistochemical staining for PLIN2, a lipid droplet protein, was conducted as described previously (Rasineni et al., 2014). Paraffin-embedded liver sections were deparaffinized, rehydrated and treated with 10 mM sodium citrate buffer (pH 6) for 20 min for antigen retrieval. Liver sections were incubated with a PLIN2 antibody (Fitzgerald#10R-A117ax) overnight followed by the appropriate Alexa Fluor secondary antibody for 1 h. Vectashield mounting medium with DAPI was used for mounting sections. Images were visualized and captured using a Keyence BZ-X series fluorescence microscope.

Western Blot Analysis

Liver homogenates were prepared in TE buffer containing protease inhibitor cocktail (#P2714, Sigma, St. Louis, MO, United States). Liver samples were subjected to SDS-PAGE, followed by blotting of proteins to nitrocellulose membranes. The proteins were detected with specific primary antibodies and fluorescently labeled secondary antibodies. The proteins were visualized and quantified using the Odyssey Infrared Imager and associated software (LI-COR Biosciences, Lincoln, NE, United States).

Messenger RNA Quantification

RNA was isolated from liver and epididymal adipose tissue using the PureLink RNA Mini Kit (Invitrogen, Carlsbad, CA, United States) and reverse-transcribed using the High Capacity cDNA Transcription Kit (Applied Biosystems, Carlsbad, CA, United States). Messenger RNAs were measured using iTaq Universal SYBR Green Supermix (Bio-Rad, Hercules, CA, United States) and primers from Integrated DNA Technologies (Coralville, IA, United States). PPARγ: Sense 5′- GAGATCCTCCTGTTGACCCAG-3′; Antisense 5′-CC ACAGAGCTGATTCCGAAGT-3′, PPARα: Sense 5′-GTCCT CTGGTTGTCCCCTTG-3′; Antisense 5′- GTCAGTTCACAGG GAAGGCA-3′, FAS: Sense 5′- TCCCAGGTCTTGCCGTGC-3′; Antisense 5′-GCGGATGCCTAGGATGTGTGC-3′, FATP2: Sense 5′- AGTACATCG GTGAACTGCTTCGGT-3′; Antisense 5′-TGCCTTCAGTGGAAGCGTAGAACT-3′, CD36: Sense 5′-AACCCAGAGGAAGTGGCAAAG-3′; Antisense 5′-GACAG TGAAGGCTCAAAGATGG-3′. Samples were analyzed using the 7500 Real Time PCR System (Applied Biosystems, Carlsbad, CA, United States). We used rat-specific primers from Applied Biosystems for mRNA analysis of monocyte chemoattractant protein-1 (MCP-1/CCL2; catalog #Rn00580555) and interleukin 1 beta (IL-1β; catalog #Rn00580432). The $\Delta\Delta$Ct method was used to determine the fold change of each transcript using β-actin or 36B4 mRNA for normalization.

Statistical Analysis

Results are expressed as mean values ± SEM. Comparison between fed and fasted animals in AFL and NAFL groups were analyzed using the Student's *t*-test. *p*-values of <0.05 were considered significant. For statistical analyses, data from ethanol-fed rats and their fasted cohorts were compared with pair-fed control rats. In the NAFL group, HFD-fed rats and their fasted cohorts were compared with chow-fed rats.

RESULTS

Liver and Adipose Weight in Fed and Fasted Rats

As shown in **Figure 1A**, with pair-feeding, we observed similar body weights in the ethanol-fed and pair-fed control rats. While we did not observe any difference in the average caloric intake per day in the NAFL model groups (chow-fed rats:100.6 ± 6.93 Kcal/day; HFD-fed rats:114.1 ± 10.94 Kcal/day; n = 8; data expressed as mean ± SEM), we did see significantly higher body weights in HFD-fed rats compared to chow-fed rats (**Figure 1B**). Forty-eight hours of fasting significantly reduced the body weights of rats in all experimental groups compared with their respective fed-counterparts, except for the HFD group. Furthermore, consistent with our previous study (Rasineni et al., 2019b), liver weights were significantly higher and adipose weights lower in ethanol-fed rats, resulting in an increased liver/body weight ratio (**Figure 1C**) and decreased adipose/body weight ratio (**Figure 1E**) as compared to their respective controls. Interestingly, in HFD-fed rats, both liver and body weights were increased, resulting in no change in the liver/body weight ratio when compared to the chow-fed rats (**Figure 1D**). However, we did observe significantly higher epididymal adipose weight and consequently higher epididymal/body weight ratios in HFD-fed rats compared with chow-fed rats (**Figure 1F**). As shown in **Figures 1C,D**, 48 h fasting decreased liver weight, resulting in a decline in liver/body weight ratio in all experimental groups. In addition, we observed a significant decrease in adipose weight with 48 h fasting in all experimental groups except ethanol-fed rats (**Figures 1E,F**).

Activity of Hepatic Injury Marker Enzymes and Lipid Concentrations in Serum

Since studies from our group and others have reported that the activity of serum hepatic injury markers increases during the development of both AFL and NAFL, we measured serum alanine aminotransferase (ALT) and alkaline phosphatase (ALP) to investigate the effect of 48 h fasting on hepatic injury. As expected, activity of serum ALT and ALP increased in

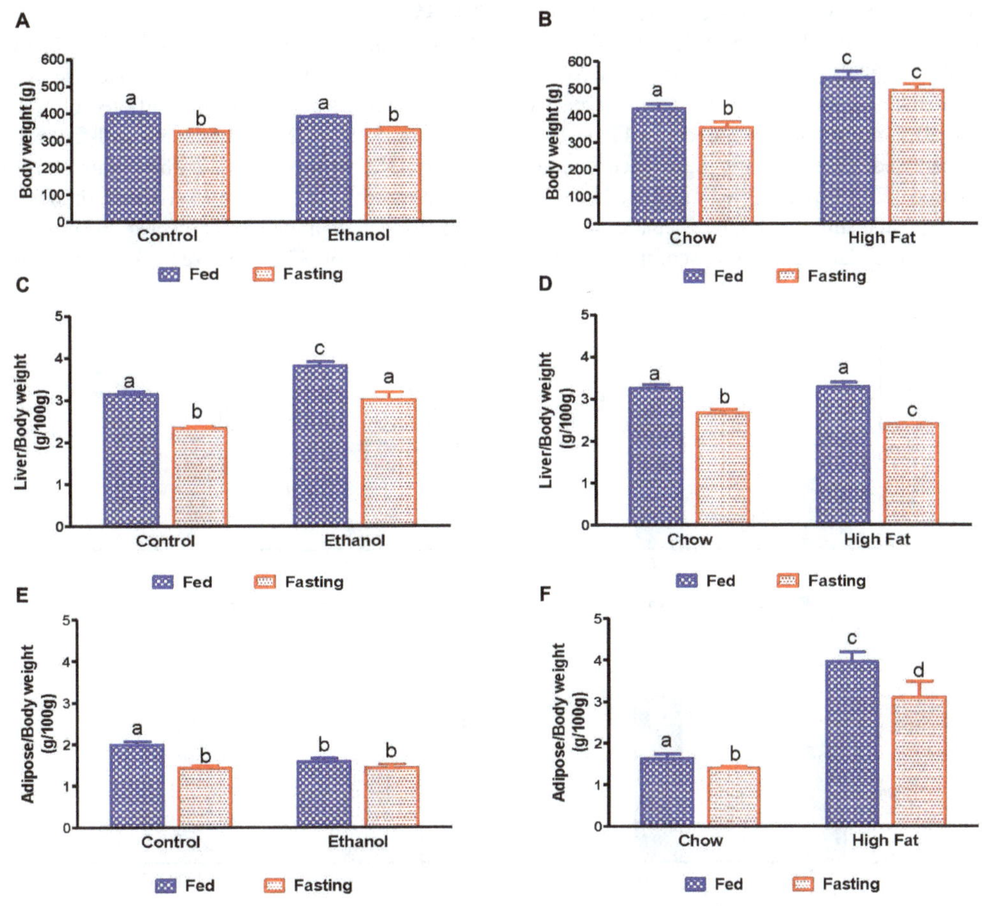

FIGURE 1 | Body, liver, and adipose weight in fed and fasting AFL and NAFL experimental animals. Body weights of **(A)** Lieber-DeCarli pair-fed control and ethanol-fed rats (AFL) and their respective fasted counterparts, **(B)** chow or high-fat diet (HFD) fed rats (NAFL) and their respective fasted groups. Liver weights of **(C)** AFL group and **(D)** NAFL group. Adipose weights of **(E)** AFL group and **(F)** NAFL group. Values are means ± SEM (n = 8). Values not sharing a common letter in each group are statistically different, $p < 0.05$.

both ethanol and HFD-fed rats compared with pair-fed control and chow-fed rats, respectively (**Figure 2**). Whereas 48 h fasting caused a significant ALT decrease in only the HFD-fed group (**Figures 2A,B**), serum ALP levels decreased in all experimental groups compared to their respective fed-counterparts (**Figures 2C,D**).

We also measured serum lipid content in all experimental groups. Serum NEFA, TG, and total cholesterol levels were higher in ethanol and HFD-fed rats compared with their respective controls (**Figures 3A–F**). As expected, 48 h fasting increased circulating NEFA levels in all experimental groups, except the ethanol group, relative to corresponding fed groups (**Figures 3A,B**). In contrast to serum NEFA levels, fasting significantly decreased serum TG and cholesterol levels in all experimental groups compared with fed groups (**Figures 3C–F**).

Morphology of Liver Tissue and Hepatic TG Levels in Fed and Fasted AFL and NAFL Rats

We collected livers from fed and fasted rats to examine fat content by both histological and biochemical assessments. The histopathological evaluations of the formalin-fixed H&E stained liver sections were consistent with previous reports in that both alcohol and HFD-fed rats showed higher hepatic fat accumulation with evidence of both micro and macrovesicular steatosis as compared with their respective controls (**Figures 4A,B**). Since we observed decreased liver/body weight ratios, we expected lower hepatic lipid accumulation in fasted rats compared with respective fed animals. However, all except ethanol-fed rats showed higher hepatic fat with predominantly microvesicular steatosis compared with respective fed groups after 48 h fasting (**Figures 4A,B**). Interestingly in ethanol-fed rats, 48 h fasting decreased hepatic lipid accumulation, showing mostly microvesicular steatosis. These histological findings were corroborated by quantification of hepatic TG levels (**Figures 5A,B**) showing, in most cases, that fasting increased TG levels in the liver. Further, we stained hepatic sections for lipid droplet associated protein, perilipin2 (PLIN2). Perilipins are one of the most abundant lipid droplet proteins (Sztalryd and Brasaemle, 2017). Among them, perilipin2 is ubiquitously expressed and exclusively associated with lipid droplets (LDs) as reported previously (Rasineni et al., 2014, 2016). As shown in **Figures 6A–D**, with quantitative analysis, we observed a marked increase in PLIN2 staining of ethanol and HFD-fed rat LDs. Apart from the ethanol-fed rats, all groups showed increased PLIN2 staining following 48 h fasting. The area of PLIN2 staining was concurrent with the histology (**Figures 4A,B**) and hepatic TG levels (**Figures 5A,B**).

Hepatic Fatty Acid Synthesis, Break Down and β-Oxidation in Fed and Fasted States

We measured mRNA that encodes fatty acid synthase (FAS), which catalyzes fatty acid synthesis. Because we observed elevated TG in the livers of alcohol and HFD-fed rats, we expected higher levels of FAS mRNA. While ethanol-fed rats showed higher FAS mRNA expression than their pair-fed controls, HFD-fed rats showed lower FAS mRNA levels than respective controls, suggesting that lipogenic pathways are upregulated during the development of AFL (**Figures 7A,B**), but not NAFL. Fasting

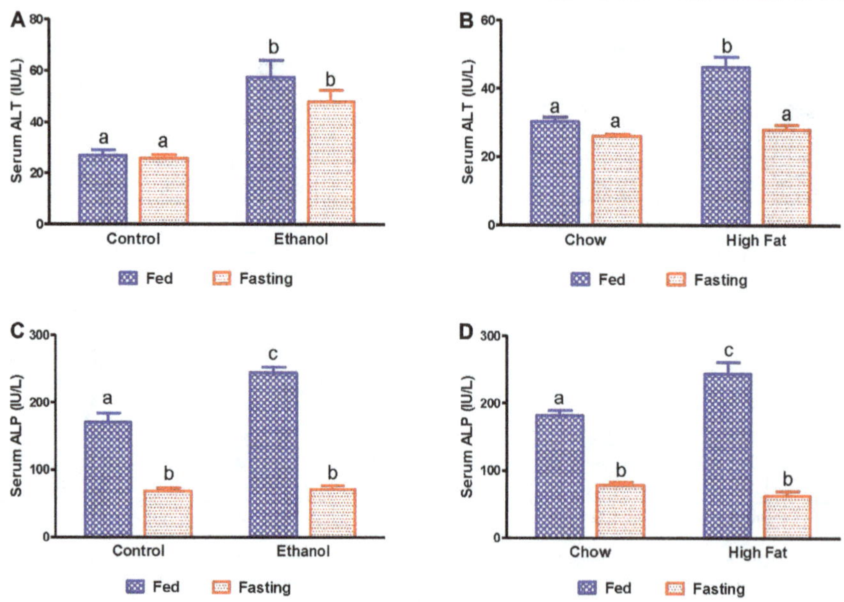

FIGURE 2 | Liver injury markers in serum of AFL and NAFL experimental groups. Hepatic injury markers ALT in **(A)** Lieber-DeCarli pair-fed control and ethanol-fed rats (AFL) and their respective fasted counterparts, **(B)** chow or high-fat diet (HFD) fed rats (NAFL) and their respective fasted groups. ALP in **(C)** AFL group and **(D)** NAFL group. Values are means ± SEM (n = 8). Values not sharing a common letter in each group are statistically different, $p < 0.05$.

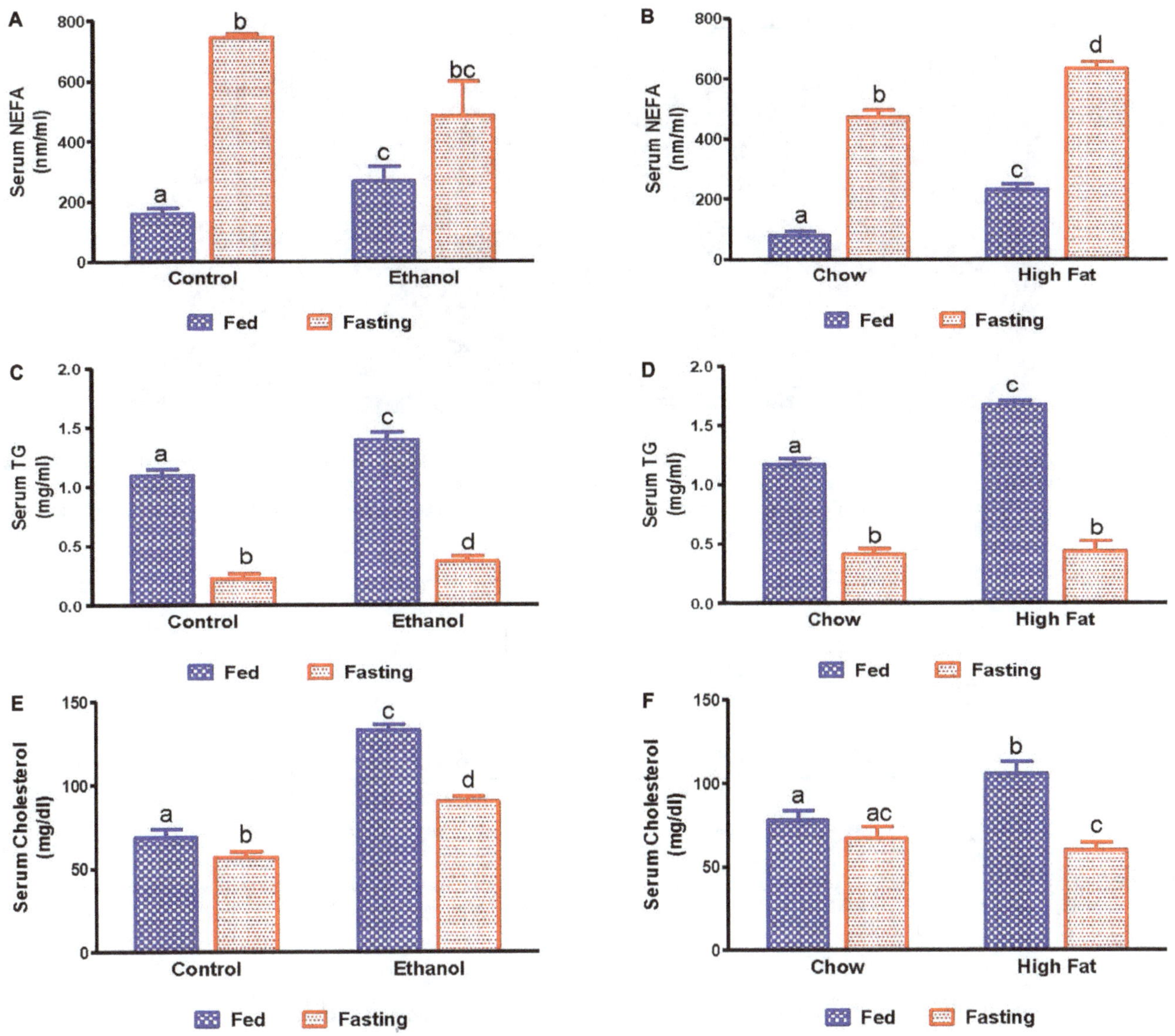

FIGURE 3 | Serum lipid content in fed and fasting states of AFL and NAFL model animals. Serum NEFA in **(A)** Lieber-DeCarli pair-fed control and ethanol-fed rats (AFL) and their respective fasted counterparts, **(B)** chow or high-fat diet (HFD) fed rats (NAFL) and their respective fasted groups. Serum TG in **(C)** AFL group and **(D)** NAFL group. Serum cholesterol in **(E)** AFL group and **(F)** NAFL group. Values are means ± SEM ($n = 8$). Values not sharing a common letter in each group are statistically different, $p < 0.05$.

significantly decreased FAS mRNA in all experimental groups (**Figures 7A,B**).

Since fat accumulation represents either increased fat synthesis and/or lower fat catabolism, we measured the activities of two main lipases, adipose triacylglycerol lipase (ATGL) and hormone sensitive lipase (HSL), which catalyzes triglyceride breakdown. Western blot analysis (**Figures 8A–J**) revealed no significant change in either total ATGL (**Figures 8C,D**) or HSL (**Figures 8G,H**) protein content in the livers of ethanol or HFD-fed rats. However, we did observe a significant decrease in the active forms of ATGL (pATGL) and HSL (pHSL) in ethanol-fed rats compared with their pair-fed controls (**Figures 8E,I**). Notably, we observed no significant changes in either pATGL or pHSL in HFD-fed rats compared to chow-fed rats (**Figures 8F,J**). Fasting significantly decreased pATGL in rats fed the Lieber-DeCarli control diet and HFD, but not in the ethanol or chow-fed rats. However, active HSL was significantly decreased in all fasted animals compared to respective fed groups. Further, we measured hepatic peroxisome proliferator-activated receptor alpha, PPARα, a ligand-activated transcription factor involved in fatty acid oxidation. As expected, PPARα in ethanol-fed rats was lower than in pair-fed controls (**Figure 9A**). In HFD-fed rats, however, we observed no significant change in PPARα expression when compared to chow-fed rats (**Figure 9B**). Since fatty acids are a major source of energy during starvation, 48 h fasting increased

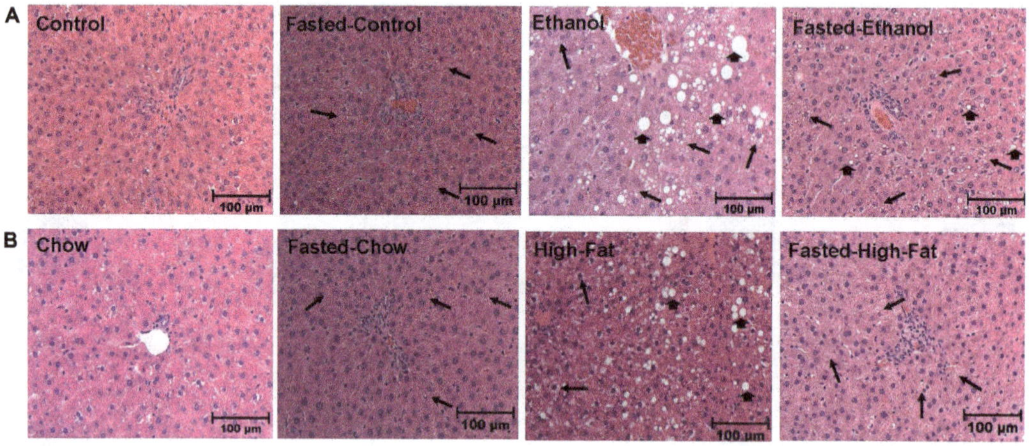

FIGURE 4 | Morphology of liver tissue. Hematoxylin and eosin staining was performed on paraffin sections of fed and fasted ethanol- and high-fat diet (HFD)-fed rats and their respective controls. Images are representative of each group (*n* = 8). Magnification, 200X. **(A)** shows Lieber-DeCarli pair-fed control and ethanol-fed rats (AFL) and their respective fasted counterparts. **(B)** shows chow or high-fat diet (HFD)-fed rats (NAFL) and their respective fasted groups. Macrovesicular steatosis is denoted by arrowhead while arrow depict microvesicular steatosis.

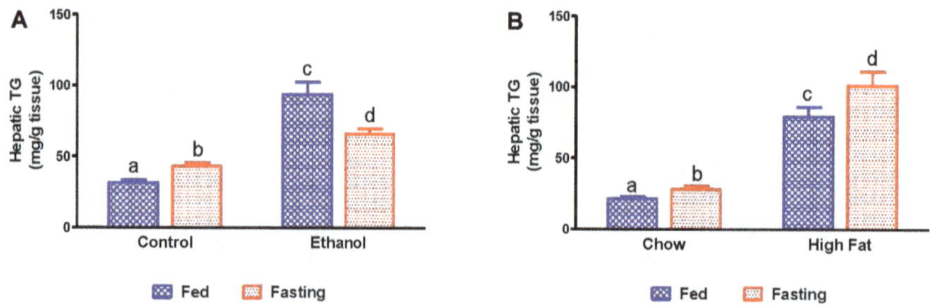

FIGURE 5 | Quantification of lipid content in liver. Hepatic TG in **(A)** pair-fed control and ethanol Lieber-DeCarli liquid diet-fed rats (AFL) and their respective fasted counterparts, **(B)** chow or high-fat diet (HFD) fed rats (NAFL) and their respective fasted groups. Values are means ± SEM (*n* = 8). Values not sharing a common letter in each group are statistically different, $p < 0.05$.

PPARα expression in all experimental groups, as expected (**Figures 9A,B**).

Hepatic Fatty Acid Uptake

Several studies have reported that adipose-derived free fatty acids are taken up by the liver and esterified to form TG, which can be utilized either for energy production, gluconeogenesis or stored in lipid droplets during fatty liver development. Several proteins are responsible for hepatic fatty acid uptake/transport, including fatty acid transport protein 2 (FATP2, a member of the FATP family of fatty acid uptake mediators) and cluster of differentiation 36 (CD36, a long-chain fatty acid-translocase). As expected, we observed increased expression of hepatic FATP2 and CD36 in ethanol and HFD-fed rats compared with pair-fed control and chow-fed rats, respectively (**Figures 10A–D**). Except for ethanol-fed rats, 48 h fasting increased circulating NEFA in parallel with a significant elevation of CD36 expression compared with respective fed-counterparts, indicating that fasting increases both adipose lipolysis and hepatic uptake of circulating fatty acids (**Figures 10A–D**). Similar increases in FATP2 were observed in all groups except for ethanol-fed animals following 48 h fasting.

Hepatic Inflammation

Since it has been reported that fatty liver can promote inflammation (Mandrekar et al., 2011), which is a key player in progression of both alcoholic and non-alcoholic liver diseases (Gao and Tsukamoto, 2016), we examined the expression of inflammatory markers, monocyte chemoattractant protein 1 (MCP-1), and interleukin 1 beta (IL-1β). As shown in **Figure 11**, we observed increased MCP-1 in alcohol and HFD-fed rats compared to respective controls. Fasting for 48 h increased MCP1 in all experimental groups relative to respective controls, except for the ethanol-fed group (**Figures 11A,B**). No significant elevation of IL-1β was observed in either the ethanol or HFD-fed rats compared to respective controls nor did 48 h fasting induce IL-1β expression in any experimental groups.

Fatty Acid Storage and Fatty Acid Breakdown in Adipose Tissue

We collected the epididymal white adipose tissue (eWAT) from fed and fasted animals to examine adipocyte size, which is representative of fat content. The histological evaluations of the

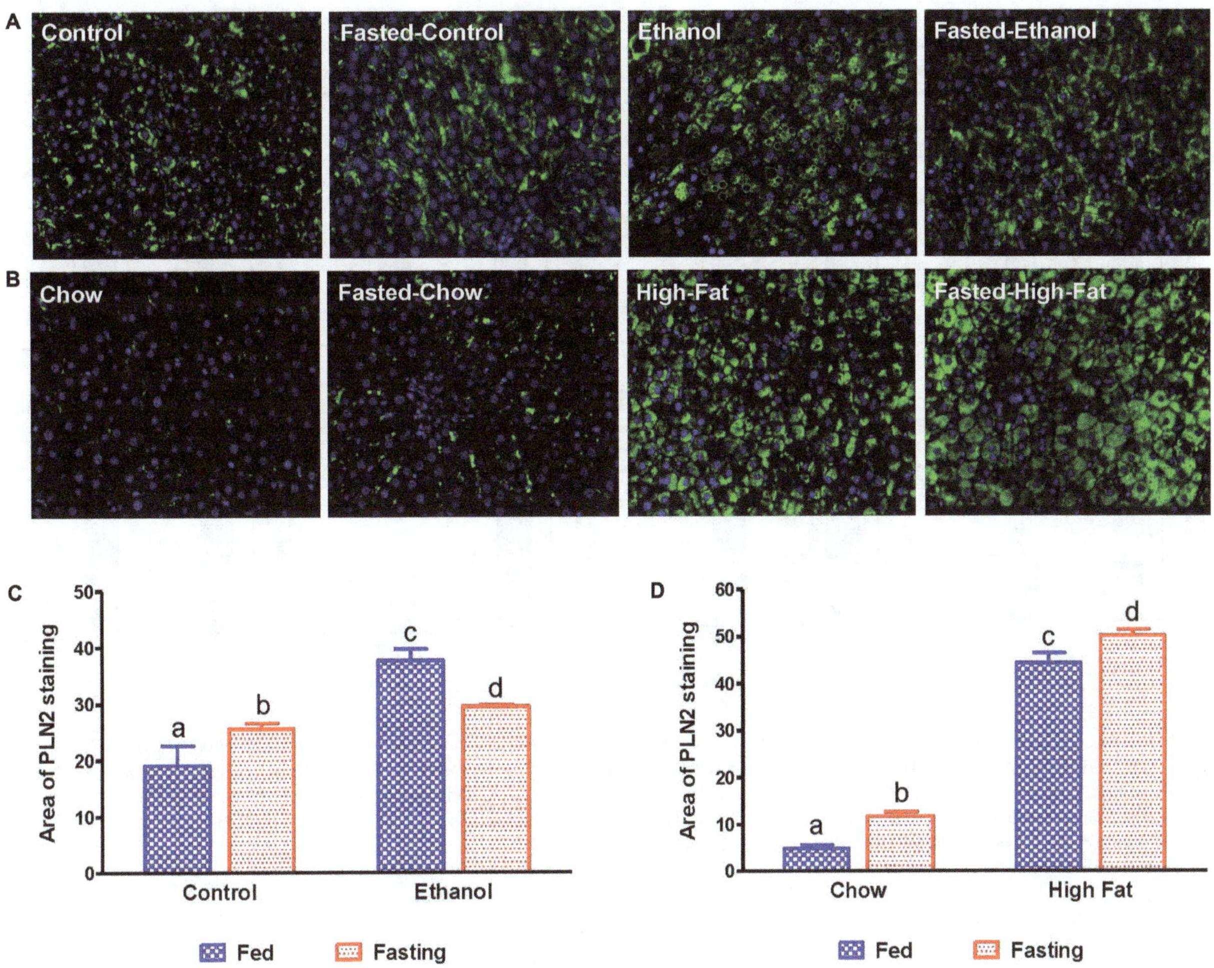

FIGURE 6 | Immunohistochemical staining for lipid droplet-associated protein PLIN2. Liver sections from animals were stained with perilipin 2 (PLIN2) antibody. **(A)** Lieber-DeCarli pair-fed control and ethanol-fed rats (AFL) and their respective fasted counterparts. **(B)** chow or high-fat diet-fed rats (NAFL) and their respective fasted groups. Images are representative of each group of $n = 8$. Magnification, 400×. The histogram represents the area of PLIN 2 staining in **(C)** AFL group and **(D)** NAFL group. Values are means ± SEM ($n = 8$). Values not sharing a common letter in each group are statistically different, $p < 0.05$.

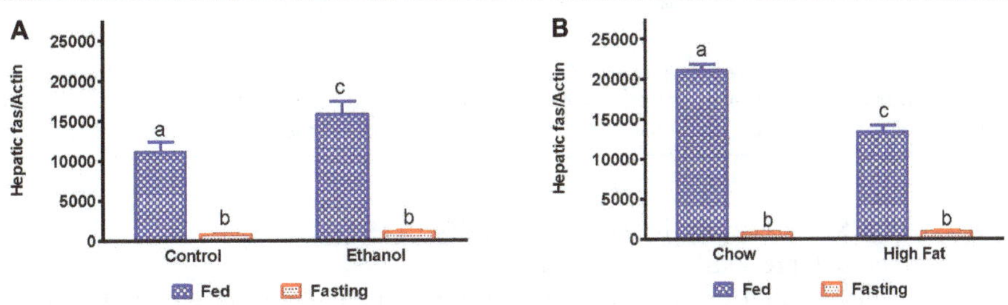

FIGURE 7 | Hepatic fatty acid synthesis in AFL and NAFL animals during fed and fasting conditions. Hepatic expression of fatty acid synthase (FAS), an enzyme which regulates fatty acid synthesis. FAS in **(A)** Lieber-DeCarli pair-fed control and ethanol-fed rats (AFL) and their respective fasted counterparts, **(B)** chow or high-fat diet (HFD) fed rats (NAFL) and their respective fasted groups. Values are means ± SEM ($n = 8$). Values not sharing a common letter in each group are statistically different, $p < 0.05$.

formalin-fixed H&E stained eWAT revealed a decrease in the adipocyte size of ethanol-fed rats compared with controls, which is consistent with previous reports (Zhong et al., 2012). HFD-fed rats showed larger adipocyte size compared to chow-fed controls as previously reported (Li et al., 2016; **Figures 12A–D**). All fasted rats showed decreased adipocyte size compared with respective fed groups (**Figures 12C,D**). Further, we measured PPARγ (a transcription factor that induces adipose differentiation and

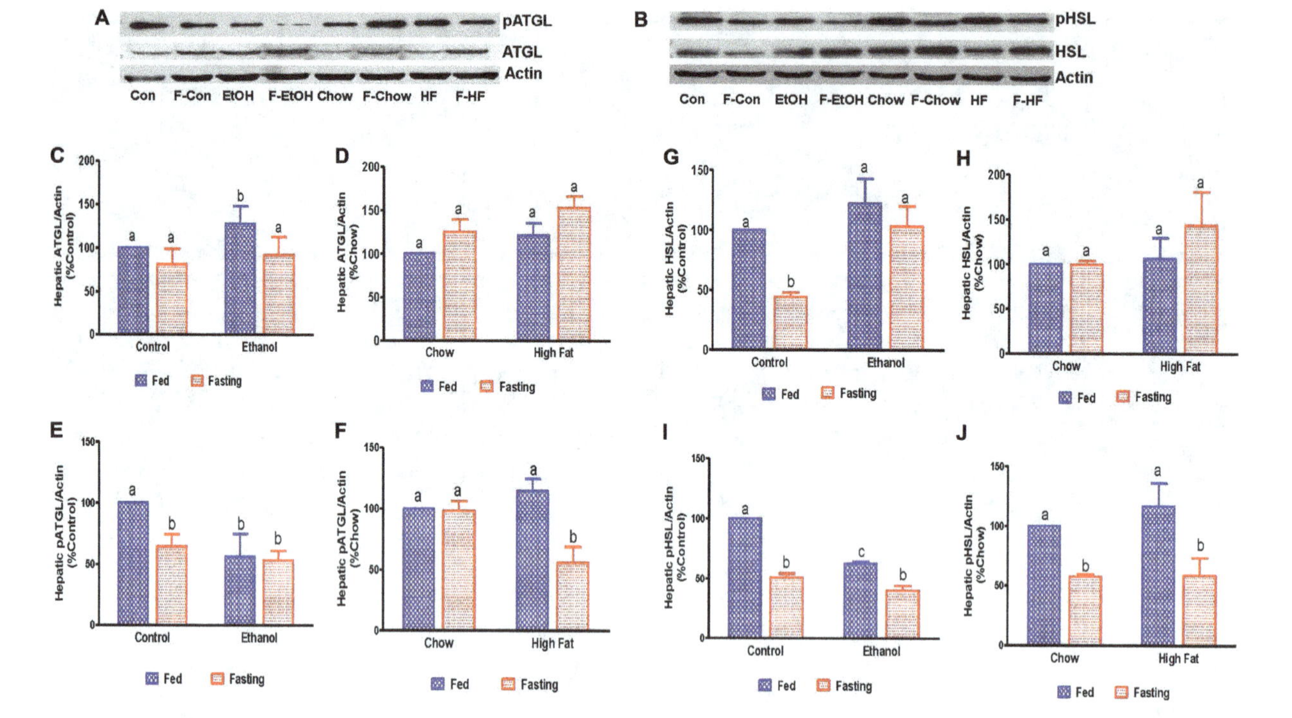

FIGURE 8 | Estimation of hepatic enzymes involved in the regulation of hepatic triglyceride breakdown. Representative Western Blot from AFL and NAFL groups for **(A)** adipose triglyceride lipase (ATGL) and **(B)** hormone-sensitive lipase (HSL). **(C–F)** Panels of densitometric values of total and active (phosphorylated) content of ATGL in AFL and NAFL groups. **(G–J)** Panels of densitometric values of total and active HSL in AFL and NAFL groups. Values are means ± SEM ($n = 6$). Values not sharing a common letter in each group are statistically different, $p < 0.05$. Con, control; F-Con, fasted control; EtOH, ethanol; F-EtOH, fasted ethanol; Chow, chow fed; F-Chow, fasted chow; HF, high-fat-fed; F-HF, fasted high-fat-fed group.

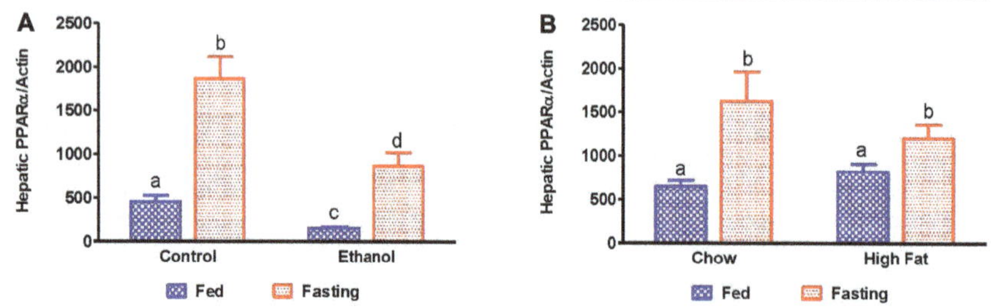

FIGURE 9 | Expression of peroxisome proliferator-activated receptor α (PPARα). qPCR analysis of hepatic gene expression related to fatty acid oxidation, PPARα. **(A)** PPARα in Lieber-DeCarli pair-fed control and ethanol-fed rats (AFL) and their respective fasted counterparts, **(B)** chow or high-fat diet (HFD) fed rats (NAFL) and their respective fasted cohorts. Values are means ± SEM ($n = 8$). Values not sharing a common letter in each group are statistically different, $p < 0.05$.

increases fat storage capacity) and HSL (an enzyme that catalyzes triglyceride breakdown). As reported previously, in ethanol-fed rats we observed lower adipose PPARγ (**Figure 13A**) and higher active HSL levels compared with pair-fed controls (**Figures 13C,D,F**). In HFD-fed rats, parallel to increased eWAT weight, we observed higher adipose PPARγ (**Figure 13B**) and HSL expression compared with chow-fed rats (**Figures 13E,G**). PPARγ expression declined in all groups after 48 h fasting. Whereas fasting significantly increased adipose HSL activity in rats fed the Lieber-DeCarli control, chow or high-fat diet, this same increase was not observed in adipose tissue of ethanol-fed rats (**Figures 13F,G**).

DISCUSSION

Fatty liver arising from either excessive alcohol consumption or over-consumption of a high-fat/high-sugar diet have similar phenotypes of hepatic lipid accumulation In our previous studies, we reported that despite showing similar phenotypic characteristics of accumulation of hepatic lipids and increased oxidative stress in livers of rats with AFL or NAFL, though there are mechanistic differences including impairment in membrane trafficking, which is observed only in AFL development (Rasineni et al., 2016). Here, we sought to evaluate the effect of fasting on lipid dynamics and metabolism

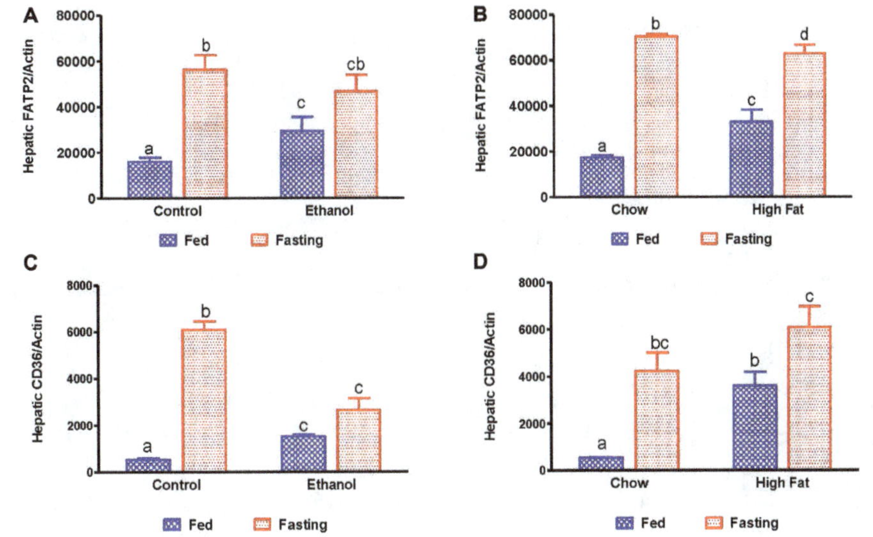

FIGURE 10 | Quantitative analysis of hepatic fatty acid uptake. Hepatic gene expression related to fatty acid uptake. Fatty acid transport protein 2 (FATP2) in **(A)** Lieber-DeCarli pair-fed control and ethanol-fed rats (AFL) and their respective fasted counterparts, **(B)** in chow or high-fat diet (HFD) fed rats (NAFL) and their respective fasted cohorts. Fatty acid translocase CD36 in **(C)** AFL group and **(D)** NAFL group. Values are means ± SEM (n = 8). Values not sharing a common letter in each group are statistically different, $p < 0.05$.

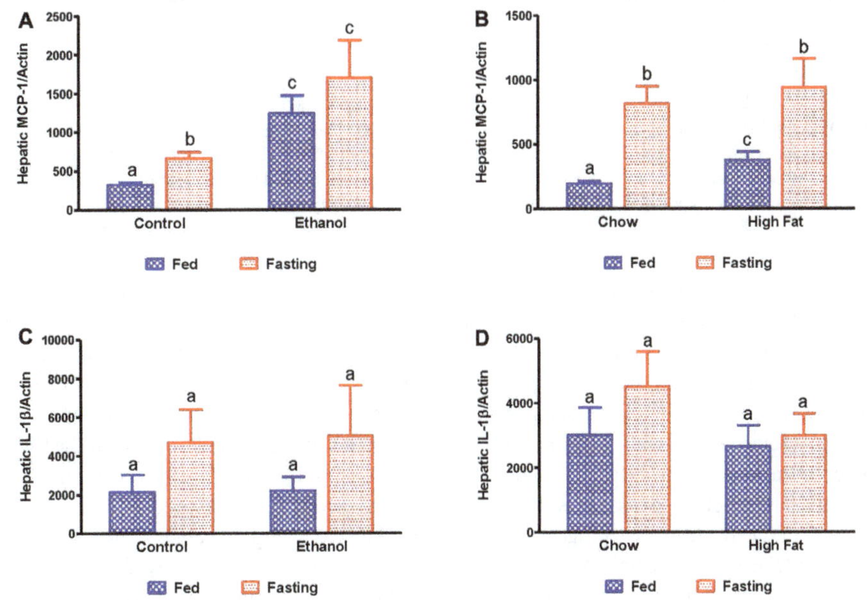

FIGURE 11 | Expression of hepatic inflammatory markers. qPCR analysis of hepatic gene expression related to inflammation and steatosis. Monocyte chemoattractant protein-1 (MCP-1/CCL2) in **(A)** Lieber-DeCarli pair-fed control and ethanol-fed rats (AFL) and their respective fasted counterparts, **(B)** chow or high-fat diet-fed rats (NAFL) and their respective fasted cohorts. Interleukin 1 beta (IL-1β) in **(C)** AFL group and **(D)** NAFL group. Values are means ± SEM (n = 8). Values not sharing a common letter in each group are statistically different, $p < 0.05$.

by focusing on the adipose-liver axis in both models of fatty liver disease.

As expected, HFD-fed rats exhibited increased body weight and adipose/body weight ratios but had no change in liver/body weight ratio compared to the chow-fed group. In the case of HFD-fed rats, excessive nutrient/caloric intake results in additional energy being stored in adipose tissue in the form of lipids. This results in an increased adipose, body weight, and adipose/body weight ratio compared with the chow group. Further, when adipose tissue exceeds its ability to store lipids, NEFA flow to other organs increases, especially to the liver, leading to increased fat deposition and liver weight (Langin, 2011). Since there was an increase in both the liver and body weight of rats fed the HFD, the liver/body weight ratio in these

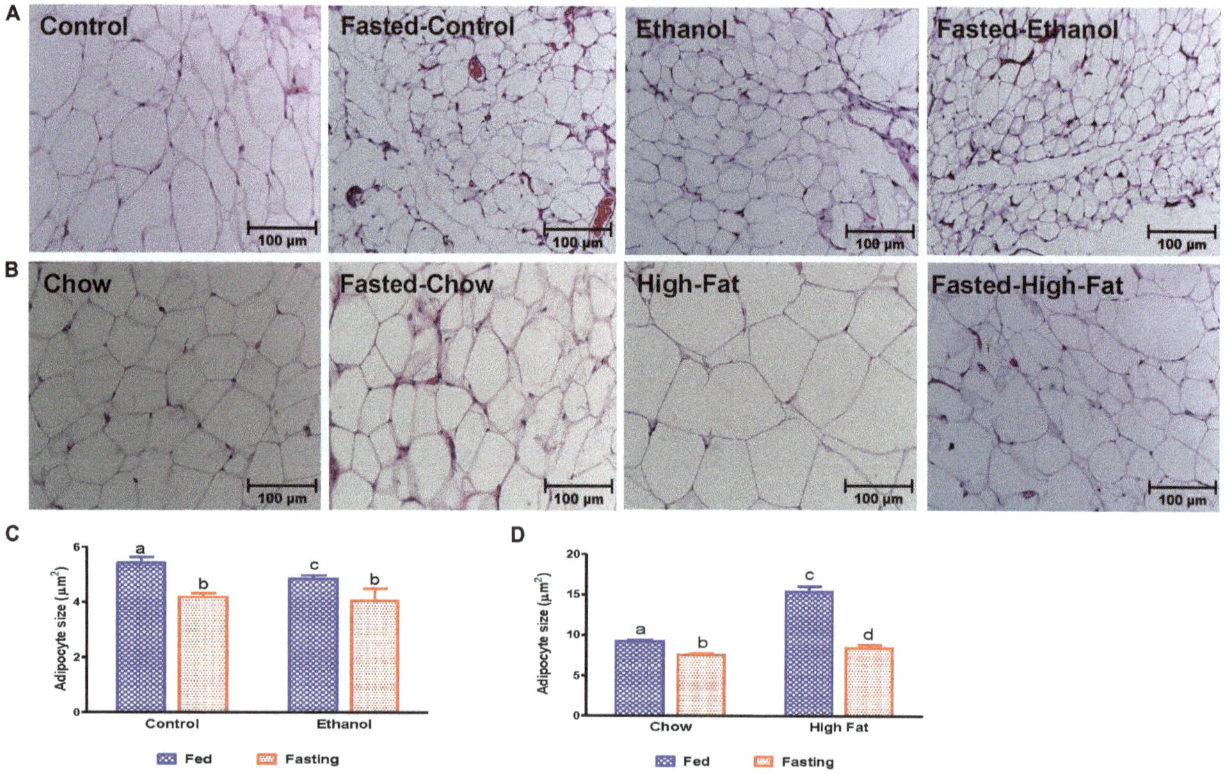

FIGURE 12 | Morphology of epididymal adipose tissue. Hematoxylin and Eosin staining was performed on paraffin sections. Images are representative of each group of $n = 8$. Magnification 200X. **(A)** Lieber-DeCarli pair-fed control and ethanol-fed rats (AFL) and their respective fasted counterparts. **(B)** chow or high-fat diet (HFD) fed rats (NAFL) and their respective fasted groups. Average adipocyte size in **(C)** AFL group and **(D)** NAFL group. ImageJ software (National Institutes of Health, Bethesda, MD, United States) was used to measure average adipocyte size. Values are means ± SEM of four randomly selected fields from each section, and data pooled from sections obtained from four animals from each experimental group. Values not sharing a common letter in each group are statistically different, $p < 0.05$.

rats did not differ from the chow-fed controls. However, despite weighing ~100 g less than HFD-fed rats, ethanol-fed rats showed similar body weights to pair-fed controls, but markedly decreased adipose/body weight ratios as adipose lipolysis increased. As a result, the ethanol-fed rats exhibited increased liver/body weight ratios partly due to protein (Kharbanda et al., 2007b) and fat accumulation in the liver compared with respective controls (Rasineni et al., 2014). The latter occurred as a result of the combined effect of alcohol-induced *de novo* lipogenesis and adipose-derived fatty acid uptake and esterification as well as decreased fatty acid oxidation and VLDL secretion (Kharbanda et al., 2009; Rasineni et al., 2019a). Fasting for 48 h caused a significant decrease in body weights of all experimental animals except HFD-fed rats, which is consistent with reports in the literature (Li and Wassner, 1984). It has been shown that the extent of weight gain and body fat accumulation in older rats can regulate body weight loss following food deprivation. Hence, percentage of body weight loss is greater in younger rats than in older rats after 24 h of starvation (Li and Wassner, 1984). Our results were more consistent with liver weights which decreased in all experimental groups after the 48 h fast. This fasting-induced decrease in liver weights is likely due to breakdown and utilization of glycogen, which is an immediate and effective energy source to maintain blood glucose during the early stages of fasting (Ohama et al., 1994; Klover and Mooney, 2004), combined with the considerable amount of glycogen-associated water loss (Sharma et al., 1985). While glycogen is utilized during early periods of starvation, 48 h fasting results in the breakdown of adipose-stored TG for energy. Indeed, adipose/body weight ratios significantly decreased following fasting, indicating increased adipose lipolysis in all experimental groups except ethanol-fed rats. This was also indicated by increased circulating NEFA levels in all fasted groups except ethanol-fed rats. This discrepancy with the ethanol-fed rats is likely due to already accelerated lipolysis and perhaps the inability of adipose tissue to respond adequately to the fasting stimulus and release NEFA to the extent observed in control, chow, and HFD-fed rats.

Serum aminotransferase increase is an index of hepatocyte injury. Consistent with our previous studies and others, we saw elevated serum ALT and ALP in animals with fatty livers (Toshikuni et al., 2013; Echeverria et al., 2018). Elevated ALT is also an indicator of insulin resistance. Fasting reduced serum ALT levels in HFD-fed rats. Such observations were reported in several studies showing improvement in liver enzymes (transaminase) after exercise and restricted diets (Vajro et al., 1994; Ueno et al., 1997). Except in HFD-fed rats, other experimental groups showed no decline in ALT levels with fasting, which is consistent with earlier reports (Krahenbuhl et al., 1991;

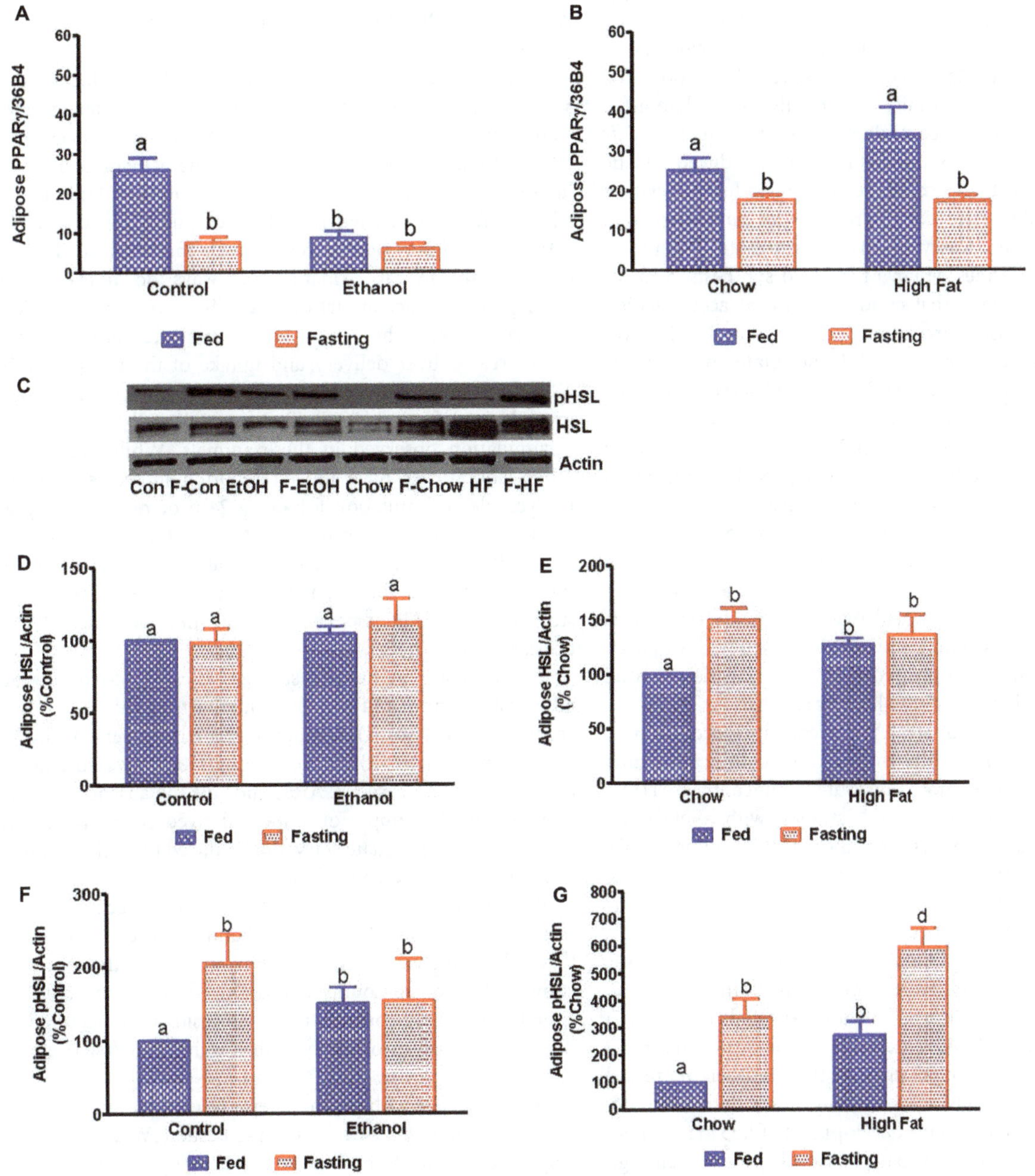

FIGURE 13 | Quantitative analysis of the adipose fatty acid breakdown. qPCR analysis of peroxisome proliferator-activated receptor γ (PPARγ) in **(A)** Lieber-DeCarli pair-fed control and ethanol-fed rats (AFL) and their respective fasted counterparts, **(B)** in chow or high-fat diet (HFD) fed rats (NAFL) and their respective fasted cohorts. For quantitative analysis of adipose lipid breakdown, we estimated total and phosphorylated hormone-sensitive lipase (HSL). **(C)** Representative Western Blot. **(D,E)** Panel of densitometric values of total HSL in AFL and NAFL groups. **(F,G)** Panel of densitometric values of active (phosphorylated) HSL in AFL and NAFL groups. Values are means ± SEM ($n = 6$). Values not sharing a common letter in each group are statistically different, $p < 0.05$. Con, control-fed; F-Con, fasted control; EtOH, ethanol-fed; F-EtOH, fasted ethanol; Chow, chow-fed; F-Chow, fasted chow; HFD, high-fat diet-fed; F-HFD, fasted high-fat diet group.

Browning et al., 2012). Fasting for 48 h reduced ALP levels in all experimental animals, as has been reported in chow-fed control and CCl4-induced cirrhotic rats (Abraira et al., 1980; Krahenbuhl et al., 1991; Restellini et al., 2013; Fazeli et al., 2015).

Histological assessment of the H&E stained liver sections showed lipid accumulation after excessive alcohol intake or HFD consumption with the two models of fatty liver disease being essentially indistinguishable. This assessment was corroborated by biochemical quantitation which revealed a nearly 2.5-fold increase in hepatic TG in both models compared with pair-fed control or chow-fed rats.

Pathomechanisms that underlie the development of hepatic steatosis include increased *de novo* lipogenesis, increased circulating fatty acid uptake by the liver coupled with decreased fatty acid oxidation and reduced fat export as VLDL (Kharbanda et al., 2009; Wei et al., 2013; Osna et al., 2017; You and Arteel, 2019). For *de novo* lipogenesis, fatty acid synthesis is regulated by the enzyme fatty acid synthase (FAS). We observed increased expression of FAS mRNA in the livers of ethanol-fed rats compared with pair-fed controls, suggesting that increased *de novo* fatty acid synthesis contributes to ethanol-induced hepatic fat accumulation. Further, alcohol metabolism-induced increases in the NADH/NAD ratio could promote *de novo* fatty acid synthesis (Rasineni and Casey, 2012) and contribute to increased fat accumulation. Besides *de novo* fatty acid synthesis, a major physiological mechanism that contributes to fat accumulation in the liver is increased circulating NEFA uptake by the liver and its esterification with glycerol-3-phosphate to form TG (Alves-Bezerra and Cohen, 2017). Here, we observed increased serum NEFA in conjunction with an increased expression of hepatic fatty acid transporters FATP2 and CD36, indicating that increased hepatic uptake of circulating NEFA contributes to fat accumulation in ethanol-fed rats. Ethanol consumption also resulted in impaired triglyceride hydrolysis and fatty acid oxidation as indicated by a decline in the activation of the two major lipases (HSL and ATGL) as well as a decrease in PPARα, which regulates fatty acid oxidation. Collectively, it is the upregulation of lipogenic pathways, increased NEFA uptake, decreased hydrolysis and impaired fatty acid oxidation that all contribute to the ethanol-induced hepatic steatosis.

We observed that FAS mRNA expression is decreased in HFD-fed rats compared with chow-fed rats, indicating that *de novo* lipogenesis does not contribute significantly to HFD-induced hepatic steatosis. Several studies with dietary fat challenge in human subjects or experimental animals have similarly reported that the source of TG in hepatic tissue is mainly dietary lipids and that very little is from *de novo* lipogenesis (Donnelly et al., 2005; Delgado et al., 2009; Oosterveer et al., 2009; Duarte et al., 2014). Furthermore, HSL and ATGL activity were similar in both chow and HFD-fed animals and instead of an expected decrease, a moderate increase in PPARα expression was seen after HFD consumption. These results suggest that neither increased lipogenesis, impaired triglyceride hydrolysis nor decreased fatty acid oxidation contribute to the development of hepatic steatosis in HFD-fed rats. Rather, hepatic steatosis occurs through increased NEFA flow from the diet or adipose tissue and heightened uptake by the liver, facilitated by the elevated levels of fatty acid transporters CD36 and FABP4, as shown here. Other factors that may contribute to hepatic steatosis after HFD consumption are direct elongation and subsequent desaturation of dietary fatty acids in the liver (Oosterveer et al., 2009; Duarte et al., 2014).

Fasting for 48 h also revealed a differential effect on hepatic steatosis induced by ethanol or HFD consumption. While rats fed Lieber-DeCarli control, chow or high-fat diet showed accumulation of liver TG after 48 h of fasting, ethanol-fed rats showed a decrease compared with their fed counterparts. The fasting-induced change in hepatic lipids followed the same pattern as serum NEFA, which increased in all experimental groups compared to respective fed-groups except the 48 h fasted ethanol rats. Fasting reduced FAS expression while it increased PPARα expression in all experimental groups compared to respective fed groups. These findings corroborate previous studies, showing that fasting-induced glucocorticoid secretion promotes PPARα activation to utilize fat as energy source during fasting (Lemberger et al., 1994; Steineger et al., 1994). We also observed a decline in the activation of hepatic lipases, ATGL and HSL, in fasted control and HFD-fed rats whereas fasted chow-fed rats showed a decrease in only HSL activation. These results reveal that increases in lipogenic or decreases in fat oxidation pathways do not contribute to hepatic fat accumulation seen in rats fed the Lieber-DeCarli control, chow or high-fat diet after fasting. Rather, the increased liver delivery and uptake of the adipose-derived NEFA and its subsequent esterification combined with reduced breakdown of stored TG likely contributed to hepatic fat accumulation observed in these animals. While studies from other laboratories have indeed reported increases in hepatic triglyceride accumulation following 24 h or more of fasting in healthy humans and control rats (Moller et al., 2008; Browning et al., 2012; Geisler et al., 2016; Pantaleao et al., 2017), ours is the first report to show that fasting for 48 h increases hepatic steatosis in an HFD-associated NAFLD (non-alcoholic fatty liver disease) animal model.

The decrease in hepatic steatosis in alcohol-fed rats after 48 h fasting compared to fed-counterparts could be due to the combined effects of (i) abstinence-related recovery of the liver and adipose tissue, (ii) an increase in liver fatty acid oxidation as evident by increased PPARα, and (iii) the absence of further increases in the supply of adipose-derived NEFA to the liver because of an inadequate starvation-induced lipolytic stimulus as observed in pair-fed control rats.

It is noteworthy that there was no further change in the hepatic p-ATGL (active form) between fed and fasted ethanol rats, and that p-HSL (active form) decreased in fasted ethanol-fed rats compared with fed-counterparts. This decrease in active HSL after fasting likely contributes to the residual fat accumulation due to deceleration of lipolysis in the livers of fasted ethanol-fed rats.

In congruence with previous reports, ethanol-fed rats showed decreased epididymal white adipose tissue (eWAT) weight and adipocyte size while both were significantly elevated in HFD-fed rats compared with their respective controls. In correlation with adipocyte size, we observed increased HSL enzyme activity and decreased expression of PPARγ, which induces adipose differentiation and increases its fat storing capacity in the eWAT of ethanol-fed rats compared with control. These ethanol-induced changes in eWAT promote adipose lipolysis, causing a rise in adipose-derived serum NEFA levels as reported in our recent study (Rasineni et al., 2019a). Fasting pair-fed control rats reduced eWAT PPARγ expression while it increased adipose p-HSL levels, thereby enhancing lipolysis, as evident by reduced adipocyte size, and subsequently, an elevation in serum NEFA levels. These results were as expected. However, this normal fasting-induced lipolytic response was absent in ethanol-fed rats, with no change in PPARγ, active HSL or serum NEFA levels between the fed and fasted states.

We observed that the dietary fat mainly contributed to the higher serum NEFA levels in HFD-fed rats compared with chow-fed rats. However, the increased HSL activation seen in eWAT of HFD-fed rats may have also contributed to the rise in NEFA. Fasting for 48 h induced similar responses in the eWAT of chow and HFD-fed rats and caused a further increase in HSL activation to promote eWAT lipolysis (as judged by the decrease in adipocyte size compared to fed-counterparts) ultimately leading to elevated adipose-derived serum NEFA levels.

Increased fat accumulation makes the liver susceptible to inflammatory mediators, thereby, promoting the development of advanced liver injury. We observed elevated levels of the chemokine MCP-1 in livers of ethanol- and HFD-fed rat which is consistent with previous reports (Ito et al., 2007; Mandrekar et al., 2011; Gao and Tsukamoto, 2016). However, we observed no histological evidence of inflammation. This may be because MCP-1 not only plays a role in macrophage recruitment and inflammation but also directly plays a significant role in the development of hepatic steatosis via affecting fatty acid metabolism (Mandrekar et al., 2011). FFAs regulate MCP-1 expression (Yeop Han et al., 2010; Asterholm et al., 2012), which we believe may be contributing to the increase in this chemokine level in livers of HFD- and ethanol-fed rats. Upon fasting, all other experimental rats, except for the ethanol-fed animals, showed increased hepatic MCP-1 levels, which is in line with the increased flow of FFAs seen in these other experimental groups after 48 h fasting.

In summary, although AFL and NAFL feeding models showed similar histology, the physiological mechanisms in fatty liver development in each are different. Increased hepatic *de novo* fatty acid synthesis, higher uptake of adipose-derived NEFA and impaired fatty acid breakdown contribute to the development of AFL. In the development of NAFL, however, increased dietary fatty acid uptake by the liver plays a major role. Likewise, the response of each model to fasting is also diverse. While hepatic steatosis decreased after fasting in ethanol-fed rats, animals with NAFL had increased hepatic steatosis compared with their fed-counterparts. This rise in hepatic steatosis after 48 h fasting of HFD-fed rats was likely due to increased delivery to the liver and enhanced hepatic uptake and esterification of adipose-derived NEFA combined with reduced TG lipolysis. The decrease in hepatic steatosis in AFL rats after 48 h fasting likely resulted from a combined effect of abstinence-related recovery, an increase in fatty acid oxidation and the absence of any further increase in the supply of adipose-derived NEFA to the liver.

AUTHOR CONTRIBUTIONS

KR: funding acquisition, conception, design of the study, data analysis and interpretation, and writing the original draft. CJ: performing the experiments, data acquisition, and data analysis. PT, JK, ES, and SS: aided in performing the experiments. GT: histological evaluation. TD: helped with interpretation of the data and editing the manuscript. MM: funding acquisition. KK: funding acquisition, data interpretation, and review and editing the manuscript. CC: funding acquisition, supervision of the project, and review and editing the manuscript. All authors contributed to the article and approved the submitted version.

REFERENCES

Abraira, C., Virupannavar, C., and Nemchausky, B. (1980). Protective effect of small amounts of glucose on abnormal liver function tests during starvation. *Metabolism* 29, 943–948. doi: 10.1016/0026-0495(80)90037-2

Alves-Bezerra, M., and Cohen, D. E. (2017). Triglyceride metabolism in the liver. *Compr. Physiol.* 8, 1–8. doi: 10.1002/cphy.c170012

Asterholm, I. W., McDonald, J., Blanchard, P. G., Sinha, M., Xiao, Q., Mistry, J., et al. (2012). Lack of "immunological fitness" during fasting in metabolically challenged animals. *J. Lipid Res.* 53, 1254–1267. doi: 10.1194/jlr.M021725

Browning, J. D., Baxter, J., Satapati, S., and Burgess, S. C. (2012). The effect of short-term fasting on liver and skeletal muscle lipid, glucose, and energy metabolism in healthy women and men. *J. Lipid Res.* 53, 577–586. doi: 10.1194/jlr.P020867

Chao, H. W., Chao, S. W., Lin, H., Ku, H. C., and Cheng, C. F. (2019). Homeostasis of glucose and lipid in non-alcoholic fatty liver disease. *Int. J. Mol. Sci.* 20:298. doi: 10.3390/ijms20020298

Cotter, T. G., Dong, L., Holmen, J., Gilroy, R., Krong, J., and Charlton, M. (2020). Nonalcoholic fatty liver disease: impact on healthcare resource utilization, liver transplantation and mortality in a large, integrated healthcare system. *J. Gastroenterol.* 55, 722–730. doi: 10.1007/s00535-020-01684-w

Cotter, T. G., and Rinella, M. (2020). Nonalcoholic fatty liver disease 2020: the state of the disease. *Gastroenterology* 158, 1851–1864. doi: 10.1053/j.gastro.2020.01.052

Cuervo, A. M., Knecht, E., Terlecky, S. R., and Dice, J. F. (1995). Activation of a selective pathway of lysosomal proteolysis in rat liver by prolonged starvation. *Am. J. Physiol.* 269(5 Pt 1), C1200–C1208. doi: 10.1152/ajpcell.1995.269.5.C1200

Delgado, T. C., Pinheiro, D., Caldeira, M., Castro, M. M., Geraldes, C. F., Lopez-Larrubia, P., et al. (2009). Sources of hepatic triglyceride accumulation during high-fat feeding in the healthy rat. *NMR Biomed.* 22, 310–317. doi: 10.1002/nbm.1327

Donnelly, K. L., Smith, C. I., Schwarzenberg, S. J., Jessurun, J., Boldt, M. D., and Parks, E. J. (2005). Sources of fatty acids stored in liver and secreted via lipoproteins in patients with nonalcoholic fatty liver disease. *J. Clin. Invest.* 115, 1343–1351. doi: 10.1172/JCI23621

Duarte, J. A., Carvalho, F., Pearson, M., Horton, J. D., Browning, J. D., Jones, J. G., et al. (2014). A high-fat diet suppresses de novo lipogenesis and desaturation but not elongation and triglyceride synthesis in mice. *J. Lipid Res.* 55, 2541–2553. doi: 10.1194/jlr.M052308

Echeverria, F., Valenzuela, R., Bustamante, A., Alvarez, D., Ortiz, M., Soto-Alarcon, S. A., et al. (2018). Attenuation of high-fat diet-induced rat liver oxidative stress and steatosis by combined hydroxytyrosol- (HT-) eicosapentaenoic acid supplementation mainly relies on HT. *Oxid. Med. Cell Longev.* 2018:5109503. doi: 10.1155/2018/5109503

Fazeli, P. K., Lun, M., Kim, S. M., Bredella, M. A., Wright, S., Zhang, Y., et al. (2015). FGF21 and the late adaptive response to starvation in humans. *J. Clin. Invest.* 125, 4601–4611. doi: 10.1172/JCI83349

Folch, J., Lees, M., and Sloane Stanley, G. H. (1957). A simple method for the isolation and purification of total lipides from animal tissues. *J. Biol. Chem.* 226, 497–509.

Gao, B., Ahmad, M. F., Nagy, L. E., and Tsukamoto, H. (2019). Inflammatory pathways in alcoholic steatohepatitis. *J. Hepatol.* 70, 249–259. doi: 10.1016/j.jhep.2018.10.023

Gao, B., and Tsukamoto, H. (2016). Inflammation in alcoholic and nonalcoholic fatty liver disease: friend or foe?". *Gastroenterology* 150, 1704–1709. doi: 10.1053/j.gastro.2016.01.025

Geisler, C. E., Hepler, C., Higgins, M. R., and Renquist, B. J. (2016). Hepatic adaptations to maintain metabolic homeostasis in response to fasting and refeeding in mice. *Nutr. Metab.* 13:62. doi: 10.1186/s12986-016-0122-x

Ito, M., Suzuki, J., Tsujioka, S., Sasaki, M., Gomori, A., Shirakura, T., et al. (2007). Longitudinal analysis of murine steatohepatitis model induced by chronic exposure to high-fat diet. *Hepatol. Res.* 37, 50–57. doi: 10.1111/j.1872-034X.

2007.00008.x

Kaushik, S., and Cuervo, A. M. (2015). Degradation of lipid droplet-associated proteins by chaperone-mediated autophagy facilitates lipolysis. *Nat. Cell Biol.* 17, 759–770. doi: 10.1038/ncb3166

Kawano, Y., and Cohen, D. E. (2013). Mechanisms of hepatic triglyceride accumulation in non-alcoholic fatty liver disease. *J. Gastroenterol.* 48, 434–441. doi: 10.1007/s00535-013-0758-5

Kharbanda, K. K., Mailliard, M. E., Baldwin, C. R., Beckenhauer, H. C., Sorrell, M. F., and Tuma, D. J. (2007a). Betaine attenuates alcoholic steatosis by restoring phosphatidylcholine generation via the phosphatidylethanolamine methyltransferase pathway. *J. Hepatol.* 46, 314–321. doi: 10.1016/j.jhep.2006.08.024

Kharbanda, K. K., Mailliard, M. E., Baldwin, C. R., Sorrell, M. F., and Tuma, D. J. (2007b). Accumulation of proteins bearing atypical isoaspartyl residues in livers of alcohol-fed rats is prevented by betaine administration: effects on protein-L-isoaspartyl methyltransferase activity. *J. Hepatol.* 46, 1119–1125. doi: 10.1016/j.jhep.2007.01.026

Kharbanda, K. K., Todero, S. L., King, A. L., Osna, N. A., McVicker, B. L., Tuma, D. J., et al. (2012). Betaine treatment attenuates chronic ethanol-induced hepatic steatosis and alterations to the mitochondrial respiratory chain proteome. *Int. J. Hepatol.* 2012:962183. doi: 10.1155/2012/962183

Kharbanda, K. K., Todero, S. L., Ward, B. W., Cannella, J. J. III, and Tuma, D. J. (2009). Betaine administration corrects ethanol-induced defective VLDL secretion. *Mol. Cell Biochem.* 327, 75–78. doi: 10.1007/s11010-009-0044-2

Klover, P. J., and Mooney, R. A. (2004). Hepatocytes: critical for glucose homeostasis. *Int. J. Biochem. Cell Biol.* 36, 753–758. doi: 10.1016/j.biocel.2003.10.002

Krahenbuhl, S., Weber, F. L. Jr., and Brass, E. P. (1991). Decreased hepatic glycogen content and accelerated response to starvation in rats with carbon tetrachloride-induced cirrhosis. *Hepatology* 14, 1189–1195.

Langin, D. (2011). "In and out: adipose tissue lipid turnover in obesity and dyslipidemia. *Cell Metab.* 14, 569–570. doi: 10.1016/j.cmet.2011.10.003

Lemberger, T., Staels, B., Saladin, R., Desvergne, B., Auwerx, J., and Wahli, W. (1994). Regulation of the peroxisome proliferator-activated receptor alpha gene by glucocorticoids. *J. Biol. Chem.* 269, 24527–24530.

Li, J., Zou, B., Yeo, Y. H., Feng, Y., Xie, X., Lee, D. H., et al. (2019). Prevalence, incidence, and outcome of non-alcoholic fatty liver disease in Asia, 1999-2019: a systematic review and meta-analysis. *Lancet Gastroenterol. Hepatol.* 4, 389–398. doi: 10.1016/S2468-1253(19)30039-1

Li, J. B., and Wassner, S. J. (1984). Effects of food deprivation and refeeding on total protein and actomyosin degradation. *Am. J. Physiol.* 246(1 Pt 1), E32–E37. doi: 10.1152/ajpendo.1984.246.1.E32

Li, X., Yang, M., Li, Z., Xue, M., Shangguan, Z., Ou, Z., et al. (2016). Fructus xanthii improves lipid homeostasis in the epididymal adipose tissue of rats fed a high-fat diet. *Mol. Med. Rep.* 13, 787–795. doi: 10.3892/mmr.2015.4628

Lieber, C. S. (2004). Alcoholic fatty liver: its pathogenesis and mechanism of progression to inflammation and fibrosis. *Alcohol* 34, 9–19. doi: 10.1016/j.alcohol.2004.07.008

Lomonaco, R., Ortiz-Lopez, C., Orsak, B., Webb, A., Hardies, J., Darland, C., et al. (2012). Effect of adipose tissue insulin resistance on metabolic parameters and liver histology in obese patients with nonalcoholic fatty liver disease. *Hepatology* 55, 1389–1397. doi: 10.1002/hep.25539

Mandrekar, P., Ambade, A., Lim, A., Szabo, G., and Catalano, D. (2011). An essential role for monocyte chemoattractant protein-1 in alcoholic liver injury: regulation of proinflammatory cytokines and hepatic steatosis in mice. *Hepatology* 54, 2185–2197. doi: 10.1002/hep.24599

Mitra, S., De, A., and Chowdhury, A. (2020). Epidemiology of non-alcoholic and alcoholic fatty liver diseases. *Transl. Gastroenterol. Hepatol.* 5:16. doi: 10.21037/tgh.2019.09.08

Moller, L., Stodkilde-Jorgensen, H. H., Jensen, F. T., and Jorgensen, J. O. (2008). Fasting in healthy subjects is associated with intrahepatic accumulation of lipids as assessed by 1H-magnetic resonance spectroscopy. *Clin. Sci.* 114, 547–552. doi: 10.1042/CS20070217

Ohama, T., Matsuki, N., Saito, H., Tsukamoto, K., Kinoshita, M., Katsuragawa, K., et al. (1994). Effect of starving and refeeding on lipid metabolism in suncus. *J. Biochem.* 115, 190–193. doi: 10.1093/oxfordjournals.jbchem.a124316

Oosterveer, M. H., van Dijk, T. H., Tietge, U. J., Boer, T., Havinga, R., Stellaard, F., et al. (2009). High fat feeding induces hepatic fatty acid elongation in mice. *PLoS One* 4:e6066. doi: 10.1371/journal.pone.0006066

Osna, N. A., Donohue, T. M. Jr., and Kharbanda, K. K. (2017). Alcoholic liver disease: pathogenesis and current management. *Alcohol. Res.* 38, 147–161.

Pantaleao, L. C., Murata, G., Teixeira, C. J., Payolla, T. B., Santos-Silva, J. C., Duque-Guimaraes, D. E., et al. (2017). Prolonged fasting elicits increased hepatic triglyceride accumulation in rats born to dexamethasone-treated mothers. *Sci. Rep.* 7:10367. doi: 10.1038/s41598-017-10642-1

Rasineni, K., and Casey, C. A. (2012). Molecular mechanism of alcoholic fatty liver. *Indian J. Pharmacol.* 44, 299–303. doi: 10.4103/0253-7613.96297

Rasineni, K., Kubik, J. L., Casey, C. A., and Kharbanda, K. K. (2019a). Inhibition of ghrelin activity by receptor antagonist [d-Lys-3] GHRP-6 attenuates alcohol-induced hepatic steatosis by regulating hepatic lipid metabolism. *Biomolecules* 9:517. doi: 10.3390/biom9100517

Rasineni, K., Thomes, P. G., Kubik, J. L., Harris, E. N., Kharbanda, K. K., and Casey, C. A. (2019b). Chronic alcohol exposure alters circulating insulin and ghrelin levels: role of ghrelin in hepatic steatosis. *Am. J. Physiol. Gastrointest. Liver Physiol.* 316, G453–G461. doi: 10.1152/ajpgi.00334.2018

Rasineni, K., McVicker, B. L., Tuma, D. J., McNiven, M. A., and Casey, C. A. (2014). Rab GTPases associate with isolated lipid droplets (LDs) and show altered content after ethanol administration: potential role in alcohol-impaired LD metabolism. *Alcohol. Clin. Exp. Res.* 38, 327–335. doi: 10.1111/acer.12271

Rasineni, K., Penrice, D. D., Natarajan, S. K., McNiven, M. A., McVicker, B. L., Kharbanda, K. K., et al. (2016). Alcoholic vs non-alcoholic fatty liver in rats: distinct differences in endocytosis and vesicle trafficking despite similar pathology. *BMC Gastroenterol.* 16:27. doi: 10.1186/s12876-016-0433-4

Restellini, S., Spahr, L., and Rubbia Brandt, L. (2013). Severe starvation-induced hepatocyte autophagy as a cause of acute liver injury in anorexia nervosa: a case report. *Case Reports Hepatol.* 2013:749169. doi: 10.1155/2013/749169

Schneider, J. L., Suh, Y., and Cuervo, A. M. (2014). Deficient chaperone-mediated autophagy in liver leads to metabolic dysregulation. *Cell Metab.* 20, 417–432. doi: 10.1016/j.cmet.2014.06.009

Sharma, M., Lal, H., and Saini, A. S. (1985). Effect of prolonged starvation and refeeding on fuel metabolism in rats. *Indian J. Physiol. Pharmacol.* 29, 107–110.

Singal, A. K., and Anand, B. S. (2013). Recent trends in the epidemiology of alcoholic liver disease. *Clin. Liver Dis.* 2, 53–56. doi: 10.1002/cld.168

Singal, A. K., Chaha, K. S., Rasheed, K., and Anand, B. S. (2013). Liver transplantation in alcoholic liver disease current status and controversies. *World J. Gastroenterol.* 19, 5953–5963. doi: 10.3748/wjg.v19.i36.5953

Steineger, H. H., Sorensen, H. N., Tugwood, J. D., Skrede, S., Spydevold, O., and Gautvik, K. M. (1994). Dexamethasone and insulin demonstrate marked and opposite regulation of the steady-state mRNA level of the peroxisomal proliferator-activated receptor (PPAR) in hepatic cells. Hormonal modulation of fatty-acid-induced transcription. *Eur. J. Biochem.* 225, 967–974. doi: 10.1111/j.1432-1033.1994.0967b.x

Sztalryd, C., and Brasaemle, D. L. (2017). The perilipin family of lipid droplet proteins: gatekeepers of intracellular lipolysis. *Biochim. Biophys. Acta Mol. Cell Biol. Lipids* 1862(10 Pt B), 1221–1232. doi: 10.1016/j.bbalip.2017.07.009

Tang, H. N., Tang, C. Y., Man, X. F., Tan, S. W., Guo, Y., Tang, J., et al. (2017). Plasticity of adipose tissue in response to fasting and refeeding in male mice. *Nutr. Metab.* 14:3. doi: 10.1186/s12986-016-0159-x

Tapper, E. B., and Parikh, N. D. (2018). Mortality due to cirrhosis and liver cancer in the United States, 1999-2016: observational study. *BMJ* 362:k2817. doi: 10.1136/bmj.k2817

Toshikuni, N., Fukumura, A., Hayashi, N., Nomura, T., Tsuchishima, M., Arisawa, T., et al. (2013). Comparison of the relationships of alcoholic and nonalcoholic fatty liver with hypertension, diabetes mellitus, and dyslipidemia. *J. Clin. Biochem. Nutr.* 52, 82–88. doi: 10.3164/jcbn.12-55

Ueno, T., Sugawara, H., Sujaku, K., Hashimoto, O., Tsuji, R., Tamaki, S., et al. (1997). Therapeutic effects of restricted diet and exercise in obese patients with fatty liver. *J. Hepatol.* 27, 103–107. doi: 10.1016/s0168-8278(97)80287-5

Vajro, P., Fontanella, A., Perna, C., Orso, G., Tedesco, M., and De Vincenzo, A. (1994). Persistent hyperaminotransferasemia resolving after weight reduction in obese children. *J. Pediatr.* 125, 239–241. doi: 10.1016/s0022-3476(94)70202-0

Wei, X., Shi, X., Zhong, W., Zhao, Y., Tang, Y., Sun, W., et al. (2013). Chronic alcohol exposure disturbs lipid homeostasis at the adipose tissue-liver axis in mice: analysis of triacylglycerols using high-resolution mass spectrometry in combination with in vivo metabolite deuterium labeling. *PLoS One* 8:e55382. doi: 10.1371/journal.pone.0055382

Wong, T., Dang, K., Ladhani, S., Singal, A. K., and Wong, R. J. (2019). Prevalence of alcoholic fatty liver disease among adults in the united states, 2001-2016. *JAMA* 321, 1723–1725. doi: 10.1001/jama.2019.2276

Yeop Han, C., Kargi, A. Y., Omer, M., Chan, C. K., Wabitsch, M., O'Brien, K. D., et al. (2010). Differential effect of saturated and unsaturated free fatty acids on the generation of monocyte adhesion and chemotactic factors by adipocytes: dissociation of adipocyte hypertrophy from inflammation. *Diabetes* 59, 386–396. doi: 10.2337/db09-0925

You, M., and Arteel, G. E. (2019). Effect of ethanol on lipid metabolism. *J. Hepatol.* 70, 237–248. doi: 10.1016/j.jhep.2018.10.037

Zhong, W., Zhao, Y., Tang, Y., Wei, X., Shi, X., Sun, W., et al. (2012). Chronic alcohol exposure stimulates adipose tissue lipolysis in mice: role of reverse triglyceride transport in the pathogenesis of alcoholic steatosis. *Am. J. Pathol.* 180, 998–1007. doi: 10.1016/j.ajpath.2011.11.017

7

Sinapic Acid Reduces Oxidative Stress and Pyroptosis via Inhibition of BRD4 in Alcoholic Liver Disease

Junyi Chu[1,2]*, Ran Yan*[1]*, Sai Wang*[1,2]*, Guoyang Li*[1,2]*, Xiaohui Kang*[2]*, Yan Hu*[1,2]*, Musen Lin*[1,2]*, Wen Shan*[1,3]*, Yan Zhao*[2]*, Zhecheng Wang*[2]*, Ruimin Sun*[2]*, Jihong Yao*[2]* *and Ning Zhang*[1]**

[1]*Department of Pharmacy, The Second Hospital of Dalian Medical University, Dalian, China,* [2]*College of Pharmacy, Dalian Medical University, Dalian, China,* [3]*Department of Pharmacy, The Third Hospital of Dalian Medical University, Dalian, China*

Correspondence:
Jihong Yao
yaojihong65@hotmail.com
Ning Zhang
zn-dl@163.com

Alcoholic liver disease (ALD) is one of the main causes of death in chronic liver disease. Oxidative stress and pyroptosis are important factors leading to ALD. Bromodomain-containing protein 4 (BRD4) is a factor that we have confirmed to regulate ALD. As a phenolic acid compound, sinapic acid (SA) has significant effects in antioxidant, anti-inflammatory and liver protection. In this study, we explored whether SA regulates oxidative stress and pyroptosis through BRD4 to play a protective effect in ALD. Male C57BL/6 mice and AML-12 cells were used for experiments. We found that SA treatment largely abolished the up-regulation of BRD4 and key proteins of the canonical pyroptosis signalling in the liver of mice fed with alcohol, while conversely enhanced the antioxidant response. Consistantly, both SA pretreatment and BRD4 knockdown inhibited oxidative stress, pyroptosis, and liver cell damage *in vitro*. More importantly, the expression levels of BRD4 and pyroptosis indicators increased significantly in ALD patients. Molecule docking analysis revealed a potent binding of SA with BRD4. In conclusion, this study demonstrates that SA reduces ALD through BRD4, which is a valuable lead compound that prevents the ALD process.

Keywords: alcoholic liver disease, sinapic acid, BRD4, oxidative stress, pyroptosis

INTRODUCTION

Long-term and excessive alcohol consumption can lead to progressive steatohepatitis and fibrosis, which further develops into liver cirrhosis and hepatocellular carcinoma. Among men, the proportion of global deaths caused by alcohol is 7.6%, among women it is 4.0%, and 139 million disability-adjusted life-years are lost due to drinking, accounting for 5.1% of the total global disease burden (Seitz et al., 2018; Singal et al., 2018). Alcohol-induced liver steatosis is initially manifested as the accumulation of small or large droplets in hepatocytes (Gao and Bataller, 2011). When alcohol continues to be overloaded, it will further aggravate liver damage, leading to inflammation, oxidative stress, and multiple pathways of programmed cell death (Rangwala et al., 2011; Ikura and Caldwell, 2015; Ma et al., 2020). Due to the complicated pathogenesis of alcohol-associated liver disease (ALD) and unclear underlying mechanism, is still there is no targeted treatment. Therefore, it is necessary to better understand the pathogenesis of ALD and develop new and safe drugs for the treatment.

Sinapic acid (SA, 4-hydroxy-3,5-dimethoxy cinnamic acid), one of the phenolic acid compounds, is the effective ingredients of traditional Chinese medicine. It is widely found in various oil crops, grains, vegetables, and berries. SA has anti-inflammatory, antioxidant, and antibacterial effects

(Chen, 2016; Huang et al., 2018; Lee, 2018; Huang et al., 2020). It has been proved that SA has a strong effect on reducing the oxidative stress of the liver and colon of rats fed high-fat diet (Yang et al., 2019) and abating the pyroptosis in diabetic atherosclerosis (Han et al., 2018). Shin et al. demonstrated that SA protected the rat liver from CCl4-induced inflammation and exhibited antifibrotic effects against DMN-induced liver injury (Shin et al., 2013b; Shin et al., 2013a). However, the efficacy of SA in prevention of alcohol-associated liver disease has not yet been studied.

Oxidative stress has been identified as a potential mechanism of ALD, which is caused by the imbalance between antioxidant capacity and reactive oxygen species (ROS) (Hsu et al., 2020). The nuclear factor-erythroid 2-related factor (Nrf2) is considered to be a cytoprotective factor, and to a certain extent it exerts anti-oxidant and anti-inflammatory effects through heme oxygenase-1 (HO-1) and their products (Loboda et al., 2016). In addition to oxidative stress, multiple forms of cell death also play the considerable role in the complicated ALD pathogenesis. Recently, pyroptosis, a new type of inflammatory programmed cell death was discovered in ALD, which also provides new ideas for the treatment of ALD (Heo et al., 2019; Kai et al., 2020).

Bromodomain-containing protein 4 (BRD4) is the most widely studied member of the bromodomain and extra terminal domain-containing (BET) protein family. Recently, we first determined that BRD4-induced inflammatory response is a split-new access for ALD (Lan et al., 2020). Studies have shown that BRD4 can be regarded as a therapeutic target in many diseases related to oxidative stress and pyroptosis, such as renal ischemia/reperfusion injury, macrophage dysfunction, acute gouty arthritis and renal cell carcinoma (Liu et al., 2019a; Hao et al., 2020; Tan et al., 2020; Zhu et al., 2020). However, the potential role of BRD4 in ALD needs to be further clarified.

In this study, we first explored whether SA can protect against ALD. Subsequently, molecular docking and biochemical evaluation were applied to verify the binding mode of SA and BRD4. It is revealed that SA targets BRD4 to alleviate the oxidative stress and pyroptosis of ALD.

MATERIALS AND METHODS

Animals and Treatments

Male C57BL/6 mice (8 weeks old) were obtained from the Animal Center of Dalian Medical University (Dalian, China). All animal procedures were performed in accordance with the Guidelines for the Care and Use of Laboratory Animals and were approved by the Institutional Ethics Committee of Dalian Medical University (Dalian, China). SA (>98% purity) and sodium carboxy methyl cellulose (CMC-Na) were separately purchased from Sigma-Aldrich (Missouri, United States) and Solarbio (Beijing, China). SA is suspended in 0.1% CMC-Na solution before use. The mice were adapted for one week before the experiment and then fed either a normal diet (control) or a Lieber-DeCarli liquid diet containing 5% ethanol (v/v) (EtOH) for 8 weeks. Liquid diets were freshly prepared before distribution. Sixty mice were equally divided into five groups, including control group, control + SA (20 mg kg^{-1} per day) group, EtOH group, and two groups of SA-treated EtOH mice that were respectively administrated (i.g.) with SA at the dosages of 10 and 20 mg kg^{-1} per day. Subsequently, blood was gathered from the abdominal aorta and liver tissues were collected for further analysis.

Human Liver Samples

Liver samples of human ALD patients were obtained from the Second Affiliated Hospital of Dalian Medical University (Dalian, China), and were handled under the approval of the Ethics Committee of Dalian Medical University. All patients signed informed consent forms. The basic biological information of controls and patients were presented in **Supplementary Table S1**.

Cell Culture and Treatment

Mouse hepatocyte cell line AML-12 cells (American Type Culture Collection (ATCC), Manassas, VA, United States) were maintained at 37 °C in a humidified atmosphere with 5% CO_2, and cultured in a 1:1 mixture of Dulbecco's modified Eagle's medium/Ham's F-12 medium (Gibco, New York, United States) containing 40 ng/ml dexamethasone, 5 μg/ml Insulin-Transferrin-Selenium (Sigma-Aldrich, Missouri, United States), and 10% fetal bovine serum (Gibco, New York, United States).

Before protein extraction, cells were pretreated with 20 μM SA for 6 h, 100 mM ethanol, or neither (control) for 24 h. Small interfering RNA (siRNA)was designed and synthesized by GenePharma (Shanghai, China). Lipofectamine 3,000 (Invitrogen) was used for transfection. The sequences of the BRD4 siRNA were as follows: sense 5′- GCCUGAGAUGAA GCCUGUATT -3′, antisense 5′- UACAGGCUUCAUCUC AGGCTT -3′. After transfection for 24 h, the cells were incubated either with or without 20 μM SA for 6 h and either with or without ethanol for 24 h. Finally, the cells were harvested and processed for protein extraction.

Cell Viability

Cell viability was quantitatively analyzed with the Cell Counting Kit-8 (CCK-8, Dojindo, Tokyo, Japan). The experiments were carried out in 96-well plates, incubated at 37 °C for 2 h, and then optical density (OD) values were measured with Thermo Multiskan FC microplate luminometerat 450 nm.

Biochemical Analysis

Alanine aminotransferase (ALT), aspartate aminotransferase (AST), total cholesterol (TC), triglyceride (TG) and alcohol dehydrogenase (ADH) levels were assayed in serum, while malondialdehyde (MDA) and glutathione (GSH) levels were determined in liver tissues by commercial kits according to the manufacturer's instructions (Nanjing Jiancheng Corp., Nanjing, China).

Histological Analysis

Isolated liver lobes were fixed in 4% paraformaldehyde at room temperature at least overnight and then embedded in paraffin for hematoxylin-eosin (H&E) or used to prepare frozen sections for Oil Red O staining. The sections were examined by light microscopy.

For immunohistochemistry, antigen retrieval was performed in a Tris/EDTA buffer (pH 9). Then, the sections were incubated with F4/80, NLRP3 or caspase-1 primary antibody (Abcam, Cambridge, United Kingdom), followed by the corresponding secondary antibody. After visualizing with 3,3-diaminobenzidine (DAB) colour-rendering solution, the sections were counterstained with hematoxylin.

Immunofluorescence Staining

Liver sections from ALD patients were incubated with anti-BRD4 primary antibody (Abcam, Cambridge, United Kingdom) overnight at 4 °C, followed by incubation with secondary antibody for 2 h at room temperature. Next, DAPI (Beyotime Institute of Biotechnology, Hangzhou, China) was used to stain nuclei.

Western Blotting

The tissues and cells were lysed in Lysis Buffer for Western with 1 mM PMSF according to the manufacturer's instructions (Beyotime, Shanghai, China). Total protein solution was separated by centrifuge at 4 °C for 10 min, and the supernatant was quantified with a BCA kit (Beyotime, Shanghai, China). Then, the supernatant was boiled for 10 min by adding loading buffer and separated by SDS-PAGE. The primary antibodies used for western blotting were as follows: BRD4, GSDMD, IL-18, Nrf2, HO-1 (all from Abcam, Cambridge, United Kingdom), caspase-1, IL-1β (both from Cell Signalling Technology, Boston, United States), NLRP3, SOD2, and *β*-actin (all from Proteintech, Wuhan, China).

Molecular Docking Assay

The BRD4 protein structure (PDB: 3P5O) was taken from the Protein Data Bank (http://www.rcsb.org/pdb). The structure sequence was analyzed by PyMOL software to remove the original ligands and water molecules. Coordinates for both the ligand (SA) and target protein (BRD4) were prepared with AutoDock Tools-1.5.6, and molecular docking analysis of ligand-protein complexes was conducted using the AutoDock4.2. The docking results are presented after mapping with Discovery Studio version4.5.

Nile Red Staining

To examine intracellular lipid accumulation, AML-12 cells were incubated with Nile red staining (Sigma, Missouri, United States). The images were observed with a fluorescence microscope.

DCFH-DA Staining

AML-12 cells were stained with 10 μM DCFH-DA staining (Sigma, Missouri, United States) for 30 min at 37 °C away from light. DCFH-DA fluorescence results were viewed using a fluorescence microscope.

Statistical Analysis

The results are expressed as the mean ± SD. GraphPad Prism (GraphPad Prism Software, CA, United States) was used to analyze the data. Student's unpaired *t*-test (two-group comparisons) and one-way ANOVA (multigroup comparisons) were executed. $p < 0.05$ was considered statistically significant.

RESULTS

SA Attenuates Chronic Alcohol-Induced Liver Injury and Steatosis

We first explored whether SA exerts a protective effect in alcohol-induced liver injury. Compared to the control, serum ALT, AST (**Figure 1A**), TC, TG (**Figure 1B**), the liver/body weight ratios (**Figure 1C**) were obviously increased after an ethanol diet, while serum ADH (**Figure 1D**) levels were decreased. SA treatment diminished the alcohol-induced liver injury in a dose-dependent manner. TNF-α mRNA levels, CYP2E1 protein expression levels and MCP-1 staining reflected the same fact (**Supplementary Figures S1A–C**). Further histology analysis by H&E staining and Oil Red O verified the effects of SA on protecting mice from alcohol-induced liver injury. The morphological and histological examination showed that the liver sizes were enlarged, the colour changed, lipid droplets accumulated in hepatocytes in the model group. SA, however, alleviated these changes and minimized the pathology. The mRNA levels of FASN, SREBP-1c, ACOX-1, and ADRP also confirmed the truth of SA regulating fatty acid metabolism (**Supplementary Figure 1D**). In addition, in immunostaining experiments, SA treatment reduced the F4/80 staining intensity of the liver of mice fed with alcohol (**Figure 1E**). These results indicate that SA effectively protects against alcohol-induced liver injury and steatosis in mice.

SA Reduces Alcohol-Induced Liver Damage by Inhibiting Oxidative Stress

Oxidative stress is a main contributor to the pathogenesis of liver damage caused by alcohol. Indeed, mice that consumed alcohol showed decreased levels of antioxidant genes including Nrf2, HO-1, and SOD2 (**Figure 2A**) and hepatic GSH (**Figure 2B**) but represented high levels of hepatic MDA (**Figure 2C**). Furthermore, SA treatment significantly reversed the alcohol-mediated downregulation of protein expressions and GSH levels, whereas caused the decrease in MDA levels. Taken together, SA regulates alcohol-associated liver damage through suppressing oxidative stress related to Nrf2/HO-1 signalling.

Alcohol-Induced Liver Damage Is Alleviated by SA Through Canonical Pyroptosis Signalling

In recent years, the key role of pyroptosis and inflammasome activation in the development of ALD has been shown by substantial evidence (Heo et al., 2019; Kai et al., 2020). Based on previous studies, the canonical pyroptosis signalling in ALD was detected. First, we examined NLRP3 inflammasome and caspase-1 expression by immunohistochemistry (IHC) staining in liver samples from ALD patients. In IHC, NLRP3 and caspase-1 staining intensities were increased in ALD patients (**Figures 3A,B**), which was further confirmed by western blot analysis in

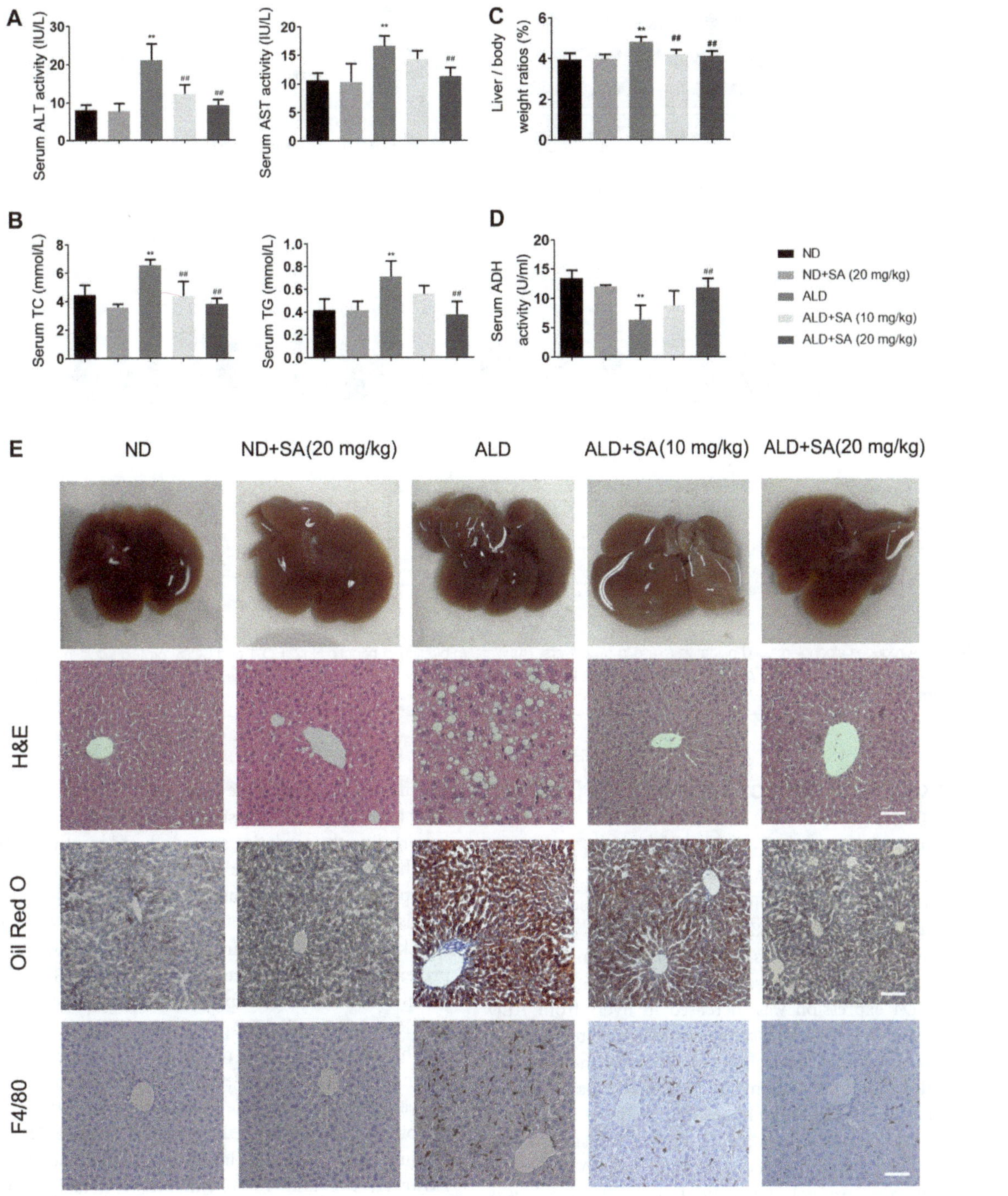

FIGURE 1 | SA diminishes alcohol-induced liver injury and steatosis in mice. **(A)** Serum levels of ALT and AST. **(B)** Serum levels of TC and TG. **(C)** Liver/body weight ratio **(D)** Serum ADH levels. The data are the mean ± SD (n = 8). **(E)** Representative morphological, H&E staining (×200), Oil Red O staining (×200) and F4/80 staining (×200) of liver sections from the different experimental groups: normal diet (ND), ND + SA (20 mg/kg), Lieber-DeCarli diet (ALD), ALD + SA (10 mg/kg), and ALD + SA (20 mg/kg). Scale bar = 50 μm $^{**}p < 0.01$ *vs* the ND group; $^{\#\#}p < 0.01$ *vs* the ALD group.

mice. The protein levels of key regulatory proteins in canonical cell pyroptosis, including NLRP3, activated caspase-1 and GSDMD were increased by ethanol and declined by SA in a dose-dependent manner. Western blot analyses also demonstrated that SA could reduce the levels of activated IL-18 and IL-1β in ALD mice, which were the substrate of caspase-1 and most commonly used pyroptosis inflammatory marker (**Figure 3C**). To sum up, the above data indicate that SA could attenuate ethanol induced pyroptosis via canonical caspase-1 pathway.

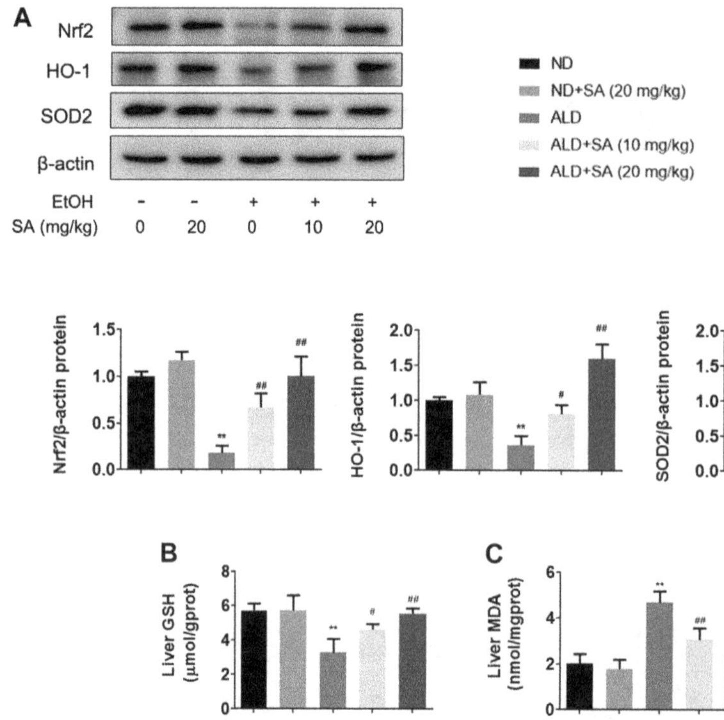

FIGURE 2 | SA reduces alcohol-induced oxidative stress in mice livers. **(A)** Western blotting of hepatic Nrf2, HO-1 and SOD2 protein levels in livers ($n = 3$). $^{**}p < 0.01$ *vs* the ND group; $^{\#}p < 0.05$, $^{\#\#}p < 0.01$ *vs* the ALD group. **(B)** Hepatic GSH levels ($n = 6$). **(C)** Hepatic MDA levels ($n = 6$). $^{**}p < 0.01$ *vs* the ND group; $^{\#}p < 0.05$, $^{\#\#}p < 0.01$ *vs* the ALD group.

The Protective Effect of SA in ALD Is Related to BRD4

Simultaneously, our previous studies have confirmed that BRD4 expression can be stimulated in ALD (Lan et al., 2020). In order to determine the biological role of BRD4 in alcohol-associated liver disease in clinical setting, BRD4 expression was compared assayed in liver biopsy samples between healthy controls and ALD patients by immunofluorescence. Consistent with previous research, BRD4 expression was increased in livers from ALD patients (**Figure 4A**). Western blotting also validated the increase of BRD4 expression levels in alcohol-exposed mice, and the dose-dependent decrease by SA treatment (**Figure 4B**). Based on the above findings, AML-12 cells were induced by EtOH for 24 h to establish the ALD model *in vitro*. AML-12 cells transfected with BRD4 siRNA, and then different concentrations of SA pretreated the cells. *In vitro* we got the same trend, 20 μM SA was determined for the following experiments (**Figure 4C**). These results indicate that BRD4 is involved in the effect of SA on ALD.

SA Prevents Alcohol-Induced Hepatocyte Injury and Steatosis Through BRD4

In AML-12 cells, after EtOH treatment, the expression of BRD4 in the cells was significantly increased, SA treatment and si-BRD4 both down-regulated the increase (**Figure 5A**). Similarly, EtOH treatment resulted the decrease of Nrf2, HO-1 and SOD2, and SA treatment upregulated the expression of Nrf2, HO-1 and SOD2. BRD4 knockdown had a similar effect as that of SA treatment in suppressing the oxidative stress induced by ethanol (**Figure 5B**). At the same time, trends of the key regulatory proteins in pyroptosis, NLRP3, caspase-1, GSDMD, IL-18 and IL-1β, were consistent with that *in vivo* experiments. Moreover, BRD4 knockdown did not further reduce the pyroptosis related proteins in AML-12 cells treated with SA (**Figure 5C**). Meanwhile, BRD4 also played a similar role in HepG2 cells and Raw 264.7 cells (**Supplementary Figures S2, 3**).

The fluorescent stain results also confirmed our hypothesis. The number of lipid droplets in the EtOH group were significantly increased observed by Nile Red staining, SA treatment and BRD4 inhibition both reduced this increase (**Figure 5D**). DCFH-DA staining also indicated increased intracellular ROS in ALD. However, SA and BRD4 inhibition notably inhibited ROS formation in ALD (**Figure 5E**). Therefore, these findings indicate that BRD4 down-regulation mediates the protective effect of SA in alcohol-induced hepatocyte injury and steatosis.

Specify Domain Interactions Between SA and BRD4

Our data suggest that SA protects alcohol-induced liver damage through BRD4 suppression, implying that SA is a BRD4-specific inhibitor. We then applied molecular docking calculation technology to study the specific binding between SA and

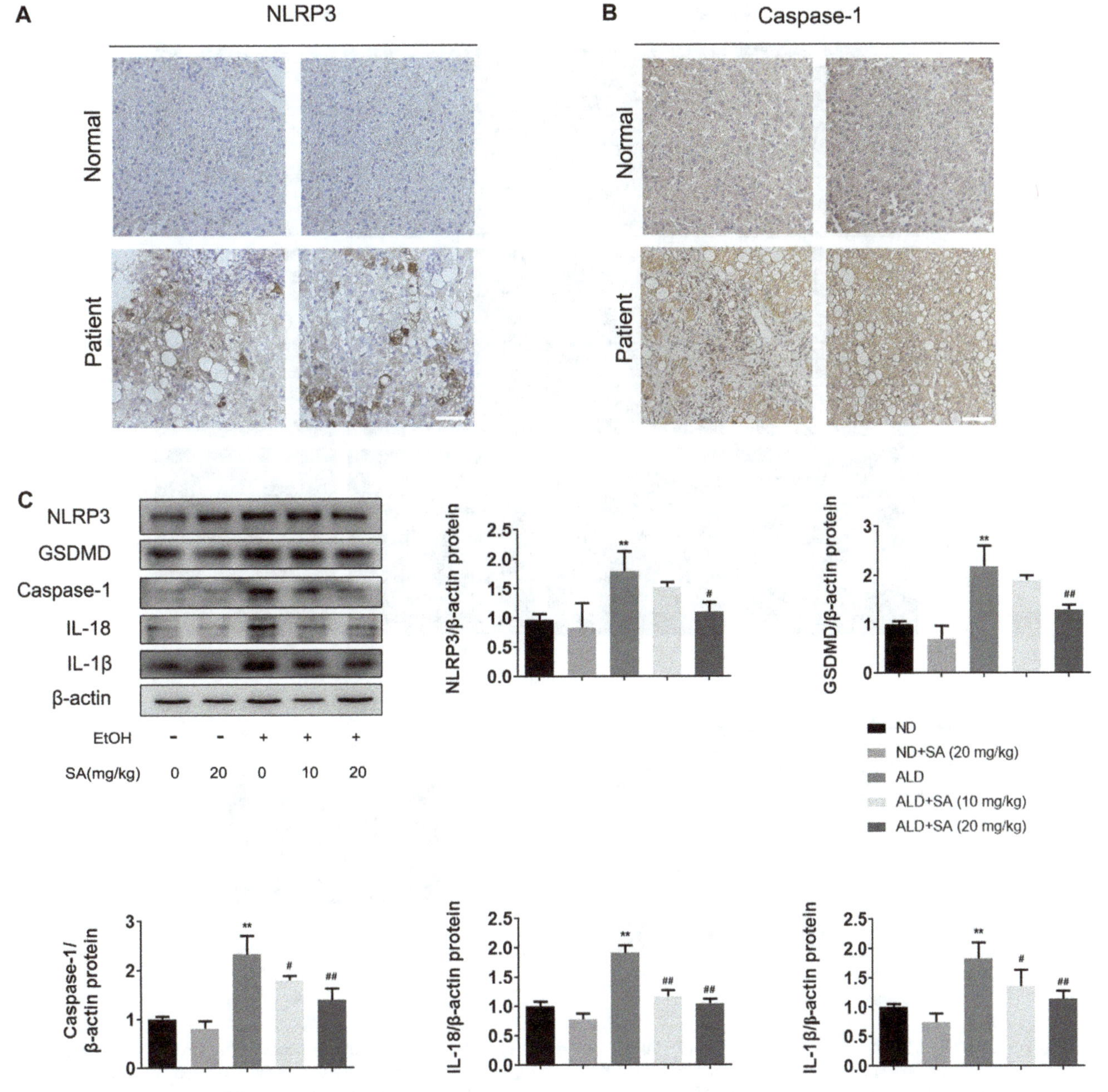

FIGURE 3 | Alcohol-induced pyroptosis is alleviated by SA **(A)** IHC staining for NLRP3 inflammasome (×200) **(B)** IHC staining for caspase-1 (×200). Scale bar = 50 μm (n = 3) **(C)** Western blotting of hepatic NLRP3, GSDMD, activated caspase-1, IL-18 and IL-1β protein levels in livers (n = 3). $^{**}p < 0.01$ *vs* the ND group; $^{\#}p < 0.05$, $^{\#\#}p < 0.01$ *vs* the ALD group.

BRD4 (**Figure 6A**). The hydrophilic -OH groups in SA formed hydrogen bonds with Asp88, Pro82 and Asn140 (**Figure 6B**). In addition to hydrogen bonds, benzene ring can form hydrophobic interactions with amino acids residues Val87, Ile146 and Cys136 through π-σ and π-alkyl interactions (**Figure 6C**). SA contacts with nearby Met132 through carbon-hydrogen bonds, and contacts with Pro86, Gln85, Trp81, Leu94, Tyr139, Tyr97, and Phe83 through van der Waals interactions (**Figure 6D**).

Consistently, research showed that most BRD4 inhibitors imitate acetyl-lysine, occupy the central hydrophobic cavity, and form hydrogen bonds with Asn140 and Tyr97 directly or indirectly. Inhibitors can also extend to the ZA ring hydrophobic region, including the Trp/Pro/Phe motif, and the ZA channel, especially Pro82 to Leu91 in BRD4 BD1 through replacing benzene ring. To sum up, the binding ability of BRD4 and SA explains the mechanism by which SA relieves alcohol-associated liver disease.

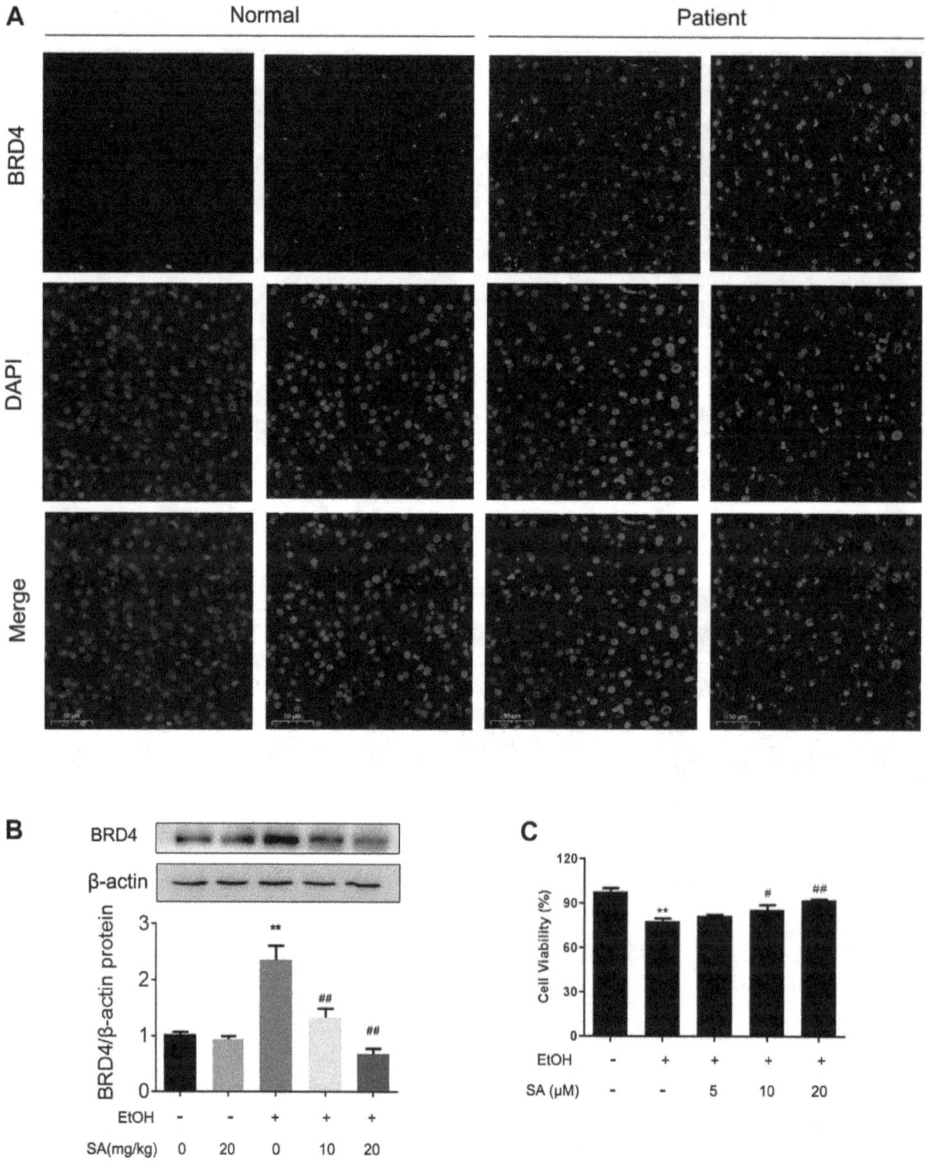

FIGURE 4 | Effects of SA on BRD4 protein level *in vivo* and *in vitro* **(A)** Immunofluorescence analysis of BRD4 protein expression in human (×200). Scale bar = 50 μm ($n = 3$). **(B)** Western blotting of hepatic BRD4 protein levels in mice ($n = 3$). $^{**}p < 0.01$ *vs* the ND group; $^{\#\#}p < 0.01$ *vs* the ALD group. **(C)** AML-12 cells were pretreated with 5, 10, or 20 μM SA for 6 h before exposure to EtOH (100 mM) for another 24 h. The viable cells were determined by the CCK8 assay. $^{**}p < 0.01$ *vs* the control group; $^{\#}p < 0.05$, $^{\#\#}p < 0.01$ *vs* the EtOH group.

DISCUSSION

The pathogenesis of ALD is complicated, involving ethanol metabolism, oxidative stress, gut microbiota imbalance, pyroptosis, lipid accumulation etc., which are widely considered to be important causes of clinical disease. Therefore, in-depth research on molecular mechanisms and effective drug treatments are necessary for the development of potential therapeutic methods. The current study presents the first attempt to demonstrate that SA contributes to the protection against ALD by reducing BRD4.

Natural compounds such as flavonoids, resveratrol, saponins, and *ß*-carotene have shown the protective effect on liver injury, through various mechanisms composed of antioxidative, anti-inflammatory, anti-apoptotic and so on (Tu et al., 2019). Our previous studies have verified that phenolic compound protocatechuic acid, salvianic acid A and salvianic acid B could reduce ALD (Zhang et al., 2017; Fu et al., 2019; Lan et al., 2020). SA is a phenolic compound commonly found in Chinese herbal medicine. In recent years, it has been reported that SA ameliorated liver disease and showed a protective effect on multiple organ diseases (Li et al., 2019; Aldubayan et al., 2020; Yun and Yang, 2020). However, whether SA treatment can relieve

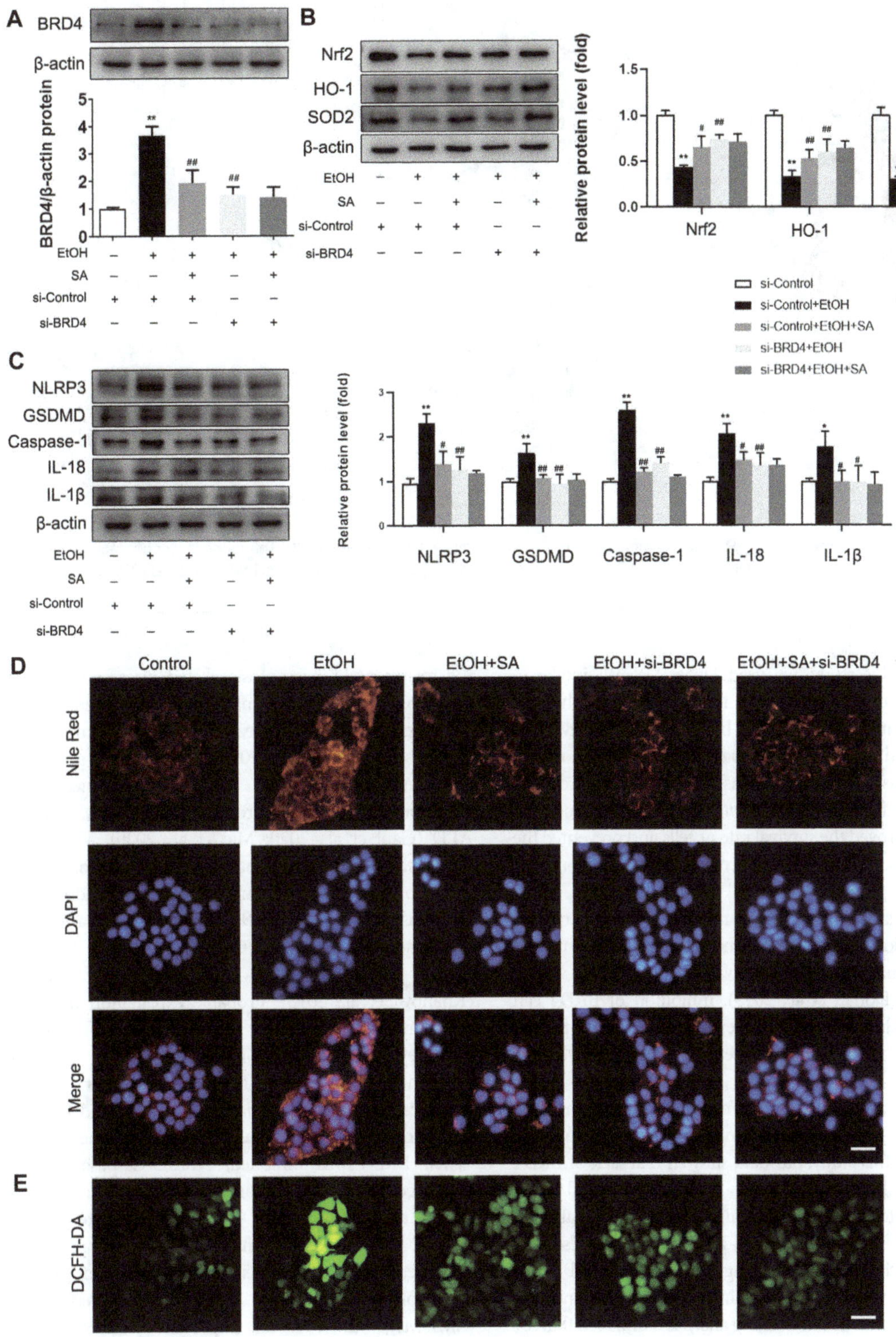

FIGURE 5 | SA ameliorates oxidative stress, pyroptosis and reduces lipid accumulation in EtOH-treated AML-12 cells by regulating BRD4. **(A)** AML-12 cells were transfected with BRD4 siRNA or control siRNA for 24 h, 20 μM SA for 6 h, before exposure to EtOH (100 mM) for 24 h or not. Expression of BRD4 was measured *in vitro* ($n = 3$). **(B)** Western blotting of Nrf2, HO-1, and SOD2 levels ($n = 3$). **(C)** Western blotting of NLRP3, GSDMD, activated caspase-1, IL-18 and IL-1β protein levels ($n = 3$). $^{*}p < 0.05$, $^{**}p < 0.01$ *vs* the control group; $^{\#}p < 0.05$, $^{\#\#}p < 0.01$ *vs* the EtOH group. **(D)** Intracellular lipid accumulation was measured by Nile Red staining (×200). Scale bar = 50 μm. **(E)** DCFH-DA staining (×200). Scale bar = 50 μm.

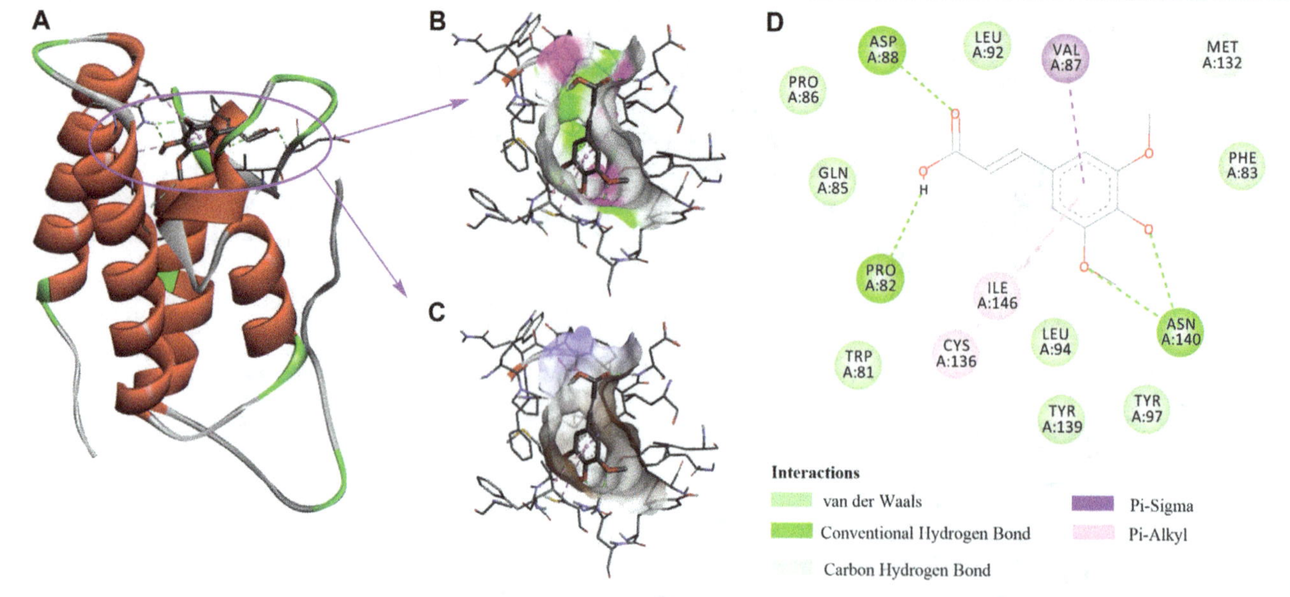

FIGURE 6 | The interactions between SA and BRD4. **(A)** 3D structure of BRD4 (PDB:3P5O) in complex with SA. **(B)** The strong hydrophilic regions are green. **(C)** The strong hydrophobic regions are orange. **(D)** The BRD4 and SA interaction network is composed of van der Waals, Hydrogen bonds, Carbon Hydrogen bond, and π-ineractions.

ALD is unclear. In this study, we used Lieber-DeCarli intake to establish an ALD model, and for the first time found that SA treatment can inhibit ALD indicated by the reduced levels of serum indicators and improved liver pathology. In addition, SA can prevent alcohol-associated liver disease by inhibiting pyroptosis and oxidative stress. Furthermore, the *in vitro* data also confirmed our above results. SA improved the survival rate of cells and prevented the progression of ALD. Therefore, we continued to explore the mechanism of SA to protect ALD.

Recent evidence shows that BRD4 not only plays a role in transcription regulation, but also has a non-transcriptional role in controlling DNA damage checkpoint activation and repair as well as telomere regulation (Donati et al., 2018). Inhibition of BRD4 can alleviate a variety of diseases, and our previous research has proved the vital role of BRD4 in chronic liver disease (Liu et al., 2019b; Hao et al., 2020; Lan et al., 2020; Tan et al., 2020; Zhu et al., 2020). Intriguingly, BRD4 could regulate the homeostasis of cardiomyocyte mitochondria and is essential for maintaining normal heart function (Kim et al., 2020). In this study, our data showed that lack of BRD4 remarkably reduced liver lipid droplets accumulation and ROS, which was similar to the results obtained after SA treatment. Therefore, we suggest that targeting BRD4 may represent a therapeutic approach for attenuating ethanol-induced liver damage. Due to strong hydrogen bonding, hydrophobic and van der Waals interactions, molecular docking analysis confirmed that SA exhibits a strong affinity for BRD4, suggesting that SA may be a promising activator by binding BRD4 in ALD.

Hepatocyte death is caused by apoptosis, necrosis, autophagy, necroptosis, pyroptosis, or the combination of its complex balance (Mazzolini et al., 2016). BRD4 positively regulates necroptosis through modulating the necroptosis executor mixed-lineage kinase domain-like (MLKL) expression and BET inhibitors have potential in the treatment of necroptosis-related diseases (Xiong et al., 2019). Pyroptosis leads to the formation of pores in the plasma membrane, cell swelling and the release of pro-inflammatory cell contents (Jorgensen and Miao, 2015). Hepatocyte pyroptosis and the inflammasome activation are also new mechanisms for the development of liver fibrosis, non-alcoholic steatohepatitis and ALD (Gaul et al., 2020; Mai et al., 2020). Moreover, Heo et al. has revealed ethanol promotes the overexpression of TXNIP and the activation of NLRP3 inflammasome, thereby inducing canonical cell pyroptosis (Heo et al., 2019), whereas Khanova et al. reported that non-canonical caspase-11/GSDMD pathway but not canonical caspase-1/IL-1β pathway is activated in alcoholic hepatitis (Khanova et al., 2018). Probable explanation may be due to the above-mentioned unclear boundary from chronic alcoholic steatohepatitis to alcoholic hepatitis and the differences in experimental conditions. In this study, our data showed that canonical pyroptosis pathway exist in our model, and the patient's immunohistochemical results are also in line with expectations. When BRD4 was inhibited, NLRP3/Caspase-1/GSDMD are all decreased, which is similar to the previous study: JQ1 inhibits BRD4 and reduces the LPS-induced acute colon injury by NLRP3/ASC/Caspase-1 inflammatory pyroptosis composition (Chen et al., 2021). Of interest, BRD4 might not participate in the activation of NLRP3 in bone marrow–derived macrophages (BMDMs), but it is an important regulator for the NLRC4 inflammasome activation in response to *S. typhimurium* infection. This is possibly due to BRD4 selectively activates a subset of NF-κB target genes (Dong et al., 2021). Nevertheless, the precise molecular mechanisms by which BRD4 promotes pyroptosis in ALD remain as an interesting open question, which is worthy of further investigation.

Oxidative stress is a process in which organisms or cells produce excessive ROS and then destroy proteins and DNA (S Narasimhan et al., 2020). Studies have shown that oxidative stress is inseparable from the pathogenesis of both acute and chronic ALD, and Nrf2/HO-1 signalling pathway takes part in oxidation resistance process. The liver protein expression of Nrf2 in ALD mice is significantly reduced (Wang et al., 2020). Similarly, ethanol administration can lead to decreased Nrf2 and HO-1 expression in livers from both chronic and acute model (Zeng et al., 2017). Interestingly, the liver expression of HO-1 in acute alcoholic liver damage may also increase in the short term (Liu et al., 2019a). In our current research, BRD4 expression as determined by western blot was increased in ALD and was greatly reduced by antioxidant SA treatment. Here we also showed that BRD4 inhibited oxidative stress in ALD, and the level of anti-oxidative stress increased after knocking down BRD4. It has been shown that NADPH oxidase 4 (Nox4) is downregulated in idiopathic pulmonary fibrosis myofibroblasts by Brd4 inhibition, (Sanders et al., 2020). In addition, BRD4 could directly associates to chromatin regulatory regions of the NADPH oxidase subunits and BET inhibitors dramatically reduces oxidative stress and ameliorates skeletal muscle homeostasis and muscle function (Segatto et al., 2020). However, additional molecular pathways involved in BRD4 anti-oxidant functions cannot be excluded, which deserves further study.

In aggregate, our results demonstrated for the first time that SA could be a promising therapeutic agent for ALD via BRD4, which reduces oxidative stress and pyroptosis. This study may provide a new strategy for the treatment of alcohol-associated liver disease.

AUTHOR CONTRIBUTIONS

JC, RY, JY and NZ designed the study. JC, RY, SW, GL, XK, YH, ML and WS performed the study. JC, YZ, ZW and RS analyzed the data. JC drafted the article.

REFERENCES

Aldubayan, M. A., Ahmed, A. S., Emara, A. M., Ahmed, A. A., and Elgharabawy, R. M. (2020). Sinapic Acid Attenuates Cardiovascular Disorders in Rats by Modulating Reactive Oxygen Species and Angiotensin Receptor Expression. *Oxidative Med. Cell Longevity* 2020, 1–14. doi:10.1155/2020/1436858

Chen, C. (2016). Sinapic Acid and Its Derivatives as Medicine in Oxidative Stress-Induced Diseases and Aging. *Oxidative Med. Cell Longevity* 2016, 1–10. doi:10.1155/2016/3571614

Chen, L., Zhong, X., Cao, W., Mao, M., Li, W., Yang, H., et al. (2021). JQ1 as a BRD4 Inhibitor Blocks Inflammatory Pyroptosis-Related Acute Colon Injury Induced by LPS. *Front. Immunol.* 12, 609319. doi:10.3389/fimmu.2021.609319

Donati, B., Lorenzini, E., and Ciarrocchi, A. (2018). BRD4 and Cancer: Going beyond Transcriptional Regulation. *Mol. Cancer* 17 (1), 164. doi:10.1186/s12943-018-0915-9

Dong, X., Hu, X., Bao, Y., Li, G., Yang, X.-d., Slauch, J. M., et al. (2021). Brd4 Regulates NLRC4 Inflammasome Activation by Facilitating IRF8-Mediated Transcription of Naips. *J. Cel Biol* 220 (3), e202005148. doi:10.1083/jcb.202005148

Fu, R., Zhou, J., Wang, R., Sun, R., Feng, D., Wang, Z., et al. (2019). Protocatechuic Acid-Mediated miR-219a-5p Activation Inhibits the P66shc Oxidant Pathway to Alleviate Alcoholic Liver Injury. *Oxidative Med. Cell Longevity* 2019, 1–15. doi:10.1155/2019/3527809

Gao, B., and Bataller, R. (2011). Alcoholic Liver Disease: Pathogenesis and New Therapeutic Targets. *Gastroenterology* 141 (5), 1572–1585. doi:10.1053/j.gastro.2011.09.002

Gaul, S., Leszczynska, A., Alegre, F., Kaufmann, B., Johnson, C. D., Adams, L. A., et al. (2021). Hepatocyte Pyroptosis and Release of Inflammasome Particles Induce Stellate Cell Activation and Liver Fibrosis. *J. Hepatol.* 74, 156–167. doi:10.1016/j.jhep.2020.07.041

Han, Y., Qiu, H., Pei, X., Fan, Y., Tian, H., and Geng, J. (2018). Low-dose Sinapic Acid Abates the Pyroptosis of Macrophages by Downregulation of lncRNA-MALAT1 in Rats With Diabetic Atherosclerosis. *J. Cardiovasc. Pharmacol.* 71 (2), 104–112. doi:10.1097/fjc.0000000000000550

Hao, K., Jiang, W., Zhou, M., Li, H., Chen, Y., Jiang, F., et al. (2020). Targeting BRD4 Prevents Acute Gouty Arthritis by Regulating Pyroptosis. *Int. J. Biol. Sci.* 16 (16), 3163–3173. doi:10.7150/ijbs.46153

Heo, M. J., Kim, T. H., You, J. S., Blaya, D., Sancho-Bru, P., and Kim, S. G. (2019). Alcohol Dysregulates miR-148a in Hepatocytes through FoxO1, Facilitating Pyroptosis via TXNIP Overexpression. *Gut* 68 (4), 708–720. doi:10.1136/gutjnl-2017-315123

Hsu, M.-F., Koike, S., Mello, A., Nagy, L. E., and Haj, F. G. (2020). Hepatic Protein-Tyrosine Phosphatase 1B Disruption and Pharmacological Inhibition Attenuate Ethanol-Induced Oxidative Stress and Ameliorate Alcoholic Liver Disease in Mice. *Redox Biol.* 36, 101658. doi:10.1016/j.redox.2020.101658

Huang, J.-F., Zheng, X.-Q., Lin, J.-L., Zhang, K., Tian, H.-J., Zhou, W.-X., et al. (2020). Sinapic Acid Inhibits IL-1β-Induced Apoptosis and Catabolism in Nucleus Pulposus Cells and Ameliorates Intervertebral Disk Degeneration. *Jir* 13, 883–895. doi:10.2147/jir.S278556

Huang, X., Pan, Q., Mao, Z., Zhang, R., Ma, X., Xi, Y., et al. (2018). Sinapic Acid Inhibits the IL-1β-Induced Inflammation via MAPK Downregulation in Rat Chondrocytes. *Inflammation* 41 (2), 562–568. doi:10.1007/s10753-017-0712-4

Ikura, Y., and Caldwell, S. H. (2015). Lipid Droplet-Associated Proteins in Alcoholic Liver Disease: a Potential Linkage with Hepatocellular Damage. *Int. J. Clin. Exp. Pathol.* 8 (8), 8699–8708.

Jorgensen, I., and Miao, E. A. (2015). Pyroptotic Cell Death Defends against Intracellular Pathogens. *Immunol. Rev.* 265 (1), 130–142. doi:10.1111/imr.12287

Kai, J., Yang, X., Wang, Z., Wang, F., Jia, Y., Wang, S., et al. (2020). Oroxylin a Promotes PGC-1α/Mfn2 Signaling to Attenuate Hepatocyte Pyroptosis via Blocking Mitochondrial ROS in Alcoholic Liver Disease. *Free Radic. Biol. Med.* 153, 89–102. doi:10.1016/j.freeradbiomed.2020.03.031

Khanova, E., Wu, R., Wang, W., Yan, R., Chen, Y., French, S. W., et al. (2018). Pyroptosis by Caspase11/4-Gasdermin-D Pathway in Alcoholic Hepatitis in Mice and Patients. *Hepatology* 67 (5), 1737–1753. doi:10.1002/hep.29645

Kim, S. Y., Zhang, X., Schiattarella, G. G., Altamirano, F., Ramos, T. A. R., French, K. M., et al. (2020). Epigenetic Reader BRD4 (Bromodomain-Containing Protein 4) Governs Nucleus-Encoded Mitochondrial Transcriptome to Regulate Cardiac Function. *Circulation* 142, 2356–2370. doi:10.1161/circulationaha.120.047239

Lan, Y., Yan, R., Shan, W., Chu, J., Sun, R., Wang, R., et al. (2020). Salvianic Acid A Alleviates Chronic Alcoholic Liver Disease by Inhibiting HMGB1 Translocation via Down-regulating BRD4. *J. Cel Mol Med* 24 (15), 8518–8531. doi:10.1111/jcmm.15473

Lee, J.-Y. (2018). Anti-inflammatory Effects of Sinapic Acid on 2,4,6-trinitrobenzenesulfonic Acid-Induced Colitis in Mice. *Arch. Pharm. Res.* 41 (2), 243–250. doi:10.1007/s12272-018-1006-6

Li, X., Lin, J., Ding, X., Xuan, J., Hu, Z., Wu, D., et al. (2019). The Protective Effect of Sinapic Acid in Osteoarthritis: *In Vitro* and *In Vivo* Studies. *J. Cel Mol Med* 23 (3), 1940–1950. doi:10.1111/jcmm.14096

Liu, H., Wang, L., Weng, X., Chen, H., Du, Y., Diao, C., et al. (2019a). Inhibition of Brd4 Alleviates Renal Ischemia/reperfusion Injury-Induced Apoptosis and Endoplasmic Reticulum Stress by Blocking FoxO4-Mediated Oxidative Stress. *Redox Biol.* 24, 101195. doi:10.1016/j.redox.2019.101195

Liu, X., Wang, Y., Wu, D., Li, S., Wang, C., Han, Z., et al. (2019b). Magnolol Prevents Acute Alcoholic Liver Damage by Activating PI3K/Nrf2/PPARγ and Inhibiting NLRP3 Signaling Pathway. *Front. Pharmacol.* 10, 1459. doi:10.3389/fphar.2019.01459

Loboda, A., Damulewicz, M., Pyza, E., Jozkowicz, A., and Dulak, J. (2016). Role of Nrf2/HO-1 System in Development, Oxidative Stress Response and Diseases: an Evolutionarily Conserved Mechanism. *Cell. Mol. Life Sci.* 73 (17), 3221 3247. doi:10.1007/s00018-016-2223-0

Ma, X.-y., Zhang, M., Fang, G., Cheng, C.-j., Wang, M.-k., Han, Y.-m., et al. (2020). Ursolic Acid Reduces Hepatocellular Apoptosis and Alleviates Alcohol-

Induced Liver Injury via Irreversible Inhibition of CASP3 *In Vivo*. *Acta Pharmacol. Sin.* doi:10.1038/s41401-020-00534-y

Mai, W., Xu, Y., Xu, J., Zhao, D., Ye, L., Yu, G., et al. (2020). Berberine Inhibits Nod-like Receptor Family Pyrin Domain Containing 3 Inflammasome Activation and Pyroptosis in Nonalcoholic Steatohepatitis via the ROS/TXNIP Axis. *Front. Pharmacol.* 11, 185. doi:10.3389/fphar.2020.00185

Mazzolini, G., Sowa, J.-P., and Canbay, A. (2016). Cell Death Mechanisms in Human Chronic Liver Diseases: a Far Cry from Clinical Applicability. *Clin. Sci. (Lond)* 130 (23), 2121–2138. doi:10.1042/cs20160035

Rangwala, F., Guy, C. D., Lu, J., Suzuki, A., Burchette, J. L., Abdelmalek, M. F., et al. (2011). Increased Production of Sonic Hedgehog by Ballooned Hepatocytes. *J. Pathol.* 224 (3), 401–410. doi:10.1002/path.2888

S Narasimhan, K. K., Devarajan, A., Karan, G., Sundaram, S., Wang, Q., van Groen, T., et al. (2020). Reductive Stress Promotes Protein Aggregation and Impairs Neurogenesis. *Redox Biol.* 37, 101739. doi:10.1016/j.redox.2020.101739

Sanders, Y. Y., Lyv, X., Zhou, Q. J., Xiang, Z., Stanford, D., Bodduluri, S., et al. (2020). Brd4-p300 Inhibition Downregulates Nox4 and Accelerates Lung Fibrosis Resolution in Aged Mice. *JCI Insight* 5 (14). doi:10.1172/jci.insight.137127

Segatto, M., Szokoll, R., Fittipaldi, R., Bottino, C., Nevi, L., Mamchaoui, K., et al. (2020). BETs Inhibition Attenuates Oxidative Stress and Preserves Muscle Integrity in Duchenne Muscular Dystrophy. *Nat. Commun.* 11 (1), 6108. doi:10.1038/s41467-020-19839-x

Seitz, H. K., Bataller, R., Cortez-Pinto, H., Gao, B., Gual, A., Lackner, C., et al. (2018). Alcoholic Liver Disease. *Nat. Rev. Dis. Primers* 4 (1), 16. doi:10.1038/s41572-018-0014-7

Shin, D.-S., Kim, K. W., Chung, H. Y., Yoon, S., and Moon, J.-O. (2013a). Effect of Sinapic Acid against Carbon Tetrachloride-Induced Acute Hepatic Injury in Rats. *Arch. Pharm. Res.* 36 (5), 626–633. doi:10.1007/s12272-013-0050-5

Shin, D.-S., Kim, K. W., Chung, H. Y., Yoon, S., and Moon, J.-O. (2013b). Effect of Sinapic Acid against Dimethylnitrosamine-Induced Hepatic Fibrosis in Rats. *Arch. Pharm. Res.* 36 (5), 608–618. doi:10.1007/s12272-013-0033-6

Singal, A. K., Bataller, R., Ahn, J., Kamath, P. S., and Shah, V. H. (2018). ACG Clinical Guideline: Alcoholic Liver Disease. *Am. J. Gastroenterol.* 113 (2), 175–194. doi:10.1038/ajg.2017.469

Tan, Y.-F., Wang, M., Chen, Z.-Y., Wang, L., and Liu, X.-H. (2020). Inhibition of BRD4 Prevents Proliferation and Epithelial-Mesenchymal Transition in Renal Cell Carcinoma via NLRP3 Inflammasome-Induced Pyroptosis. *Cell Death Dis* 11 (4), 239. doi:10.1038/s41419-020-2431-2

Tu, Y., Zhu, S., Wang, J., Burstein, E., and Jia, D. (2019). Natural Compounds in the Chemoprevention of Alcoholic Liver Disease. *Phytotherapy Res.* 33 (9), 2192–2212. doi:10.1002/ptr.6410

Wang, C., Zheng, L., Liu, S., Guo, X., Qu, Y., Gao, M., et al. (2020). A Novel Acidic Polysaccharide from the Residue of Panax Notoginseng and its Hepatoprotective Effect on Alcoholic Liver Damage in Mice. *Int. J. Biol. Macromolecules* 149, 1084–1097. doi:10.1016/j.ijbiomac.2020.02.034

Xiong, Y., Li, L., Zhang, L., Cui, Y., Wu, C., Li, H., et al. (2019). The Bromodomain Protein BRD4 Positively Regulates Necroptosis via Modulating MLKL Expression. *Cell Death Differ* 26 (10), 1929–1941. doi:10.1038/s41418-018-0262-9

Yang, C., Deng, Q., Xu, J., Wang, X., Hu, C., Tang, H., et al. (2019). Sinapic Acid and Resveratrol Alleviate Oxidative Stress with Modulation of Gut Microbiota in High-Fat Diet-Fed Rats. *Food Res. Int.* 116, 1202–1211. doi:10.1016/j.foodres.2018.10.003

Yun, U. J., and Yang, D. K. (2020). Sinapic Acid Inhibits Cardiac Hypertrophy via Activation of Mitochondrial Sirt3/SOD2 Signaling in Neonatal Rat Cardiomyocytes. *Antioxidants* 9 (11), 1163. doi:10.3390/antiox9111163

Zeng, X., Li, X., Xu, C., Jiang, F., Mo, Y., Fan, X., et al. (2017). Schisandra Sphenanthera Extract (Wuzhi Tablet) Protects against Chronic-Binge and Acute Alcohol-Induced Liver Injury by Regulating the NRF2-ARE Pathway in Mice. *Acta Pharmaceutica. Sinica. B* 7 (5), 583–592. doi:10.1016/j.apsb.2017.04.002

Zhang, N., Hu, Y., Ding, C., Zeng, W., Shan, W., Fan, H., et al. (2017). Salvianolic Acid B Protects against Chronic Alcoholic Liver Injury via SIRT1-Mediated Inhibition of CRP and ChREBP in Rats. *Toxicol. Lett.* 267, 1–10. doi:10.1016/j.toxlet.2016.12.010

Zhu, F., Xiong, F., He, J., Liu, K., You, Y., Xu, Q., et al. (2020). Brd4 Inhibition Ameliorates Pyocyanin-Mediated Macrophage Dysfunction via Transcriptional Repression of Reactive Oxygen and Nitrogen Free Radical Pathways. *Cel Death Dis* 11 (6), 459. doi:10.1038/s41419-020-2672-0

8

Alcohol and Liver Clock Disruption Increase Small Droplet Macrosteatosis, Alter Lipid Metabolism and Clock Gene mRNA Rhythms and Remodel the Triglyceride Lipidome in Mouse Liver

*Jennifer A. Valcin[1], Uduak S. Udoh[1], Telisha M. Swain[1], Kelly K. Andringa[2], Chirag R. Patel[3], Sameer Al Diffalha[3], Paul R. S. Baker[4], Karen L. Gamble[5] and Shannon M. Bailey[1]**

[1]Division of Molecular and Cellular Pathology, Department of Pathology, University of Alabama at Birmingham, Birmingham, AL, United States, [2]Division of Nephrology, Department of Medicine, University of Alabama at Birmingham, Birmingham, AL, United States, [3]Division of Anatomic Pathology, Department of Pathology, University of Alabama at Birmingham, Birmingham, AL, United States, [4]Avanti Polar Lipids, Inc., Alabaster, AL, United States, [5]Department of Psychiatry and Behavioral Neurobiology, University of Alabama at Birmingham, Birmingham, AL, United States

***Correspondence:**
Shannon M. Bailey
shannonbailey@uabmc.edu

Heavy alcohol drinking dysregulates lipid metabolism, promoting hepatic steatosis – the first stage of alcohol-related liver disease (ALD). The molecular circadian clock plays a major role in synchronizing daily rhythms in behavior and metabolism and clock disruption can cause pathology, including liver disease. Previous studies indicate that alcohol consumption alters liver clock function, but the impact alcohol or clock disruption, or both have on the temporal control of hepatic lipid metabolism and injury remains unclear. Here, we undertook studies to determine whether genetic disruption of the liver clock exacerbates alterations in lipid metabolism and worsens steatosis in alcohol-fed mice. To address this question, male liver-specific *Bmal1* knockout (LKO) and flox/flox (Fl/Fl) control mice were fed a control or alcohol-containing diet for 5 weeks. Alcohol significantly dampened diurnal rhythms of mRNA levels in clock genes *Bmal1* and *Dbp*, phase advanced *Nr1d1*/REV-ERBα, and induced arrhythmicity in *Clock*, *Noct*, and *Nfil3*/E4BP4, with further disruption in livers of LKO mice. Alcohol-fed LKO mice exhibited higher plasma triglyceride (TG) and different time-of-day patterns of hepatic TG and macrosteatosis, with elevated levels of small droplet macrosteatosis compared to alcohol-fed Fl/Fl mice. Diurnal rhythms in mRNA levels of lipid metabolism transcription factors (*Srebf1*, *Nr1h2*, and *Ppara*) were significantly altered by alcohol and clock disruption. Alcohol and/or clock disruption significantly altered diurnal rhythms in mRNA levels of fatty acid (FA) synthesis and oxidation (*Acaca/b*, *Mlycd*, *Cpt1a*, *Fasn*, *Elovl5/6*, and *Fads1/2*), TG turnover (*Gpat1*, *Agpat1/2*, *Lpin1/2*, *Dgat2*, and *Pnpla2/3*), and lipid droplet (*Plin2/5*, *Lipe*, *Mgll*, and *Abdh5*) genes, along with protein abundances of p-ACC, MCD, and FASN. Lipidomics analyses showed that alcohol, clock disruption, or both significantly altered FA saturation and remodeled the FA composition of the hepatic TG pool, with higher percentages of several long and very long chain FA in livers of alcohol-fed LKO mice. In conclusion, these results show that the liver clock is important for maintaining temporal control of hepatic lipid metabolism and that disrupting the liver clock exacerbates alcohol-related hepatic steatosis.

Keywords: liver, alcohol, circadian clock, BMAL1, steatosis, triglyceride, fatty acid, lipidomics

INTRODUCTION

Alcohol use is a top 10 cause of preventable death in the United States, with alcohol-related liver disease (ALD) the number one cause of death from excessive alcohol consumption (Minino et al., 2006; Danaei et al., 2009). Hepatic steatosis, the accumulation of triglyceride (TG)-rich lipid droplets in the cytosol of hepatocytes, is the first response that occurs in the liver following heavy alcohol drinking. Alcohol metabolism increases the hepatic NADH/NAD$^+$ ratio (Bailey and Cunningham, 1998), which inhibits mitochondrial fatty acid oxidation (FAO; Cederbaum et al., 1975; Salaspuro et al., 1981) and increases *de novo* lipogenesis (You and Arteel, 2019). Moreover, alcohol impacts lipid metabolism at the transcriptional level by affecting SREBP-1c (You et al., 2002), PPARα and γ (Abdelmegeed et al., 2011; Zhang et al., 2016b, 2018), and LXR-mediated pathways (Sengupta et al., 2018). Alcohol also impairs lipid droplet turnover and lipophagy, which contribute to the development of hepatic steatosis (Orlicky et al., 2011; Carr et al., 2013; Yang et al., 2019). Steatosis is recognized as a crucial first step in the initiation and progression of ALD by sensitizing hepatocytes to additional metabolic stressors, leading to cell death and disease (Spach et al., 1991; Jou et al., 2008; Zelickson et al., 2011).

Steatosis is divided into two types - macrosteatosis and microsteatosis. Macrosteatosis is characterized by the presence of large lipid droplets, whereas microsteatosis is characterized by the presence of many tiny cytosolic lipid droplets giving hepatocytes a foamy-like appearance (Brunt, 2007; Yeh and Brunt, 2014). Macrosteatosis occurs with acute and chronic alcohol consumption in humans and experimental animal models (Sakhuja, 2014). In contrast, microsteatosis is more rare and observed during severe clinical situations, such as acute fatty liver of pregnancy (Brady, 2020), Reyes syndrome in children (Glasgow and Middleton, 2001), and drug-induced hepatotoxicity (Begriche et al., 2011) in response to significant mitochondrial damage and impaired FAO (Fromenty and Pessayre, 1995; Fromenty and Pessayre, 1997). Microsteatosis is also found in ALD patients, but is uncommon (Theise, 2013). Recent guidelines suggest that macrosteatosis be classified as a mixture of large and small lipid droplets. In small droplet macrosteatosis, smaller droplets of varying sizes are present in the cytosol with the nucleus remaining in the center of hepatocytes. On the other hand, in large droplet macrosteatosis, the nucleus is displaced to one side of the cell by a large unilocular lipid droplet (Mostafa et al., 2020). As highlighted by Mostafa et al. (2020), this classification is highly important as small droplet macrosteatosis is commonly mistaken for microsteatosis by researchers. Importantly, the molecular events underpinning these different steatosis phenotypes and their pathological significance are poorly understood. One possible reason for this is that there are still large gaps in knowledge regarding lipid metabolism, including an incomplete understanding regarding how alcohol affects diurnal regulation of lipid metabolism, including effects on the molecular circadian clock, a key regulator of metabolism (Filiano et al., 2013; Zhou et al., 2014; Zhang et al., 2018).

Biological circadian rhythms are regulated by interactions of multiple inputs from sources that are external (light/dark and feeding/fasting cycles) and internal (molecular clock). The clock is a hierarchal system comprised of molecular oscillators found throughout the body that synchronize daily rhythms in behavior, metabolism, and physiology to maintain normal organ function and overall whole body health (Bailey et al., 2014; Takahashi, 2017; Koronowski et al., 2019). Circadian rhythms are generated at the molecular level by a system of transcriptional-translational feedback loops. In the first loop, the transcription factors brain and muscle ARNT-like 1 (BMAL1) and circadian locomotor output cycles kaput (CLOCK) hetero-dimerize and bind to gene promoter E-box motifs to activate transcription of *Period 1*, *2*, or *3* (*Per1–3*) and *Cryptochrome 1* or *2* (*Cry1–2*) genes, whose protein products (PER1–3, CRY1–2) feedback to inhibit BMAL1-CLOCK and their own transcription (Ko and Takahashi, 2006). A second feedback loop is formed by the retinoid-related orphan receptors (ROR) and nuclear receptor subfamily 1 group D members 1 and 2 (NR1D1 and 2; a.k.a., REV-ERBα and β), which activate and inhibit *Bmal1* transcription, respectively (Preitner et al., 2002; Sato et al., 2004). BMAL1-CLOCK also drives diurnal rhythms in mRNA levels of numerous non-clock and metabolic genes in the liver, e.g., approximately 10% of transcripts oscillate in a BMAL1-dependent manner in livers of normal wild-type mice (Koronowski et al., 2019).

Disruption in circadian clocks and their metabolic and functional outputs lead to pathology. For example, whole-body *Bmal1* knockout mice and *Clock*$^{\Delta19/\Delta19}$ mutant mice have severe dyslipidemia (Turek et al., 2005; Shimba et al., 2011). Altered lipid and cholesterol metabolism also occur in mice with liver-specific deletion of *Bmal1* and *Nr1d1*/REV-ERBα (Bugge et al., 2012; Cho et al., 2012; Zhang et al., 2014). Both genetic (*Clock*$^{\Delta19/\Delta19}$ mice) and environmental (chronic phase shifts of the light/dark cycle) circadian disruption exacerbate alcohol-related pathologies, including increased intestinal permeability and hepatic inflammation (Summa et al., 2013; Voigt et al., 2016). Similarly, we have reported that liver clock disruption (by *Bmal1* deletion in hepatocytes) significantly disrupts 24 h rhythms in mRNA levels of glycogen and glucose metabolism genes and glycogen content in livers of alcohol-fed mice (Udoh et al., 2017). Based on this, we hypothesized that genetic disruption of the liver clock would exacerbate alcohol-related impairments in lipid metabolism and worsen steatosis in the liver. To test this hypothesis, we determined clock and lipid metabolism mRNA levels, hepatic and plasma TG levels, liver injury, and the fatty acid (FA) profile of the hepatic TG pool, i.e., TG lipidome, in mice with liver-specific knockout of *Bmal1* fed a control or alcohol-containing diet.

MATERIALS AND METHODS

Chronic Alcohol Feeding Procedure

Eight to ten week old male liver-specific *Bmal1* knockout mice (LKO mice: $Alb^{Cre+/-}$; $Bmal1^{Fl/Fl}$) and control littermates (Fl/Fl mice: $Alb^{Cre-/-}$; $Bmal1^{Fl/Fl}$) on a C57BL/6J background were weight-matched into pairs and then assigned into a control or alcohol (ethanol) diet feeding group as described in our previous study (Udoh et al., 2017). Mice were pair-fed iso-caloric (1 kcal/ml) liquid diets (control diet: F1259SP and ethanol diet: F1258SP) from Bio-Serv (Frenchtown, NJ; Filiano et al., 2013). Mice in the alcohol-fed group were acclimated to the diet by gradually increasing the concentration of alcohol in the diet from 0 to 3% (w/v) over a 1 week period and maintained at this level for 4 weeks (Udoh et al., 2017). This concentration of alcohol (3%, w/v) in the diet is equivalent to 22% total daily caloric intake. This alcohol-feeding protocol is widely used and well accepted as a model of the earliest stage of ALD - hepatic steatosis (Lieber et al., 1989; Brandon-Warner et al., 2012). Mice were single-housed in standard cages with bedding and kept in a temperature-, humidity-, and light-controlled room with a 12-h light:12-h dark (12-h L:D) schedule. The amount of liquid diet consumed by each mouse was measured every 24 h with diets replaced daily between zeitgeber time (ZT) 10–12 (ZT 0 = beginning of lights on/inactive period and ZT 12 = beginning of lights off/active period). At the end of the feeding study, mice were euthanized by decapitation every 4 h at ZT 3, 7, 11, 15, 19, and 23. During the dark period (ZT 12–24), an infrared viewer was used for tissue collection at ZT 15, 19, and 23 with photic input to the suprachiasmatic nucleus (SCN) prevented by removing the eyes prior to light exposure (Filiano et al., 2013). Blood was collected in EDTA-treated tubes and placed on ice before centrifugation to obtain plasma. Livers were quickly divided into portions and placed into liquid nitrogen, RNA*later*™ stabilization solution (Invitrogen, Carlsbad, CA), or 10% buffered formalin. All procedures were approved by the UAB IACUC and compliant with the NIH Guide for the Care and Use of Laboratory Animals (8th ed., National Academy of Sciences, 2011).

RNA Isolation and Real Time-PCR

Total RNA was isolated from liver using TRI-Reagent® (Sigma-Aldrich, St. Louis, MO). Isolated RNA was DNase treated with DNA-*free*™ DNase Treatment and Removal Reagents (Thermo Fisher Scientific, Waltham, MA) and the DNase-treated RNA (260/280 ratio > 1.8) was converted to cDNA using the High-Capacity cDNA Reverse Transcription Kit (Thermo Fisher Scientific, Waltham, MA). Measurements of mRNA levels were done by Real Time PCR (RT-PCR) using commercially available gene-specific TaqMan™ primers from Thermo Fisher Scientific (Waltham, MA) with either an Applied Biosystems 7900HT Real-time PCR or QuantStudio6 Flex Real-time PCR system (Thermo Fisher Scientific, Waltham, MA). Relative levels of mRNA for each gene were determined using the $\Delta\Delta$Ct method (Livak and Schmittgen, 2001) with values normalized to either glyceraldehyde-3-phosphate dehydrogenase (*Gapdh*) or peptidyl-prolyl isomerase A (*Ppia*). Data are presented as fold-change set to the control diet-Fl/Fl mice group trough (Udoh et al., 2017). A list of gene primers is provided in the supplemental data section (**Supplementary Table 13**).

Plasma and Liver TG Measurements

Plasma TG was determined using reagents from Pointe Scientific (Canton, MI) and reported as mg TG/dL. For hepatic TG content, lipids were extracted by methods described previously (Filiano et al., 2013), TG was quantified using L-Type Triglyceride M colorimetric assay reagents (FUJIFILM Wako Diagnostics, Mountain View, CA) and reported as μg TG/mg liver.

Liver Histopathology and Scoring

Liver was collected every 4 h at ZT 3, 7, 11, 15, 19, and 23 and a small piece of liver was dissected from the large outer right lobe of all mice, placed into 10% buffered formalin, and embedded in paraffin before being sectioned at a 5 μm thickness. Liver was mounted onto slides and stained with hematoxylin and eosin (H and E) according to accepted guidelines (Kleiner et al., 2005). Slides from each experimental group and for all time-points were coded with a unique number designation for unbiased examination and scoring by pathologists. Steatosis (percentage of hepatocytes containing lipid droplets), lobular inflammation (number of inflammatory foci), ballooning, and fibrosis were scored by pathologists blinded to the experimental design using the NAFLD activity scoring (NAS) protocol (Brunt et al., 1999). While the NAS protocol is not intended for ALD, we applied this system to assign a histopathology score to cases in this experimental animal study. Steatosis was scored as 0, <5%; 1, 5–33%; 2, >34–65%; and 3, >66% of hepatocytes containing lipid droplets. Lobular inflammation was scored as: 0, no foci; 1, <2 foci; 2, 2–4 foci, and 3, >4 foci. Ballooned hepatocytes were rare and fibrosis was undetectable; thus, histopathology scores reported in **Table 1** largely reflect steatosis and inflammation. Pathologists also recorded the percentage of hepatocytes containing large and small droplet macrosteatosis.

Western Blotting

Livers were homogenized in 0.25 M sucrose buffer, pH 7.4, supplemented with protease and phosphatase inhibitor cocktails (Sigma-Aldrich, St. Louis, MO) and equal amounts of protein were separated on 4–20% Criterion™ TGX™ Precast Gels (Bio-Rad Laboratories, Hercules, CA) from all time-points of tissue collection (Udoh et al., 2015, 2017). Proteins were

TABLE 1 | Statistical analyses of liver histopathology scores.

Histology variable	Control Fl/Fl mice (*N* = 35)	Ethanol Fl/Fl mice (*N* = 33)	Control LKO mice (*N* = 30)	Ethanol LKO mice (*N* = 31)	*p*
Histopathology score					
0	23 (65.7)[a]	22 (66.7)	20 (66.7)	12 (38.7)	0.020[b]
1	7 (20.0)	6 (18.2)	5 (16.7)	11 (35.5)	
2	2 (5.7)	4 (12.1)	3 (10.0)	3 (9.7)	
3	2 (5.7)	1 (3.0)	1 (3.3)	3 (9.7)	
4	1 (2.9)	0 (0)	0 (0)	1 (3.2)	
5	0 (0)	0 (0)	1 (3.3)	1 (3.2)	
Steatosis grade					
0 – <5%	33 (94.3)	27 (81.8)	27 (90.0)	16 (51.6)	0.660[c]
1 – 5–33%	1 (2.85)	6 (18.2)	3 (10.0)	12 (38.7)	0.016[d]
2 – 34–66%	1 (2.85)	0 (0)	0 (0)	3 (9.7)	
3 – >66%	0 (0)	0 (0)	0 (0)	0 (0)	
Lobular inflammation					
0 – none	20 (57.1)	24 (72.7)	21 (70.0)	19 (61.3)	0.314[e]
1 – <2	9 (25.7)	7 (21.2)	7 (23.3)	10 (32.3)	0.427[f]
2 – 2–4	5 (14.3)	1 (3.0)	0 (0)	1 (3.2)	
3 – >4	1 (2.9)	1 (3.0)	2 (6.7)	1 (3.2)	
Ballooning					
0 – none	35 (100)	33 (100)	27 (90)	29 (93.5)	0.093[g]
1 – few	0 (0)	0 (0)	3 (10)	3 (9.7)	0.108[h]
2 – many	0 (0)	0 (0)	0 (0)	0	

[a]*Values are N (%).*
[b]*Values of p are from an ordinal contingency analysis for each parameter; significant Genotype X Diet Interaction.*
[c]*Values of p for steatosis are from a Fisher's Exact Test comparing absence (steatosis grade 0) and presence (grade 1 + 2) in control-fed Fl/Fl vs. control-fed LKO mice.*
[d]*Values of p for steatosis are from a Fisher's Exact Test comparing absence (steatosis grade 0) and presence (1 + 2) in alcohol-fed Fl/Fl vs. alcohol-fed LKO mice.*
[e]*Values of p for lobular inflammation are from a Fisher's Exact Test comparing presence (1–3) or absence (0) of lobular inflammation in control-fed Fl/Fl vs. control-fed LKO mice.*
[f]*Values of p for lobular inflammation are from a Fisher's Exact Test comparing presence (1–3) or absence (0) of lobular inflammation in alcohol-fed Fl/Fl vs. alcohol-fed LKO mice.*
[g]*Values of p for hepatocyte ballooning are from a Fisher's Exact Test comparing presence or absence of ballooned hepatocytes in control-fed Fl/Fl vs. control-fed LKO mice.*
[h]*Values of p for hepatocyte ballooning are from a Fisher's Exact Test comparing presence or absence of ballooned hepatocytes in alcohol-fed Fl/Fl vs. alcohol-fed LKO mice.*

transferred from gels to nitrocellulose membranes and membranes were incubated at room temperature for 1 h in LI-COR® Blocking Buffer (LI-COR® Biosciences, Lincoln, NE). Membranes were incubated with primary antibodies overnight at 4°C: total ACC, 1:1,000 (cat. no. 3676, Cell Signaling Technologies, Danvers, MA); phospho-ACC-Ser79, 1:1,000 (cat. no. 11818, Cell Signaling Technology, Danvers, MA); FASN, 1:1,000 (cat no. 3180S, Cell Signaling Technology, Danvers, MA); and MCD, 1:1,000 (cat. no. PA5-22081, Thermo Fisher Scientific, Waltham, MA). An anti-β-actin antibody (cat. no. A5441, Sigma-Aldrich, St. Louis, MO) was used as the loading control (1:5,000). Membranes were washed and incubated in secondary antibodies from LI-COR® Biosciences (Lincoln, NE) for 1 h at room temperature. The secondary antibody used for total and phospho-ACC was IRDye 680RD (rabbit, cat. no. 926-68071), for MCD and FASN was 800CW (rabbit, cat. no. 926-32213), and for β-actin was 800CW (mouse, cat. no. 926-32210) or IRDye 680 RD (mouse, cat. no. 926-68070). Fluorescence was detected and densitometry of protein bands was quantified using the LI-COR Odyssey® CLx imaging system (Udoh et al., 2015, 2017). Data are presented as the average of protein densitometry across all time-points normalized to β-Actin for each treatment group as done in (Hatori et al., 2012). The antibodies used for total and phospho-ACC detect both ACC1 (265 kDa) and ACC2 (280 kDa) isoforms. Due to the close proximity of isoform bands on images, values represent the combined densitometry for total ACC1 and 2 and phospho-ACC1 and 2, respectively.

Lipidomics

Lipidomics analysis was performed on liver lipid extracts collected at ZT 3 and ZT 15 from control and alcohol-fed Fl/Fl and LKO mice. Lipids were extracted from tissue using a modified Bligh and Dyer method (Bligh and Dyer, 1959). Briefly, 50–100 mg of frozen liver tissue was homogenized in 0.9 ml of dichloromethane and 2.0 ml of methanol (Honeywell Burdick and Jackson, Muskegon, MI). After homogenization, 10 μl of EquiSPLASH LIPIDOMIX Quantitative Mass Spec internal standard (cat. no. 330731, Avanti Polar Lipids, Alabaster, AL) was added and samples were incubated at room temperature for 30 min. One milliliter of liquid chromatography-mass spectrometry grade water (Honeywell Burdick and Jackson, Muskegon, MI) and 0.9 ml of dichloromethane were added, samples were centrifuged at 1200 rpm for 10 min at 4°C to separate phases, and the bottom hydrophobic organic phase containing lipids was collected and placed into a fresh glass test tube. The remaining upper hydrophilic phase was re-extracted with dichloromethane and the two organic phases were combined and dried under a stream of nitrogen. Lipids were re-solubilized in 300 μl injection solvent (dichloromethane:methanol, 50:50, with 5 mM ammonium acetate) and MS/MS^{ALL} mass spectrometric analysis and lipid species identification was performed as previously described in (Gajenthra Kumar et al., 2018) using a SCIEX Triple-TOF 6600+ (SCIEX, Framingham, MA) in the positive ion mode. Lipid species based on precursor fragment ion pairs were determined using the LipidView comprehensive target list (SCIEX, Framingham, MA) and the detected lipid species present in the TG pool (**Supplementary Table 8**) were compiled into a spreadsheet for statistical analyses. From these results, the percent TG FA saturation and percent TG FA composition were determined for the hepatic TG pool. The percent TG FA saturation was determined by dividing the sum of saturated fatty acids (SFA), monounsaturated fatty acids (MUFA), diunsaturated fatty acids (DUFA), or polyunsaturated fatty acids (PUFA) by the sum of all TG FA in the samples and multiplying by 100. Similarly, the percent TG FA composition was determined by dividing the sum of the most abundant individual TG FA species (12:0, 12:1, 14:0, 14:1, 16:0, 16:1, 18:1, 18:2, 20:0, 20:1, 20:2, 20:4, 22:1, and 22:6) by the sum of all TG FA in the samples and multiplying by 100.

Statistical Analyses

Two or three-factor ANOVA, where indicated, were used to determine statistical significance of main effects of genotype, diet, time, and/or interactions with Tukey's HSD test for *post hoc* analyses. To measure variation over time of day, cosinor analysis was performed to determine whether experimental measures fit a 24 h rhythm. For this, data were fitted to a cosine wave equation, $f(t)$ = mesor + amplitude * $\cos[(2\pi t/T)$ + acrophase], in SPSS (IBM) using a non-linear regression module (Filiano et al., 2013; Udoh et al., 2015, 2017). The mesor (midline estimating statistic of rhythm) = mean of the rhythm; amplitude = 1/2 the distance between the peak and trough; t = time-point (ZT 3, 7, 11, 15, 19, or 23); T = the period (fixed to 24 h); and acrophase = ZT time of the peak of the rhythm, i.e., cosine maximum. Rhythmicity was determined using a linear regression model $f(t) = M + \cos(2\pi t/T) + \sin(2\pi t/T)$, and data were considered rhythmic if the p of the R^2 was ≤ 0.05. Student's t-test was used to compare parameter estimates among the experimental treatment groups when the overall R^2 was significant. Data that significantly fit a cosine function (rhythmic) are represented in graphs by solid lines, whereas non-significant data (arrhythmic) are represented by dashed lines. Sample sizes are included in figure legends with statistical significance set at $p \leq 0.05$. Liver and plasma TG measurements were analyzed using non-parametric algorithm JTK_CYCLE in R (Hughes et al., 2010), with the period set to 24 h to test for rhythmicity in which statistical significance was set at $p \leq 0.05$. Significant interactions of diet and genotype for the histopathology score was determined by ordinal contingency analysis comparing each treatment group, collapsed across ZTs. Steatosis grade, inflammation, and hepatocyte ballooning were assessed for significant differences in Fl/Fl vs. LKO control and alcohol-fed mice using Fisher's Exact Test. For macrosteatosis, Fl/Fl control and LKO mice were compared across circadian time within diet groups. Hepatocytes containing small and large lipid droplets (macrosteatosis) were counted and quantified as a percentage of total hepatocytes in each image. Large droplet macrosteatosis percentages in both control diet groups were too low to warrant analysis. Distributions for large and small droplet macrosteatosis were positively skewed, which is often the case for count and percentage data. Positive skew for the small droplet macrosteatosis percentages within the alcohol group was corrected by a square root transformation. As a result, small droplet macrosteatosis data for alcohol-fed Fl/Fl and LKO mice were analyzed *via* cosinor analysis after square root transformation. For genotype comparisons of small droplet macrosteatosis percentages within the control diet group, transformation did not correct the positive skew. Thus, data were stratified by genotype and a negative binomial regression (Dupont, 2002) with linearized cosine functions as fixed factors $[(\cos(2\pi t/24))$ and $\sin(\cos(2\pi t/24))]$ was performed in SPSS (IBM) followed by planned *post hoc* comparisons between groups at each ZT. Likewise, large droplet macrosteatosis data were positively skewed and were analyzed similarly *via* negative binomial regression. For lipidomics analysis, we performed three-factor ANOVA to determine main effects of genotype, diet, time, and/or interactions with Tukey's HSD for *post hoc* pairwise comparisons between each group. Two-factor ANOVA was performed for TG FA, where indicated, in cases that showed significant two-way interaction by three-factor ANOVA, but did not significantly show three-way interactions (**Supplementary Tables 9–12**).

RESULTS

This study is a follow-up from our previous work showing that alcohol and liver clock disruption differentially alter hepatic glycogen content and diurnal mRNA rhythms in glycogen and glucose metabolism genes (Udoh et al., 2017). In our previous paper, we validated the *Bmal1* LKO mouse model showing liver-specific absence of BMAL1 protein, and significant attenuation in transcript rhythms of *Bmal1* and the clock-controlled output gene D site of albumin promoter binding protein (*Dbp*) in the liver, whereas high amplitude mRNA rhythms in these genes and other clock genes were unaffected in extra-hepatic tissues (Udoh et al., 2017). Furthermore, we found no difference in alcohol intake, blood alcohol, and body weight gain between LKO and littermate control Fl/Fl mice (Udoh et al., 2017). Here, we extend our studies by investigating the combined effect of alcohol and liver clock disruption on temporal variations in diurnal mRNA rhythms in clock and lipid metabolism genes, hepatic and plasma TG levels, liver histopathology, and the FA composition of the hepatic TG pool.

Circadian Clock Genes

Consistent with our previous findings (Filiano et al., 2013), chronic alcohol consumption significantly altered rhythmicity of clock gene mRNA levels in the liver (Cosinor analysis; **Figure 1** and **Supplementary Table 1**). Specifically, alcohol decreased the midline estimating statistic of rhythm (mesor) and amplitude of *Bmal1* in liver of Fl/Fl mice (**Figure 1A**). A low amplitude *Bmal1* rhythm persists in livers of LKO mice that is most likely due to non-hepatocyte cell types in liver that do not express Cre recombinase (**Figure 1B**). Compared to control-fed mice, alcohol abolished rhythmic mRNA levels

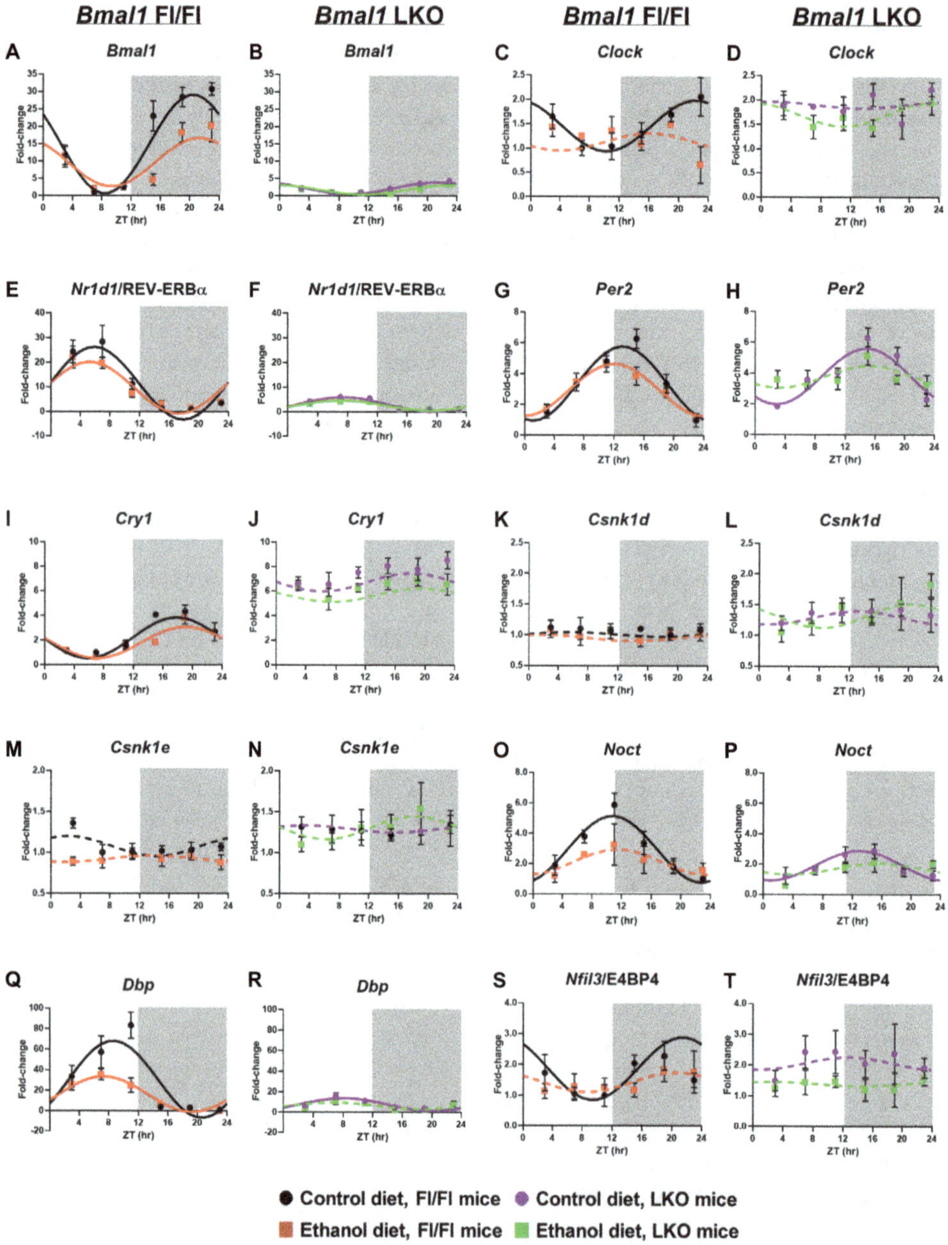

FIGURE 1 | Chronic alcohol and liver clock disruption alter 24 h mRNA rhythms in molecular clock genes in the liver. Diurnal mRNA profiles of Brain and Muscle ARNT-like 1 (*Bmal1*; **A,B**), Circadian Locomotor Output Cycles Kaput (*Clock*; **C,D**), Nuclear Receptor Subfamily 1 Group D Member 1 (*Nr1d1*/Rev-Erbα; **E,F**), Period 2 (*Per2*; **G,H**), Cryptochrome 1 (*Cry1*; **I,J**), Casein Kinase 1 Delta (*Csnk1d*; **K,L**), Casein Kinase 1 Epsilon (*Csnk1e*; **M,N**), Nocturnin (*Noct*; **O,P**), D site of Albumin Promoter Binding Protein (*Dbp*; **Q,R**) and Nuclear Factor, Interleukin 3 Regulated (*Nfil3*/E4BP4; **S,T**) were measured in livers of control-fed (black) and alcohol-fed (red) *Bmal1* Flox/Flox (Fl/Fl) and control-fed (purple) and alcohol-fed (green) *Bmal1* liver-specific knockout (LKO) mice at ZT 3, 7, 11, 15, 19, and 23 (ZT 0: lights on/inactive period, ZT 12: lights off/active period, gray area) by real time (RT)-PCR. Data are presented as a fold-change to the *Bmal1* Fl/Fl control diet trough time-point and normalized to *Gapdh*. Cosinor analysis was performed using a nonlinear regression module in SPSS. Data are expressed as mean ± SEM for n = 4–8 mice/genotype/diet/time-point. Solid lines indicate rhythmic mRNA levels and a significant cosine fit, whereas dashed lines indicate arrhythmicity and a non-significant cosine fit. Results for Cosinor and ANOVA analyses are provided in **Supplementary Tables 1** and **2**, respectively.

of the other positive regulator, *Clock*, in livers of Fl/Fl mice (**Figure 1C**). Diet had no effect on arrhythmic mRNA levels of *Clock* in livers from LKO mice (**Figure 1D**).

Nr1d1/REV-ERBα forms an important secondary feedback loop that regulates the clock *via Bmal1* transcriptional repression (Preitner et al., 2002). Rhythmic mRNA levels of *Nr1d1*/REV-ERBα were evident in livers from all four groups (**Supplementary Table 1**). In Fl/Fl mice, alcohol induced a significant ~3 h phase advance compared to control-fed mice (**Figure 1E**). Liver clock disruption significantly phase delayed and reduced the amplitude of *Nr1d1*/REV-ERBα rhythms in livers from LKO mice fed either diet compared to Fl/Fl mice (**Figures 1E,F**). LKO livers showed a ~5-fold reduction in *Nr1d1* amplitude compared to Fl/Fl mice (**Figure 1F**; **Supplementary Table 1**).

We next examined rhythmic transcription of *Per2* and *Cry1*, negative regulators of the clock (Kume et al., 1999; Zheng et al., 1999). Although alcohol had a minimal effect on diurnal rhythms in mRNA levels of *Per2* and *Cry1* in livers of Fl/Fl mice (**Figures 1G,I**), the combination of liver clock disruption and alcohol resulted in arrhythmic *Per2* mRNA levels (**Figure 1H**). *Per2* mRNA levels remained rhythmic in livers of control-fed LKO mice, albeit with a significant phase delay in the peak of *Per2* compared to control-fed Fl/Fl mice (**Figure 1H**). *Cry1* mRNA levels were arrhythmic in livers of LKO mice (**Figure 1J**).

Other factors that regulate the clock, or are themselves regulated by the clock, may also be affected by alcohol and/or liver clock disruption. For example, casein kinase 1 delta and epsilon (*Csnk1d* and *Csnk1e*) are two kinases that regulate clock timing through phosphorylation of core clock proteins (Vielhaber et al., 2000; Etchegaray et al., 2009; Lee et al., 2009). Measurements of mRNA levels for these genes were arrhythmic and unaffected by alcohol (**Figures 1K–N**). However, several important clock-controlled genes showed sensitivity to alcohol or the combination of alcohol and liver clock disruption. Both nocturnin (*Noct*; an mRNA deadenylase; Kojima et al., 2012) and *Dbp* (a D-box binding b-ZIP transcription factor) showed rhythmic mRNA levels in livers of control-fed mice; however, amplitude was significantly reduced in LKO mice compared to Fl/Fl mice (**Figures 1O–R**). Importantly, alcohol altered the diurnal rhythms in mRNA levels of *Noct* and *Dbp* in livers from mice of either genotype (**Figures 1O–R**). Although *Dbp* in livers of alcohol-fed Fl/Fl mice was still rhythmic, the amplitude was decreased by more than half (**Figure 1Q**). While control-fed LKO mice exhibited low amplitude *Dbp* and *Noct* rhythms, these rhythms were lost when LKO mice were fed alcohol (**Figures 1P,R**). Another D-box binding b-ZIP transcription factor, *Nfil3*/E4BP4 (interleukin 3 regulated/E4 promoter-binding protein 4; Mitsui et al., 2001; Ripperger and Schibler, 2006) displayed a significant diurnal rhythm in livers of control-fed Fl/Fl mice that was anti-phase to *Nr1d1*/REV-ERBα and *Dbp* (**Figure 1S**). Alcohol, liver clock disruption, or both, abolished *Nfil3*/E4BP4 rhythmicity (**Figures 1S,T**). Together, these results extend our previous findings and show that genetic disruption of the liver clock exacerbates the circadian rhythm-impairing effects of alcohol.

In order to assess whether alcohol-induced effects on overall clock mRNA levels depend on genotype (independent of time), we performed two-factor ANOVA on clock and clock-controlled genes (**Supplementary Table 2**). Alcohol reduced overall levels of *Bmal1*, *Clock*, *Cry1*, *Nfil3*/E4BP4, and *Dbp*, regardless of genotype (main effect of diet). In addition, livers from LKO mice generally had higher mRNA levels of *Clock*, *Per2*, *Cry1*, *Csnk1d*, and *Csnk1e*, as well as lower expression of *Bmal1*, *Dbp*, and *Nr1d1*/REV-ERBα, compared to livers from Fl/Fl mice (main effect of genotype). Although no Genotype X Diet interactions reached significance, there was a trend for *Bmal1*, *Dbp*, and *Nfil3*/E4BP4. Specifically, alcohol-fed Fl/Fl mice had lower mRNA levels of *Bmal1* and *Dbp*, whereas LKO mice on either diet had minimal levels of mRNA for these genes (**Figures 1B,R**). Higher *Nfil3*/E4BP4 mRNA levels in livers of control-fed LKO mice tended to be reduced when mice were fed alcohol (**Figures 1S,T**).

Liver and Plasma TG Levels

TG was significantly elevated in livers of alcohol-fed Fl/Fl and LKO mice (**Figures 2B,D**) compared to control diet counterparts (**Figures 2A,C**). Two-factor ANOVA showed significant interaction of Genotype X Diet for liver TG (**Figure 2I**). Plasma TG were also increased by alcohol in both genotypes (**Figures 2F,H**) compared to control diet mice (**Figures 2E,G**) with the highest overall levels of plasma TG observed in alcohol-fed LKO mice (**Figure 2H**). Plasma TG were rhythmic in control-fed Fl/Fl and LKO mice (Fl/Fl, $p = 0.049$; LKO, $p = 0.0005$; JTK cycle). Similar to liver TG, two-factor ANOVA for plasma TG shows a significant interaction of Genotype X Diet (**Figure 2I**). Taken together, these data illustrate differential impacts of liver clock disruption on TG metabolism in alcohol-fed mice.

Liver Histopathology

A significantly greater percentage of livers from alcohol-fed LKO mice had higher overall histopathology scores (one or more) compared to the other three groups (**Table 1**). Steatosis was analyzed by comparing livers scored at grade 0 to those scored at grades 1 + 2 in control-fed and alcohol-fed mice. There was a statistically significant difference in steatosis grade in livers of alcohol-fed mice with increased numbers of livers exhibiting grade 1 + 2 compared to grade 0, and there was no effect in control-fed mice (**Table 1**). We observed no significant differences in lobular inflammation between groups. Ballooned hepatocytes were only seen in livers of LKO mice that were collected during the inactive period (ZT 0–12) of the day (**Table 1**). Mildly reactive Kupffer cells were also rare and only detected in livers of two alcohol-fed LKO mice.

We also examined livers for temporal differences in both large and small droplet macrosteatosis (**Figure 3**). Representative images are presented for livers collected at ZT 15 (**Figures 3I–L**). Both large (**Figures 3A–D**) and small droplet (**Figures 3E–H**) macrosteatosis were present; however, small droplet macrosteatosis was more prevalent with the highest levels seen in livers of alcohol-fed mice (**Figures 3F,H**). Low levels of large and small droplet macrosteatosis were observed in livers of some control-fed Fl/Fl mice (**Figures 3A,E**), with higher levels in livers of control-fed LKO mice (**Figures 3C,G**). In alcohol-fed mice, large droplet macrosteatosis displayed a significant 24 h rhythm (**Figure 3B**; $\chi^2(5) = 12.8$, $p = 0.005$) in livers of Fl/Fl mice but not in livers of LKO mice (**Figure 3D**; $\chi^2(5) = 1.23$, $p = 0.805$). Specifically, large droplet macrosteatosis in livers of alcohol-fed Fl/Fl mice were significantly less likely to be observed at ZT 3, 7, and 19 compared to ZT 11 (**Figure 3B**; $\chi^2(5) = 12.7$, $p = 0.03$). In LKO mice fed a control diet, livers had a decreased likelihood of large droplet macrosteatosis at ZT 3, 7, 15, 19, and 23 compared to ZT 11 (**Figure 3C**; $\chi^2(5) = 53.6$, $p = 2.5E\text{-}10$).

We also examined temporal dynamics of small droplet macrosteatosis. Cosinor analysis revealed that small droplet macrosteatosis exhibited a 24 h rhythm in livers of alcohol-fed Fl/Fl mice (**Figure 3F**; $R^2 = 0.29$; $p = 0.006$; peak phase = ZT 14.44) but not in livers of alcohol-fed LKO mice (**Figure 3H**; $R^2 = 0.15$; $p = 0.11$). In contrast, small droplet macrosteatosis was rhythmic in livers of control-fed LKO mice (**Figure 3G**; $\chi^2(5) = 48.1$, $p = 3.3E\text{-}9$), but not in livers of control-fed Fl/Fl mice (**Figure 3E**; $\chi^2(5) = 8.0$, $p = 0.16$). Livers of control-fed LKO mice had a decreased likelihood of small droplet macrosteatosis specifically at ZT 3, 15, 19, and 23 compared to ZT 7 and ZT 11 (**Figure 3G**; $\chi^2(5) = 25.3$, $p < 0.05$). Together, these results show that alcohol-induced macrosteatosis varies over the 24h day in a liver-clock dependent manner.

Lipid Metabolism Transcription Factors

Sterol regulatory element binding transcription factor 1/protein 1C (*Srebf1*/SREBP-1C) mRNA levels were rhythmic, peaking in the inactive period of the day in livers of control-fed Fl/Fl mice with alcohol inducing arrhythmicity (**Figure 4A**). *Srebf1*/SREBP-1C was arrhythmic in livers of LKO mice (**Figure 4B**). MLX interacting protein like/carbohydrate-responsive element binding protein (*Mlxipl*/ChREBP) was arrhythmic in all groups (**Figures 4C,D**). Nuclear receptor subfamily 1 group H member 3/Liver X receptor α (*Nr1h3*/LXRα) was also arrhythmic in all groups (**Figures 4E,F**), whereas *Nr1h2*/LXRβ was rhythmic in livers of control-fed Fl/Fl mice, but arrhythmic in livers of alcohol-fed Fl/Fl (**Figure 4G**) and LKO mice (**Figure 4H**). Peroxisome proliferator-activated receptor alpha (PPARα), a transcription factor that activates expression of many FAO and FA transport genes, was surprisingly arrhythmic in livers of control-fed Fl/Fl mice, but rhythmic in livers of alcohol-fed Fl/Fl mice (**Figure 4I**). *Ppara* was also arrhythmic in livers of LKO mice (**Figure 4J**). Results of cosinor analyses for lipid metabolism transcription factors are included in **Supplementary Table 3**.

Two-factor ANOVA was performed to determine significant main effects of alcohol and genotype on mRNA levels of lipid metabolism transcription factors, regardless of time (**Supplementary Table 4**). Independent of genotype, alcohol-fed mice generally displayed reduced mRNA levels of *Srebf1*/SREBP-1C, *Nr1h3*/LXRα, *Nr1h2*/LXRβ, and *Ppara*. Further, genetic disruption of the liver clock resulted in increased mRNA levels of *Srebf1*/SREBP-1C and *Nr1h2*/LXRβ, while decreasing mRNA levels of *Mlxipl*/ChREBP and *Ppara* (main effect of genotype). We also observed a trend toward a significant interaction of Genotype X Diet for *Mlxipl*/ChREBP.

Fatty Acid Metabolism

Acetyl CoA carboxylase alpha/1 (*Acaca*/ACC1), an enzyme that catalyzes the formation of malonyl-CoA (substrate for *de novo* FA synthesis) by the carboxylation of acetyl-CoA (Thampy and Wakil, 1988), was rhythmic in livers of control-fed

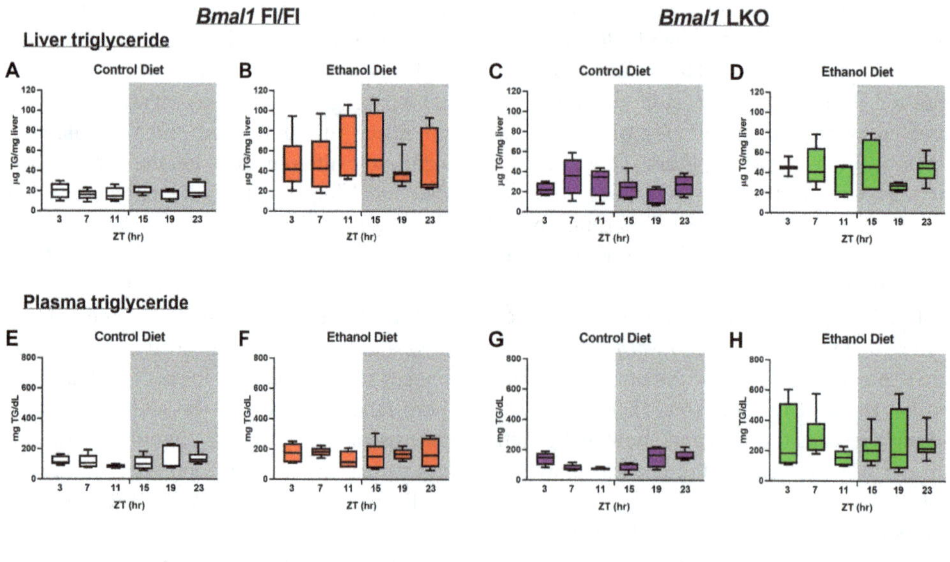

I

	Genotype		Diet		G X D	
	F	p-value	F	p-value	F	p-value
Liver TG	0.3	0.62	50.5	7.2E-11	5.4	0.02
Plasma TG	5.1	0.03	30.1	2.2E-7	7.7	0.01

FIGURE 2 | Chronic alcohol and liver clock disruption alter diurnal variations in liver and plasma triglyceride levels. Liver **(A–D)** and plasma **(E–F)** triglyceride (TG) were measured in samples collected from control-fed (**A,E** white) and alcohol-fed (**B,F** red) *Bmal1* Flox/Flox (Fl/Fl) and control-fed (**C,G** purple) and alcohol-fed (**D,H** green) *Bmal1* liver-specific knockout (LKO) mice at ZT 3, 7, 11, 15, 19, and 23 (ZT 0: lights on/inactive period, ZT 12: lights off/active period, gray area). Data are shown as min to max box and whisker plots for n = 3–8 mice/genotype/diet/time-point. Results from two-factor ANOVA are provided in **(I)**.

Fl/Fl mice and arrhythmic in livers of alcohol-fed Fl/Fl mice and LKO mice (**Figures 5A,B**). *Acacb*/ACC2 also catalyzes the generation of malonyl-CoA, which acts as an allosteric inhibitor of FAO by decreasing FA uptake into mitochondria by carnitine palmitoyltransferse-1A (CPT1A) activity (Abu-Elheiga et al., 2000). *Acacb*/ACC2 mRNA levels were rhythmic in livers of control and alcohol-fed Fl/Fl mice (**Figure 5C**) with alcohol significantly decreasing the mesor. While *Acacb*/ACC2 was rhythmic in livers of control-fed LKO mice (**Figure 5D**), the mesor was decreased and the peak was phase delayed in livers of control-fed LKO mice compared to Fl/Fl mice. *Acacb*/ACC2 was arrhythmic in livers of alcohol-fed LKO mice (**Figure 5D**). Malonyl CoA decarboxylase (*Mlycd*/MCD), an enzyme that catalyzes malonyl-CoA degradation to acetyl-CoA, was rhythmic in livers of control and alcohol-fed Fl/Fl mice (**Figure 5E**); however, alcohol feeding significantly decreased the mesor and induced a phase delay. *Mlycd*/MCD was rhythmic in livers of control-fed LKO mice (**Figure 5F**) with increased mesor and delayed peak mRNA levels compared to livers of control-fed Fl/Fl mice. *Mlycd*/MCD was arrhythmic in livers of alcohol-fed LKO mice (**Figure 5F**). *Cpt1a* was rhythmic in livers of Fl/Fl mice (**Figure 5G**) and alcohol-fed LKO mice (**Figure 5H**) with peak mRNA levels phase advanced in livers of alcohol-fed LKO mice compared to alcohol-fed Fl/Fl mice.

Fatty acid synthase (*Fasn*), a multi-functional enzyme that uses acetyl-CoA and malonyl-CoA to eventually produce palmitic acid (16:0), was rhythmic in livers of control and alcohol-fed Fl/Fl mice with peak mRNA levels occurring in the early active period (**Figure 5I**). *Fasn* was arrhythmic in livers of LKO mice (**Figure 5J**). FA elongation and biosynthesis of MUFA and PUFA is catalyzed through actions of stearoyl CoA desaturase 1 (*Scd1*), fatty acid desaturase 1 (*Fads1*), *Fads2*, and fatty acid elongase 5 (*Elovl5*) and *Elovl6* (Zhang et al., 2016a). *Scd1*, the rate-limiting step in the synthesis of MUFA, was arrhythmic in all groups (**Figures 5K,L**). *Elovl5* was rhythmic in livers of Fl/Fl mice (**Figure 5M**), but arrhythmic in livers of LKO mice (**Figure 5N**). Interestingly, diurnal rhythms in *Elovl6* mRNA levels were anti-phase to *Elovl5* mRNA levels when comparing control-fed Fl/Fl mice (**Figures 5M,O**) and was arrhythmic in livers of alcohol-fed Fl/Fl mice (**Figure 5O**) and livers of LKO mice (**Figure 5P**). *Fads1* mRNA levels were arrhythmic in all groups (**Figures 5Q,R**), whereas *Fads2* mRNA levels were rhythmic only in livers of control-fed Fl/Fl mice (**Figures 5S,T**). Results of cosinor analyses for these FA metabolism genes are provided in **Supplementary Table 5**.

Two-factor ANOVA (**Supplementary Table 4**) revealed that the overall mRNA levels of *Acaca*, *Acacb*, *Mlycd*, *Elovl6*, *Fads1*, and *Fads2* had significant main effects of genotype, independent of diet. In LKO mice, we observed overall increased mRNA

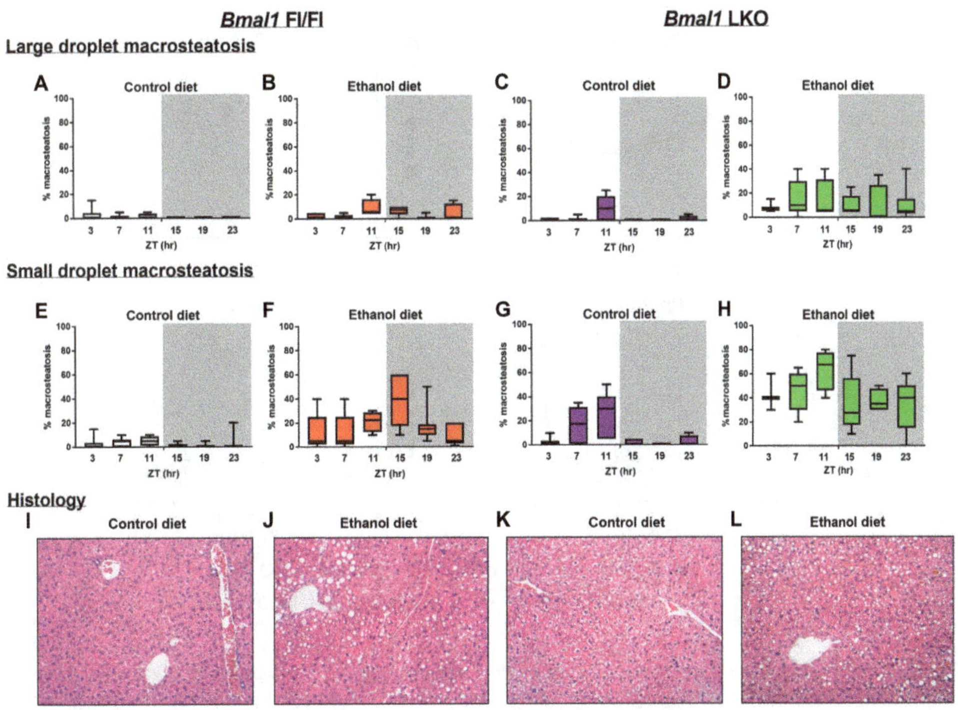

FIGURE 3 | Chronic alcohol and liver clock disruption enhance liver histopathology. Large droplet **(A–D)** and small droplet **(E–H)** macrosteatosis were assessed in H and E-stained liver sections prepared from control-fed **(A,E** white) and alcohol-fed **(B,F** red) *Bmal1* Flox/Flox (Fl/Fl) and control-fed **(C,G** purple) and alcohol-fed **(D,H** green) *Bmal1* liver-specific knockout (LKO) mice at ZT 3, 7, 11, 15, 19, and 23 (ZT 0: lights on/inactive period, ZT 12: lights off/active period, gray area). Liver sections were scored at multiple magnifications. Data represent the percentage of hepatocytes containing large and small droplet macrosteatosis per section. Results shown as min to max box and whisker plots for n = 3–8 mice/genotype/diet/time-point. **(I–L)** Representative H and E stained histology images from each group at ZT 15 (20X mag). Results for statistical analyses are provided in **Table 1**.

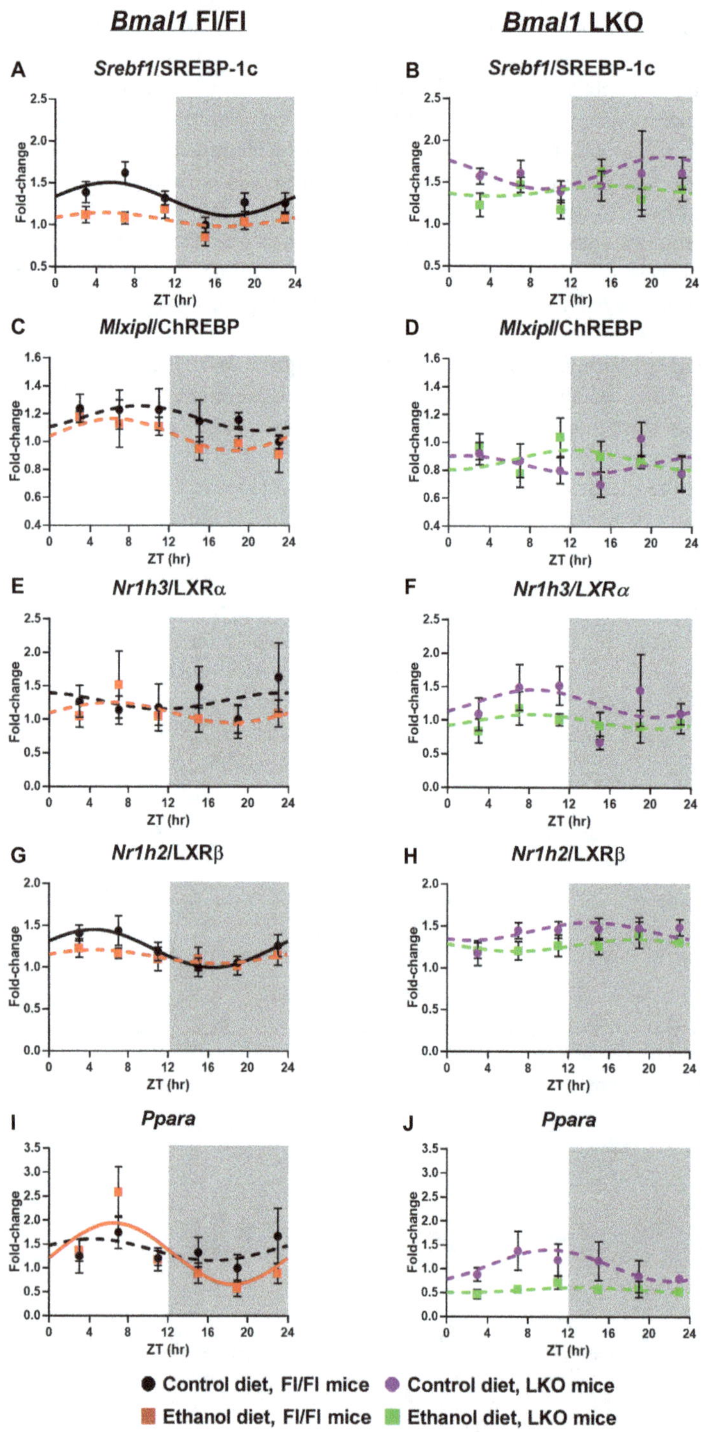

FIGURE 4 | Chronic alcohol and liver clock disruption alter diurnal mRNA rhythms of lipid metabolism transcription factors in the liver. Diurnal mRNA profiles of Sterol regulatory element binding transcription factor 1 (*Srebf1*/SREBP-1C; **A,B**), MLX-interacting protein-like/Carbohydrate-responsive element-binding protein (*Mlxipl*/ChREBP; **C,D**), Nuclear receptor subfamily 1, group H, member 3/Liver X receptor alpha (*Nr1h3*/ LXRα; **E,F**), Nuclear receptor subfamily 1, group H, member 2/Liver X receptor beta (*Nr1h2*/LXRβ; **G,H**), Peroxisome proliferator-activated receptor alpha (*Pparα*; **I,J**) were measured in livers of control-fed (black) and alcohol-fed (red) *Bmal1* Flox/Flox (Fl/Fl) and control-fed (purple) and alcohol-fed (green) *Bmal1* liver-specific knockout (LKO) mice at ZT 3, 7, 11, 15, 19, and 23 (ZT 0: lights on/inactive period, ZT 12: lights off/active period, gray area) by RT-PCR. Data are presented as a fold-change to the *Bmal1* Fl/Fl control diet trough time-point and normalized to *Ppia*. Cosinor analysis was performed using a nonlinear regression module in SPSS. Data are expressed as mean ± SEM for n = 4–8 mice/genotype/diet/time point. Solid lines indicate rhythmic mRNA levels and a significant cosine fit, whereas dashed lines indicate arrhythmicity and a non-significant cosine fit. Results for Cosinor and ANOVA analyses are provided in **Supplementary Tables 3** and **4**, respectively.

levels of *Acaca*, *Mlycd*, and decreased *Acacb*, *Elovl6*, *Fads1*, *Fads2*, and *Scd1*. Independent of genotype, alcohol decreased overall mRNA levels of *Acacb* and *Mlycd* and increased mRNA levels of *Elovl6*. A significant interaction of Genotype X Diet was detected for *Acacb* where alcohol decreased *Acacb* in Fl/Fl, but not LKO mice. In contrast, alcohol increased *Fasn* mRNA levels in livers of LKO, but not Fl/Fl mice. In addition, a trend toward a significant interaction was observed for *Acaca* and *Mlycd*. Specifically, in LKO mice, mRNA levels of *Mlycd* tended to be decreased and *Acaca* mRNA levels increased by alcohol feeding.

We also examined protein abundance and phosphorylation for a small set of FA metabolism enzymes, ACC, MCD, and FASN, to complement gene expression analyses. As no time-of-day differences were detected, results were analyzed by pooling all time points for each treatment group, as done in previous studies (Hatori et al., 2012). While the antibodies used for total and phospho-ACC detect both ACC1 (265 kDa) and ACC2 (280 kDa) isoforms, our data largely showed the presence of the lower molecular weight lipogenic ACC1 isoform in liver (**Figure 6**), which is in agreement with other studies in rodents (Bianchi et al., 1990). Total ACC was unchanged in all treatment groups (**Figure 6A**), whereas p-ACC levels were significantly lower in livers of alcohol-fed LKO mice compared to levels measured in control-fed LKO mice (**Figure 6B**). Two-factor ANOVA showed a significant main effect of diet for p-ACC and a trend toward a significant Genotype X Diet interaction ($p = 0.07$). MCD was significantly lower in livers of LKO mice compared to Fl/Fl mice (**Figure 6C**) with a significant effect of genotype. Similarly, FASN was lower in livers of alcohol-fed Fl/Fl mice and LKO mice compared to control-fed Fl/Fl mice (**Figure 6D**). Two-factor ANOVA showed a significant genotype effect for FASN.

Triglyceride Metabolism

Previous studies report diurnal rhythms in mRNA levels of TG metabolism genes (**Figure 7A**) in the liver (Adamovich et al., 2014); however, the impact alcohol and liver clock disruption have on these day/night differences is unknown. Glycerol-3-phosphate acyltransferase 1 (*Gpat1*), the first enzyme of TG synthesis that catalyzes acylation of glycerol-3-phosphate (G3P) to lysophosphatidic acid (LPA; Coleman and Mashek, 2011), was

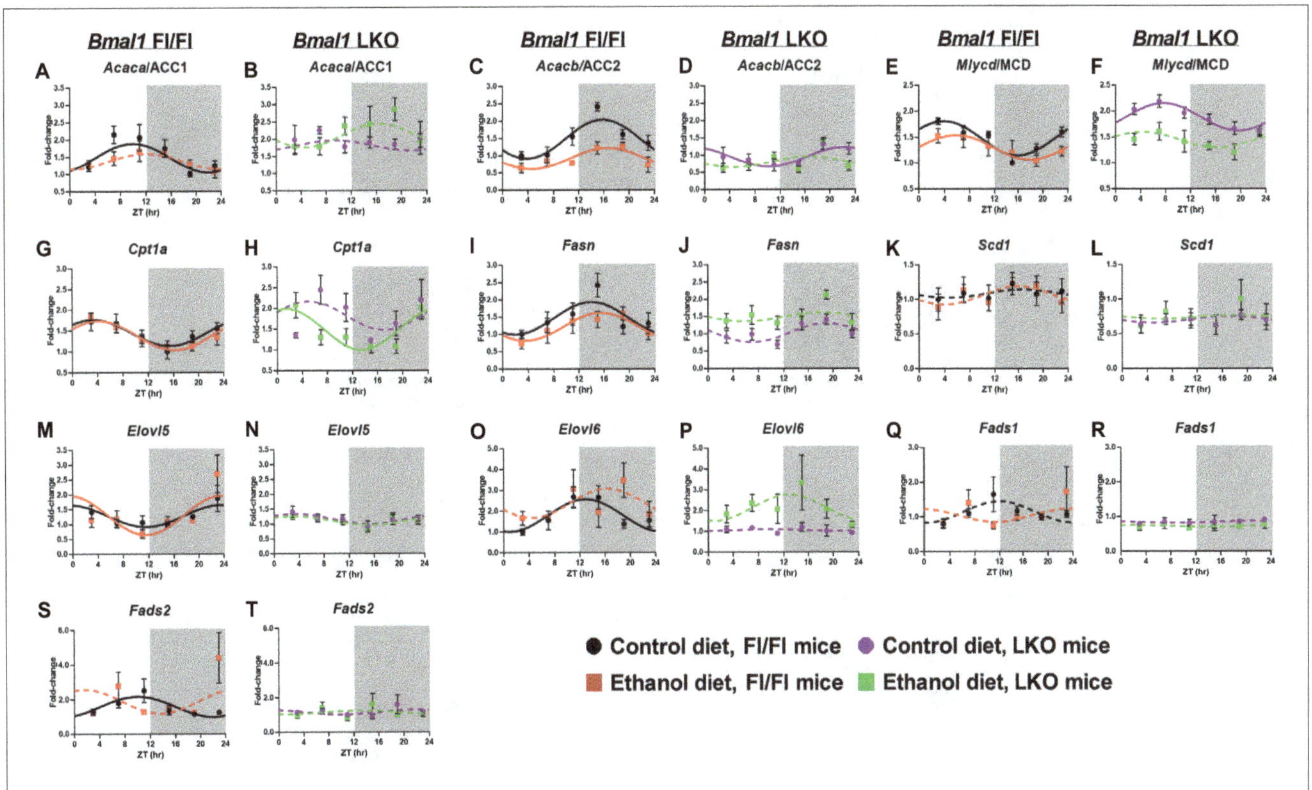

FIGURE 5 | Chronic alcohol and liver clock disruption alter diurnal mRNA rhythms of fatty acid metabolism genes. Diurnal mRNA profiles of Acetyl-CoA carboxylase 1 (*Acaca*/ACC1; **A,B**), Acetyl-CoA carboxylase 2 (*Acacb*/ACC2; **C,D**), Malonyl-CoA decarboxylase (*Mlycd*/MCD; **E,F**), Carnitine-palmitoyl transferase 1A (*Cpt1a*; **G,H**), Fatty acid synthase (*Fasn*; **I,J**), Stearyl-CoA desaturase 1 (*Scd1*; **K,L**), Elongation of very long chain fatty acids protein 5 (*Elovl5*; **M,N**), Elongation of very long chain fatty acid protein 6 (*Elovl6*; **O,P**), Fatty acid desaturase 1 (*Fads1*; **Q,R**), and Fatty acid desaturase 2 (*Fads2*; **S,T**) were measured in livers of control-fed (black) and alcohol-fed (red) *Bmal1* Flox/Flox (Fl/Fl) and control-fed (purple) and alcohol-fed (green) *Bmal1* liver-specific knockout (LKO) mice at ZT 3, 7, 11, 15, 19, and 23 (ZT 0: lights on/inactive period, ZT 12: lights off/active period, gray area) by RT-PCR. Data are presented as a fold-change to the *Bmal1* Fl/Fl control diet trough time-point and normalized to *Ppia*. Data are expressed as mean ± SEM for $n = 4$–8 mice/genotype/diet/time point. Solid lines indicate rhythmic mRNA levels and a significant cosine fit, whereas dashed lines indicate arrhythmicity and a non-significant cosine fit. Results for Cosinor and ANOVA analyses are provided in **Supplementary Tables 4** and **5**, respectively.

rhythmic in livers of control-fed Fl/Fl and LKO mice, whereas mRNA levels were arrhythmic in livers of alcohol-fed mice (**Figures 7B,C**). The next step in TG synthesis involves 1-acyl-sn-glycerol-3-phosphate acyltransferase 1 and 2 (AGPAT1, 2) that transfer an additional FA to LPA producing phosphatidate (PA). *Agpat1* was rhythmic in livers of both control-fed Fl/Fl and LKO mice (**Figures 7D,E**) with peak *Agpat1* mRNA levels phase delayed in livers of LKO mice. *Agpat1* was arrhythmic in livers of alcohol-fed Fl/Fl mice, but rhythmic in livers of alcohol-fed LKO mice (**Figures 7D,E**). *Agpat2* mRNA levels were rhythmic in livers of Fl/Fl mice (**Figure 7F**), as well as livers of control-fed LKO mice, but not livers of alcohol-fed LKO mice (**Figure 7G**). The peak of *Agpat2* was phase advanced ~3.5 h in livers of control-fed LKO compared to control-fed Fl/Fl mice. Lipins catalyze diglyceride (DG) formation through phosphatidate phosphatase-1 activity (Reue and Wang, 2019). *Lpin1* displayed a high amplitude rhythm in livers of control-fed Fl/Fl mice that was significantly lower in livers of alcohol-fed Fl/Fl mice (**Figure 7H**) and control-fed LKO mice (**Figure 7I**). *Lpin1* was arrhythmic in livers of alcohol-fed LKO mice (**Figure 7I**). *Lpin2* mRNA levels were also rhythmic in livers of control-fed Fl/Fl mice, but arrhythmic in livers of alcohol-fed Fl/Fl mice (**Figure 7J**) and LKO mice (**Figure 7K**).

The last step of TG synthesis is the conversion of DG to TG by diacylglycerol O-acyltransferase (DGAT) enzymes. *Dgat2* mRNA levels were rhythmic in livers of control and alcohol-fed Fl/Fl mice (**Figure 7L**) and control-fed LKO mice (**Figure 7M**), but arrhythmic in livers of alcohol-fed LKO mice (**Figure 7M**).

We also measured 24 h rhythms in mRNA levels for patatin like phospholipase domain containing 2/adipose triglyceride lipase (*Pnpla2*/ATGL) and *Pnpla3*, which are lipases that mediate the first step in TG breakdown (**Figure 7A**; Trepo et al., 2016; Schreiber et al., 2019). *Pnpla2*/ATGL mRNA levels were rhythmic in livers of both control-fed and alcohol-fed Fl/Fl mice; however, alcohol feeding significantly decreased the mesor and amplitude of *Pnpla2*/ATGL (**Figure 7N**). Lower mRNA levels of *Pnpla2*/ATGL were also seen in livers of control-fed LKO mice with alcohol inducing arrhythmicity (**Figure 7O**). *Pnpla3* exhibited a high amplitude rhythm in livers of control-fed Fl/Fl mice that was significantly decreased by alcohol feeding (**Figure 7P**). *Pnpla3* was arrhythmic in livers of LKO mice (**Figurer 7Q**). Cosinor analyses results for TG metabolism genes are included in **Supplementary Table 6**.

Assessment of mRNA levels of TG metabolism genes was next performed by two-factor ANOVA to determine whether

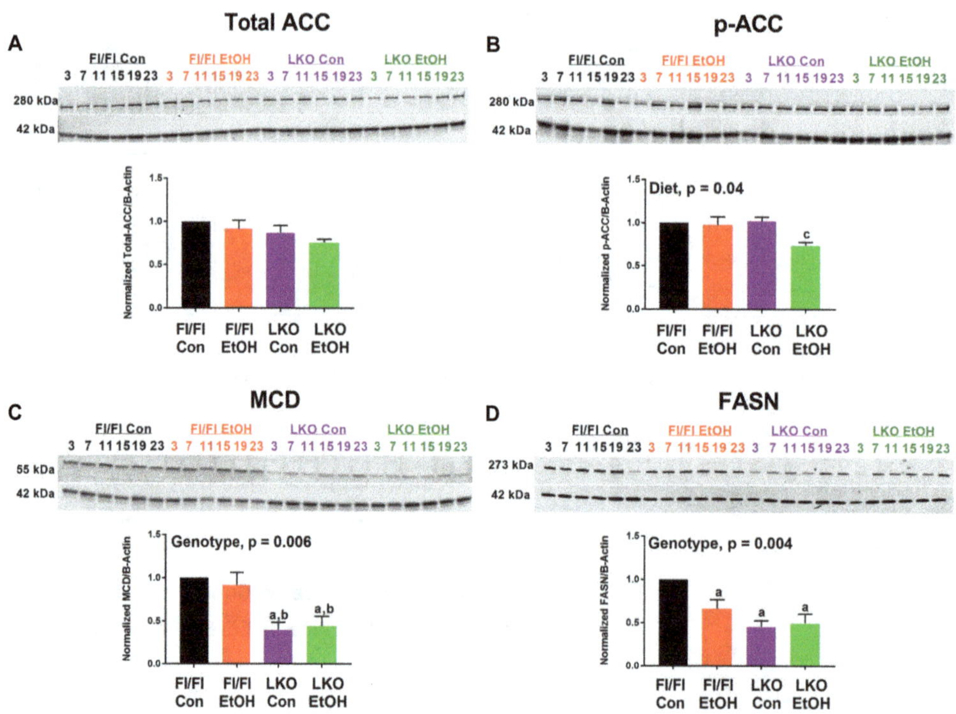

FIGURE 6 | Chronic alcohol and liver clock disruption alter abundance and phosphorylation state of select fatty acid metabolism proteins. Diurnal protein abundances of total acetyl CoA carboxylase (Total ACC; **A**), phosphorylated acetyl CoA carboxylase (p-ACC; **B**), malonyl-CoA decarboxylase (MCD; **C**), and fatty acid synthase (FASN; **D**) were determined by western blotting using liver homogenates of control-fed (black) and alcohol-fed (red) *Bmal1* Flox/Flox (Fl/Fl) and control-fed (purple) and alcohol-fed (green) *Bmal1* liver-specific knockout (LKO) mice from ZT 3, 7, 11, 15, 19, and 23 (ZT 0: lights on/inactive period, ZT 12: lights off/active period). Protein abundances were detected using the LI-COR Odyssey® digital imaging system. A representative image is presented for each protein of interest showing a full time course. The bar graphs indicate the average protein abundance calculated over the 24 h day normalized to β-actin, and levels are displayed as a fold-change from the control-fed Fl/Fl group. Data are shown as mean ± SEM n = 3–4 mice/genotype/diet. Significant two-factor ANOVA results are included in graphs. Letters indicate statistically significant differences ($p < 0.05$) for comparisons to control-fed Fl/Fl mice (a), alcohol-fed Fl/Fl mice (b), and control-fed LKO mice (c).

the observed effects of alcohol were dependent on genotype, regardless of time of day (**Supplementary Table 4**). Alcohol decreased mRNA levels of *Agpat1*, *Lpin1*, *Lpin2*, and *Pnpla2*/ATGL and *Pnpla3*. Significant main effects of genotype were found for *Agpat1* and *Agpat2*, which were generally increased in livers of LKO mice. In contrast, *Pnpla3* mRNA levels were significantly decreased in livers of LKO mice. We also observed a significant interaction of Genotype X Diet for *Pnpla3*, due to the dramatic alcohol-induced decrease in *Pnpla3* mRNA levels observed in Fl/Fl mice.

Lipid Droplet-Associated Components

Lipid droplet turnover is regulated by the coordinated actions of multiple proteins located on the lipid droplet surface (**Figure 8K**). First, we measured 24 h rhythms in mRNA levels of two members of the perilipin (PLIN) family, *Plin2* and *Plin5*, which recruit lipases to the lipid droplet surface initiating lipolysis (Itabe et al., 2017). *Plin2* mRNA levels were rhythmic in livers of Fl/Fl mice (**Figure 8A**) and arrhythmic in LKO mice (**Figure 8B**). In contrast, *Plin5* was arrhythmic in livers of Fl/Fl mice (**Figure 8C**), but rhythmic in livers of LKO mice (**Figure 8D**). Abhydrolase domain containing 5/comparative gene identification-58 (*Abdh5*/CGI-58), postulated to activate *Pnpla2*/ATGL and start TG hydrolysis (Lass et al., 2006), was arrhythmic in all groups (**Figures 8E,F**). Lipase E/hormone sensitive type (*Lipe*/HSL), which catalyzes DG hydrolysis, was rhythmic in livers of control-fed Fl/Fl mice, but arrhythmic in livers of alcohol-fed Fl/Fl mice (**Figure 8G**) and livers of LKO mice (**Figure 8H**). The final step in lipolysis is catalyzed by monoacylglycerol lipase (*Mgll*), which works in concert with *Lipe*/HSL to hydrolyze DG to FA and glycerol (Fredrikson et al., 1986). *Mgll* was rhythmic in livers of control and alcohol-fed Fl/Fl mice (**Figure 8I**), but arrhythmic in livers of LKO mice (**Figure 8J**). Results of cosinor analyses for lipid droplet-associated genes are included in **Supplementary Table 7**.

We examined genotype and alcohol-induced effects on mRNA levels of lipid droplet components by two-factor ANOVA, independent of time (**Supplementary Table 4**). Livers of LKO mice generally exhibited increased mRNA levels of *Plin5* and *Abdh5*/CGI-58 and decreased *Lipe*/HSL and *Mgll* (main effect of genotype). Alcohol decreased mRNA levels of *Plin2*, *Plin5*, *Lipe*/HSL, and *Abdh5*/CGI-58, independent of genotype (main

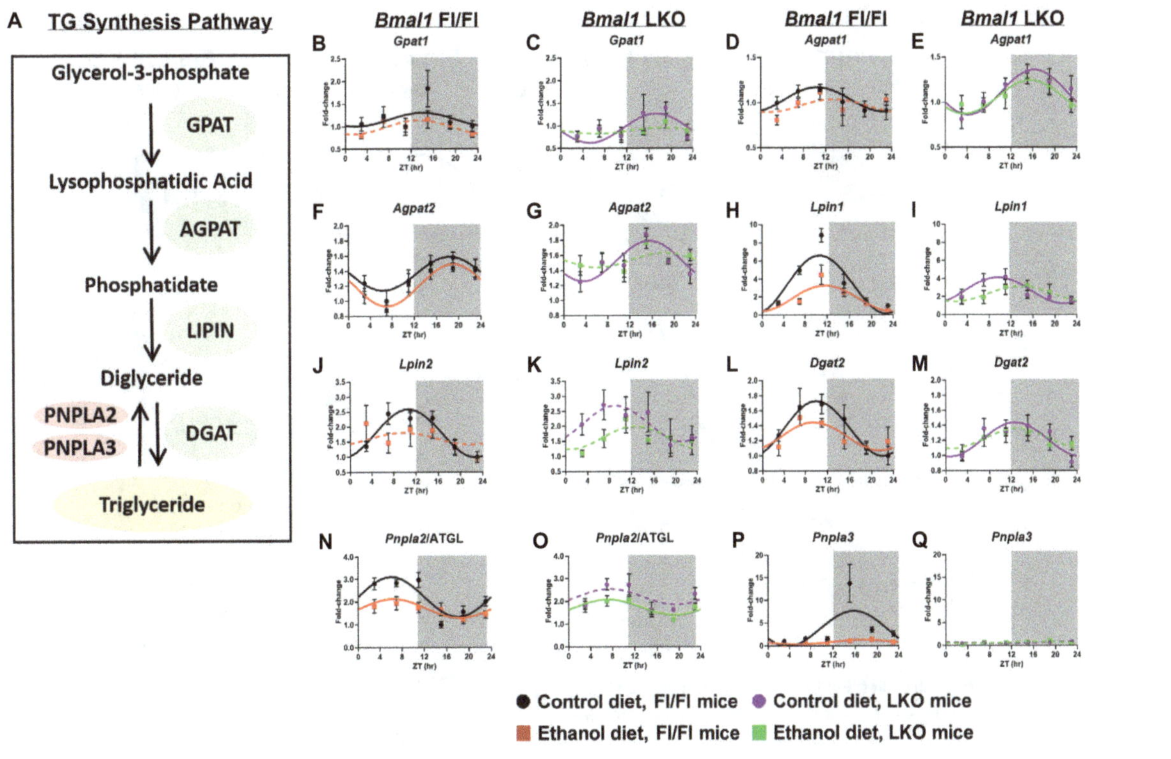

FIGURE 7 | Chronic alcohol and liver clock disruption alter diurnal mRNA rhythms of triglyceride metabolism genes. Pathway for triglyceride synthesis/breakdown **(A)**. Diurnal mRNA profiles of Glycerol-3-phosphate acyltransferase (*Gpat1*; **B,C**), 1-acyl-sn-glycerol-3-phosphate acyltransferase alpha (*Agpat1*; **D,E**), 1-acyl-sn-glycerol-3-phosphate acyltransferase beta (*Agpat2*; **F,G**), Lipin-1 (*Lpin1*; **H,I**), Lipin-2 (*Lpin2*; **J,K**), Diacylglycerol o-acyltransferase 2 (*Dgat2*; **L,M**), Patatin-like phospholipase domain-containing protein 2/Adipose Triglyceride Lipase (*Pnpla2*/ATGL; **N,O**), Patatin-like phospholipase domain-containing protein 3 (*Pnpla3*; **P,Q**) were measured in livers of control-fed (black) and alcohol-fed (red) *Bmal1* Flox/Flox (Fl/Fl) and control-fed (purple) and alcohol-fed (green) *Bmal1* liver-specific knockout (LKO) mice at ZT 3, 7, 11, 15, 19, and 23 (ZT 0: lights on/inactive period, ZT 12: lights off/active period, gray area) by RT-PCR. Data are presented as a fold-change to the *Bmal1* Fl/Fl control diet trough time-point and normalized to *Ppia*. Data are expressed as mean ± SEM for $n = 4–8$ mice/genotype/diet/time point. Solid lines indicate rhythmic mRNA levels and a significant cosine fit, whereas dashed lines indicate arrhythmicity and a non-significant cosine fit. Results for Cosinor and ANOVA analyses are provided in **Supplementary Tables 4** and **6**, respectively.

effect of diet). *Plin2* mRNA levels were lower in livers of alcohol-fed LKO mice, with a significant Genotype X Diet interaction. A trend toward a significant Genotype X Diet interaction was found for *Plin5* and *Abdh5*/CGI-58, where increased mRNA levels of these genes in livers of LKO mice tended to be decreased by alcohol.

Lipidomics

Finally, to gain greater insight into the effects alcohol and liver clock disruption have on lipid metabolism we conducted a lipidomics analysis on livers collected at ZT 3 and ZT 15. A complete list of the TG species detected in livers is provided in **Supplementary Table 8** and these results were used to calculate the percent TG FA saturation and percent TG FA composition in the hepatic TG pool. First, we analyzed for effects on FA saturation. Hepatic TG FA were grouped accordingly to the saturation state (SFA, MUFA, DUFA, or PUFA) and data were analyzed by three-factor ANOVA (**Supplementary Table 9**). Alcohol significantly decreased the percentage of TG SFA in livers of Fl/Fl and LKO mice compared to control diet mice (**Figure 9A**) with significant main effects of genotype and diet. In contrast, TG MUFA are increased in livers of alcohol-fed mice (vs. control-fed mice) and at ZT 15 (vs. ZT 3; **Figure 9B**) with significant main effects of diet and time. Alcohol also increased TG DUFA levels (compared to control-fed mice) and livers from LKO mice had higher TG DUFA than livers from Fl/Fl mice (main effects of genotype and diet; **Figure 9C**). TG PUFA made up the smallest percentage of FA detected in the hepatic TG pool. Alcohol decreased the percentage of TG PUFA (main effect of diet; **Figure 9D**).

Next, we analyzed lipidomics results to look for effects on the individual FA species in the hepatic TG pool (**Figure 10A**). Results for three-factor ANOVA are provided in **Supplementary Table 9**. The significant interaction of Genotype X Diet X Time was observed for several long chain FA with 20 or more carbons. Specifically, pair-wise comparisons (**Supplementary Table 10**) show that the combination of alcohol and liver clock disruption significantly increased liver content of arachidic acid (20:0; **Figure 10J**), eicosadienoic acid (20:2; **Figure 10L**), and docosenoic acid (22:1; **Figure 10N**), especially at ZT 15. In contrast, alcohol and liver clock disruption significantly decreased arachidonic acid (20:4), specifically at ZT 3 (**Figure 10M**).

Significant main effects of genotype, diet, or time were also found for several FA species. Independent of genotype and time (main effect of diet; **Supplementary Table 9**),

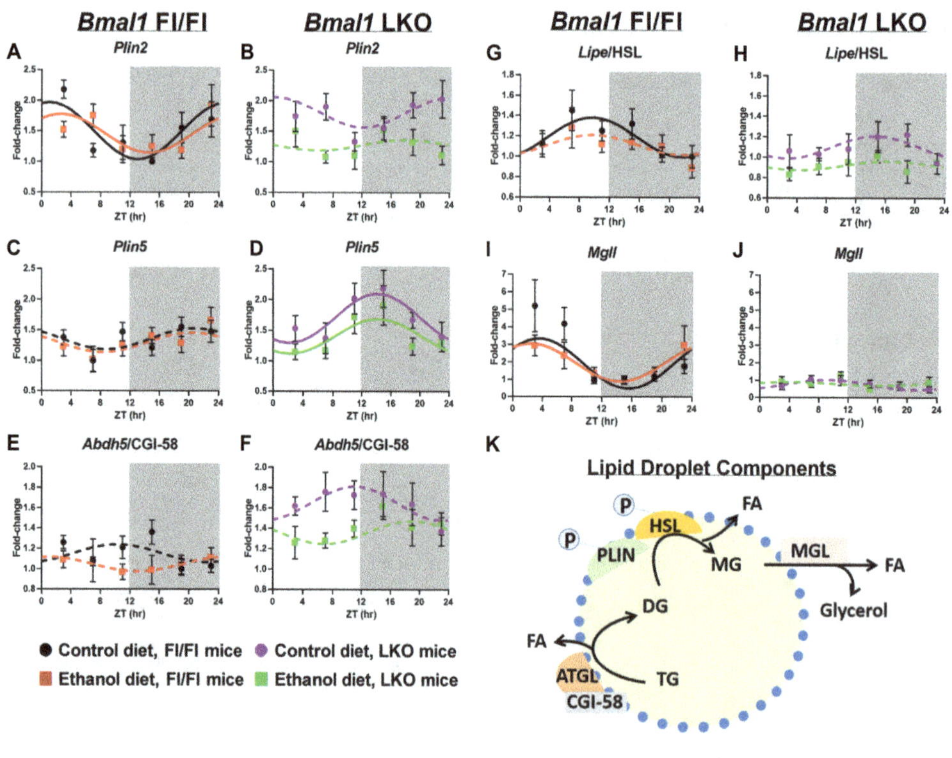

FIGURE 8 | Chronic alcohol and liver clock disruption alter diurnal mRNA rhythms of lipid droplet-associated genes. Diurnal mRNA profiles of lipid droplet genes Perilipin 2 (*Plin2*; **A,B**), Perilipin 5 (*Plin5*; **C,D**), Abhydrolase domain containing 5/Comparative Gene Interaction-58 (*Abdh5*/CGI-58; **E,F**), Hormone sensitive lipase (*Lipe*/HSL; **G,H**), and Monoacylglycerol lipase (*Mgll*; **I,J**) were measured in livers of control-fed (black) and alcohol-fed (red) *Bmal1* Flox/Flox (Fl/Fl) and control-fed (purple) and alcohol-fed (green) *Bmal1* liver-specific knockout (LKO) mice at ZT 3, 7, 11, 15, 19, and 23 (ZT 0: lights on/inactive period, ZT12: lights off/active period, gray area) by RT-PCR. Data are presented as a fold-change to the *Bmal1* Fl/Fl control diet trough time-point and normalized to *Ppia*. Data are expressed as mean ± SEM for n = 4–8 mice/genotype/diet/time point. Solid lines indicate rhythmic mRNA levels and a significant cosine fit, whereas dashed lines indicate arrhythmicity and a non-significant cosine fit. Diagram of a lipid droplet and lipid droplet-associated turnover proteins and enzymes **(K)**. After phosphorylation, PLIN recruits lipases to the surface of the lipid droplet to initiate TG breakdown to glycerol and FA. Results for Cosinor and ANOVA analyses are provided in **Supplementary Tables 4** and **7**, respectively.

alcohol significantly increased lauric acid (12:0; **Figure 10B**), lauroleic acid (12:1; **Figure 10C**), and the most abundant FA, oleic acid (18:1; **Figure 10H**). The PUFA docosahexanoic acid (22:6) also tended to be increased in livers of alcohol-fed mice compared to control-fed mice (**Figure 10O**). Interestingly, alcohol induced an overall decrease in palmitic acid (16:0), the enzymatic product of FASN and a long chain FA precursor, compared to mice fed the control diet (**Figure 10F**). Genetic disruption of the liver clock alone (main effect of genotype; **Supplementary Table 9**) induced an overall increase in lauric acid (12:0; **Figure 10B**), lauroleic acid (12:1; **Figure 10C**) and linoleic acid (18:2; **Figure 10I**). We also observed a general decrease in the levels of palmitic acid (16:0; **Figure 10F**) in livers of LKO mice compared to Fl/Fl mice (main effect of genotype; **Supplementary Table 9**). A time-of-day difference was observed for the overall level of myristoleic acid (14:1; **Figure 10E**), which was higher at ZT 3 regardless of genotype or diet (main effect of time; **Supplementary Table 9**).

Where significant two-factor interactions (Genotype X Diet or Diet X Time) and no three-factor interaction was present, we conducted two-factor ANOVA with pairwise comparisons between groups. Specifically, corresponding data were collapsed together across time for a Genotype X Diet interaction or across genotype for a Diet X Time interaction. No Genotype X Time interactions were present. These additional analyses revealed that independent of time there was a significant interaction of Genotype X Diet (**Supplementary Tables 9** and **11**) for myristic acid (14:0; **Supplementary Figure 1A**) and myristoleic acid (14:1 **Supplementary Figure 1B**). Alcohol significantly increased overall levels of myristic acid (14:0) in livers of Fl/Fl mice (**Supplementary Figure 1A**); however, pair-wise comparisons did not reach significance (**Supplementary Figure 1C**). Pair-wise comparison revealed increased levels of myristoleic acid (14:1) in livers of control-fed LKO mice compared to control-fed Fl/Fl mice and alcohol-fed LKO mice (**Supplementary Figures 1B,C**). Time-of-day dependent effects of alcohol feeding (significant interaction of Diet X Time; **Supplementary Table 8**) were observed for linoleic acid (18:2) and eicosenoic acid (20:1), regardless of genotype. Specifically, at ZT 3 alcohol-fed mice have increased linoleic acid levels, whereas alcohol feeding has no significant effect at ZT 15 (**Supplementary Figures 2A,C**). Conversely, higher levels of eicosenoic acid are present in livers of alcohol-fed mice compared to control-fed mice at ZT 15, but not ZT 3 (**Supplementary Figures 2B,C**). Collectively, these exciting new lipidomics findings indicate that chronic alcohol consumption and liver clock disruption differentially affect FA saturation and composition of the hepatic TG pool.

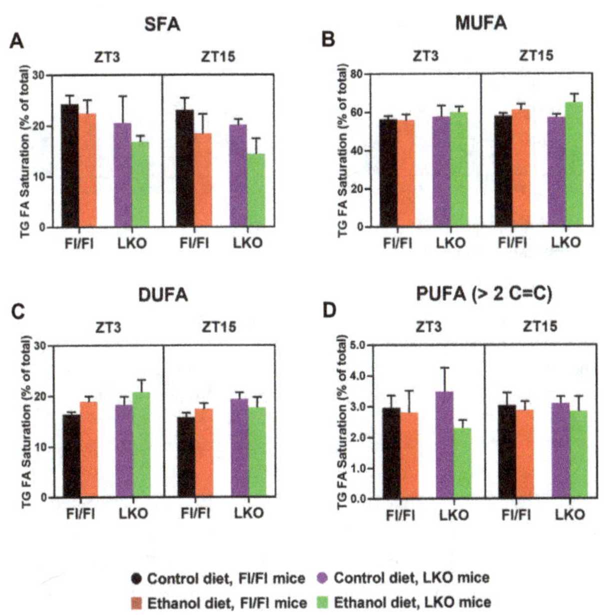

FIGURE 9 | Chronic alcohol and liver clock disruption differentially alter triglyceride fatty acid saturation in the liver. Triglyceride (TG) fatty acid (FA) saturation as a percentage of total saturated fatty acids (SFA, **A**), monounsaturated fatty acids (MUFA, **B**), diunsaturated fatty acids (DUFA, **C**), and polyunsaturated fatty acids (PUFA, **D**) was determined in liver lipid extracts from control-fed (black) and alcohol-fed (red) *Bmal1* Flox/Flox (Fl/Fl) and control-fed (purple) and alcohol-fed (green) *Bmal1* liver-specific knockout (LKO) mice at ZT 3 and ZT 15 (ZT = 0: lights on/inactive active, ZT = 12: lights offs/active period) using MS/MS^{ALL}. Data are mean ± SEM for n = 3–4 mice/genotype/diet/time-point. Results for ANOVA analyses are provided in **Supplementary Table 9**.

DISCUSSION

In this study, we provide a temporal analysis of hepatic lipid metabolism at multiple levels (mRNA, protein abundance, metabolite, and histology) in livers of mice with an intact (Fl/Fl) or disrupted liver clock (LKO) fed either a control or alcohol-containing diet. Several novel findings regarding lipid metabolism were revealed in these studies. First, small droplet macrosteatosis and plasma TG are higher in alcohol-fed LKO mice compared to Fl/Fl mice. Second, LKO mice exhibit different time-of-day patterns of hepatic TG and steatosis type compared to Fl/Fl mice. Third, alcohol or clock disruption alone significantly alters 24 h rhythms in mRNA levels of clock and lipid metabolism genes, with some genes differentially impacted by alcohol in livers of LKO mice. Finally, lipidomics revealed novel changes in TG FA content in livers of alcohol-fed and clock-disrupted mice in a time-of-day dependent manner. In summary, these new findings show that the liver clock is important for maintaining diurnal control of lipid metabolism and that disrupting the liver clock exacerbates alcohol-related hepatic steatosis.

Previously, we found that alcohol consumption disrupts 24 h rhythms in mRNA levels of clock genes and induces circadian misalignment between the master clock in the SCN of the hypothalamus and the peripheral liver clock in wild-type mice (Filiano et al., 2013). These findings were replicated in subsequent alcohol studies from other laboratories (Zhou et al., 2014; Zhang et al., 2018). In this current paper, we observed similar changes in rhythmic mRNA levels of

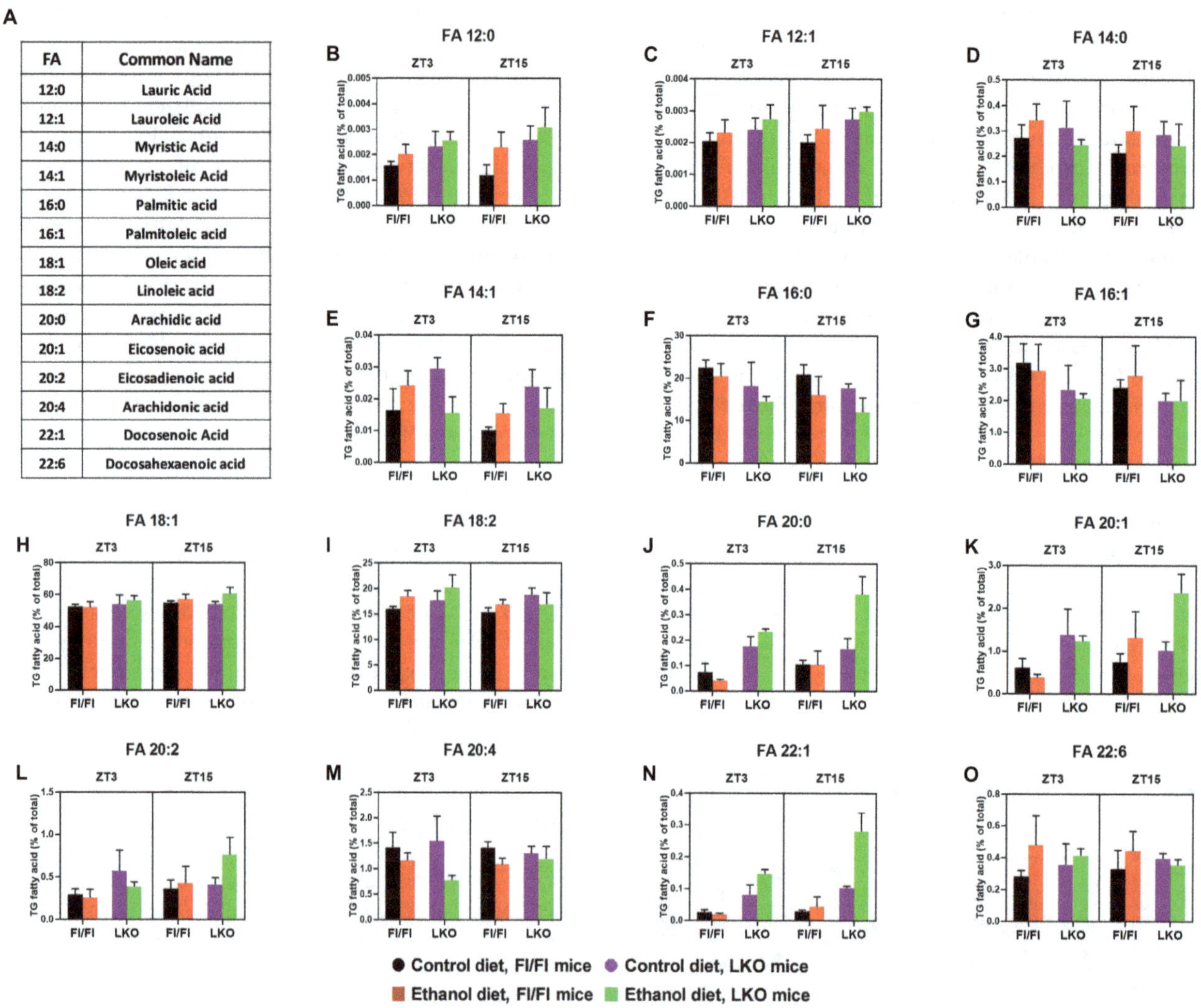

FIGURE 10 | Chronic alcohol and liver clock disruption differentially alter triglyceride fatty acid composition in the liver. Fatty acids (FA, **B–O**) as a percentage of the total triglyceride (TG) FA pool was determined in liver lipid extracts from control-fed (black) and alcohol-fed (red) *Bmal1* Flox/Flox (Fl/Fl) and control-fed (purple) and alcohol-fed (green) *Bmal1* liver-specific knockout (LKO) mice at ZT 3 and ZT 15 (ZT 0: lights on/inactive period, ZT 12: lights offs/active period) using MS/MS^{ALL}. FA common names and structure are shown in panel **(A)**. Data are mean ± SEM for n = 3–4 mice/genotype/diet/time-point. Results for ANOVA analyses and relevant pair-wise comparisons are provided in **Supplementary Tables 9–12**, respectively.

clock genes in livers of alcohol-fed Fl/Fl mice. Alcohol dampened diurnal rhythms in mRNA levels of *Bmal1*, *Per2*, and *Nr1d1*/REV-ERBα and the clock-controlled transcription factor *Dbp*. Interestingly, alcohol induced arrhythmic *Clock*, *Noct*, and *Nfil3*/E4BP4 mRNA levels. A recent RNA-seq analysis from global *Nfil3*/E4BP4 knockout mice shows that this b-ZIP transcription factor represses liver mRNA rhythms (Yoshitane et al., 2019), suggesting that *Nfil3*/E4BP4 (a repressor) might work in concert with BMAL1 (an activator) to temporally regulate liver metabolism. While *Nfil3*/E4BP4 has mostly been studied in immune cells (Male et al., 2012), emerging work points to a pivotal role of *Nfil3*/E4BP4 in regulating liver metabolism, including *de novo* lipogenesis (Tong et al., 2016; Zheng et al., 2016), gluconeogenesis (Kang et al., 2017), and FGF21 (Tong et al., 2010, 2013) – pathways implicated in ALD.

For the first time, the present study also assessed 24 h mRNA levels of clock genes in mice with a non-functional liver clock – LKO mice (Udoh et al., 2017). As expected, we observed arrhythmic or dampened mRNA levels for most of the clock and clock-controlled genes in livers of LKO mice compared to Fl/Fl mice, with alcohol further decreasing rhythmic amplitude. We also observed differential effects on mRNA levels of clock genes between genotypes. For example, *Bmal1*, *Nr1d1*/REV-ERBα, *Dbp*, and *Noct* have a lower mesor in livers of LKO mice compared to Fl/Fl mice. Conversely, *Clock*, *Cry1*, and *Csnk1d/e*, while arrhythmic in livers of LKO mice, have higher overall mRNA levels compared to Fl/Fl mice. While the significance of these opposing changes is not clear, we propose that these distinct responses in mRNA levels of clock (*Bmal1*, *Clock*, and *Nr1d1*/REV-ERBα) and clock-controlled (*Nfil3*/E4BP4,

Noct, and *Dbp*) genes most likely underpins many of the intriguing outcomes in lipid metabolism we observed in livers of LKO mice exposed to alcohol.

Only a handful of studies investigating ALD have considered the temporal nature of lipid metabolism and the molecular clock (Kudo et al., 2009; Filiano et al., 2013; Zhou et al., 2014; Zhang et al., 2018). Therefore, we first measured hepatic and plasma TG levels over a 24 h period. Expectedly, hepatic TG is higher in alcohol compared to control-fed mice over the course of the 24 h day. We also found a modest elevation in plasma TG in alcohol-fed Fl/Fl mice. Given that previous studies show dyslipidemia in mice with genetically altered clocks (Turek et al., 2005; Shimba et al., 2011; Bugge et al., 2012; Cho et al., 2012), we predicted that 24 h TG levels would be higher in livers from alcohol-fed LKO mice. Surprisingly, hepatic TG levels in alcohol-fed LKO mice were not dramatically elevated over levels measured in alcohol-fed Fl/Fl mice. We did however see higher and more variable levels of plasma TG in LKO mice fed alcohol compared to alcohol-fed Fl/Fl mice, supporting the hypothesis that the liver clock is important for consolidating hepatic TG export/uptake to particular times of day (Pan and Hussain, 2007; Pan et al., 2010). Interestingly, some of our findings differ from those reported in other studies. For example, alcohol-fed *Clock*$^{\Delta19/\Delta19}$ mutant mice have elevated hepatic, but unchanged plasma TG levels over the course of the day compared to wild-type mice fed alcohol (Kudo et al., 2009). Similarly, Zhang et al. (2018) reported higher TG in livers of LKO compared to wild-type mice when using the short-term "chronic + binge" alcohol model; however, hepatic TG was only reported at one time of day. Reasons for these disparate results likely include differences in the genetic mouse models of clock disruption, alcohol feeding protocol, and/or sex. Female mice were used in some of these studies (Kudo et al., 2009; Zhang et al., 2018). Female sex is associated with increased sensitivity to alcohol toxicity (Eagon 2010; Wagnerberger et al., 2013) and sex differences in clock gene rhythms are also known (Yang et al., 2009; Kuljis et al., 2013); thus, use of only male mice in our study may explain why we did not see higher TG content in livers of alcohol-fed LKO mice.

Accumulating evidence suggests that there may be time-of-day differences in susceptibility to alcohol-related liver injury. Voigt et al. (2017) showed diurnal variation in the integrity of the intestinal barrier and liver injury in mice subjected to alcohol "binges" (large one-time oral dose) given at different times of the day. Given this, we histologically examined livers to determine whether clock disruption increases markers of alcohol-related injury (e.g., steatosis, lobular inflammation, and hepatocyte ballooning) in a time-of-day dependent manner. We found that alcohol-fed LKO mice had the highest histopathology score with ballooned hepatocytes only detected in LKO mice. Mice with a disrupted liver clock also had a much higher percentage of hepatocytes containing lipid droplets as compared to Fl/Fl mice. Interestingly, alcohol induced more small vs. large droplet macrosteatosis, with the highest levels of small droplet macrosteatosis seen in livers of alcohol-fed LKO mice. The higher prevalence of small vs. large droplet macrosteatosis in livers of LKO mice likely explains the similarity in overall hepatic TG content in LKO and Fl/Fl mice, and highlights the importance of using both biochemical and histological measurements of steatosis in assessing fatty liver injury. Moreover, one limitation of only using H and E-stained liver sections in assessing steatosis is that lipid droplets are detected in the form of optically "empty" vacuoles in the tissue. Moving forward, it will be important to use neutral lipid (i.e., TG) staining reagents, such as BODIPY 493/503 to facilitate more rigorous visualization and quantification of lipid droplets in steatotic liver (Rasineni et al., 2014).

Notably, small droplet macrosteatosis is associated with reduced hepatic ATP content and poorer outcomes in liver transplant patients, suggesting a link to mitochondrial dysfunction (Ferri et al., 2019). Previously, we have shown that alcohol impairs mitochondrial bioenergetics (Young et al., 2006; King et al., 2014) and damages mtDNA (Venkatraman et al., 2004), with other studies reporting clock control of mitochondrial function (Peek et al., 2013; Jacobi et al., 2015). Thus, enhanced mitochondrial damage from the double "hit" of alcohol and clock disruption likely explains increased small droplet macrosteatosis in livers of alcohol-fed LKO mice.

We also observed time-of-day differences in steatosis. Small droplet macrosteatosis peaked in livers of alcohol-fed Fl/Fl mice during the early active period, whereas higher levels were seen in the inactive period for LKO mice. The inactive period of the day was also where we observed ballooned hepatocytes in livers of LKO mice, suggesting time-of-day dependent susceptibility to cell death. Ballooned hepatocytes are a hallmark feature of steatohepatitis, characterized by cell swelling, ubiquitinated protein accumulation, and intermediate cytoskeleton filament keratin 8/18 loss (Lackner et al., 2008; Mostafa et al., 2020). Interestingly, immune responsiveness and inflammation show day/night differences that are gated by the molecular clock (Keller et al., 2009; Nguyen et al., 2013; Curtis et al., 2015). Voigt et al. (2017) found diurnal variations in immune cell trafficking, with higher numbers of immune cells present in livers of alcohol-fed mice during the inactive period of the day. Taken together, these results support the concept that the degree of alcohol-related liver injury may be time-of-day dependent and/or influenced by the timing of alcohol consumption.

While transcriptomic studies indicate that mRNA levels of many lipid metabolism genes exhibit day/night differences (Adamovich et al., 2014; Aviram et al., 2016), the influence alcohol and liver clock disruption have on these diurnal rhythms in mRNA levels is not known. Therefore, we determined 24 h rhythms in mRNA levels for multiple lipid metabolism genes implicated in ALD. The first set of genes we examined were the canonical lipid metabolism transcription factors *Srebf1*/SREBP-1c, *Mlxipl*/ChREBP, *Nr1h3*/LXRα, *Nr1h2*/LXRβ, and *Ppara*. Arrhythmic mRNA levels were found in livers of LKO mice, suggesting clock-regulation of these transcription factors. We observed arrhythmic mRNA levels of *Srebf1*/SREBP-1c in livers of alcohol-fed Fl/Fl mice, leading to disrupted diurnal rhythms in mRNA levels for the SREBP-1c target genes *Acaca*/ACC1 and *Fasn*. Gaucher et al. (2019) also found that *Srebf1*/SREBP-1c and targets were repressed by 6 weeks of alcohol consumption. While it might be predicted that *Srebf1*/SREBP-1c mRNA levels would be elevated in alcohol-induced fatty liver, You et al. (2002) reported that alcohol increases *de novo* lipogenesis post-transcriptionally by increasing translocation of the mature form of SREBP-1c protein into the nucleus. Attempts to assess time-of-day rhythms in SREBP-1c protein translocation in the current study were unsuccessful due to poor antibody specificity (data not shown). Like *Srebf1*/SREBP-1c, *Nr1h2*/LXRβ was also rhythmic in livers of control-fed Fl/Fl, but arrhythmic in livers of alcohol-fed Fl/Fl mice. We propose that the alcohol-mediated loss of rhythmic *Nr1h2*/LXRβ mRNA levels drive arrhythmic *Srebf1*/SREBP-1c, a known target of LXRα/β (Repa et al., 2000). Significant main effects of genotype and diet were observed for both *Sreb1f*/SREBP-1c and *Nr1h2*/LXRβ in livers of LKO compared to Fl/Fl mice, further suggesting crosstalk between these two main lipid metabolism transcription factors in alcohol-exposed liver.

We also assessed diurnal rhythms in mRNA levels of *Ppara*, a transcriptional regulator of genes involved in multiple energy metabolism pathways, including FA transport and oxidation (Pawlak et al., 2015). Interestingly, *Ppara* mRNA levels were rhythmic in livers of alcohol-fed Fl/Fl mice, but arrhythmic in livers of control-fed Fl/Fl mice. With this said, the overall mRNA levels of *Ppara* were significantly lower in livers of alcohol-fed Fl/Fl mice and LKO mice, suggesting alcohol-related suppression of the hepatic FAO pathway. This finding is supported by other studies showing that acetaldehyde, the oxidative product of alcohol metabolism, inhibits DNA binding and transcriptional activity of PPARα and decreases FAO (Galli et al., 2001). Zhang et al. (2018) showed that treatment with fenofibrate, a synthetic PPARα ligand, and overexpression of ChREBP alleviate alcohol-related steatosis by activating FAO. Here, we found alcohol and clock-related decreases in the mesor of *Mlxpil*/ChREBP in the liver. Taken together, we propose that the combined effects of alcohol and clock disruption on *Srebf1*/SREBP-1c, *Nr1h2*/LXRβ, and/or *Ppara* rhythms impair oscillations of target FA and TG metabolism genes, contributing to steatosis.

A key regulatory node for partitioning lipids is the intersection of reactions involved in FA synthesis and oxidation, namely ACC1, ACC2, and MCD. *Acaca*/ACC1 catalyzes the generation of malonyl-CoA, which serves as the substrate for FA synthesis (McGarry et al., 1978b). In contrast, malonyl-CoA synthesized by *Acacb*/ACC2 functions as an allosteric inhibitor of CPT1a by inhibiting FA transport into mitochondria for FAO (McGarry et al., 1978a). These complementary enzymes help ensure that FA synthesis and oxidation do not occur simultaneously. In keeping with this, we found that *Acaca*/ACC1 and *Acacb*/ACC2 rhythms have different peaks in livers of control-fed Fl/Fl mice. *Acaca*/ACC1 peaks during the inactive period, whereas *Acacb*/ACC2 peaks during the active period of the day. We also observed that alcohol significantly dampened rhythms of both genes. At the protein level, AMPK phosphorylates and inactivates ACC, blocking malonyl-CoA production (Munday et al., 1988; Fullerton et al., 2013). Importantly, alcohol inhibits AMPK (Garcia-Villafranca et al., 2008), which is predicted to increase ACC activity and malonyl-CoA production, resulting in increased FA synthesis and decreased FAO – two potential mechanisms of steatosis. Therefore, we chose to assess both total and phosphorylated ACC1 and ACC2. Unfortunately, the results from these studies were equivocal. First, a p-ACC2 antibody is not available, thus, we had to use an antibody that detects both p-ACC1 and p-ACC2. Second, because these two proteins have high molecular weights of similar size (e.g., ACC1 = 265 kDa and ACC2 = 280 kDa), we were not able to achieve sufficient separation of proteins to analyze each band separately for densitometry. Therefore, bands were analyzed together. A significant main effect of diet was found for p-ACC1/2 with significantly lower levels in livers of alcohol-fed LKO mice. Accordingly, we predict that ACC1/2 activity and malonyl-CoA levels would be increased. We also assessed mRNA and proteins levels of *Mlycd*/MCD, the enzyme responsible for decarboxylation of malonyl-CoA back to acetyl-CoA (Saggerson, 2008). *Mlycd*/MCD mRNA levels were rhythmic in livers of control-fed Fl/Fl mice, with alcohol inducing a significant 3.6 h phase delay in the peak of the rhythm. MCD protein levels were stable throughout the day; however, there was a significant main effect of genotype with 50% less MCD protein in livers of LKO mice compared to Fl/Fl mice. Thus, these results predict higher levels of malonyl-CoA in livers of alcohol-fed LKO mice that will increase FA synthesis and/or decrease FAO oxidation, leading to steatosis. Previous studies show that *Mlycd*/MCD is a PPARα target, as decreased MCD mRNA levels/activity and FAO are present in hearts of PPARα knockout mice (Campbell et al., 2002). Future studies are planned to determine whether temporal dysregulation in a PPARα-ACC1/2-MCD-malonyl-CoA axis promotes alcohol-induced steatosis, especially in circadian clock disrupted livers.

Adamovich et al. (2014) reported that the enzymes involved in TG synthesis and breakdown exhibit diurnal variations in mRNA levels. Our results are consistent with these findings, showing significant diurnal rhythms in mRNA levels for *Gpat1*, *Agpat1/2*, *Lpin1/2*, *Dgat2*, and *Pnpla2/3* in livers of control-fed Fl/Fl mice, with changed rhythms in livers of LKO mice. We predicted alcohol feeding would increase mRNA levels of TG synthesis genes; however, we largely observed dampening of rhythms. Importantly, alcohol significantly decreased the mesor and amplitude of *Pnpla2*/ATGL and *Pnpla3* rhythms. *Pnpla2*/ATGL is regarded as the rate-limiting enzyme in TG breakdown where it translocates to the surface of lipid droplets, binds *Abdh5*/CGI-58, and catalyzes the breakdown of TG to DG. Similarly, *Pnpla3* is a TG hydrolase with LPA transacylase activity (Jenkins et al., 2004; Lake et al., 2005; He et al., 2010); however, the physiological relevance of *Pnpla3* in TG metabolism remains ambiguous as targeted deletion of *Pnpla3* does not impair TG hydrolysis or promote steatosis (Basantani et al., 2011). In contrast, a missense genetic variant in PNPLA3 (I148M) in humans is strongly associated with fatty liver disease (Romeo et al., 2008) by reduced hydrolase activity (Huang et al., 2011) and disruption of *Pnpla2*/ATGL function on the lipid droplet surface (BasuRay et al., 2019; Wang et al., 2019). Interestingly, *Pnpla3* mRNA levels were dramatically reduced and arrhythmic in livers of LKO mice, which is similar to findings using *Per1/2* double knockout mice (Adamovich et al., 2014), suggesting a strong role of the clock in regulating *Pnpla3* mRNA levels in the liver.

The lipid droplet structure is maintained by PLIN1–5 with PLIN2 being the most abundant PLIN in liver (Itabe et al., 2017).

Briefly, phosphorylation of PLIN2 by protein kinase A recruits PNPLA2/ATGL and PNPLA3 to the lipid droplet surface and initiates TG hydrolysis to DG, with subsequent breakdown reactions catalyzed by *Lipe*/HSL and *Mgll*, resulting in release of glycerol and FA (Zechner et al., 2009). We observed significant diurnal rhythms for *Plin2*, *Lipe*, and *Mgll*, but not *Plin5* and *Abdh5*/CGI-58 in livers of control-fed Fl/Fl mice. A role for PLIN2 in ALD is supported by studies showing alcohol-related increases in PLIN2 mRNA and protein in liver (Carr et al., 2013; Rasineni et al., 2014) and *Plin2* knockout mice are protected from ALD (Carr et al., 2014). Here, we found lower and higher levels of *Plin2* at ZT 3 and ZT 7, respectively, in livers of alcohol-fed Fl/Fl mice compared to control-fed Fl/Fl mice, suggesting alcohol-related dysregulation in mRNA levels of *Plin2*. This finding also highlights the importance of assessing 24 h rhythms in mRNA levels vs. only one time point during the day as a completely different alcohol-related response in mRNA levels were observed in only a 4 h time window for *Plin2*. PLIN5 is proposed to facilitate FA uptake from lipid droplets to mitochondria for FAO (Wang et al., 2011). Live cell imaging shows reduced contact between mitochondria and lipid droplets and decreased FAO in hepatocytes from *Plin5* knockout mice (Keenan et al., 2019). Here, *Plin5* mRNA levels were arrhythmic in livers of Fl/Fl mice, but rhythmic in livers of LKO mice with peak phase occurring at ZT 14. This finding suggests that *Plin5* mRNA levels may entrain to the feeding/fasting cycle in the absence of a functional liver clock; however, additional studies are needed to verify this finding. In contrast, *Plin2*, *Abdh5*/CGI-58, *Lipe*/HSL, and *Mgll* were all arrhythmic in livers of LKO mice. These novel findings suggest an important role of the circadian clock in maintaining temporal control of lipid droplet dynamics in hepatocytes.

In addition to lipolysis, lipophagy significantly contributes to lipid droplet catabolism by selectively targeting lipid droplets to lysosomes for degradation (Singh et al., 2009). In fact, several of the lipid droplet components we measured in this current study also participate in lipophagy. For example, PLIN2 functions as a substrate for chaperone-mediated lipophagy by recruiting *Pnpla2*/ATGL and autophagy-related proteins to the lipid droplet (Kaushik and Cuervo, 2015). *Pnpla2*/ATGL-mediated signaling through SIRT1 also stimulates lipophagy in hepatocytes (Sathyanarayan et al., 2017). It is also well-known that chronic alcohol impairs lipophagy, which along with lipolysis inhibition promotes developments of steatosis (Schulze et al., 2017; Chao and Ding, 2019). Interestingly, new work shows differential morphology in lipid droplet size when inhibiting lipolysis or lipophagy in hepatocytes (Schott et al., 2019). Specifically, inhibition of *Pnpla2*/ATGL with atglistatin results in accumulation of large lipid droplets, whereas inhibition of the lysosomal lipophagy pathway with chloroquine results in accumulation of small lipid droplets enriched in autophagic (LC3) and lysosomal (LAMP2A) markers in hepatocytes (Schott et al., 2019). While beyond the scope of this current paper, it will be important that future studies determine if impairment in lipophagy underpins increased small droplet macrosteatosis in livers of mice with a disrupted liver clock.

Previous studies have reported that alcohol alters the profile of multiple lipid species in the liver, including glycerolipids, glycerophospholipids, sphingolipids, and ceramides (see review Clugston et al., 2017). Important for this current study is work showing that the majority of oscillating lipids in the liver are TG species (Adamovich et al., 2014). Based on this, we used an MS/MS^{ALL}-based lipidomics approach (Gajenthra Kumar et al., 2018) to provide novel mechanistic insights into how alcohol and clock disruption affect TG metabolism and steatosis. Specifically, we defined two characteristics of the hepatic TG pool – the overall TG FA saturation state and TG FA composition at ZT 3 and ZT 15 as these times generally corresponded to the nadir and peak of total TG content in livers of alcohol-fed Fl/Fl mice. First, we found lower and higher percentages of TG SFA and TG DUFA, respectively, in livers of alcohol-fed Fl/Fl mice. These findings coincide with data from other labs reporting decreases in SFA and increases in MUFA and PUFAs in livers of alcohol-fed mice and rats, representing a shift toward FA unsaturation (Clugston et al., 2011; Fernando et al., 2011). Accordingly, livers from alcohol-fed LKO mice also had higher TG MUFA and TG DUFA content, but lower TG PUFA content, especially at ZT 3. It should also be pointed out that FA saturation is likely linked to the composition of the Lieber-DeCarli diet that is high in unsaturated FA (Lieber et al., 1989).

Regarding FA composition, we found that alcohol and liver clock disruption differentially affect the FA profile of the hepatic TG pool in a time-of-day dependent manner. The most abundant FA detected in the TG pool were palmitic acid (16:0), oleic acid (18:1), and linoleic acid (18:2). Interestingly, palmitic acid (16:0) was significantly decreased in livers of alcohol-fed LKO mice at both time points compared to Fl/Fl mice, which likely correlates with much lower FASN levels in livers of LKO mice. Interestingly, Chakravarthy et al. (2005) found that a lack of FASN (by liver-specific FASN KO) did not protect against the development of hepatic steatosis, but rather increased steatosis due to reduced mitochondrial FAO in response to increased malonyl-CoA levels. As mentioned earlier, malonyl-CoA inhibits CPT1, the enzyme responsible for entry of fatty acyl-CoA into mitochondria for oxidation. Similarly, they hypothesized that newly FASN-synthesized palmitic acid functions as an endogenous ligand for PPARα, which would have the effect of increasing FAO in mitochondria. In support of this hypothesis, other studies have reported that saturated FA like palmitic acid bind to PPARα with affinities similar to those of unsaturated fatty acids (Kliewer et al., 1997; Xu et al., 1999). Taken together, these findings indicate that an alcohol-dependent decrease in MCD, FASN, and FASN-derived palmitic acid likely contributes to hepatic steatosis by decreasing mitochondrial FAO in the liver.

In contrast, we observed increased linoleic acid (18:2) in livers of alcohol-fed LKO mice at ZT 3. Other studies have also shown alcohol-related increases in 18 carbon FA of varying saturation in the total liver lipid pool (Puri et al., 2016). Importantly, Kirpich and colleagues have found that linoleic acid (18:2) increases alcohol-related liver injury in mice through production of oxidized linoleic acid metabolites that activate pro-inflammatory macrophages (Warner et al., 2017). Thus, it is possible that this mechanism contributed to increased injury in LKO mice. We also found large increases in the lower abundant 20 carbon FA, arachidic acid (20:0), eicosanoid acid (20:1), and eicosadienoic acid (20:2) in livers of alcohol-fed LKO at ZT 15, indicating a time-dependent shift in accumulation. We also observed interesting effects on arachidonic acid (20:4), an important precursor for synthesis of eicosanoids and other biologically active metabolites involved in cellular signaling and inflammatory response (Calder, 2012). Here, we found significantly lower levels of arachidonic acid (20:4) in livers of alcohol-fed mice, specifically in LKO mice at ZT 3, which is consistent with other studies in mice (Bradford et al., 2008; Loftus et al., 2011). However, alcohol increases arachidonic acid (20:4) in livers of alcohol-fed rats, suggesting species differences in FA turnover (Loftus et al., 2011). We also observed the highest levels of docosenoic acid (22:1) in livers of LKO mice that were further elevated at ZT 15. Finally, we observed a trend toward increased docosahexanoic acid (DHA, 22:6) in livers of alcohol-fed mice. Other studies have reported alcohol-related increases in DHA (Clugston et al., 2011; Puri et al., 2016), an important omega-3 PUFA with anti-inflammatory properties (Calder, 2012).

Based on these lipidomics finding, we would have predicted to have found a more pronounced disruption in the time-of-day patterns in mRNA levels of FA biosynthesis genes *Scd1*, *Elovl5/6*, and *Fads1/2*. We did however observe arrhythmic mRNA levels for all genes in livers of LKO mice, and alcohol-related alterations in *Elovl6* and *Fads2* rhythms in livers of Fl/Fl mice. These changes may have contributed to differences in TG FA composition between genotypes. Moving forward, future studies should incorporate assessments at the protein level as posttranslational modifications like phosphorylation and acetylation are important determinants of FA metabolism enzyme activity. Additionally, assessing TG FA composition over the entire 24 h period will provide a more complete picture of the dynamic nature of the hepatic lipidome.

CONCLUDING REMARKS

In conclusion, the current study provides several novel observations regarding alcohol-related changes in lipid metabolism that may be of relevance in ALD. These studies reveal that liver clock disruption increases small droplet macrosteatosis in livers of alcohol-fed mice and significantly disrupts 24 h rhythms in mRNA levels of multiple clock and lipid metabolism genes in the liver. Importantly, we also found that alcohol, liver clock disruption, or both conditions in combination significantly remodeled the FA profile of the hepatic TG pool lipidome. Taken together, these novel findings highlight the importance of a functional liver molecular clock in maintaining hepatic lipid homeostasis, and suggest that circadian clock disruption may be an important risk factor in the pathogenesis of ALD.

AUTHOR CONTRIBUTIONS

JV, UU, TS, and KA performed research. CP and SD performed histology scoring. JV and PB performed mass spectrometry. JV, KG, and SB performed statistical analyses. KG and SB designed study. JV and SB wrote manuscript with co-author input and review. All authors contributed to the article and approved the submitted version.

ACKNOWLEDGMENTS

The authors thank Dr. Martin Young, University of Alabama at Birmingham, Birmingham, AL, USA for his assistance in generating the Bmall LKO mouse model.

REFERENCES

Abdelmegeed, M. A., Yoo, S. H., Henderson, L. E., Gonzalez, F. J., Woodcroft, K. J., and Song, B. J. (2011). PPARalpha expression protects male mice from high fat-induced nonalcoholic fatty liver. *J. Nutr.* 141, 603–610. doi: 10.3945/jn.110.135210

Abu-Elheiga, L., Brinkley, W. R., Zhong, L., Chirala, S. S., Woldegiorgis, G., and Wakil, S. J. (2000). The subcellular localization of acetyl-CoA carboxylase 2. *Proc. Natl. Acad. Sci. U. S. A.* 97, 1444–1449.

Adamovich, Y., Rousso-Noori, L., Zwighaft, Z., Neufeld-Cohen, A., Golik, M., Kraut-Cohen, J., et al. (2014). Circadian clocks and feeding time regulate the oscillations and levels of hepatic triglycerides. *Cell Metab.* 19, 319–330. doi: 10.1016/j.cmet.2013.12.016

Aviram, R., Manella, G., Kopelman, N., Neufeld-Cohen, A., Zwighaft, Z., Elimelech, M., et al. (2016). Lipidomics analyses reveal temporal and spatial lipid organization and uncover daily oscillations in intracellular organelles. *Mol. Cell* 62, 636–648. doi: 10.1016/j.molcel.2016.04.002

Bailey, S. M., and Cunningham, C. C. (1998). Acute and chronic ethanol increases reactive oxygen species generation and decreases viability in fresh, isolated rat hepatocytes. *Hepatology* 28, 1318–1326. doi: 10.1002/hep.510280521

Bailey, S. M., Udoh, U. S., and Young, M. E. (2014). Circadian regulation of metabolism. *J. Endocrinol.* 222, R75–R96. doi: 10.1530/JOE-14-0200

Basantani, M. K., Sitnick, M. T., Cai, L., Brenner, D. S., Gardner, N. P., Li, J. Z., et al. (2011). Pnpla3/Adiponutrin deficiency in mice does not contribute to fatty liver disease or metabolic syndrome. *J. Lipid Res.* 52, 318–329. doi: 10.1194/jlr.M011205

BasuRay, S., Wang, Y., Smagris, E., Cohen, J. C., and Hobbs, H. H. (2019). Accumulation of PNPLA3 on lipid droplets is the basis of associated hepatic steatosis. *Proc. Natl. Acad. Sci. U. S. A.* 116, 9521–9526. doi: 10.1073/pnas.1901974116

Begriche, K., Massart, J., Robin, M. A., Borgne-Sanchez, A., and Fromenty, B. (2011). Drug-induced toxicity on mitochondria and lipid metabolism: mechanistic diversity and deleterious consequences for the liver. *J. Hepatol.* 54, 773–794. doi: 10.1016/j.jhep.2010.11.006

Bianchi, A., Evans, J. L., Iverson, A. J., Nordlund, A. C., Watts, T. D., and Witters, L. A. (1990). Identification of an isozymic form of acetyl-CoA carboxylase. *J. Biol. Chem.* 265, 1502–1509.

Bligh, E. G., and Dyer, W. J. (1959). A rapid method of total lipid extraction and purification. *Can. J. Biochem. Physiol.* 37, 911–917. doi: 10.1139/o59-099

Bradford, B. U., O'Connell, T. M., Han, J., Kosyk, O., Shymonyak, S., Ross, P. K., et al. (2008). Metabolomic profiling of a modified alcohol liquid diet model for liver injury in the mouse uncovers new markers of disease. *Toxicol. Appl. Pharmacol.* 232, 236–243. doi: 10.1016/j.taap.2008.06.022

Brady, C. W. (2020). Liver disease in pregnancy: what's new. *Hepatol. Commun.* 4, 145–156. doi: 10.1002/hep4.1470

Brandon-Warner, E., Schrum, L. W., Schmidt, C. M., and McKillop, I. H.

(2012). Rodent models of alcoholic liver disease: of mice and men. *Alcohol* 46, 715–725. doi: 10.1016/j.alcohol.2012.08.004

Brunt, E. M. (2007). Pathology of fatty liver disease. *Mod. Pathol.* 20 (Suppl. 1), S40–S48. doi: 10.1038/modpathol.3800680

Brunt, E. M., Janney, C. G., Di Bisceglie, A. M., Neuschwander-Tetri, B. A., and Bacon, B. R. (1999). Nonalcoholic steatohepatitis: a proposal for grading and staging the histological lesions. *Am. J. Gastroenterol.* 94, 2467–2474. doi: 10.1111/j.1572-0241.1999.01377.x

Bugge, A., Feng, D., Everett, L. J., Briggs, E. R., Mullican, S. E., Wang, F., et al. (2012). Rev-erbalpha and Rev-erbbeta coordinately protect the circadian clock and normal metabolic function. *Genes Dev.* 26, 657–667. doi: 10.1101/gad.186858.112

Calder, P. C. (2012). Long-chain fatty acids and inflammation. *Proc. Nutr. Soc.* 71, 284–289. doi: 10.1017/S0029665112000067

Campbell, F. M., Kozak, R., Wagner, A., Altarejos, J. Y., Dyck, J. R., Belke, D. D., et al. (2002). A role for peroxisome proliferator-activated receptor alpha (PPARalpha) in the control of cardiac malonyl-CoA levels: reduced fatty acid oxidation rates and increased glucose oxidation rates in the hearts of mice lacking PPARalpha are associated with higher concentrations of malonyl-CoA and reduced expression of malonyl-CoA decarboxylase. *J. Biol. Chem.* 277, 4098–4103. doi: 10.1074/jbc.M106054200

Carr, R. M., Dhir, R., Yin, X., Agarwal, B., and Ahima, R. S. (2013). Temporal effects of ethanol consumption on energy homeostasis, hepatic steatosis, and insulin sensitivity in mice. *Alcohol. Clin. Exp. Res.* 37, 1091–1099. doi: 10.1111/acer.12075

Carr, R. M., Peralta, G., Yin, X., and Ahima, R. S. (2014). Absence of perilipin 2 prevents hepatic steatosis, glucose intolerance and ceramide accumulation in alcohol-fed mice. *PLoS One* 9:e97118. doi: 10.1371/journal.pone.0097118

Cederbaum, A. I., Lieber, C. S., Beattie, D. S., and Rubin, E. (1975). Effect of chronic ethanol ingestion on fatty acid oxidation in hepatic mitochondria. *J. Biol. Chem.* 250, 5122–5129.

Chakravarthy, M. V., Pan, Z., Zhu, Y., Tordjman, K., Schneider, J. G., Coleman, T., et al. (2005). "New" hepatic fat activates PPARalpha to maintain glucose, lipid, and cholesterol homeostasis. *Cell Metab.* 1, 309–322. doi: 10.1016/j.cmet.2005.04.002

Chao, X., and Ding, W. X. (2019). Role and mechanisms of autophagy in alcohol-induced liver injury. *Adv. Pharmacol.* 85, 109–131. doi: 10.1016/bs.apha.2019.01.008

Cho, H., Zhao, X., Hatori, M., Yu, R. T., Barish, G. D., Lam, M. T., et al. (2012). Regulation of circadian behaviour and metabolism by REV-ERB-alpha and REV-ERB-beta. *Nature* 485, 123–127. doi: 10.1038/nature11048

Clugston, R. D., Gao, M. A., and Blaner, W. S. (2017). The hepatic lipidome: a gateway to understanding the pathogenes is of alcohol-induced fatty liver. *Curr. Mol. Pharmacol.* 10, 195–206. doi: 10.2174/1874467208666150817111419

Clugston, R. D., Jiang, H., Lee, M. X., Piantedosi, R., Yuen, J. J., Ramakrishnan, R., et al. (2011). Altered hepatic lipid metabolism in C57BL/6 mice fed alcohol: a targeted lipidomic and gene expression study. *J. Lipid Res.* 52, 2021–2031. doi: 10.1194/jlr.M017368

Coleman, R. A., and Mashek, D. G. (2011). Mammalian triacylglycerol metabolism: synthesis, lipolysis, and signaling. *Chem. Rev.* 111, 6359–6386. doi: 10.1021/cr100404w

Curtis, A. M., Fagundes, C. T., Yang, G., Palsson-McDermott, E. M., Wochal, P., McGettrick, A. F., et al. (2015). Circadian control of innate immunity in macrophages by miR-155 targeting Bmal1. *Proc. Natl. Acad. Sci. U. S. A.* 112, 7231–7236. doi: 10.1073/pnas.1501327112

Danaei, G., Ding, E. L., Mozaffarian, D., Taylor, B., Rehm, J., Murray, C. J., et al. (2009). The preventable causes of death in the United States: comparative risk assessment of dietary, lifestyle, and metabolic risk factors. *PLoS Med.* 6:e1000058. doi: 10.1371/journal.pmed.1000058

Dupont, W. D. (2002). *Statistical modeling for biomedical researchers: A simple introduction to the analysis of complex data.* New York: Cambridge University Press.

Eagon, P. K. (2010). Alcoholic liver injury: influence of gender and hormones. *World J. Gastroenterol.* 16, 1377–1384. doi: 10.3748/wjg.v16.i11.1377

Etchegaray, J. P., Machida, K. K., Noton, E., Constance, C. M., Dallmann, R., Di Napoli, M. N., et al. (2009). Casein kinase 1 delta regulates the pace of the mammalian circadian clock. *Mol. Cell. Biol.* 29, 3853–3866. doi: 10.1128/MCB.00338-09

Fernando, H., Bhopale, K. K., Kondraganti, S., Kaphalia, B. S., and Shakeel Ansari, G. A. (2011). Lipidomic changes in rat liver after long-term exposure to ethanol. *Toxicol. Appl. Pharmacol.* 255, 127–137. doi: 10.1016/j.taap.2011.05.022

Ferri, F., Lai, Q., Molinaro, A., Poli, E., Parlati, L., Lattanzi, B., et al. (2019). Donor small-droplet macrovesicular steatosis affects liver transplant outcome in HCV-negative recipients. *Can. J. Gastroenterol. Hepatol.* 2019, 1–13. doi: 10.1155/2019/5862985

Filiano, A. N., Millender-Swain, T., Johnson, R. Jr., Young, M. E., Gamble, K. L., and Bailey, S. M. (2013). Chronic ethanol consumption disrupts the core molecular clock and diurnal rhythms of metabolic genes in the liver without affecting the suprachiasmatic nucleus. *PLoS One* 8:e71684. doi: 10.1371/journal.pone.0071684

Fredrikson, G., Tornqvist, H., and Belfrage, P. (1986). Hormone-sensitive lipase and monoacylglycerol lipase are both required for complete degradation of adipocyte triacylglycerol. *Biochim. Biophys. Acta* 876, 288–293.

Fromenty, B., and Pessayre, D. (1995). Inhibition of mitochondrial beta-oxidation as a mechanism of hepatotoxicity. *Pharmacol. Ther.* 67, 101–154. doi: 10.1016/0163-7258(95)00012-6

Fromenty, B., and Pessayre, D. (1997). Impaired mitochondrial function in microvesicular steatosis. Effects of drugs, ethanol, hormones and cytokines. *J. Hepatol.* 26(Suppl. 2), 43–53.

Fullerton, M. D., Galic, S., Marcinko, K., Sikkema, S., Pulinilkunnil, T., Chen, Z. P., et al. (2013). Single phosphorylation sites in Acc1 and Acc2 regulate lipid homeostasis and the insulin-sensitizing effects of metformin. *Nat. Med.* 19, 1649–1654. doi: 10.1038/nm.3372

Gajenthra Kumar, N., Contaifer, D. Jr., Baker, P. R. S., Ekroos, K., Jefferson, K. K., and Wijesinghe, D. S. (2018). Untargeted lipidomic analysis to broadly characterize the effects of pathogenic and non-pathogenic staphylococci on mammalian lipids. *PLoS One* 13:e0206606. doi: 10.1371/journal.pone.0206606

Galli, A., Pinaire, J., Fischer, M., Dorris, R., and Crabb, D. W. (2001). The transcriptional and DNA binding activity of peroxisome proliferator-activated receptor alpha is inhibited by ethanol metabolism. A novel mechanism for the development of ethanol-induced fatty liver. *J. Biol. Chem.* 276, 68–75. doi: 10.1074/jbc.M008791200

Garcia-Villafranca, J., Guillen, A., and Castro, J. (2008). Ethanol consumption impairs regulation of fatty acid metabolism by decreasing the activity of AMP-activated protein kinase in rat liver. *Biochimie* 90, 460–466. doi: 10.1016/j.biochi.2007.09.019

Gaucher, J., Kinouchi, K., Ceglia, N., Montellier, E., Peleg, S., Greco, C. M., et al. (2019). Distinct metabolic adaptation of liver circadian pathways to acute and chronic patterns of alcohol intake. *Proc. Natl. Acad. Sci. U. S. A.* 116, 25250–25259. doi: 10.1073/pnas.1911189116

Glasgow, J. F., and Middleton, B. (2001). Reye syndrome—insights on causation and prognosis. *Arch. Dis. Child.* 85, 351–353. doi: 10.1136/adc.85.5.351

Hatori, M., Vollmers, C., Zarrinpar, A., DiTacchio, L., Bushong, E. A., Gill, S., et al. (2012). Time-restricted feeding without reducing caloric intake prevents metabolic diseases in mice fed a high-fat diet. *Cell Metab.* 15, 848–860. doi: 10.1016/j.cmet.2012.04.019

He, S., McPhaul, C., Li, J. Z., Garuti, R., Kinch, L., Grishin, N. V., et al. (2010). A sequence variation (I148M) in PNPLA3 associated with nonalcoholic fatty liver disease disrupts triglyceride hydrolysis. *J. Biol. Chem.* 285, 6706–6715. doi: 10.1074/jbc.M109.064501

Huang, Y., Cohen, J. C., and Hobbs, H. H. (2011). Expression and characterization of a PNPLA3 protein isoform (I148M) associated with nonalcoholic fatty liver disease. *J. Biol. Chem.* 286, 37085–37093. doi: 10.1074/jbc.M111.290114

Hughes, M. E., Hogenesch, J. B., and Kornacker, K. (2010). JTK_CYCLE: an efficient nonparametric algorithm for detecting rhythmic components in genome-scale data sets. *J. Biol. Rhythm.* 25, 372–380. doi: 10.1177/0748730410379711

Itabe, H., Yamaguchi, T., Nimura, S., and Sasabe, N. (2017). Perilipins: a diversity of intracellular lipid droplet proteins. *Lipids. Health. Dis.* 16:83. doi: 10.1186/s12944-017-0473-y

Jacobi, D., Liu, S., Burkewitz, K., Kory, N., Knudsen, N. H., Alexander, R. K., et al. (2015). Hepatic Bmal1 regulates rhythmic mitochondrial dynamics and promotes metabolic fitness. *Cell Metab.* 22, 709–720. doi: 10.1016/j.cmet.2015.08.006

Jenkins, C. M., Mancuso, D. J., Yan, W., Sims, H. F., Gibson, B., and Gross, R. W. (2004). Identification, cloning, expression, and purification of three novel human calcium-independent phospholipase A2 family members possessing triacylglycerol lipase and acylglycerol transacylase activities. *J. Biol. Chem.*

279, 48968–48975. doi: 10.1074/jbc.M407841200

Jou, J., Choi, S. S., and Diehl, A. M. (2008). Mechanisms of disease progression in nonalcoholic fatty liver disease. *Semin. Liver Dis.* 28, 370–379. doi: 10.1055/s-0028-1091981

Kang, G., Han, H. S., and Koo, S. H. (2017). NFIL3 is a negative regulator of hepatic gluconeogenesis. *Metabolism* 77, 13–22. doi: 10.1016/j.metabol.2017.08.007

Kaushik, S., and Cuervo, A. M. (2015). Degradation of lipid droplet-associated proteins by chaperone-mediated autophagy facilitates lipolysis. *Nat. Cell Biol.* 17, 759–770. doi: 10.1038/ncb3166

Keenan, S. N., Meex, R. C., Lo, J. C. Y., Ryan, A., Nie, S., Montgomery, M. K., et al. (2019). Perilipin 5 deletion in hepatocytes remodels lipid metabolism and causes hepatic insulin resistance in mice. *Diabetes* 68, 543–555. doi: 10.2337/db18-0670

Keller, M., Mazuch, J., Abraham, U., Eom, G. D., Herzog, E. D., Volk, H. D., et al. (2009). A circadian clock in macrophages controls inflammatory immune responses. *Proc. Natl. Acad. Sci. U. S. A.* 106, 21407–21412. doi: 10.1073/pnas.0906361106

King, A. L., Swain, T. M., Mao, Z., Udoh, U. S., Oliva, C. R., Betancourt, A. M., et al. (2014). Involvement of the mitochondrial permeability transition pore in chronic ethanol-mediated liver injury in mice. *Am. J. Physiol. Gastrointest. Liver Physiol.* 306, G265–G277. doi: 10.1152/ajpgi.00278.2013

Kleiner, D. E., Brunt, E. M., Van Natta, M., Behling, C., Contos, M. J., Cummings, O. W., et al. (2005). Design and validation of a histological scoring system for nonalcoholic fatty liver disease. *Hepatology* 41, 1313–1321. doi: 10.1002/hep.20701

Kliewer, S. A., Sundseth, S. S., Jones, S. A., Brown, P. J., Wisely, G. B., Koble, C. S., et al. (1997). Fatty acids and eicosanoids regulate gene expression through direct interactions with peroxisome proliferator-activated receptors alpha and gamma. *Proc. Natl. Acad. Sci. U. S. A.* 94, 4318–4323.

Ko, C. H., and Takahashi, J. S. (2006). Molecular components of the mammalian circadian clock. *Hum. Mol. Genet.* 15, R271–R277. doi: 10.1093/hmg/ddl207

Kojima, S., Sher-Chen, E. L., and Green, C. B. (2012). Circadian control of mRNA polyadenylation dynamics regulates rhythmic protein expression. *Genes Dev.* 26, 2724–2736. doi: 10.1101/gad.208306.112

Koronowski, K. B., Kinouchi, K., Welz, P. S., Smith, J. G., Zinna, V. M., Shi, J., et al. (2019). Defining the independence of the liver circadian clock. *Cell* 177, 1448–1462.e14. doi: 10.1016/j.cell.2019.04.025

Kudo, T., Tamagawa, T., and Shibata, S. (2009). Effect of chronic ethanol exposure on the liver of clock-mutant mice. *J. Circadian Rhythms* 7:4. doi: 10.1186/1740-3391-7-4

Kuljis, D. A., Loh, D. H., Truong, D., Vosko, A. M., Ong, M. L., McClusky, R., et al. (2013). Gonadal- and sex-chromosome-dependent sex differences in the circadian system. *Endocrinology* 154, 1501–1512. doi: 10.1210/en.2012-1921

Kume, K., Zylka, M. J., Sriram, S., Shearman, L. P., Weaver, D. R., Jin, X., et al. (1999). mCRY1 and mCRY2 are essential components of the negative limb of the circadian clock feedback loop. *Cell* 98, 193–205. doi: 10.1016/S0092-8674(00)81014-4

Lackner, C., Gogg-Kamerer, M., Zatloukal, K., Stumptner, C., Brunt, E. M., and Denk, H. (2008). Ballooned hepatocytes in steatohepatitis: the value of keratin immunohistochemistry for diagnosis. *J. Hepatol.* 48, 821–828. doi: 10.1016/j.jhep.2008.01.026

Lake, A. C., Sun, Y., Li, J. L., Kim, J. E., Johnson, J. W., Li, D., et al. (2005). Expression, regulation, and triglyceride hydrolase activity of Adiponutrin family members. *J. Lipid Res.* 46, 2477–2487. doi: 10.1194/jlr.M500290-JLR200

Lass, A., Zimmermann, R., Haemmerle, G., Riederer, M., Schoiswohl, G., Schweiger, M., et al. (2006). Adipose triglyceride lipase-mediated lipolysis of cellular fat stores is activated by CGI-58 and defective in Chanarin-Dorfman syndrome. *Cell Metab.* 3, 309–319. doi: 10.1016/j.cmet.2006.03.005

Lee, H., Chen, R., Lee, Y., Yoo, S., and Lee, C. (2009). Essential roles of CKIdelta and CKIepsilon in the mammalian circadian clock. *Proc. Natl. Acad. Sci. U. S. A.* 106, 21359–21364. doi: 10.1073/pnas.0906651106

Lieber, C. S., DeCarli, L. M., and Sorrell, M. F. (1989). Experimental methods of ethanol administration. *Hepatology* 10, 501–510. doi: 10.1002/hep.1840100417

Livak, K. J., and Schmittgen, T. D. (2001). Analysis of relative gene expression data using real-time quantitative PCR and the 2(-Delta Delta C(T)) method. *Methods* 25, 402–408. doi: 10.1006/meth.2001.1262

Loftus, N., Barnes, A., Ashton, S., Michopoulos, F., Theodoridis, G., Wilson, I., et al. (2011). Metabonomic investigation of liver profiles of nonpolar metabolites obtained from alcohol-dosed rats and mice using high mass accuracy MSn analysis. *J. Proteome Res.* 10, 705–713. doi: 10.1021/pr100885w

Male, V., Nisoli, I., Gascoyne, D. M., and Brady, H. J. (2012). E4BP4: an unexpected player in the immune response. *Trends Immunol.* 33, 98–102. doi: 10.1016/j.it.2011.10.002

McGarry, J. D., Leatherman, G. F., and Foster, D. W. (1978a). Carnitine palmitoyltransferase I. The site of inhibition of hepatic fatty acid oxidation by malonyl-CoA. *J. Biol. Chem.* 253, 4128–4136.

McGarry, J. D., Takabayashi, Y., and Foster, D. W. (1978b). The role of malonyl-coa in the coordination of fatty acid synthesis and oxidation in isolated rat hepatocytes. *J. Biol. Chem.* 253, 8294–8300.

Minino, A. M., Heron, M. P., and Smith, B. L. (2006). Deaths: preliminary data for 2004. *Natl. Vital Stat. Rep.* 54, 1–49.

Mitsui, S., Yamaguchi, S., Matsuo, T., Ishida, Y., and Okamura, H. (2001). Antagonistic role of E4BP4 and PAR proteins in the circadian oscillatory mechanism. *Genes Dev.* 15, 995–1006. doi: 10.1101/gad.873501

Mostafa, M., Abdelkader, A., Evans, J. J., Hagen, C. E., and Hartley, C. P. (2020). Fatty liver disease: a practical approach. *Arch. Pathol. Lab. Med.* 144, 62–70. doi: 10.5858/arpa.2019-0341-RA

Munday, M. R., Campbell, D. G., Carling, D., and Hardie, D. G. (1988). Identification by amino acid sequencing of three major regulatory phosphorylation sites on rat acetyl-CoA carboxylase. *Eur. J. Biochem.* 175, 331–338. doi: 10.1111/j.1432-1033.1988.tb14201.x

Nguyen, K. D., Fentress, S. J., Qiu, Y., Yun, K., Cox, J. S., and Chawla, A. (2013). Circadian gene Bmal1 regulates diurnal oscillations of Ly6C(hi) inflammatory monocytes. *Science* 341, 1483–1488. doi: 10.1126/science.1240636

Orlicky, D. J., Roede, J. R., Bales, E., Greenwood, C., Greenberg, A., Petersen, D., et al. (2011). Chronic ethanol consumption in mice alters hepatocyte lipid droplet properties. *Alcohol. Clin. Exp. Res.* 35, 1020–1033. doi: 10.1111/j.1530-0277.2011.01434.x

Pan, X., and Hussain, M. M. (2007). Diurnal regulation of microsomal triglyceride transfer protein and plasma lipid levels. *J. Biol. Chem.* 282, 24707–24719. doi: 10.1074/jbc.M701305200

Pan, X., Zhang, Y., Wang, L., and Hussain, M. M. (2010). Diurnal regulation of MTP and plasma triglyceride by CLOCK is mediated by SHP. *Cell Metab.* 12, 174–186. doi: 10.1016/j.cmet.2010.05.014

Pawlak, M., Lefebvre, P., and Staels, B. (2015). Molecular mechanism of PPARalpha action and its impact on lipid metabolism, inflammation and fibrosis in non-alcoholic fatty liver disease. *J. Hepatol.* 62, 720–733. doi: 10.1016/j.jhep.2014.10.039

Peek, C. B., Affinati, A. H., Ramsey, K. M., Kuo, H. Y., Yu, W., Sena, L. A., et al. (2013). Circadian clock NAD^+ cycle drives mitochondrial oxidative metabolism in mice. *Science* 342:1243417. doi: 10.1126/science.1243417

Preitner, N., Damiola, F., Lopez-Molina, L., Zakany, J., Duboule, D., Albrecht, U., et al. (2002). The orphan nuclear receptor REV-ERBalpha controls circadian transcription within the positive limb of the mammalian circadian oscillator. *Cell* 110, 251–260. doi: 10.1016/S0092-8674(02)00825-5

Puri, P., Xu, J., Vihervaara, T., Katainen, R., Ekroos, K., Daita, K., et al. (2016). Alcohol produces distinct hepatic lipidome and eicosanoid signature in lean and obese. *J. Lipid Res.* 57, 1017–1028. doi: 10.1194/jlr.M066175

Rasineni, K., McVicker, B. L., Tuma, D. J., McNiven, M. A., and Casey, C. A. (2014). Rab GTPases associate with isolated lipid droplets (LDs) and show altered content after ethanol administration: potential role in alcohol-impaired LD metabolism. *Alcohol. Clin. Exp. Res.* 38, 327–335. doi: 10.1111/acer.12271

Repa, J. J., Liang, G., Ou, J., Bashmakov, Y., Lobaccaro, J. M., Shimomura, I., et al. (2000). Regulation of mouse sterol regulatory element-binding protein-1c gene (SREBP-1c) by oxysterol receptors, LXRalpha and LXRbeta. *Genes Dev.* 14, 2819–2830. doi: 10.1101/gad.844900

Reue, K., and Wang, H. (2019). Mammalian lipin phosphatidic acid phosphatases in lipid synthesis and beyond: metabolic and inflammatory disorders. *J. Lipid Res.* 60, 728–733. doi: 10.1194/jlr.S091769

Ripperger, J. A., and Schibler, U. (2006). Rhythmic CLOCK-BMAL1 binding to multiple E-box motifs drives circadian Dbp transcription and chromatin transitions. *Nat. Genet.* 38, 369–374. doi: 10.1038/ng1738

Romeo, S., Kozlitina, J., Xing, C., Pertsemlidis, A., Cox, D., Pennacchio, L. A., et al. (2008). Genetic variation in PNPLA3 confers susceptibility to nonalcoholic fatty liver disease. *Nat. Genet.* 40, 1461–1465. doi: 10.1038/ng.257

Saggerson, D. (2008). Malonyl-CoA, a key signaling molecule in mammalian cells. *Annu. Rev. Nutr.* 28, 253–272. doi: 10.1146/annurev.nutr.28.061807.155434

Sakhuja, P. (2014). Pathology of alcoholic liver disease, can it be differentiated from nonalcoholic steatohepatitis? *World J. Gastroenterol.* 20, 16474–16479. doi: 10.3748/wjg.v20.i44.16474

Salaspuro, M. P., Shaw, S., Jayatilleke, E., Ross, W. A., and Lieber, C. S. (1981). Attenuation of the ethanol-induced hepatic redox change after chronic alcohol consumption in baboons: metabolic consequences *in vivo* and *in vitro*. *Hepatology* 1, 33–38. doi: 10.1002/hep.1840010106

Sathyanarayan, A., Mashek, M. T., and Mashek, D. G. (2017). ATGL promotes autophagy/lipophagy via SIRT1 to control hepatic lipid droplet catabolism. *Cell Rep.* 19, 1–9. doi: 10.1016/j.celrep.2017.03.026

Sato, T. K., Panda, S., Miraglia, L. J., Reyes, T. M., Rudic, R. D., McNamara, P., et al. (2004). A functional genomics strategy reveals Rora as a component of the mammalian circadian clock. *Neuron* 43, 527–537. doi: 10.1016/j.neuron.2004.07.018

Schott, M. B., Weller, S. G., Schulze, R. J., Krueger, E. W., Drizyte-Miller, K., Casey, C. A., et al. (2019). Lipid droplet size directs lipolysis and lipophagy catabolism in hepatocytes. *J. Cell Biol.* 218, 3320–3335. doi: 10.1083/jcb.201803153

Schreiber, R., Xie, H., and Schweiger, M. (2019). Of mice and men: the physiological role of adipose triglyceride lipase (ATGL). *Biochim. Biophys. Acta Mol. Cell Biol. Lipids* 1864, 880–899. doi: 10.1016/j.bbalip.2018.10.008

Schulze, R. J., Drizyte, K., Casey, C. A., and McNiven, M. A. (2017). Hepatic lipophagy: new insights into autophagic catabolism of lipid droplets in the liver. *Hepatol. Commun.* 1, 359–369. doi: 10.1002/hep4.1056

Sengupta, M., Griffett, K., Flaveny, C. A., and Burris, T. P. (2018). Inhibition of hepatotoxicity by a LXR inverse agonist in a model of alcoholic liver disease. *ACS Pharmacol. Transl. Sci.* 1, 50–60. doi: 10.1021/acsptsci.8b00003

Shimba, S., Ogawa, T., Hitosugi, S., Ichihashi, Y., Nakadaira, Y., Kobayashi, M., et al. (2011). Deficient of a clock gene, brain and muscle Arnt-like protein-1 (BMAL1), induces dyslipidemia and ectopic fat formation. *PLoS One* 6:e25231. doi: 10.1371/journal.pone.0025231

Singh, R., Kaushik, S., Wang, Y., Xiang, Y., Novak, I., Komatsu, M., et al. (2009). Autophagy regulates lipid metabolism. *Nature* 458, 1131–1135. doi: 10.1038/nature07976

Spach, P. I., Herbert, J. S., and Cunningham, C. C. (1991). The interaction between chronic ethanol consumption and oxygen tension in influencing the energy state of rat liver. *Biochim. Biophys. Acta* 1056, 40–46. doi: 10.1016/S0005-2728(05)80070-2

Summa, K. C., Voigt, R. M., Forsyth, C. B., Shaikh, M., Cavanaugh, K., Tang, Y., et al. (2013). Disruption of the circadian clock in mice increases intestinal permeability and promotes alcohol-induced hepatic pathology and inflammation. *PLoS One* 8:e67102. doi: 10.1371/journal.pone.0067102

Takahashi, J. S. (2017). Transcriptional architecture of the mammalian circadian clock. *Nat. Rev. Genet.* 18, 164–179. doi: 10.1038/nrg.2016.150

Thampy, K. G., and Wakil, S. J. (1988). Regulation of acetyl-coenzyme A carboxylase. I. Purification and properties of two forms of acetyl-coenzyme A carboxylase from rat liver. *J. Biol. Chem.* 263, 6447–6453.

Theise, N. D. (2013). Histopathology of alcoholic liver disease. *Clin. Liver Dis.* 2, 64–67. doi: 10.1002/cld.172

Tong, X., Li, P., Zhang, D., VanDommelen, K., Gupta, N., Rui, L., et al. (2016). E4BP4 is an insulin-induced stabilizer of nuclear SREBP-1c and promotes SREBP-1c-mediated lipogenesis. *J. Lipid Res.* 57, 1219–1230. doi: 10.1194/jlr.M067181

Tong, X., Muchnik, M., Chen, Z., Patel, M., Wu, N., Joshi, S., et al. (2010). Transcriptional repressor E4-binding protein 4 (E4BP4) regulates metabolic hormone fibroblast growth factor 21 (FGF21) during circadian cycles and feeding. *J. Biol. Chem.* 285, 36401–36409. doi: 10.1074/jbc.M110.172866

Tong, X., Zhang, D., Buelow, K., Guha, A., Arthurs, B., Brady, H. J., et al. (2013). Recruitment of histone methyltransferase G9a mediates transcriptional repression of Fgf21 gene by E4BP4 protein. *J. Biol. Chem.* 288, 5417–5425. doi: 10.1074/jbc.M112.433482

Trepo, E., Romeo, S., Zucman-Rossi, J., and Nahon, P. (2016). PNPLA3 gene in liver diseases. *J. Hepatol.* 65, 399–412. doi: 10.1016/j.jhep.2016.03.011

Turek, F. W., Joshu, C., Kohsaka, A., Lin, E., Ivanova, G., McDearmon, E., et al. (2005). Obesity and metabolic syndrome in circadian clock mutant mice. *Science* 308, 1043–1045. doi: 10.1126/science.1108750

Udoh, U. S., Swain, T. M., Filiano, A. N., Gamble, K. L., Young, M. E., and Bailey, S. M. (2015). Chronic ethanol consumption disrupts diurnal rhythms of hepatic glycogen metabolism in mice. *Am. J. Physiol. Gastrointest. Liver Physiol.* 308, G964–G974. doi: 10.1152/ajpgi.00081.2015

Udoh, U. S., Valcin, J. A., Swain, T. M., Filiano, A. N., Gamble, K. L., Young, M. E., et al. (2017). Genetic deletion of the circadian clock transcription factor BMAL1 and chronic alcohol consumption differentially alter hepatic glycogen in mice. *Am. J. Physiol. Gastrointest. Liver Physiol.* 314, G431–G447. doi: 10.1152/ajpgi.00281.2017

Venkatraman, A., Landar, A., Davis, A. J., Chamlee, L., Sanderson, T., Kim, H., et al. (2004). Modification of the mitochondrial proteome in response to the stress of ethanol-dependent hepatotoxicity. *J. Biol. Chem.* 279, 22092–22101. doi: 10.1074/jbc.M402245200

Vielhaber, E., Eide, E., Rivers, A., Gao, Z. H., and Virshup, D. M. (2000). Nuclear entry of the circadian regulator mPER1 is controlled by mammalian casein kinase I epsilon. *Mol. Cell. Biol.* 20, 4888–4899. doi: 10.1128/MCB.20.13.4888-4899.2000

Voigt, R. M., Forsyth, C. B., Shaikh, M., Zhang, L., Raeisi, S., Aloman, C., et al. (2017). Diurnal variations in intestinal barrier integrity and liver pathology in mice: implications for alcohol binge. *Am. J. Physiol. Gastrointest. Liver Physiol.* 314, G131–G141. doi: 10.1152/ajpgi.00103.2017

Voigt, R. M., Summa, K. C., Forsyth, C. B., Green, S. J., Engen, P., Naqib, A., et al. (2016). The circadian clock mutation promotes intestinal dysbiosis. *Alcohol. Clin. Exp. Res.* 40, 335–347. doi: 10.1111/acer.12943

Wagnerberger, S., Fiederlein, L., Kanuri, G., Stahl, C., Millonig, G., Mueller, S., et al. (2013). Sex-specific differences in the development of acute alcohol-induced liver steatosis in mice. *Alcohol. Alcohol.* 48, 648–656. doi: 10.1093/alcalc/agt138

Wang, Y., Kory, N., BasuRay, S., Cohen, J. C., and Hobbs, H. H. (2019). PNPLA3, CGI-58, and inhibition of hepatic triglyceride hydrolysis in mice. *Hepatology* 69, 2427–2441. doi: 10.1002/hep.30583

Wang, H., Sreenivasan, U., Hu, H., Saladino, A., Polster, B. M., Lund, L. M., et al. (2011). Perilipin 5, a lipid droplet-associated protein, provides physical and metabolic linkage to mitochondria. *J. Lipid Res.* 52, 2159–2168. doi: 10.1194/jlr.M017939

Warner, D. R., Liu, H., Miller, M. E., Ramsden, C. E., Gao, B., Feldstein, A. E., et al. (2017). Dietary linoleic acid and its oxidized metabolites exacerbate liver injury caused by ethanol via induction of hepatic proinflammatory response in mice. *Am. J. Pathol.* 187, 2232–2245. doi: 10.1016/j.ajpath.2017.06.008

Xu, H. E., Lambert, M. H., Montana, V. G., Parks, D. J., Blanchard, S. G., Brown, P. J., et al. (1999). Molecular recognition of fatty acids by peroxisome proliferator-activated receptors. *Mol. Cell* 3, 397–403. doi: 10.1016/S1097-2765(00)80467-0

Yang, L., Yang, C., Thomes, P. G., Kharbanda, K. K., Casey, C. A., McNiven, M. A., et al. (2019). Lipophagy and alcohol-induced fatty liver. *Front. Pharmacol.* 10:495. doi: 10.3389/fphar.2019.01685

Yang, X., Zhang, Y. K., Esterly, N., Klaassen, C. D., and Wan, Y. J. (2009). Gender disparity of hepatic lipid homoeostasis regulated by the circadian clock. *J. Biochem.* 145, 609–623. doi: 10.1093/jb/mvp018

Yeh, M. M., and Brunt, E. M. (2014). Pathological features of fatty liver disease. *Gastroenterology* 147, 754–764. doi: 10.1053/j.gastro.2014.07.056

Yoshitane, H., Asano, Y., Sagami, A., Sakai, S., Suzuki, Y., Okamura, H., et al. (2019). Functional D-box sequences reset the circadian clock and drive mRNA rhythms. *Commun. Biol.* 2:300. doi: 10.1038/s42003-019-0522-3

You, M., and Arteel, G. E. (2019). Effect of ethanol on lipid metabolism. *J. Hepatol.* 70, 237–248. doi: 10.1016/j.jhep.2018.10.037

You, M., Fischer, M., Deeg, M. A., and Crabb, D. W. (2002). Ethanol induces fatty acid synthesis pathways by activation of sterol regulatory element-binding protein (SREBP). *J. Biol. Chem.* 277, 29342–29347. doi: 10.1074/jbc.M202411200

Young, T. A., Bailey, S. M., Van Horn, C. G., and Cunningham, C. C. (2006). Chronic ethanol consumption decreases mitochondrial and glycolytic production of ATP in liver. *Alcohol. Alcohol.* 41, 254–260. doi: 10.1093/alcalc/agl017

Zechner, R., Kienesberger, P. C., Haemmerle, G., Zimmermann, R., and Lass, A. (2009). Adipose triglyceride lipase and the lipolytic catabolism of cellular fat stores. *J. Lipid Res.* 50, 3–21. doi: 10.1194/jlr.R800031-JLR200

Zelickson, B. R., Benavides, G. A., Johnson, M. S., Chacko, B. K., Venkatraman, A., Landar, A., et al. (2011). Nitric oxide and hypoxia exacerbate alcohol-induced mitochondrial dysfunction in hepatocytes. *Biochim. Biophys. Acta* 1807, 1573–1582. doi: 10.1016/j.bbabio.2011.09.011

Zhang, J. Y., Kothapalli, K. S., and Brenna, J. T. (2016a). Desaturase and elongase-limiting endogenous long-chain polyunsaturated fatty acid biosynthesis. *Curr. Opin. Clin. Nutr. Metab. Care* 19, 103–110. doi: 10.1097/MCO.0000000000000254

Zhang, W., Sun, Q., Zhong, W., Sun, X., and Zhou, Z. (2016b). Hepatic peroxisome proliferator-activated receptor gamma signaling contributes to alcohol-induced hepatic steatosis and inflammation in mice. *Alcohol. Clin. Exp. Res.* 40, 988–999. doi: 10.1111/acer.13049

Zhang, D., Tong, X., Arthurs, B., Guha, A., Rui, L., Kamath, A., et al. (2014). Liver clock protein BMAL1 promotes de novo lipogenesis through insulin-mTORC2-AKT signaling. *J. Biol. Chem.* 289, 25925–25935. doi: 10.1074/jbc.M114.567628

Zhang, D., Tong, X., Nelson, B. B., Jin, E., Sit, J., Charney, N., et al. (2018). The hepatic BMAL1/AKT/Lipogenesis axis protects against alcoholic liver disease via promoting PPARalpha pathway. *Hepatology* 68, 883–896. doi: 10.1002/hep.29878

Zheng, Z., Kim, H., Qiu, Y., Chen, X., Mendez, R., Dandekar, A., et al. (2016). CREBH couples circadian clock with hepatic lipid metabolism. *Diabetes* 65, 3369–3383. doi: 10.2337/db16-0298

Zheng, B., Larkin, D. W., Albrecht, U., Sun, Z. S., Sage, M., Eichele, G., et al. (1999). The mPer2 gene encodes a functional component of the mammalian circadian clock. *Nature* 400, 169–173. doi: 10.1038/22118

Zhou, P., Ross, R. A., Pywell, C. M., Liangpunsakul, S., and Duffield, G. E. (2014). Disturbances in the murine hepatic circadian clock in alcohol-induced hepatic steatosis. *Sci. Rep.* 4:3725. doi: 10.1038/srep03725

9

Dietary Copper Plays an Important Role in Maintaining Intestinal Barrier Integrity During Alcohol-Induced Liver Disease Through Regulation of the Intestinal HIF-1α Signaling Pathway and Oxidative Stress

Hongwei Lin[1†], Dazhi Chen[2†], Qianjing Du[1], Tongtong Pan[1], Hanxiao Tu[1], Yuedong Xu[1], Teng Teng[1], Jingjing Tu[1], Ji Li[1], Zhuo Lin[1], Xiaodong Wang[1], Lanman Xu[1] and Yong-Ping Chen[1*]*

[1] Department of Infectious Diseases, The First Affiliated Hospital of Wenzhou Medical University, Zhejiang Provincial Key Laboratory for Accurate Diagnosis and Treatment of Chronic Liver Diseases, Hepatology Institute of Wenzhou Medical University, Wenzhou, China, [2] Department of Gastroenterology, Peking University First Hospital, Beijing, China

***Correspondence:**
Lanman Xu
13587646315@163.com
Yong-Ping Chen
13505777281@163.com

[†] These authors have contributed equally to this work

Impaired intestinal barrier function and oxidative stress injury play critical roles in the pathogenesis of alcoholic liver disease (ALD), and recent investigations have revealed a role for dietary copper in the liver and intestinal barrier function. Therefore, the current study investigates the mechanisms and role of dietary copper in alcohol induced liver diseases. C57BL/6 mice were used to create an alcoholic liver disease model with a Lieber-DeCarli diet containing 5% alcohol and were fed with different concentrations of dietary copper of adequate (6 ppm, CuA), marginal (1.5 ppm, CuM), or supplemental (20 ppm, CuS) amounts. Caco-2 cells were also exposed to ethanol and different concentrations of copper. Damages of the liver and intestine were evaluated by transaminases, histology staining, and protein and mRNA level, as well as cell proliferation, oxidative stress, and mitochondrial membrane potential. In animal experiments, the results indicate that an alcohol diet causes liver injury and disruption of intestinal barrier function as well as decreasing the expression of genes such as HIF-1α, occludin, SOD1, and GPX1. Supplemental dietary copper can revert these changes except for SOD1, but marginal dietary copper can worsen these changes. The *in vitro* cell experiments showed that proper copper supplementation can promote cell growth and reduce reactive oxygen species (ROS) production. In conclusion, supplemental dietary copper has beneficial effects on alcohol-induced intestine and liver injury, and marginal dietary copper shows detrimental effects on these parameters.

Keywords: copper, HIF-1α, alcoholic liver injury, intestinal barrier, Caco-2

INTRODUCTION

Alcoholic liver disease (ALD) arises due to excess use of alcohol for a long period of time and ranges from hepatic steatosis to steatohepatitis, cirrhosis, and even hepatocellular carcinoma (Seitz et al., 2018). ALD is a leading cause of morbidity and mortality worldwide, but its targeted therapy is limited (Bajaj, 2019; Ge et al., 2019). Therefore, research on mechanisms and treatment methods is urgently needed. Although the pathogenesis of ALD may involve many aspects (Rao, 2009; Gao and Bataller, 2011; Orman et al., 2013; Chen et al., 2016), recent studies have suggested that gut barrier dysfunction induced by alcohol, such as increased intestinal permeability, bacterial translocation, and release of bacteria-derived endotoxin into circulation, may play an important role in ALD development.

The barrier function of intestinal epithelial cells is regulated by a variety of factors, including oxygen (Rath et al., 2018). Moreover, alcohol-induced oxidative stress and inflammatory reactions can aggravate tissue hypoxia (Louvet and Mathurin, 2015). Since hypoxia-inducible factor-1α (HIF-1α) is a regulatory subunit of the hypoxia-inducible factor (HIF), which regulates a wide range of genes involved in cellular responses to hypoxia and other tissue environmental cues (Prabhakar and Semenza, 2012), HIF-1α should play an important role in maintaining barrier functions of intestinal epithelial cells. In addition, HIF-1α was significantly increased in hepatic fibrotic tissues and activated hepatic stellate cells (HSCs) (Moon et al., 2009), which are the consequences of alcoholic diseases. However, the role of HIF-1α in alcoholic diseases still remains to be investigated.

An adequate supply of copper is essential for healthy life, as chronic copper deficiency can elicit anemia, leucopenia, myelopathy, or skin abnormalities (Altarelli et al., 2019). Moreover, copper deficiency in rodent shows an adverse effect on lipid metabolism (Al-Othman et al., 1992, 1993). Furthermore, several investigations revealed that copper might be involved in the regulation of gut microbiota and gut barrier function (Song et al., 2018). For example, copper has been used as an antimicrobial agent throughout the ages (Hodgkinson and Petris, 2012), and the response to copper stress varies greatly among different bacterial species (Pontel and Soncini, 2009; Solioz et al., 2010). However, there are no copper-related drugs for the clinical treatment of alcoholic liver. In addition, low copper availability was observed in NAFLD patients, and a copper-deficient diet induces fatty liver in rodents (Aigner et al., 2008, 2010). However, whether and how dietary copper contributes to the development of ALD through altering gut barrier function and oxidative stress remain unknown. Therefore, in this research, we employed mice and Caco-2 cells to investigate the role of dietary copper in the development of alcoholic hepatic steatosis and intestinal epithelial functions.

MATERIALS AND METHODS

Animal Experiments

As shown in **Figure 1**, seventy-two C57BL/6 wild type (WT) mice (6 weeks of age, male) from the Shanghai Laboratory Animal Center (Shanghai, China) were fed (ad lib.) with the Lieber-DeCarli control diet (Trophic Animal Feed High-tech Co., Jiangsu, China) with a defined copper content in the form of cupric carbonate (Bertola et al., 2013). In order to adapt the animals from solid feed to liquid feed, the mice received 1.5, 6.0, or 20 ppm of copper as marginal, adequate, or supplemental doses, respectively, for 5 days. They were then divided into two groups: a control group (C) and an alcoholic steatosis model group (M). For the purpose of reducing the impact of alcohol on animal function and decreasing mortality, mice were fed a mixed diet of which the ratio (Lieber-DeCarli alcohol diet: Lieber-DeCarli control diet) changed from 2:1 to 1:1 to 1:2 at days 2, 4, and 6, respectively, for 1 week in the model group and were then fed with the Lieber-DeCarli alcohol diet to general steatosis model. In the control group, mice were fed with the Lieber-DeCarli control diet with the same copper content as mice in the model group for 6 weeks. On the 28th day, a bolus of ethanol (5 g/kg body weight, 40%) or isocaloric dextrin (8.9 g/kg body weight) was gavaged in the model and control groups, respectively. After 10 h of gavage, all mice were euthanized to collect blood, liver, and intestinal tissue. Mice were treated according to the protocols reviewed and approved by the Institutional Ethics Committee of Wenzhou Medical University, which were in accordance with the Guiding Principles for the Care and Use of Laboratory Animals in China.

Measurement of Serum Copper, ALT, and AST Levels

The collected blood was centrifuged at 1500 rpm for 10 min to obtain serum. The levels of serum copper, ALT, and AST were measured by using an automated biochemical analyzer (Abbott Laboratories, Chicago, IL, United States) in the clinical biochemical laboratory of the First Affiliated Hospital of Wenzhou Medical University.

Liver and Small Intestine Histopathology

Harvested liver and upper small intestine samples were fixed in 4% paraformaldehyde and embedded in paraffin, then cut into 4-μm sections and processed for staining with hematoxylin and eosin (H&E). Moreover, sections of the liver were quickly frozen and then cut into 4-μm sections and stained with Oil Red O. Both were analyzed by light microscopy.

Real-Time Reverse Transcriptase-Polymerase Chain Reaction (RT-PCR) Assay

Total RNA in tissues was separately extracted according to the instructions of the RNA extraction kit (Aidlab Biotechnologies Co., Beijing, China), and 1 μg total RNA was reverse-transcribed into cDNA using the PrimeScriptTM RTreagent Kit (Perfect Real Time; Aidlab Biotechnologies Co., Beijing, China). Genes related to HIF-1α and small intestine functions (Occludin, SOD1, and GPX1) were examined. The relevant cDNA was then amplified using the SYBR PremixExTaq II (TOYOBO, Osaka, Japan) with specific primers as listed in **Table 1**. RT-PCR was performed by a 7500 Real-Time PCR System (Applied

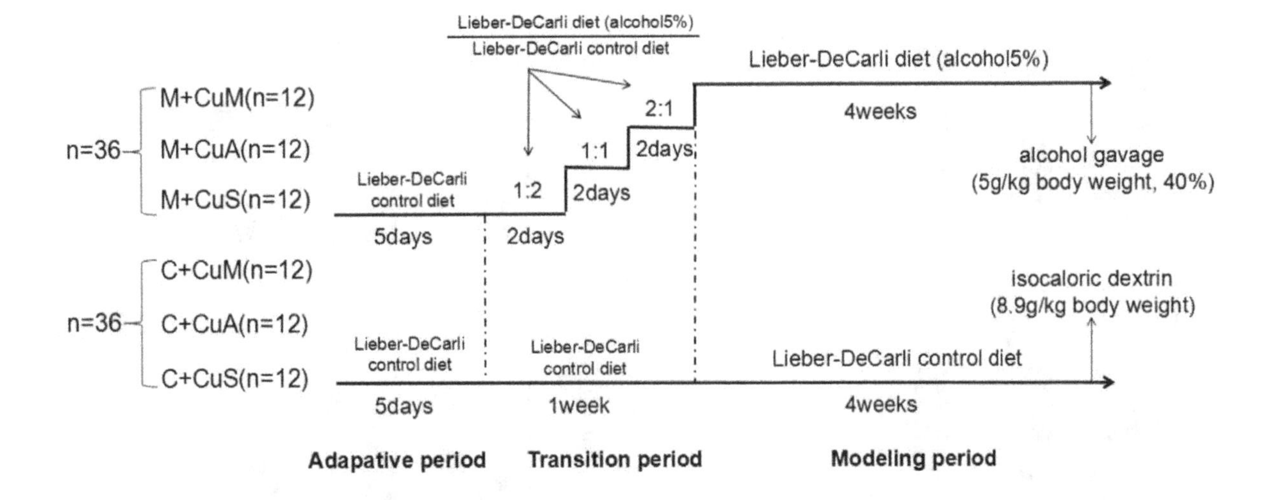

FIGURE 1 | Animal feeding schedule. M + CuM: model group + marginal Cu level, M + CuA: model group + adequate Cu level, M + CuS: model group + supplemental Cu level, C + CuM: control group + marginal Cu level, C + CuA: control group + adequate Cu level, C + CuS: control group + supplemental Cu level.

TABLE 1 | Primer sequences used in RT-PCR.

Name	Primer sequences	Tm	Length of product
HIF-1α	Forward primer: ATGCTAAATCGGAGGGTA Reverse primer: TCCTGGAAACGAGTGAAA	60	88
Occludin	Forward prime: CCATCTTTCTTCGGGTTT Reverse primer: TGGATCTATGTACGGCTCAC	60	203
SOD1	Forward primer: GGACCTCATTTTAATCCTCACTCTA Reverse primer: CACACGATCTTCAATGGACACA	60	129
GPx1	Forward primer: GAAGGTAAAGAGCGGGTGA Reverse primer: CAGAATGGCAAGAATGAAGAG	60	132
GAPDH	Forward primer: AAGAAGGTGGTGAAGCAGG Reverse primer: GAAGGTGGAAGAGTGGGAGT	60	111

Biosystems, Life Technologies, Waltham, MA, United States). Each mRNA expression was calculated based on glyceraldehyde-3-phosphate dehydrogenation (GAPDH) as a reference gene. The final mRNA expression was analyzed by the $2^{-\Delta\Delta Ct}$ method.

Western Blot Analysis

Total protein from tissues was extracted in a mixture of ice-cold RIPA (Beyotime Biotechnology, China) and protease inhibitor. Proteins were separated by 10% SDS-PAGE and electro-transferred to PVDF membrane (Millipore, Burlington, MA, United States). The membranes were blocked for 2 h at room temperature with 5% BSA in TBST solution and then incubated with primary antibodies of anti-HIF-1α (1:1000, Abcam), anti-Occludin (1:1000, Proteintech), anti-SOD1 (1:1000, Proteintech), anti-GPX1 (1:1000, Affity) and anti-βactin (1:1000, Abcam), respectively, at 4°C overnight. After being washed with TBST, the membranes were incubated with the secondary antibody (goat anti-rabbit) (1:5000, Biosharp) for 1 h and were then washed three times with TBST. The bands were then detected and analyzed by Western Bright ECL (Advansta, San Jose, CA, United States) and Image Lab 4.1 software (Bio-Rad).

Caco-2 Cell Culture

Caco-2 cells were obtained from the Cell Bank of the Chinese Academy of Sciences (Shanghai, China) and cultured in DMEM (Gibco, United States) containing 10% fetal bovine serum (Gibco, United States), penicillin (100 U/ml), and streptomycin (100 U/ml) in a 5% CO_2 humidified incubator at 37°C. The medium was changed every 2 days, and the growth of the cells was observed with an inverted microscope. The cell monolayer was used after 24 days of culture, at which time the cells have differentiated and matured. The cells were exposed to 100 mmol/L alcohol and Cu (added as $CuSO_4.5H_2O$; Macklin, Shanghai, China) with different concentrations (0, 3.125, 6.25, 12.5, and 25 μ M).

Proliferation Assay

The effect of different concentrations of copper on Caco-2 proliferation was determined using real-time cellular analysis (RTCA). After 24 h stimulation, cells (8×10^3 cells/well) were seeded in several E-Plate 16 dishes (ACEA Biosciences Inc., CA, United States) for proliferation assays. The plates were kept in the cell incubator at 37°C with 5% CO_2 for 3–4 days. The cell index and growth curves were automatically recorded on the xCELLigence RTCA System (ACEA Biosciences Inc., CA, United States).

Mitochondrial Membrane Potential Determination

The mitochondrial membrane potential ($\Delta\Psi m$) was detected according to the manual of the JC-1 Assay Kit (Beyotime, Jiangsu, China). Briefly, the cells were suspended in 1 ml PBS after 48 h

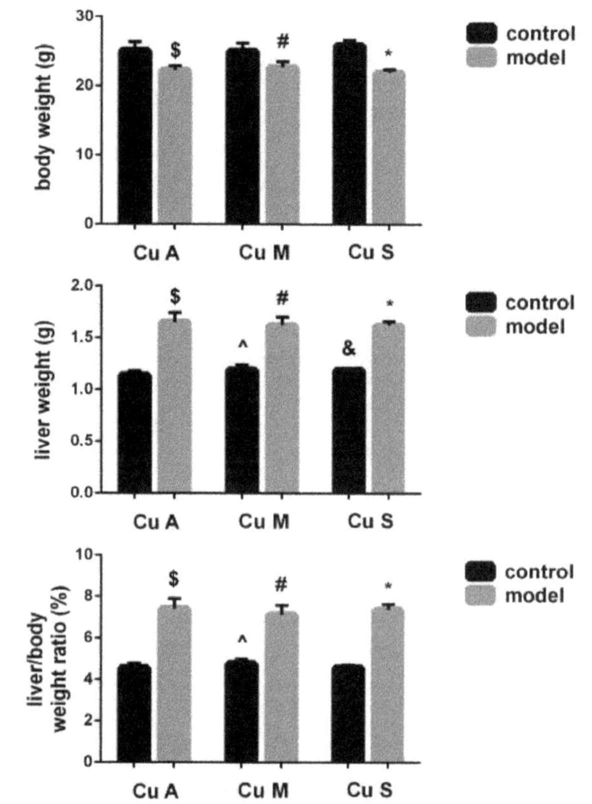

FIGURE 2 | Effects of different doses of dietary copper on body weight, liver weight, and liver/body weight ratio in mice. Comparisons between multiple sets of data were performed using one-way analysis of variance (ANOVA). Data are presented as the mean ± SD (n = 12) of three independent experiments. Statistical significance was set at $p < 0.05$. $: M + CuA versus C + Cu A; #: M + CuM versus C + CuM; *: C + CuS versus C + CuS; ^: C + CuM versus C + CuA; &: C + CuS versus C + CuA; + : M + CuM versus M + CuA; ± : M + CuS versus M + CuA.

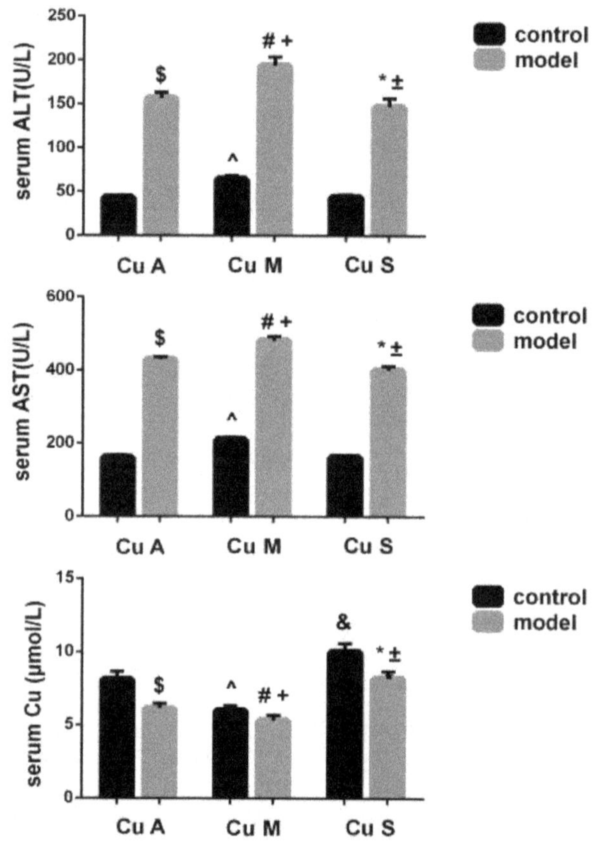

FIGURE 3 | Serum copper, ALT, and AST levels in response to different dietary doses of copper feeding, with or without alcohol. Comparisons between multiple sets of data were performed using one-way analysis of variance (ANOVA). Data are presented as the mean ± SD (n = 12) of three independent experiments. Statistical significance was set at $p < 0.05$. $: M + CuA versus C + CuA; #: M + CuM versus C + CuM; *: C + CuS versus C + Cu S; ^: C + CuM versus C + CuA; &: C + CuS versus C + CuA; + : M + CuM versus M + CuA; ± : M + CuS versus M + CuA.

of stimulation at approximately 1×10^6 cells/mL and were incubated with 2 μM of JC-1 for 15 min at 37°C. The cells were washed and resuspended in 500 μL PBS and then analyzed on a flow cytometer with 488 nm excitation and emission at 590 nm (red) and 540 nm (green).

Cellular Total ROS Level Measurement

The relative level of cellular total reactive oxygen species (ROS) level was detected according to the Reactive Oxygen Species Assay Kit (Beyotime, Jiangsu, China). The cells were collected and incubated with DCFH-DA probe solution in a 37°C, 5% CO_2 incubator for 20 min (final concentration is 10 μM). Next, they were centrifuged at 1000 rpm for 4 min and then washed three times with FBS-free DMEM to remove the residual probe. Finally, cell samples were resuspended in FBS-free DMEM and subjected to flow cytometry analysis. The mean value of fluorescence intensity indicates the relative level of cellular total ROS level.

Both mitochondrial membrane potential and cellular total ROS level were examined by using a BD Accuri C6 (BD Biosciences, Franklin Lakes, NJ, United States) flow cytometer.

Statistics and Data Analysis

Comparisons between multiple sets of data were performed using one-way analysis of variance (ANOVA), LSD, and Dunnett T3 tests in SPSS 22.0 software. Data are expressed as mean ± SD. $P < 0.05$ was considered statistically significant.

RESULTS

Effects of Different Doses of Dietary Copper on Body Weight, Liver Weight, and Liver/Body Weight Ratio in Mice

As shown in **Figure 2**, alcohol feeding resulted in a significant decrease in body weight but a significant increase in liver weight and liver/body weight ratio. In addition, although the marginal copper diet significantly increased liver weight and the liver/body weight ratio in the control group, this has little practical significance. However, there was no obvious

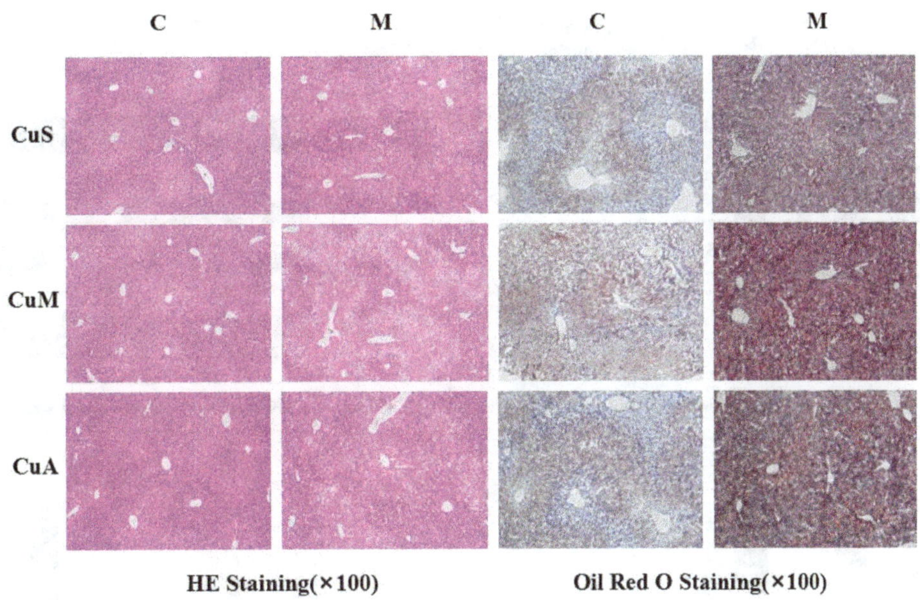

FIGURE 4 | Histology of liver stained with HE and Oil Red O. CuM: marginal Cu level (1.5 ppm); CuA: adequate Cu level (6 ppm); CuS: supplemental Cu level (20 ppm). C: control group; M: model group.

effect of copper on body weight or the liver/body weight ratio in the model group. The results showed that alcohol could damage the liver and cause liver fat deposition but that a beneficial effect of copper supplementation in the diet was not obvious. In the control group, the marginal copper diet was harmful to the liver.

Serum Copper, ALT, and AST Levels in Response to Different Doses of Dietary Copper in Mice

Liver ALT and AST were significantly increased and the serum copper was decreased in the model group (**Figure 3**). Whether in the control group or the model group, the marginal copper diet can increase ALT and AST and reduce serum copper compared to an adequate copper diet. In contrast, in the model group, copper-supplemented mice had lower ALT and AST values, and serum copper increased. Therefore, alcohol could disrupt the homeostasis of serum copper, damage the liver, and cause elevated aminotransferases. In the model group and the control group, supplemental levels of copper in the diet caused a significant improvement, while marginal copper had a harmful effect.

Effect of Different Doses of Dietary Copper on Liver Histology in Mice

Liver injury was evaluated by liver histology in mice, as shown in **Figure 4**. Significant liver injury and lipid deposition were observed in the liver of model mice as compared with that in control mice. Moreover, copper supplementation could slightly alleviate liver lipid deposition, while marginal copper exacerbated this change in the control and model groups. The results showed that the damage done by alcohol to the liver was obvious and that copper supplementation in the diet could appropriately alleviate this change, whereas a marginal copper diet exacerbated the situation.

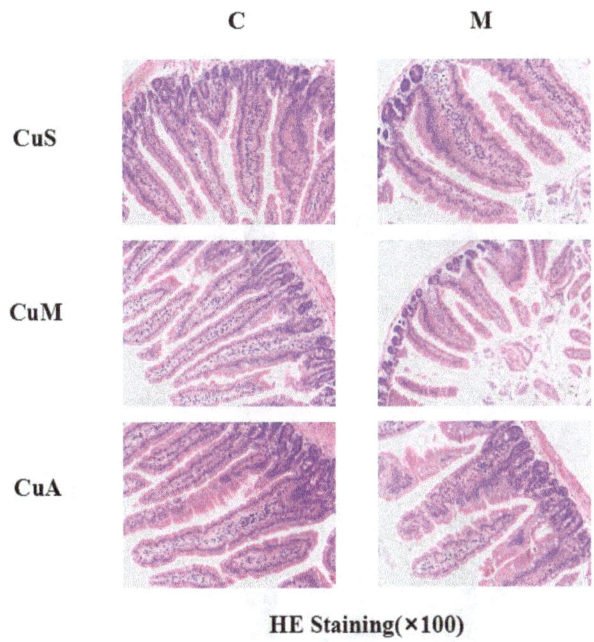

FIGURE 5 | Histology of small intestine stained with HE. CuM: marginal Cu level (1.5 ppm); CuA: adequate Cu level (6 ppm); CuS: supplemental Cu level (20 ppm). C: control group; M: model group.

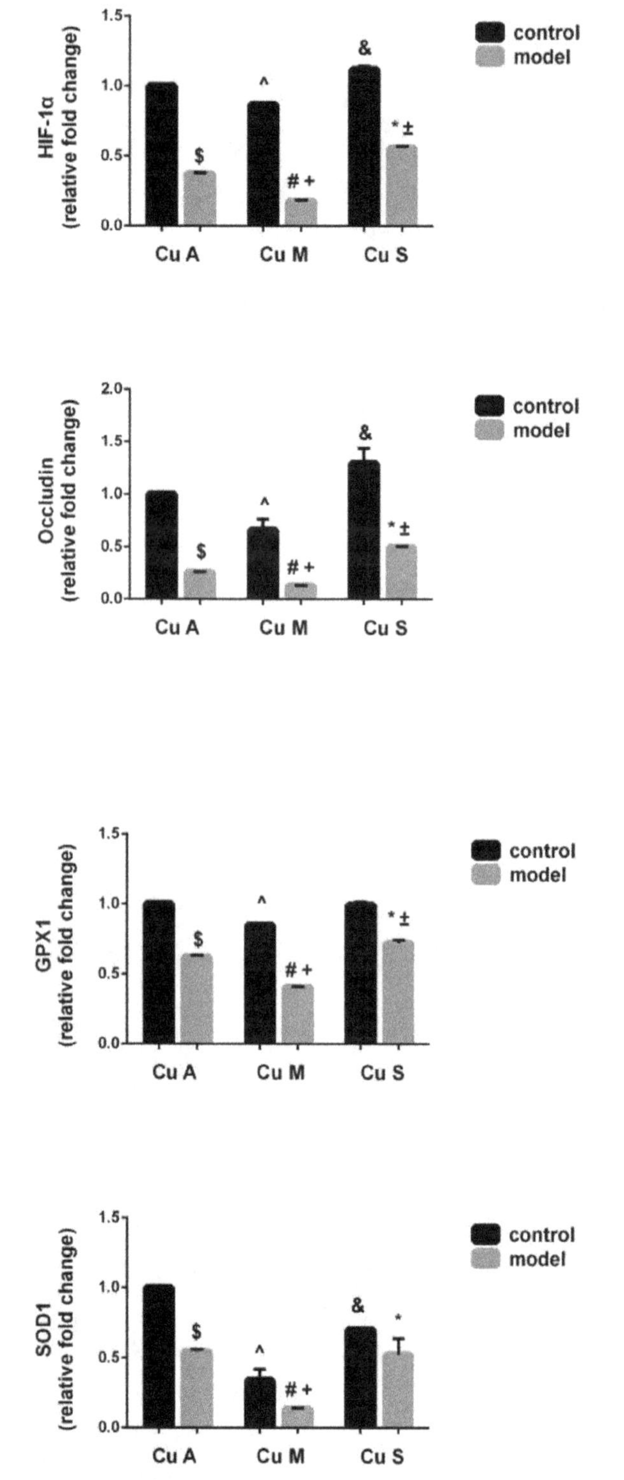

FIGURE 6 | mRNA levels of intestinal HIF-1α, Occludin, GPX1, and SOD1 evaluated by RT-PCR, normalized to the levels of GAPDH. Comparisons between multiple sets of data were performed using one-way analysis of variance (ANOVA). Data are presented as the mean ± SD (n = 12) of three independent experiments. Statistical significance was set at $p < 0.05$. $: M + CuA versus C + CuA; #: M + CuM versus C + CuM; *: C + CuS versus C + CuS; ^: C + CuM versus C + CuA; &: C + CuS versus C + CuA; + : M + CuM versus M + CuA; ± : M + CuS versus M + CuA.

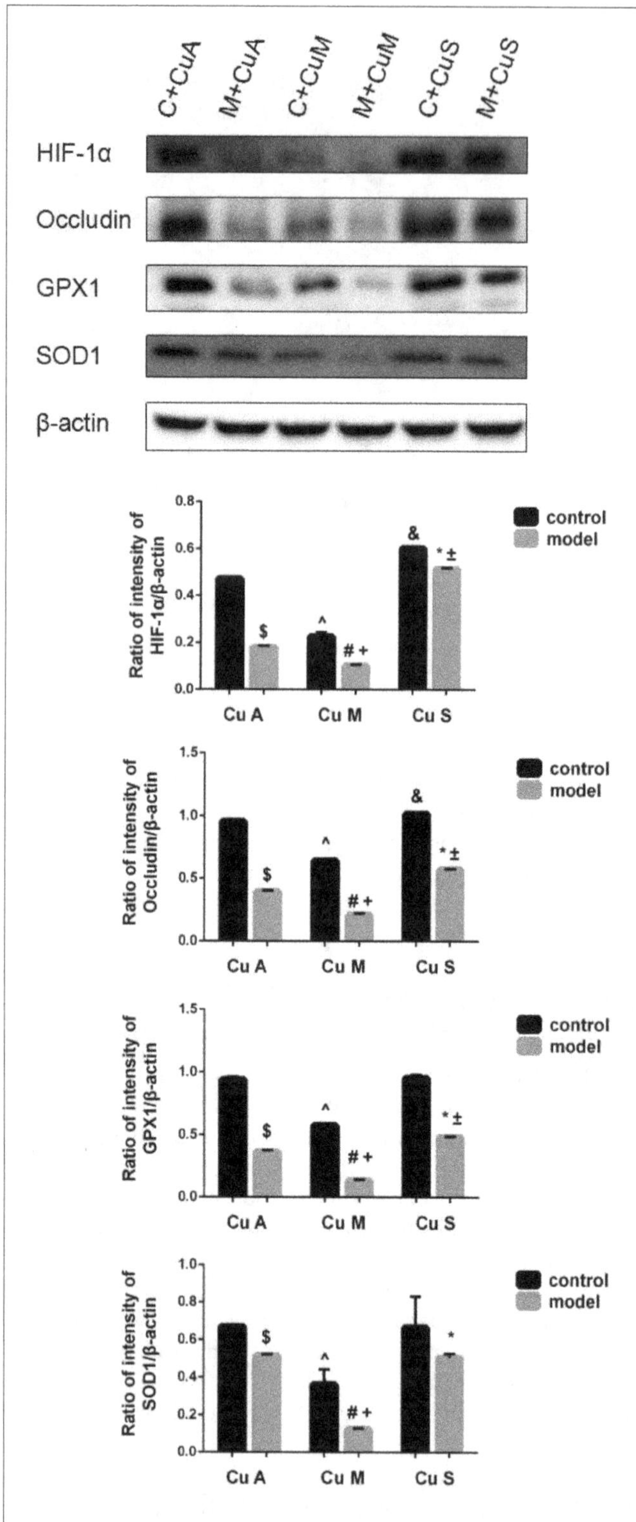

FIGURE 7 | Protein levels of intestinal HIF-1α, Occludin, GPX1, and SOD1 evaluated by WB, normalized to the levels of β-actin. Comparisons between multiple sets of data were performed using one-way analysis of variance (ANOVA). Data are presented as the mean ± SD (n = 12) of three independent experiments. Statistical significance was set at $p < 0.05$. $: M + CuA versus C + CuA; #: M + CuM versus C + CuM; *: C + CuS versus C + CuS; ^: C + CuM versus C + CuA; &: C + CuS versus C + CuA; + : M + CuM versus M + CuA; ± : M + CuS versus M + CuA.

Effect of Different Doses of Dietary Copper on the Histology and Gene Expression of Small Intestine

The histology of small intestine and gene expression in small intestine are shown in **Figures 5–7**. As shown in **Figure 5**, alcohol intake caused the intestinal villi to become thinner, shorter, and more irregular. Moreover, in the model group, the marginal copper diet exacerbated the alcohol-induced intestinal villus destruction, while the supplemental copper diet alleviated it. In the control group, the marginal copper diet also induced changes in intestinal villi, but the supplemental copper diet had no obvious impact on intestinal villi. The genes related to intestinal barrier function and HIF-1α were evaluated, as shown in **Figures 6, 7**. Alcohol intake resulted in a significant decrease in protein and mRNA levels of occludin, GPX1, and SOD1. The marginal copper diet exacerbated the change, and the supplemental copper diet ameliorated it, except for SOD1 protein expression in the model group. Moreover, alcohol decreased the HIF-1α gene expression in intestine, which suggests a role for HIF-1α in alcohol-induced intestinal injury. The mRNA and protein levels of HIF-1α were lowest in mice fed with the marginal copper diet in both the control and model groups, while the supplemental copper diet appeared to restore the HIF-1α level. The above research results showed that alcohol could damage the intestine by down-regulating the HIF-1α pathway and reducing occludin, SOD1, and GPX1 expression. Copper supplementation in the diet could alleviate these changes, except for that in SOD1, and the marginal copper diet would aggravate all these changes.

Effect of Different Doses of Dietary Copper on Caco-2 Cells

Since different concentrations of dietary copper can affect liver steatosis and small intestinal barrier function, further investigation of the effects of dietary copper was performed on small intestinal cells (Caco-2 cell line). As shown in **Figure 8A**, with an increase in the concentration of dietary copper, there was an increase in cell proliferation in an almost dose-dependent manner. Copper also affects ROS production and mitochondrial membrane potential in Caco-2 cells. As shown in **Figure 8B**, copper decreased ROS production in Caco-2 cells in an almost dose-dependent manner. The same observation was found in mitochondrial membrane potential (**Figure 8C**). The above results showed that *in vitro* experiments, proper copper supplementation was beneficial for small intestinal cells (Caco-2 cell line) but harmful to mitochondrial membrane potential.

DISCUSSION

The liver is one of the most important organs of the human body and plays an extremely important role in metabolism (Lackner and Tiniakos, 2019). Since Marshall proposed the concept of the intestinal hepatic axis in 1998, research on the relationship between intestinal and liver diseases has attracted more and more attention (Tripathi et al., 2018). It is currently believed that the intestine and the liver interact with each other, and protection of intestinal mucosal barrier integrity has been a major focus for the development of new treatments for liver diseases (Bird, 2012; Llopis et al., 2016).

The intestines are rich in blood vessels and are therefore susceptible to diseases associated with reduced blood flow and concomitant tissue hypoxia (Taylor and Colgan, 1999; Furuta et al., 2001). Hypoxia-inducible factor 1α (HIF-1α) has been implicated in transcriptional regulation of intestinal barrier integrity and inflammation (Shao et al., 2018). Disruption of epithelial HIF-1α can lead to increased epithelial permeability (Karhausen et al., 2004). Metabolism in the intestine is very active, and thus it is highly vulnerable to oxidative stress (Glover et al., 2016; Rath et al., 2018). Superoxide dismutase 1 (SOD1) and glutathione peroxidase 1 (GPX1) are the most important antioxidant enzymes in cells (Weydert and Cullen, 2010). Tight junction (TJ) is the main means of connection between intestinal epithelial cells and has a major effect on maintaining the polarity of epithelial cells and regulating the permeability of the intestinal barrier (Umeda et al., 2006). Occludin is one of the most important protein molecules in TJ (Du et al., 2010).

In the current study, we found that alcohol intake could induce liver injury and impair gut barrier function. Alcohol caused intestinal villi to become thinner and disordered, decreased the expression of genes such as HIF-1α, occludin, GPX1, and SOD1, and impaired intestinal barrier function. Disorders in intestinal morphology and functions induced by alcohol can be alleviated with supplemental dietary copper and exacerbated with marginal dietary copper. However, supplementation with copper did not produce the expected ameliorative effect on SOD1; it may not be sensitive to increased copper content and may only be more sensitive to copper reduction.

Copper is a necessary mineral element in the diet and has been shown to play roles in antioxidant defense, lipid peroxidation, and mitochondrial function (Al-Othman et al., 1992, 1993). Copper deficiency has been linked to atherogenic dyslipidemia (Aigner et al., 2010). Systemic copper deficiency can also cause mitochondrial dysfunction in mice (Nose et al., 2006), and similar morphological and functional alterations have also been described in human NAFLD (Wei et al., 2008). In the current study, we also found that mice fed with marginal dietary copper also showed damage to the liver and gut without alcohol intake. However, the effect of supplemental dietary copper on control mice was still unclear; it might have a positive effect on the intestine but had no effect on oxidative stress. All of these findings indicated that dietary copper could alter intestinal barrier function through regulation of the intestinal HIF-1α signaling pathway and oxidative stress in mice.

ROS is formed as a natural by-product of the normal metabolism of oxygen and plays an important role in cell signaling and homeostasis. When cell homeostasis is disrupted, ROS levels increase dramatically. This can cause severe

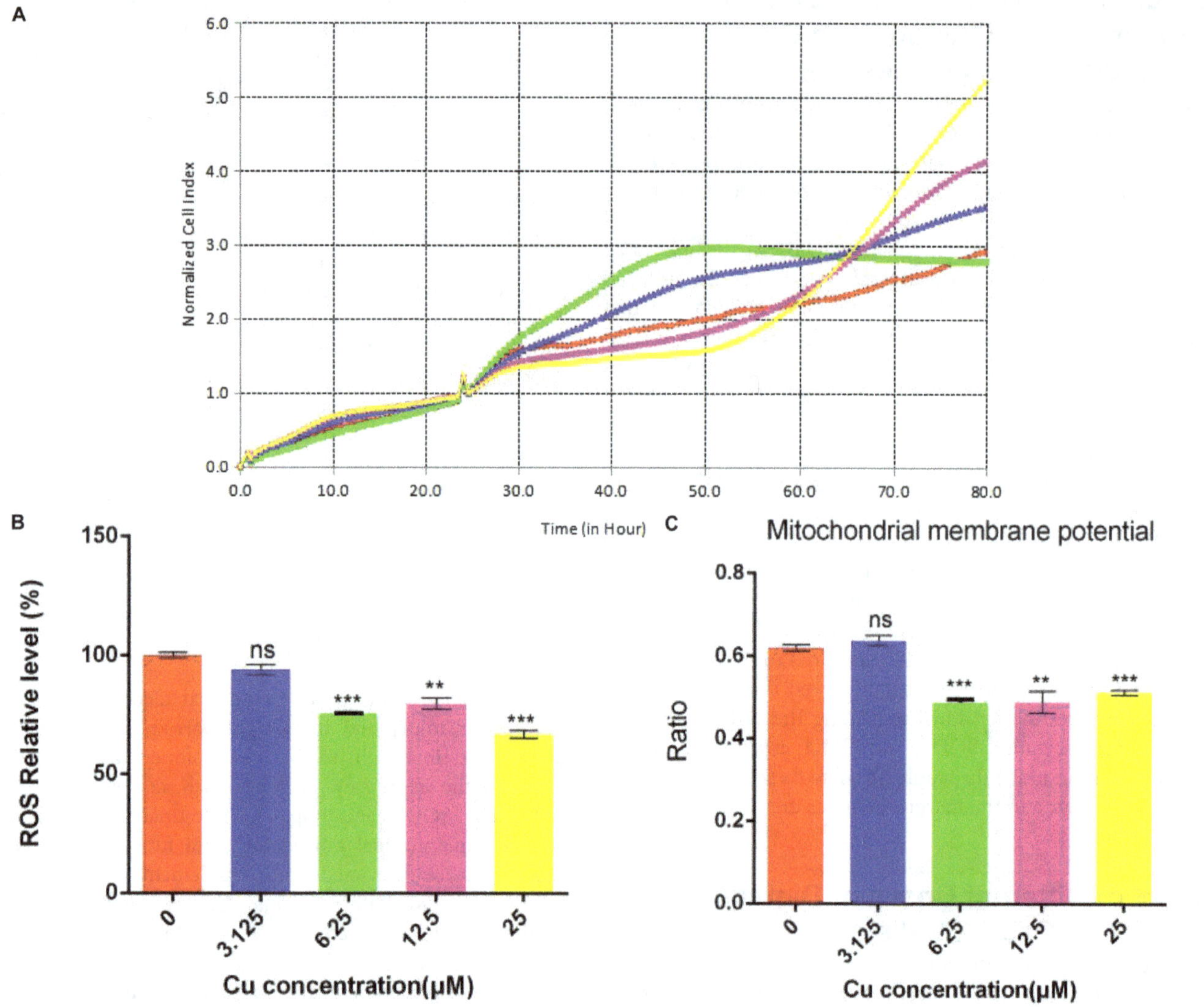

FIGURE 8 | Evaluation of functional mitochondria. **(A)** Proliferation assay real-time cellular analysis (RTCA), **(B)** Cellular total ROS level measurement, **(C)** Mitochondrial membrane potential determination. Comparisons between multiple sets of data were performed using one-way analysis of variance (ANOVA). Data are presented as the mean ± SD ($n = 12$) of three independent experiments. Statistical significance was set at $^{**}P < 0.05$, $^{***}P < 0.01$. ns: not significant.

damage to the cell structure, which is called oxidative stress. Normal MMP is a prerequisite for maintaining oxidative phosphorylation of mitochondria and producing adenosine triphosphate. The stability of MMP is conducive to maintaining the normal physiological functions of cells. The *in vitro* cell experiments demonstrated an important role of copper in cell proliferation, ROS production, and mitochondrial membrane potential. With an increase in copper concentration, there was an increase in cell proliferation but a decrease in cellular total ROS level. This means that copper could reduce ROS production and promote cell proliferation. Although there is a slight increase in mitochondrial membrane potential at low copper concentration (3.125 μM), a significant decrease in mitochondrial membrane potential was observed with increases in copper concentration. However, the functioning of mitochondria remained intact, which suggested that the membrane potential was more sensitive to changes in the concentration of copper. However, further investigations are needed to understand the relationship between copper and mitochondrial functions.

In summary, our current study provides novel discovery of the pathogenesis of ALD, which indicates that copper homeostasis is critical in maintaining gut barrier integrity and plays an important role in the prevention of ALD. The mechanism by which copper prevents ALD may be related to its regulation of intestinal HIF-1α gene expression and oxidative stress.

AUTHOR CONTRIBUTIONS

LX and Y-PC designed the protocol. HL and DC performed the experiments and edited the manuscript. QD and TP directed and participated in the sample detection. HT, YX, TT, and JT analyzed the data. HL wrote the manuscript, which was also edited by DC. All authors read and approved the final manuscript.

ACKNOWLEDGMENTS

We heartily appreciate all those who contributed to this research.

REFERENCES

Aigner, E., Strasser, M., Haufe, H., Sonnweber, T., Hohla, F., Stadlmayr, A., et al. (2010). A role for low hepatic copper concentrations in nonalcoholic Fatty liver disease. *Am. J. Gastroenterol.* 105, 1978–1985.

Aigner, E., Theurl, I., Haufe, H., Seifert, M., Hohla, F., Scharinger, L., et al. (2008). Copper availability contributes to iron perturbations in human nonalcoholic fatty liver disease. *Gastroenterology* 135, 680–688.

Al-Othman, A. A., Rosenstein, F., and Lei, K. Y. (1992). Copper deficiency alters plasma pool size, percent composition and concentration of lipoprotein components in rats. *J. Nutr.* 122, 1199–1204.

Al-Othman, A. A., Rosenstein, F., and Lei, K. Y. (1993). Copper deficiency increases in vivo hepatic synthesis of fatty acids, triacylglycerols, and phospholipids in rats. *Proc. Soc. Exp. Biol. Med.* 204, 97–103.

Altarelli, M., Ben-Hamouda, N., Schneider, A., and Berger, M. M. (2019). Copper deficiency: causes, manifestations, and treatment. *Nutr. Clin. Pract.* 34, 504–513.

Bajaj, J. S. (2019). Alcohol, liver disease and the gut microbiota. *Nat. Rev. Gastroenterol. Hepatol.* 16, 235–246.

Bertola, A., Mathews, S., Ki, S. H., Wang, H., and Gao, B. (2013). Mouse model of chronic and binge ethanol feeding (the NIAAA model). *Nat. Protoc.* 8, 627–637.

Bird, L. (2012). Gut microbiota influences liver disease. *Nat. Rev. Immunol.* 12:153.

Chen, R. C., Xu, L. M., Du, S. J., Huang, S. S., Wu, H., Dong, J.-J., et al. (2016). Lactobacillus rhamnosus GG supernatant promotes intestinal barrier function, balances Treg and TH17 cells and ameliorates hepatic injury in a mouse model of chronic-binge alcohol feeding. *Toxicol. Lett.* 241, 103–110.

Du, D., Xu, F., Yu, L., Zhang, C., Lu, X., Yuan, H., et al. (2010). The tight junction protein, occludin, regulates the directional migration of epithelial cells. *Dev. Cell* 18, 52–63.

Furuta, G. T., Turner, J. R., Taylor, C. T., Hershberg, R. M., Comerford, K., Narravula, S., et al. (2001). Hypoxia-inducible factor 1-dependent induction of intestinal trefoil factor protects barrier function during hypoxia. *J. Exp. Med.* 193, 1027–1034.

Gao, B., and Bataller, R. (2011). Alcoholic liver disease: pathogenesis and new therapeutic targets. *Gastroenterology* 141, 1572–1585.

Ge, L., Chen, D., Chen, W., Cai, C., Tao, T., Lin, Z., et al. (2019). Pre-activation of TLR3 enhances the therapeutic effect of BMMSCs through regulation the intestinal HIF-2alpha signaling pathway and balance of NKB cells in experimental alcoholic liver injury. *Int. Immunopharmacol.* 70, 477–485.

Glover, L. E., Lee, J. S., and Colgan, S. P. (2016). Oxygen metabolism and barrier regulation in the intestinal mucosa. *J. Clin. Invest.* 126, 3680–3688.

Hodgkinson, V., and Petris, M. J. (2012). Copper homeostasis at the host-pathogen interface. *J. Biol. Chem.* 287, 13549–13555.

Karhausen, J., Furuta, G. T., Tomaszewski, J. E., Johnson, R. S., Colgan, S. P., Haase, V. H., et al. (2004). Epithelial hypoxia-inducible factor-1 is protective in murine experimental colitis. *J. Clin. Invest.* 114, 1098–1106.

Lackner, C., and Tiniakos, D. (2019). Fibrosis and alcohol-related liver disease. *J. Hepatol.* 70, 294–304.

Llopis, M., Cassard, A. M., Wrzosek, L., Boschat, L., Bruneau, A., Ferrere, G., et al. (2016). Intestinal microbiota contributes to individual susceptibility to alcoholic liver disease. *Gut* 65, 830–839.

Louvet, A., and Mathurin, P. (2015). Alcoholic liver disease: mechanisms of injury and targeted treatment. *Nat. Rev. Gastroenterol. Hepatol.* 12, 231–242.

Moon, J. O., Welch, T. P., Gonzalez, F. J., and Copple, B. L. (2009). Reduced liver fibrosis in hypoxia-inducible factor-1alpha-deficient mice. *Am. J. Physiol. Gastrointest. Liver Physiol.* 296, G582–G592.

Nose, Y., Kim, B. E., and Thiele, D. J. (2006). Ctr1 drives intestinal copper absorption and is essential for growth, iron metabolism, and neonatal cardiac function. *Cell Metab.* 4, 235–244.

Orman, E. S., Odena, G., and Bataller, R. (2013). Alcoholic liver disease: pathogenesis, management, and novel targets for therapy. *J. Gastroenterol. Hepatol.* 28(Suppl. 1), 77–84.

Pontel, L. B., and Soncini, F. C. (2009). Alternative periplasmic copper-resistance mechanisms in Gram negative bacteria. *Mol. Microbiol.* 73, 212–225.

Prabhakar, N. R., and Semenza, G. L. (2012). Adaptive and maladaptive cardiorespiratory responses to continuous and intermittent hypoxia mediated by hypoxia-inducible factors 1 and 2. *Physiol. Rev.* 92, 967–1003.

Rao, R. (2009). Endotoxemia and gut barrier dysfunction in alcoholic liver disease. *Hepatology* 50, 638–644.

Rath, E., Moschetta, A., and Haller, D. (2018). Mitochondrial function - gatekeeper of intestinal epithelial cell homeostasis. *Nat. Rev. Gastroenterol. Hepatol.* 15, 497–516.

Seitz, H. K., Bataller, R., Cortez-Pinto, H., Gao, B., Gual, A., Lackner, C., et al. (2018). Alcoholic liver disease. *Nat. Rev. Dis. Primers* 4:16.

Shao, T., Zhao, C., Li, F., Gu, Z., Liu, L., Zhang, L., et al. (2018). Intestinal HIF-1alpha deletion exacerbates alcoholic liver disease by inducing intestinal dysbiosis and barrier dysfunction. *J. Hepatol.* 69, 886–895.

Solioz, M., Abicht, H. K., Mermod, M., and Mancini, S. (2010). Response of gram-positive bacteria to copper stress. *J. Biol. Inorg. Chem.* 15, 3–14.

Song, M., Li, X., Zhang, X., Shi, H., Vos, M. B., Wei, X., et al. (2018). Dietary copper-fructose interactions alter gut microbial activity in male rats. *Am. J. Physiol. Gastrointest. Liver Physiol.* 314, G119–G130.

Taylor, C. T., and Colgan, S. P. (1999). Therapeutic targets for hypoxia-elicited pathways. *Pharm. Res.* 16, 1498–1505.

Tripathi, A., Debelius, J., Brenner, D. A., Karin, M., Loomba, R., Schnabl, B., et al. (2018). The gut-liver axis and the intersection with the microbiome. *Nat. Rev. Gastroenterol. Hepatol.* 15, 397–411.

Umeda, K., Ikenouchi, J., Katahira-Tayama, S., Furuse, K., Sasaki, H., Nakayama, M., et al. (2006). ZO-1 and ZO-2 independently determine where claudins are polymerized in tight-junction strand formation. *Cell* 126, 741–754.

Wei, Y., Rector, R. S., Thyfault, J. P., and Ibdah, J. A. (2008). Nonalcoholic fatty liver disease and mitochondrial dysfunction. *World J. Gastroenterol.* 14, 193–199.

Weydert, C. J., and Cullen, J. J. (2010). Measurement of superoxide dismutase, catalase and glutathione peroxidase in cultured cells and tissue. *Nat. Protoc.* 5, 51–66.

10

Similarities and Differences: A Comparative Review of the Molecular Mechanisms and Effectors of NAFLD and AFLD

Pengyi Zhang [1†], Weiya Wang [1,2†], Min Mao [3], Ruolin Gao [1], Wenting Shi [1], Dongmei Li [4], Richard Calderone [4], Bo Sui [1], Xuewen Tian [1] and Xiangjing Meng [2*]*

[1] School of Sports and Health, Shandong Sport University, Jinan, China, [2] Shandong Academy of Pharmaceutical Science, Jinan, China, [3] Department of Allied Health, University of North Carolina at Chapel Hill, Chapel Hill, NC, United States, [4] Department of Microbiology and Immunology, Georgetown University Medical Center, Washington, DC, United States

***Correspondence:**
Pengyi Zhang
zhangpengyi@sdpei.edu.cn
Xiangjing Meng
fredamxj@163.com

† These authors have contributed equally to this work

Non-alcoholic fatty liver disease (NAFLD) and alcoholic fatty liver disease (AFLD) are the most prevalent metabolic liver diseases globally. Due to the complex pathogenic mechanisms of NAFLD and AFLD, no specific drugs were approved at present. Lipid accumulation, oxidative stress, insulin resistance, inflammation, and dietary habits are all closely related to the pathogenesis of NAFLD and AFLD. However, the mechanism that promotes disease progression has not been fully elucidated. Meanwhile, the gut microbiota and their metabolites also play an important role in the pathogenesis and development of NAFLD and AFLD. This article comparatively reviewed the shared and specific signaling pathways, clinical trials, and potential intervention effectors of NAFLD and AFLD, revealing their similarities and differences. By comparing the shared and specific molecular regulatory mechanisms, this paper provides mutual reference strategies for preventing and treating NAFLD, AFLD, and related metabolic diseases. Furthermore, it provides enlightenment for discovering novel therapies of safe and effective drugs targeting the metabolic liver disease.

Keywords: NAFLD, AFLD, signaling pathway, clinical trials, effectors, similarities and differences

Non-alcoholic fatty liver disease (NAFLD) and alcoholic fatty liver disease (AFLD) are the main metabolic liver diseases that are prevalent worldwide. Metabolic liver disease seriously affects human health and quality of life, leading to major public health problems and huge medical burdens (Estes et al., 2018; Sarin et al., 2020). NAFLD is associated with metabolic syndromes (MS) such as obesity, type 2 diabetes mellitus (T2DM), and dyslipidemia (Younossi and Henry, 2016; Zhang X. et al., 2018). The liver histology of NAFLD showed macrovesicular steatosis, mild lobular inflammation, and non-alcoholic ballooned hepatocytes (Loomba et al., 2021). NAFLD affects ∼25% of the global adult population (Younossi et al., 2019). AFLD is associated with excessive alcohol consumption and accounts for 47.9% of cirrhosis deaths worldwide. AFLD has become the most common indication for liver transplantation in the United States (Rehm et al., 2013; Johnston et al., 2020). Lipid accumulation, oxidative stress, insulin resistance (IR), inflammation, and dietary habits are all closely related to the pathogenesis of NAFLD and AFLD. However, the mechanisms that drive disease progression have not been fully elucidated. Due to the complex pathogenic mechanisms of NAFLD and AFLD, there are no approved specific drugs at present. The clinical treatment mainly controls the disease progression and risk factors by lipid-regulating and anti-inflammatory drugs, antioxidants, weight loss, and hypoglycemia. The prevention and treatment strategies for these two diseases are very limited in type and efficacy. Therefore, this article systematically reviewed and comparatively analyzed the shared and specific molecular mechanisms and intervention effectors of NAFLD and AFLD, to fully understand their pathogenic mechanisms and provide ideas for screening and discovering novel prevention strategies and therapeutic targets of metabolic fatty liver disease.

INTRODUCTION

NAFLD and AFLD are public health issues worldwide. These two diseases have a similar pathological spectrum, from simple hepatic steatosis to steatohepatitis with or without fibrosis, to cirrhosis and liver cancer. NAFLD is one of the main causes of chronic hepatitis, and it is also the only cause of a steady increase of the global liver disease incidence over time, especially in developing countries such as the Middle East or South America (Younossi et al., 2018). It is estimated that by 2030, the prevalence of the end-stage liver disease will increase by 2–3 times in Western countries and several Asian countries (Estes et al., 2017, 2018). The pathogenesis of NAFLD involves several risk factors, including obesity, IR, hyperglycemia, diabetes, hypertension, dyslipidemia, aging, and decreased physical activity, among which obesity is the most important risk factor for the development of NAFLD (Schwimmer, 2007). The prevalence of NAFLD in obese people can reach 57.5–74%, which is 4.6 times that of people with normal weight (Angulo and Lindor, 2002). The risk of NAFLD and non-alcoholic steatohepatitis (NASH) is also increased due to the imbalance of gut microbiota, increased intestinal permeability, and translocation of intestinal microbes (Chu et al., 2018). Therefore, the changes of gut microbiota diversity and abundance may be another important factor causing metabolic syndrome (Bashiardes et al., 2016). The elevated fasting plasma ethanol level was suggested to be critical for the development of NAFLD. On the one hand, it is due to the increased synthesis of endogenous alcohol in the intestine. It is reported that *Klebsiella pneumoniae* was found in a considerable proportion of fatty liver patients, which can produce a large amount of alcohol in their intestines. The endogenous alcohol produced by these bacteria is an important inducer of NAFLD (Shellito et al., 2001). On the other hand, in a study of children with early signs of NAFLD, the fasting plasma ethanol levels were positively associated with measures of IR in children with NAFLD compared with the control group. *In vivo* experiments showed that ADH activity was significantly lower in liver of ob/ob mice. Thus, the impaired insulin-dependent ADH activity in liver led to increased plasma ethanol levels in NAFLD patients, rather than increased endogenous ethanol synthesis (Engstler et al., 2016). AFLD is a fatty liver disease with fat accumulation and inflammation caused by excessive alcohol consumption, affecting more than two million people in the United States. The prevalence of AFLD is not only affected by alcohol abuse, gut microbiota, immunity, gender, genetic defects, and other environmental factors also play an important role in the progression of AFLD patients (Tilg and Mathurin, 2016).

SIGNALING PATHWAY OF NAFLD AND AFLD

The pathogenesis of NAFLD is regulated by many molecular mechanisms (Friedman et al., 2018), which is usually caused by multiple factors such as lipid metabolic dysfunction, oxidative stress, IR, and inflammation (Hardy and Mann, 2016; Eslam et al., 2018). In AFLD, excessive alcohol consumption produces a large amount of acetaldehyde, which accumulates when acetaldehyde dehydrogenase (ALDH) is relatively deficient. Excess acetaldehyde will produce more reactive oxygen species (ROS), leading to oxidative stress and hepatocyte damage. At the same time, it can form various proteins and DNA complexes, which act as antigens to activate adaptive immunity and increase inflammation (Lackner et al., 2016; Xu et al., 2017; Anty and Gual, 2019). Ethanol can also cause dyslipidemia and lipid accumulation to form lipid droplets (LDs). Excessive LDs are susceptible to the attack of ROS produced by ethanol metabolism, thereby synergistically aggravating oxidative stress and liver damage. Through systematic review and comparative analysis of the signaling pathways of NAFLD and AFLD, the common and specific signal pathways of both are revealed, and novel therapeutic strategies are provided for the treatment of NAFLD and AFLD.

NAFLD SIGNALING PATHWAY

This paper mainly introduces six signaling pathways that regulate NAFLD: ① Nrf2/FXR/LXRα/RXR/SREBP-1c signaling pathway is an important pathway that maintains the intracellular redox balance and regulates lipid metabolism. NF-E2-related factor 2 (Nrf2) is an important upstream transcription factor that regulates oxidative stress, and it is also a central regulator of intracellular redox homeostasis. The regulation of its expression is an important antioxidant defense mechanism of the body (Dodson et al., 2019). Nrf2 recruits p300 to promote the deacetylation of farnesoid X receptor (FXR) in primary hepatocytes isolated from wild-type male C57/BL6 mice. Then small heteredodimer partner (SHP) was induced by deacetylated FXR to inhibit liver X receptor α (LXRα)-dependent gene transcription. In human steatosis, Nrf2, FXR, and SHP have negative regulatory effects on LXRα and sterol regulatory element binding protein-1c (SREBP-1c). LXRα and its target SREBP-1c transcriptionally regulate fatty acid synthesis. The activation of Nrf2 suppresses the transcription of LXRα, SREBP-1c, and LXRα-dependent hepatic steatosis through FXR activation and FXR-mediated induction of SHP (Kay et al., 2011; Fan et al., 2021). LXRα and Retinoid X receptor (RXR) can form a heterodimer, which further activates SREBP-1c. SREBP-1c is the main transcription factor regulating fatty acid synthesis. It participates in the regulation of lipid and cholesterol homeostasis by positively regulating the transcription of acetyl-CoA carboxylase (ACC) and fatty acid synthase (FAS)

(Chávez-Talavera et al., 2017; Hiebl et al., 2018). On the other hand, tissue-restricted FXR agonists can improve insulin sensitivity and reduce hepatic steatosis in HFD mice and non-diabetic NAFLD patients (Carino et al., 2017; Traussnigg et al., 2021). FXR is a ligand-activated transcriptional factor. The release of bile acids (BAs) during meals selectively activates intestinal FXR. The intestinal-restricted FXR agonist fexaramine (Fex) induces intestinal fibroblast growth factor 15 (FGF15), which changes the composition of BAs but does not activate FXR target genes in the liver. In HFD mice treated with Fex (100 mg kg^{-1} d^{-1} p.o. for 5 weeks), Fex improves diet-induced body weight gain, systemic inflammation, and the lipid metabolism of liver by activating FXR (Fang et al., 2015). The activation of FXR is beneficial for the homeostasis of lipid and glucose, energy metabolism, hepatic steatosis (Gai et al., 2018), cell stress, and the intake of intestinal Bas (Han et al., 2018). FXR is also an important gene that regulates lipid metabolism in AFLD. The intestine-specific FXR knockout ($FXRint^{-/-}$) mice were more likely to cause hepatic steatosis and inflammation under alcohol induction (Huang M. et al., 2020). However, the results are not completely consistent between animal models and human research. The changes in the diversity, abundance and metabolites of gut microbiota are one potential reason worth investigating (Adorini et al., 2012; Arab et al., 2017; McIlvride et al., 2019).

② PI3K/AKT/SREBP-1c signaling pathway is an important pathway for regulating lipid metabolism, which can reduce mitochondrial oxidative stress, inhibit adipogenesis, delay excessive lipid deposition, and alleviate hepatic steatosis (Abood et al., 2018; Liao et al., 2018; Pan et al., 2018). The PI3K/AKT signaling pathway even reprograms cell carcinogenesis by regulating lipid and protein biosynthesis in mouse liver (Palian et al., 2014). Poly ADP-ribose polymerase 1(PARP-1) expressed in the nucleus is a key regulatory enzyme for DNA repair and chromatin structure maintenance. Under pathological stimulation, PARP-1 overactivation may cause cell damage, accompanied by energy depletion, mitochondrial dysfunction, and β-oxidation disruption in mouse leukemia cells (Cantó and Auwerx, 2011). The PI3K/AKT signaling pathway can be activated by the inhibition of PARP-1. AKT is an important downstream effector molecule of PI3K. Puerarin can activate this signaling pathway to down-regulate the lipid synthesis-related gene SREBP-1c, thereby reducing lipid biosynthesis and achieving the effect of improving fatty liver disease in C57BL/6J mice fed with a high-fat high-sucrose (HFHS) diet (Wang et al., 2019). PARP-1 not only directly affects the expression of liver adipose gene through transcriptional regulation, but also indirectly regulates the energy metabolism by affecting liver nicotinamide adenine dinucleotide (NAD^+) consumption and Sirtuin 1 (SIRT1) activity. The inhibition of PARP-1 can increase NAD^+ content and SIRT1 activity, enhance lipid metabolism, and improve hepatic steatosis in hepatocytes under oxidative stress and mice fed a high-fat diet (Kraus and Hottiger, 2013). ③ Amp-activated protein kinase (AMPK)/Sarcoendoplasmic reticulum Ca^{2+}-ATPase 2b (SERCA2b) pathway mediates suppression of endoplasmic reticulum (ER) stress to improve hepatic steatosis. In the case of hyperlipidemia, the reduction of ER stress in hepatocytes is the most common therapy to inhibit lipid accumulation. When AMPK is activated by maresin 1, it positively regulates the activation of SERCA2B. SERCA2B re-uptake Ca^{2+} from the cytoplasm into the ER cavity, alleviating the ER stress of hepatocytes under hyperlipidemia and maintaining ER homeostasis, thereby inhibiting lipid accumulation (Jung et al., 2018). Conversely, the inhibition of AMPKα1 promoted the development of NAFLD in HFD mice through increasing adipocyte-mediated CD36-containing exosomes release. The CD36-containing exosomes induced lipid accumulation and inflammation in hepatocytes, which could be reversed by metformin (Yan et al., 2021). ④ LILRB4/SHP1/TRAF6/NF-κB/MAPK signaling pathway can improve the development of NAFLD and related metabolic complications. Leukocyte immunoglobulin-like receptor (LILRB4) is the major receptor in the immunoglobulin superfamily, mainly located on the membrane of immune cells (Katz, 2007). The activation of LILRB4 contributes to the improvement of inflammation. LILRB4 negatively regulates protein tyrosine phosphatase (SHP1), inhibits the ubiquitination of TNF receptor associated factor 6 (TRAF6), and prevents the activation of nuclear factor kappa-B (NF-κB) and mitogen-activated protein kinase (MAPK) signaling pathways. Thus, IR, glucose metabolism imbalance, liver lipid accumulation, hepatic steatosis, and systemic inflammation in mice fed a high-fat diet could be reversed (Lu et al., 2018). ⑤ The lipid metabolism can be improved by inhibiting TXNIP/NLRP3 signaling pathway. Thioredoxin intervening protein (TXNIP), as an important mediator of redox homeostasis, was overexpressed in the liver of streptozotocin-induced diabetic rats. The high expression of TXNIP is closely related to the occurrence of oxidative stress and inflammation in the liver. The reduction of its expression can effectively inhibit the production of intracellular ROS (Zhou and Chng, 2013). NOD-like receptor protein 3 (NLRP3) inflammasome is a multi-protein complex composed of intracellular innate immune receptor NLRP3, adaptor protein ASC, and protease caspase-1, which can induce the maturation and secretion of pro-inflammatory factors IL-1β and IL-18, and promote the inflammatory response (Jiang H. et al., 2017). Inhibiting the overexpression of TXNIP can inhibit the activation of NLRP3 inflammasomes, reduce the secretion of pro-inflammatory factors, and then regulate the expression of lipid metabolism genes in rat BRL-3A hepatocytes treated with sodium palmitate (SP) (Xiao et al., 2016). NLRP3 inflammasome is crucial for the initiation of hepatic inflammatory response and the progression from hepatic steatosis to NASH. The inhibition of its endogenous activation can delay the progression of NAFLD in female Sprague-Dawley rat fed a high-fat diet (Henao-Mejia et al., 2012). ⑥ TAZ/Ihh signaling pathway: The transcription expression of hippo transcription regulator-Tafazzin (TAZ) and its downstream target hepatic stellate cell fibrosis gene activator-Indian Hedgehog (Ihh) is significantly increased in the livers of NASH patients. This phenomenon has also been verified in mouse models. TAZ promotes hepatocyte fibrosis by inducing Ihh in NASH mice. Silencing TAZ can prevent and reverse NASH, especially liver fibrosis, but not hepatic steatosis (Wang

X. et al., 2016). p62/Sqstm1 was another TAZ target gene downstream, which played an important role in inflammatory and hepatocyte injury in NASH mice. TAZ was able to regulate the expression of p62/Sqstm1 to alleviate NASH both *in vitro* and *in vivo* (Yang et al., 2021).

In addition, plasminogen activator inhibitor-1 (PAI-1) is a serine protease inhibitor and a major inhibitor of the endogenous fibrinolytic system. The expression of plasma PAI-1 was increased in people with obesity, IR, and metabolic syndromes (Cesari et al., 2010). The plasma PAI-1 level had a positive correlation with hepatic steatosis, lobular inflammation, balloonosis, and fibrosis in children with NAFLD. PAI-1 is also significantly correlated with blood lipids and IR index. PAI-1 can be used as a potential diagnostic marker and drug target for determining the progression of NAFLD (Jin et al., 2018). The animal models of NAFLD induced by HFD had very similar pathological changes to human diseases, such as obesity, dyslipidemia and IR, but only led to very little fibrosis. In fact, the therapeutic effects obtained in animal models of NAFLD were not completely consistent with human clinical trials (Tarantino et al., 2019). Nevertheless, *in vitro* and *in vivo* experiments contribute to discover and understand the multiple molecular mechanisms of NAFLD, and provide potential candidate strategies for human trials, clinical treatments and new drug screening.

AFLD SIGNALING PATHWAY

Ethanol can lead to the disorder of liver lipid metabolism and the production of inflammatory cytokines. The study of the pathogenesis and potential signal transduction pathways of AFLD has important clinical research value in preventing hepatic steatosis patients from developing more severe steatohepatitis, liver fibrosis/cirrhosis, and eventually hepatocellular carcinoma (HCC). For this reason, our paper focuses on six signaling pathways that regulate AFLD: ① SIRT1/AMPK/Lipin-1 signaling pathway: The signal transduction mechanism of AFLD involves a upstream signaling regulation system SIRT1/AMPK, with Lipin-1 as a downstream key regulator. Lipin-1 is a phospholipid acid phosphatase (PAP) that plays a dual role in promoting triglyceride (TG) synthesis during lipid metabolism and acting as a transcriptional auxiliary regulator in the nucleus. Firstly, ethanol can increase the gene and protein expression of Lipin-1, induce Lipin-1-PAP activity and nucleocytoplasmic shuttling, inhibit Lipin-1-mediated fatty acid oxidation and VLDL-TG secretion in the liver, disrupt SIRT1-SFRS10 axis to affect Lpin1 alternative splicing, interfere with Lipin-1/NF-κB/NFATc4 axis, induce the production of pro-inflammatory cytokines, and finally lead to the development of AFLD in cultured hepatocytes and in mouse livers with alcoholic hepatitis (You et al., 2017). Secondly, ethanol seriously impaired liver peroxisome proliferator-activated receptor-γ coactivator-1α (PGC-1α)/peroxisome proliferator-activated receptor α (PPARα) signal transduction and aggravated steatohepatitis in several mouse models of AFLD. Lipin-1 was transferred to the nucleus, where it co-activated PGC-1α and PPARα, enhancing the expression of mitochondrial genes involved in fatty acid oxidation. Consequently, hepatic steatosis induced by ethanol exposure was prevented (Fischer et al., 2003; Nakajima et al., 2004). In addition, ethanol-induced endoplasmic reticulum (ER) stress and SIRT1-AMPK signaling system damage caused the activation of mTORC1-nuclear lipin-1-SREBP-1 signaling pathway in AFLD mice (You et al., 2004). In hepatocytes, nuclear Lipin-1 is the key component of mTORC1-SREBP-1 pathway (Bakan and Laplante, 2012). Lipin-1 is a nucleocytoplasmic shuttling protein. The nuclear-located Lipin-1 depends on its PAP activity to inhibit the function of SREBP-1, thus reducing diet-induced hepatic steatosis. A better understanding of the regulatory mechanism of Lipin-1 under the action of ethanol will facilitate the development of novel pharmacological or nutritional therapies for the treatment of alcoholic steatosis/steatohepatitis patients (Peterson et al., 2011). ② PI3K/AKT/Nrf2/PPARγ signaling pathway: The excessive consumption of alcohol produces large amounts of ROS. The oxidative stress induced by ROS down-regulates the expression of PI3K and AKT, thus inhibiting its downstream target Nrf2 in male BALB/c mice (Liu et al., 2019; Wang et al., 2021). NRF2 and peroxisome proliferator-activated receptor γ (PPARγ) are two signaling pathways that regulate each other with positive feedback (Reddy and Standiford, 2010). Under oxidative stress, the expression of PPAR γ in Nrf2 knockout mice decreased significantly (Lee, 2017). PPARγ alleviates inflammation and oxidative stress by inhibiting the expression of NLRP3 in AFLD mice (Haneklaus and O'Neill, 2015; Hughes and O'Neill, 2018; Meng et al., 2019). ③ p62/Nrf2/KEAP1 signaling pathway: NRF2 has become a key site for the treatment of AFLD. It plays a role in the regulation of heme oxygenase 1 (HO-1) and glutathione (GSH) (Gyamfi and Wan, 2010; Li et al., 2015). The activated Nrf2 enters the nucleus, binds to the antioxidant element ARE, and then activates the expression of HO-1 and antioxidant proteases to resist internal and external stimuli in AML12 hepatocyte cells (Ge et al., 2017; Jiang L. et al., 2017). Nrf2 mediates the expression of p62 gene induced by oxidative stress, and p62 protein also contributes to the activation of Nrf2, forming a positive feedback loop (Jain et al., 2010). ARE, the antioxidant component of p62 promoter, induces oxidative stress through NRF2. Also, p62 connects to the Kelch-repeat domain of Kelch-like ECH-associated protein 1 (KEAP1) in the cytoplasm through the Keap1 interaction region (KIR), blocking the binding of KEAP1 and NRF2, leading to ubiquitination and degradation of transcription factors. The interaction between KEAP1 and p62 leads to the accumulation and autophagy degradation of endogenous KEAP1, which regulates the activation of Nrf2 (Qiu et al., 2017; Zhao et al., 2021). ④ STING-IRF3-Bax signaling pathway induces inflammation, ER stress, and apoptosis to cause hepatocyte injury and dysfunction. AFLD could be improved by inhibiting the expression of this pathway. Innate immunity is one of the driving factors of AFLD. As a mediator of innate immune signaling pathways, the stimulator of interferon genes (STING) connects the upstream DNA sensors with the downstream interferon regulatory factor 3 (IRF3). When ER stress was induced by ethanol, it caused the binding of STING, ER adapter, and IRF3. The phosphorylation of IRF3 activated B-cell lymphoma 2 (Bcl2)-associated X protein (Bax), leading to the apoptosis of hepatocytes in mice fed 4-week ethanol (Ishikawa and Barber, 2008; Petrasek et al., 2013). ⑤ C3/CYP2E1/Gly-tRF/SIRT1 complement regulation system: The C3 complement activation product C3a regulates CYP2E1 (a member of the cytochrome P450 mixed function oxidase system) to restore the expression of glycine transfer (t) RNA-derived fragments (Gly-tRF). The expression of Gly-tRF was increased in ALD patients to down-regulate the expression of downstream SIRT1, which promoted adipogenesis and inhibit fatty acid β oxidation. The complement regulation system plays a key role in the development of hepatic steatosis (Zhong et al., 2019). ⑥ LRP6/Wnt/β-catenin/CYP2E1 signaling pathway: CYP2E1 produces ROS under the action of ethanol, which leads to lipid peroxidation and DNA damage in hepatocytes of rats fed ethanol for 1 month (French, 2013). Low density lipoprotein receptor-related protein6 (LRP6) is a key protein that regulates the Wnt/β-catenin signaling pathway (Go, 2015). LRP6 can regulate the expression of CYP2E1 through the Wnt/β-catenin signaling pathway studied in liver-specific Lrp5/6 KO (Lrp-LKO) and conditional Wntless (Wls) KO mice (Yang et al., 2014), thereby affecting the susceptibility of individuals to alcoholic hepatic injury, which were investigated in AFLD patients. The results were verified in LRP6$^{(+/-)}$ mice fed with 2.4 or 4 g/kg ethanol every 7 days for 28 days (Xu et al., 2019).

In addition, p66Shc, a subtype of the shcA adaptor protein family, is an inducible oxidoreductase that regulates the production of ROS and H_2O_2. In the presence of ethanol, p66Shc can cause oxidative damage to hepatocytes (Giorgio et al., 2005; Berniakovich et al., 2008). The bioinformatics analysis indicated that p66Shc was a potential target gene of miR-219a-5p. In *in vivo* and *in vitro* experiments, miR-219a-5p can directly inhibit the expression of p66Shc to improve oxidative stress in Male Sprague-Dawley rats and AML12 hepatocyte cells (Fu et al., 2019).

SHARED SIGNALING PATHWAY OF NAFLD AND AFLD

As an upstream signaling system, the SIRT1/AMPK signaling pathway is responsible for regulating hepatic lipid metabolism. SIRT1/AMPK regulates each other and shares many molecular mechanisms, playing an important role in lipid metabolism in mice with streptozotocin/nicotinamide-induced diabetes and db/db mice fed on a high-fat diet (Chen et al., 2012). The deacetylation activity of SIRT1 is driven by NAD^+ levels. A significant increase in the ratio of NAD^+/NADH activates the expression of SIRT1, and then SIRT1 activates the phosphorylation of AMPK. AMPK is a sensor of the cellular energy state, which is activated by AMP and inhibited by ATP. AMPK is also activated by phosphorylation of the liver kinase B1 (LKB1). An increase in the ratio of NAD^+/NADH, results in the phosphorylation of LKB1 and AMPK which can activate the SIRT1/AMPK signaling pathway, inhibit adipogenesis and promote lipid oxidation, and reduce NAFLD symptoms and IR in HFD mice (Park et al., 2016). Insulin was able to activate SREBP-1c directly and increase the activity of mTORC1 to regulate SREBP-1c indirectly. In addition, SREBP-1c also regulated hepatic lipid synthesis independently of insulin (Loomba et al., 2021). On the other hand, the activation of SREBP-1 by ethanol can also be partially inhibited by AMPK. In the process of fatty acid metabolism, the phosphorylation of AMPK inhibits the activation of SREBP-1 and positively regulates the expression of PPARα, thereby regulating lipid metabolism homeostasis and improving AFLD in rat hepatic cells and in the livers of mice fed with ethanol (Zhou et al., 2001; You et al., 2004; Berger et al., 2005). Activated PPARα up-regulates the transcription of carnitine palmitoyl transferase 1 (CPT-1) and acyl coenzyme A oxidase 1 (ACOX1). As an inhibitor of fatty acid oxidation in mitochondria, CPT-1 can regulate the uptake of fatty acids. ACOX1 is a key enzyme in the oxidation of peroxisomal β. The down-regulation of this gene leads to the dysfunction of long-chain fatty acids oxidation and hepatic steatosis in HepG2 cells (Zeng et al., 2016). In HFD-induced NAFLD mice and oleic acid-induced FL83B cells, fisetin (a natural flavonoid derived from fruits and vegetables), significantly increased phosphorylation of AMPKα, production of Sirt1, and β-oxidation in hepatocytes, decreased lipid accumulation. Fisetin improved NAFLD by regulating the SIRT1/AMPK pathway and fatty acid β oxidation (Liou et al., 2018).

Also, SIRT1-AMPK is a central target of ethanol in the liver, regulating the expression of adiponectin (ADPN), a key factor in AFLD. ADPN has a protective effect on AFLD. In AFLD, the expression of ADPN and its receptors are decreased, leading to damage to the hepatic adiponectin signaling pathway in ethanol-fed mice (You and Rogers, 2009). In addition, ethanol exposure also causes ER stress, and SIRT1-AMPK is driven to regulate the expression of Lipin-1. The increase in Lipin-1 transcription and expression is related to the oxidation of fatty acid, the secretion of VLDL-TG, and the reduction of pro-inflammatory factors and lipid accumulation in cultured hepatocyte cells and in the livers of rodents (You et al., 2017). SIRT1/AMPK/SREBP-1c is a key pathway for regulating lipid metabolism in both NAFLD and AFLD (Chen et al., 2012; Quan et al., 2013). SREBP-1c is activated by ER stress and positively regulates the transcription of stearoyl-CoA desaturase 1 (SCD1), FAS, acetyl-CoA carboxylase (ACC), and ATP citrate lyase (Acly), which directly catalyze adipogenesis (Ferré and Foufelle, 2010; Fortin et al., 2017). Acly is responsible for the synthesis of Acetyl-CoA, and ACC converts Acetyl-CoA to Malonyl-CoA through carboxylation. FAS is responsible for the synthesis of long-chain fatty acids from Acetyl-CoA and Malonyl-CoA, while SCD1 is responsible for the synthesis of unsaturated fatty acids (Chirala et al., 2001; Huang et al., 2013). SCD1 is a lipogenic enzyme found in the ER, which plays a key role in energy metabolism. It can catalyze the conversion of palmitoyl-CoA and stearoyl-CoA into palmitoyl-CoA and oleoyl and oleoyl-CoA. Palmitoyl-CoA and oleoyl-CoA can be used as substrates to synthesize palmitoleic acid and oleic acid. Palmitoleic acid and oleic acid are the major components of TG, membrane phospholipids, and cholesterol esters (Ozols, 1997; Ntambi et al., 2002; Kato et al., 2006; Sampath and Ntambi, 2014; ALJohani et al., 2017). SCD1 is critical to the improvement of weight gain and IR caused by a high-fat diet in rats and mice (Gutiérrez-Juárez et al., 2017). Insulin sensitivity was increased, and body fat was decreased in

SCD1 knockout mice (Ntambi et al., 2002). SREBP-1c is also up-regulated by insulin receptor substrate 1 (IRS-1) to promote fatty acid synthesis and accumulation in hepatocytes. At the same time, IRS-2 down-regulates forkhead box protein A2 (Foxa2), a positive regulator of fatty acid oxidation. Foxa2 could be activated by the inhibition of IRS-2 to promote fatty acid oxidation in NAFLD patients (Kohjima et al., 2008).

The PI3K/AKT signaling pathway also regulates lipid metabolism and insulin signal transduction (Huang et al., 2014; Abood et al., 2018; Liao et al., 2018; Pan et al., 2018). The expression of PI3K and AKT proteins in the liver of NAFLD rats was significantly lower than those of normal rats (Liu et al., 2012; Matsuda et al., 2013). The p85 subunit of PI3K can bind to IRS and anchor in the cell membrane, and then activate the p110 subunit to regulate the transduction of glucose uptake signal in adipocytes and hepatocytes (Foster et al., 2003). AKT inhibits the expression of fatty acid oxidation genes and regulates glucose and lipid metabolism in the liver (Li et al., 2007). PARP-1 is an upstream regulator of PI3K/AKT signaling pathway. Its' over activation can lead to the inhibition of fatty acid β-oxidation (Cantó and Auwerx, 2011). The inhibition of PARP-1 can activate the PI3K/AKT pathway to down-regulate the expression of the fat synthesis gene SREBP-1c, reduce lipid synthesis and accumulation, and improve fatty liver disease in HFHS diet mice (Wang et al., 2019). In addition, inhibition of PARP-1 can also increase NAD^+ content and SIRT1 activity, enhance lipid metabolism, and improve hepatic steatosis in mice fed a high-fat diet (Kraus and Hottiger, 2013). Meanwhile, the PI3K/AKT signaling pathway also plays an important regulatory role in AFLD. Ethanol intake produces excessive ROS. The imbalance of ROS can lead to cellular oxidative stress. Oxidative stress down-regulates the expression of PI3K/AKT, and then inhibits the expression of its downstream target Nrf2 (Liu et al., 2019). The inhibition of Nrf2 down-regulates the expression of PPARγ (Lee, 2017). PPARγ can reduce the secretion of pro-inflammatory factors by inhibiting the activation of NLRP3 inflammasomes, which then interfere with lipid metabolism. NLRP3 inflammasomes are critical for the initiation of liver inflammation and the progression from hepatic steatosis to NASH. The inhibition of NLRP3 inflammasomes improves the inflammation and oxidative stress levels in AFLD mice (Haneklaus and O'Neill, 2015; Hughes and O'Neill, 2018; Meng et al., 2019).

THERAPIES OF NAFLD AND AFLD

Exercise Intervention and Abstinence

Aerobic exercise has been suggested as a potential non-clinical strategy to improve NAFLD. Eight-weeks of aerobic training could alleviate the hepatic steatosis of NAFLD mice by activating AMPK-PPAR-α signaling pathway in obese mice (Diniz et al., 2020). Irisin is derived from mouse skeletal muscles in response to exercises. It decreased body weight and fat mass of diet-induced obesity mice in a dose dependent manner. This effector reduced the concentrations of blood glucose and blood lipid, and eventually reversed hepatic steatosis (Tarantino et al., 2019). In patients with AFLD, the clinical trials showed that abstinence may reverse hepatic steatohepatitis and fibrosis, achieve compensation for liver cirrhosis, and improve survival rate of patients with advanced stage (Pár and Pár, 2019). And NAFLD patients, even if alcohol intake within safe threshold, were still at higher risk of liver disease progression. NAFLD patients should also maintain long-term abstinence (Petroni et al., 2019).

CLINICAL TREATMENT

The antioxidant treatment in NAFLD is still controversial. A short-term study of vitamin E supplementation in obese mice induced by high fat diet suggested that the concentration of ROS should be maintained at a reasonable level *in vivo*, rather than excessive or premature elimination, which can maintain the balance of intracellular energy metabolism, lipid metabolism, and insulin signal transduction (Alcala et al., 2017). There is a certain correlation between vitamin D deficiency and NAFLD. However, the effect of vitamin D was limited in clinical trials. In a systematic analysis of six trials, only two trials showed improved results, and the biomarkers of oxidative stress and inflammation decreased in three trials (Sharifi and Amani, 2019). In a vitamin D supplementation trial of 50 patients with metabolic syndromes, there were no significant differences in TG, high-density lipoprotein (HDL) cholesterol, low-density lipoprotein (LDL) cholesterol, and fasting glucose between experimental and control patients (Makariou et al., 2017). Statins reduced the expression of Perilipin 5 (Plin5) through regulating liver lipid metabolism. Atorvastatin reduced the concentration of TG in the liver by up-regulating PKA-mediated phosphorylation of Plin5 (Gao et al., 2017). Aspirin can improve the levels of serum TG, HDL cholesterol and alanine aminotransferase (ALT) in rabbits fed a cholesterol diet. Aspirin enhanced lipolysis and inhibited lipid synthesis and inflammation by activating PPARδ-AMPK-PGC-1α in HepG2 cells and vascular endothelial cells (Han et al., 2020). The glucagon-like peptide-1 (GLP-1) analog/receptor agonists is a class of drugs used for the treatment of adult T2DM, including exenatide, lixisenatide, liraglutide (LRG), albiglutide, dulaglutide, and semaglutide. Although metformin is still the first-line therapy for the treatment of T2DM, and it also has favorable effects on inflammation control in non-obese patients with T2DM and NAFLD (Mitrovic et al., 2021). But the clinical treatment of GLP-1 analogs or receptor agonists may be considered in patients with contraindications or intolerance to metformin, and in patients whose hemoglobin A1c exceeds the target value by more than 1.5% (Collins and Costello, 2020; Tarantino and Balsano, 2020). LRG can alleviate the hepatic lipid accumulation in HFD mice by increasing the phosphorylation of AMPK and ACC and inhibiting the expression of SREBP1. High-dose LRG has been approved by the FDA as a treatment for obesity in overweight patients with comorbidities. Semaglutide is also approved for the treatment of obesity, which is the most potential risk factor of NAFLD. Compared to LRG treatment, semaglutide treatment showed greater mean placebo-corrected weight reductions than LRG in participant population (12.4 vs. 4.5%). In addition, the dose and frequency of semaglutide injection was lower and the effect was persisted longer than LRG. However, the subject populations above were not the same between the two, which reduced the comparability of the two molecular drugs (He et al., 2016; Hao et al., 2019; Newsome et al., 2021; Wilding et al., 2021).

POTENTIAL EFFECTORS OF NAFLD AND AFLD

Natural compounds extracted from plants are the main sources for screening bioactive substances that are beneficial to the prevention and treatment of human diseases. Flavonoids are a group of natural substances with different phenolic structures, which are found in many fruits, vegetables, grains, and medicinal plants. Many of these natural extracts have been shown to improve hepatic lipid metabolism and inhibit the occurrence and development of NAFLD and AFLD (Zhang et al., 2013). Here, we discuss some representative natural products with potential therapeutic effects on NAFLD and AFLD (**Table 1**).

NAFLD EFFECTORS

Flavonoids have been shown to improve NAFLD in short-term randomized trials and animal studies. In a prospective study involving 2,694 adults, the intake of flavonoid-rich foods was gradually correlated with a decrease in the risk of NAFLD progression mediated by reductions in serum cholesterol and HOMA-IR (Zhong et al., 2021). Fisetin can activate the SIRT1/AMPK pathway to decrease lipid accumulation and increase fatty acid β-oxidation in hepatocytes (Liou et al., 2018). Apple polyphenol extract (APE) could activate SIRT1/AMPK pathway to regulate the autophagy in HepG2 cells, which alleviated the free-fatty-acid-induced lipid accumulation (Li et al., 2021). Vine tea polyphenol (VTP) extracted from Chinese herb *Ampelopsis grossedentata* reduced serum cholesterol and TG levels and decreased hepatic lipid accumulation in male C57BL/6N mice fed a western diet (WD). VTP inhibits lipogenesis by activating phosphorylation of AMPKα and PPARα and reducing the levels of SREBP1 and FAS. At the same time, it was found that VTP can also activate Nrf2-mediated HO-1 and quinone oxidoreductase (NQO1) expression and reduce liver thiobarbituric acid reactive substance (TBARS) levels to prevent liver oxidative stress. Dihydromyricetin (DMY), which is rich in VTP, is a potential bioactive compound to prevent NAFLD (Xie et al., 2020). Oleuropein (Ole) can activate autophagy to improve hepatic steatosis in mice. Ole was able to up-regulate the phosphorylation of Unc-51-like-kinasel (ULK1) depend on AMPK to induce the autophagy (Porcu et al., 2018). Apigenin (API), a peroxisomal proliferator-activated receptor γ modulator (PPARM), improves the lipid accumulation and oxidative stress of NAFLD by regulating Nrf2 and PPARγ in mice (Panda and Kar, 2007; Tong and Pelling, 2013; Feng et al., 2017). Puerarin is a bioactive isoflavone compound isolated from puerarin root. Puerarin can protect against hepatic steatosis, inflammation, and fibrosis, and improve NAFLD by regulating PARP-1/PI3K/AKT signaling pathway in male C57BL/6J mice (Wang S. et al., 2016). Curcumin is a kind of natural polyphenol, which improves anti-inflammation, anti-oxidation, and lipid metabolism (Um et al., 2013; Wang L. et al., 2016). In a randomized controlled trial of 45 patients with NAFLD, curcumin significantly reduced body weight, waist circumference, body fat percent, and body mass index (BMI) comparing with the placebo group (Mirhafez et al., 2021). Curcumin inhibits hepatic lipid synthesis and promotes bile acid metabolism through NRF2 /FXR/LXRα pathway, and effectively improves NAFLD induced by high-fat and high-fructose diet in C57BL/6 mice (Yan et al., 2018). Rosmarinic acid (RA) is a phenolic compound, which improves NAFLD through by down-regulating TAZ both in male SD rats fed a high fat diet and L02 cells stimulated with oleic acid (Luo et al., 2021).

AFLD EFFECTORS

Magnolol is a phenolic active substance extracted from the traditional Chinese medicine *Magnolia officinalis*. Magnolol can inhibit oxidative stress by up-regulating the phosphorylation of PI3K and AKT and increasing the expression of downstream Nrf2, HO-1, and PPARγ in male BALB/c mice. Magnolol can also inhibit the activation of NLRP3 inflammasome to reduce the inflammatory response. Magnolol may activate PI3K/AKT/NRF2/PPARγ pathway and inhibit the NLRP3 inflammasome to prevent and improve AFLD in mice (Liu et al., 2019). Dihydromyricetin (DMY) is a kind of flavonoid extracted from *Ampelopsis grossedentata*. DMY has the effects of anti-oxidation, anti-inflammation, anti-bacterial, and improving IR of skeletal muscle (Shen et al., 2012; Jiang et al., 2014; Shi et al., 2015). For ethanol-induced liver injury, DMY can promote the activation of Nrf2 and efficiently induce Keap-1 degradation by regulating p62. DMY can reduce hepatic steatosis and inflammation response in the pathological process of AFLD in male C57BL/6 mice (Qiu et al., 2017). The *Gentianae macrophyllae* root extract (GME) was the main source of gentiopicroside and swertiamarin (Huang R. et al., 2020). These two secoiridoid compounds have been shown to prevent and improve cellular inflammatory responses in rats (Saravanan et al., 2014; Zhao et al., 2015). In ethanol-induced AFLD mice, GME significantly inhibited the expression of pro-inflammatory cytokines TNF- α, IL-1, and IL-6 by inhibiting the phosphorylation of JNK and P38 (Cui et al., 2019). Moreover, the ameliorative effect of GME on AFLD was achieved in a dose-dependent manner. In ethanol-induced AFLD C57BL/6J mice, the expression of fat synthesis-related genes SREBP1, FAS and ACCα were increased, and the expression of lipolytic genes ATGL and Sirt1 were decreased. Blueberry polyphenols significantly reverse this process by promoting hepatocyte autophagy, accelerating lipolysis, and reducing lipid accumulation, but it did not change the expression of these genes in healthy control mice (Zhuge et al., 2020). Excessive alcohol consumption and a high-fat diet (HFD) can promote steatohepatitis, leading to comorbidities of NAFLD and AFLD. An *in vivo* model was established by HFD with a single dose of ethanol in male ICR mice, and an *in vitro* model was established by inducing lipid accumulation in HepG2 cells with oleic

TABLE 1 | Potential effectors shown to protect the liver from NAFLD and AFLD.

	Effectors	Treatment	Experimental model
NAFLD	Fisetin	20 mg/kg bw/twice a week for 10 weeks	HFD-induced NAFLD mice
	Apple polyphenol extract (APE)	20 μg/ml APE for 24 h	HepG2 cells
	Vine tea polyphenol (VTP)	0.5, 1, and 2% VTP for 12 weeks	Male C57BL/6N mice fed a western diet
	Oleuropein (Ole)	3% Ole for 16 weeks	HFD C57BL/6J mice
	Apigenin (API)	30 mg/kg bw/daily intraperitoneal injection for 3 weeks	Male C57BL/6J mice
	Puerarin	100 and 200 mg/kg bw/daily intraperitoneal injection for 4 weeks	Male C57BL/6J mice
	Curcumin	50 and 100 mg/kg bw/daily by oral gavage for 4 weeks	C57BL/6 mice fed high-fat and high-fructose diet
		250 mg/day for 8 weeks	NAFLD patients
	Rosmarinic acid (RA)	200 mg/kg/day for 10 weeks	Male SD rats fed a high fat diet
		5, 10, 20 μg/ml for 24 h	L02 cells with oleic acid
AFLD	Magnolol	5, 10, and 20 mg/kg BW/day intraperitoneal injection for 3 days	Male BALB/c mice
	Dihydromyricetin (DMY)	75 and 150 mg/kg bw/day for 6 weeks	Male C57BL/6 mice
	Gentianae macrophyllae root extract (GME)	20, 40, and 100 mg/kg bw/day gastric gavage for 19 days	Adult male and female Kunming mice
	Blueberry polyphenol	100 and 200 mg/kg bw/day for 1 month	Male C57BL/6J
	Taxifolin (TAX)	1, 5, and 25 mg/kg bw/day for 4 weeks	Male ICR mice
		25, 50, 100, and 200 μM for 1 h	HepG2 cells

acid or palmitic acid. Taxifolin (TAX) is a dihydroxyflavonoid compound that regulated lipid synthesis by inhibiting the expression of SREBP1 and up-regulating the level of PPARγ. In addition, TAX also inhibited the inflammatory response caused by caspase-1 activation. TAX showed a potential therapeutic effect on NAFLD and AFLD caused by ethanol combined with HFD-induced steatohepatitis (Zhan et al., 2021).

PROBIOTICS/PREBIOTICS

The gut microbiota played an important role in host metabolism, nutrient absorption, energy utilization, and immune function (Tarantino et al., 2019). The disruption of commensal homeostasis of gut microbiota-host may generate a series of chronic metabolism diseases, such as obesity, T2DM, and NAFLD (Zhang P. et al., 2018). The ecological imbalance of gut microbiota can stimulate liver fat storage by regulating intestinal permeability, dietary choline metabolism, bile acid metabolism, and the production of mild inflammation and endogenous ethanol (Arslan, 2014). NAFLD patients showed an overgrowth of gut microbiota, increased intestinal permeability and paracellular leakage of intestinal lumen antigens, which promotned the development of NASH. Increased *Proteobacteria*, *E. coli*, and *Negativicutes*, and decreased *Firmicutes* were observed in the intestines of patients with advanced fibrosis and NAFLD (Arslan, 2014). NAFLD mice were treated with *Lactobacillus bulgaricus*, *Lactobacillus casei*, *Lactobacillus helveticus*, and *Pediococcus* Kid7, either alone or in combination. The results demonstrated that probiotics had a positive effect on NAFLD by regulating gut microbiota, interfering with inflammatory response, tumor necrosis factor α (TNFα), and interleukin 1β (IL-1β) (Lee et al., 2020). The increase in the proportion of lactic acid bacteria in the feces of NAFLD mice is closely related to the reduction of intestinal inflammation and the increase of GLP-1 concentration. GLP-1 affects obesity by delaying gastric emptying decreasing food intake, and modulates glucose homeostasis by stimulating insulin secretion. A meta-analysis showed that probiotic therapies can improve NAFLD by reducing AST, ALT, total cholesterol, TNF-α, and IR in four randomized trials involving 134 NAFLD and NASH patients (Kanda et al., 2020). Because obesity is one of the main driving factors of NAFLD, in the study of probiotics to improve NAFLD, it is necessary to specifically evaluate the changes of body fat rate, TG, insulin sensitivity, fat inflammation, and various metabolic parameters to determine its function (Ahn et al., 2019). In a study of lean donor fecal microbiota transplantation (FMT), although the experiment proved to be safe, it did not reduce the BMI of patients with obesity and other metabolic diseases. Therefore, the strategy of treating chronic metabolic diseases with probiotics still needs to be carefully evaluated (Zhang et al., 2019). VTP was able to increase the relative abundance of intestinal *Akkermansia* (*AKK*) and decrease the ratio of *Firmicutes/Bacteroidetes* in mice fed a WD. VTP may prevent WD-induced NAFLD by balancing lipid metabolism, liver oxidative stress and gut microbiota (Xie et al., 2020). In addition, compared to healthy people, the decreased abundance of *AKK* in the gut microbiota of alcoholic hepatitis patients was positively correlated with the severity of AFLD. *AKK* can increase the thickness of intestinal mucus and the expression of tight junction protein to prevent alcohol-induced gastro-intestinal leakage.

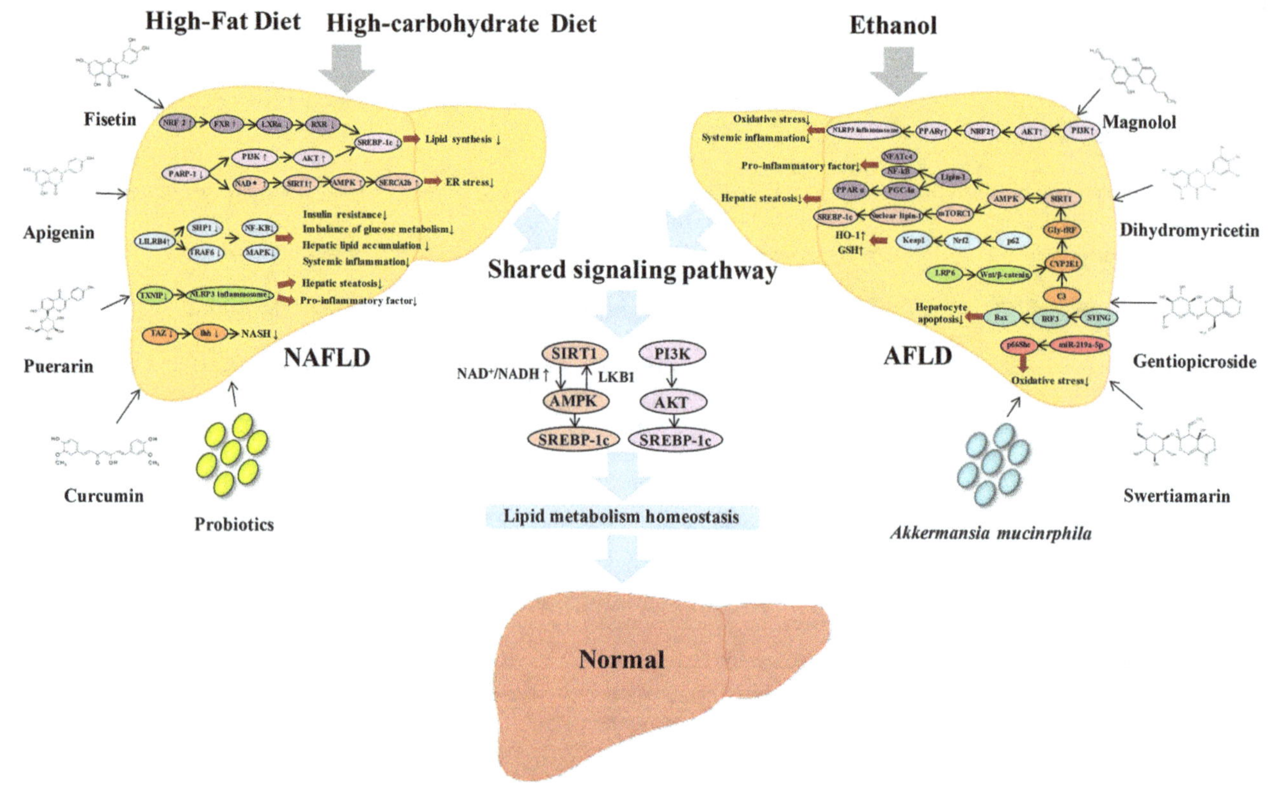

FIGURE 1 | Graphical representation of the comparative review of NAFLD and AFLD signaling pathway and effectors. High fat and high carbohydrate diet-induced NAFLD can be modulated by Nrf2/FXR/LXRα/RXR/SREBP-1c, PI3K/AKT/SREBP-1c, AMPK/SERCA2b, LILRB4/SHP1/TRAF6/NF-κB/MAPK, and TAZ/Ihh signaling pathways. Ethanol-induced AFLD can be modulated by STING-IRF3-Bax, C3 /CYP2E1/Gly-tRF/SIRT1, LRP6/Wnt/β-catenin/CYP2E1, and miR-219a-5p/p66Shc signaling pathways. NAFLD and AFLD share two signaling pathways, SIRT1/AMPK/SREBP-1c and PI3K/AKT/SREBP-1c, while other pathways are owned by each other specifically. A variety of natural flavonoids can improve NAFLD, including fisetin, apigenin, puerarin, and curcumin; and AFLD, including magnolol, dihydromyricetin, gentiopicroside, and swertiamarin. In addition, NAFLD and AFLD can also be improved by probiotics and *Akkermansia muciniphila*. Ultimately, NAFLD and AFLD could be reversed to achieve a homeostasis of lipid metabolism.

The increased abundance of *AKK* can improve the neutrophil infiltration and liver injury in AFLD patients. Exogenous supplementation of *AKK* or promoting the proliferation of *AKK* through the diet may be a potential strategy for the treatment of AFLD (Grander et al., 2018).

CONCLUSION

NAFLD and AFLD are the most prevalent metabolic liver diseases worldwide. Their complex pathogenesis restricts the progress of prevention, diagnosis, and treatment. The prevalence of NAFLD in China (22.4%) is similar to that in the United States (24.13%) and Europe (23.71%), with an estimated 173–338 million people affected by NAFLD. The prevalence of ALD in China is 4.5%, slightly lower than that in the United States (6.2%) and Europe (6%), and higher than that in Japan (1.56–2.34%), with 62 million people that are affected by AFLD. The high prevalence of metabolic liver diseases such as NAFLD and ALD has provoked concern (Xiao et al., 2019). In order to prevent the rapid rise of the incidence of metabolic liver disease, we urgently need safe and effective drug intervention and treatment. Major economies in the world have invested a lot of research funds to promote high-quality basic/clinical research and transformation. Currently, despite hundreds of promising pharmacological trials in progress, no registered drugs have been approved for the treatment of metabolic liver diseases, including NAFLD and AFLD. From 2009 to 2017, none of the new drugs approved by the CFDA were for metabolic liver disease. During the same period, 59 new drugs for liver diseases were approved by the United States Food and Drug Administration (FDA, USA), the European Medicines Agency (EMA, EU), and the Medicines and Medical Devices Agency (PMDA, Japan), almost all of which were for the treatment of viral hepatitis and cirrhosis.

It has been suggested that NAFLD is an early physiological adaptation of human liver under adverse living conditions, and it is only a physiological response (Tarantino et al., 2019). However, it has caused more serious pathological metabolic diseases in the modern lifestyle (Muñoz-Garach et al., 2016). A comprehensive understanding of NAFLD and AFLD signaling pathways and clinical treatment will help identify biomarkers and therapeutic targets for early detection and management. Although NAFLD and AFLD are major challenging public health problems, they are preventable. In daily life, lifestyle changes are still the first-line treatment for NAFLD and AFLD. Dietary ingredients and exercises that reduce the risk of NALFD can effectively reverse early fatty liver disease. AFLD can also be reversed by stopping alcohol intake and changing lifestyle. The current basic/clinical studies on NAFLD and AFLD are mainly focused on: ① Anti-inflammatory, anti-oxidant, and anti-fibrotic treatments; ② Improve insulin resistance; ③ Improve lipid metabolism and increase fatty acid β-oxidation; ④ Reduce oxidative stress, hepatic gluconeogenesis, lipid synthesis, and hepatic steatosis; ⑤ Activation and inhibitors of key targets in the glucose and lipid metabolism pathway. By comparing the specific and shared molecular regulatory mechanisms, clinical treatments, and potential effectors of NAFLD and AFLD, we provide mutual reference strategies for the prevention and treatment of NAFLD, AFLD, and their related metabolic diseases (**Figure 1**). Furthermore, it provides enlightenment and ideas for the discovery and development of safe and effective drugs in the field of metabolic liver disease.

AUTHOR CONTRIBUTIONS

PZ and XM contributed to the conception, design, and manuscript writing. WW, RG, MM, WS, DL, RC, BS, and XT contributed substantially to the writing and revision of the manuscript and approved its final version. All authors contributed to the article and approved the submitted version.

REFERENCES

Abood, S., Veisaga, M. L., López, L. A., and Barbieri, M. A. (2018). Dehydroleucodine inhibits mitotic clonal expansion during adipogenesis through cell cycle arrest. *Phytother. Res.* 32, 1583–1592. doi: 10.1002/ptr.6089

Adorini, L., Pruzanski, M., and Shapiro, D. (2012). Farnesoid X receptor targeting to treat nonalcoholic steatohepatitis. *Drug Discov. Today* 17, 988–997. doi: 10.1016/j.drudis.2012.05.012

Ahn, S. B., Jun, D. W., Kang, B. K., Lim, J. H., Lim, S., and Chung, M. J. (2019). Randomized, double-blind, placebo-controlled study of a multispecies probiotic mixture in nonalcoholic fatty liver disease. *Sci. Rep.* 9:5688. doi: 10.1038/s41598-019-42059-3

Alcala, M., Calderon-Dominguez, M., Serra, D., Herrero, L., Ramos, M. P., and Viana, M. (2017). Short-term vitamin E treatment impairs reactive oxygen species signaling required for adipose tissue expansion, resulting in fatty liver and insulin resistance in obese mice. *PLoS ONE* 12:e0186579. doi: 10.1371/journal.pone.0186579

ALJohani, A. M., Syed, D. N., and Ntambi, J. M. (2017). Insights into stearoyl-CoA desaturase-1 regulation of systemic metabolism. *Trends Endocrinol. Metab.* 28, 831–842. doi: 10.1016/j.tem.2017.10.003

Angulo, P., and Lindor, K. D. (2002). Non-alcoholic fatty liver disease. *J. Gastroenterol. Hepatol.* 17, 186–190. doi: 10.1046/j.1440-1746.17.s1.10.x

Anty, R., and Gual, P. (2019). Pathogenesis of non-alcoholic fatty liver disease. *Presse Med.* 48, 1468–1483. doi: 10.1016/j.lpm.2019.09.051

Arab, J. P., Karpen, S. J., Dawson, P. A., Arrese, M., and Trauner, M. (2017). Bile acids and nonalcoholic fatty liver disease: molecular insights and therapeutic perspectives. *Hepatology* 65, 350–362. doi: 10.1002/hep.28709

Arslan, N. (2014). Obesity, fatty liver disease and intestinal microbiota. *World J. Gastroenterol.* 20, 16452–16463. doi: 10.3748/wjg.v20.i44.16452

Bakan, I., and Laplante, M. (2012). Connecting mTORC1 signaling to SREBP-1 activation. *Curr. Opin. Lipidol.* 23, 226–234. doi: 10.1097/MOL.0b013e328352dd03

Bashiardes, S., Shapiro, H., Rozin, S., Shibolet, O., and Elinav, E. (2016). Non-alcoholic fatty liver and the gut microbiota. *Mol. Metab.* 5, 782–794. doi: 10.1016/j.molmet.2016.06.003

Berger, J. P., Akiyama, T. E., and Meinke, P. T. (2005). PPARs: therapeutic targets for metabolic disease. *Trends Pharmacol. Sci.* 26, 244–251. doi: 10.1016/j.tips.2005.03.003

Berniakovich, I., Trinei, M., Stendardo, M., Migliaccio, E., Minucci, S., Bernardi, P., et al. (2008). p66Shc-generated oxidative signal promotes fat accumulation. *J. Biol. Chem.* 283, 34283–34293. doi: 10.1074/jbc.M804362200

Cantó, C., and Auwerx, J. (2011). Targeting sirtuin 1 to improve metabolism: all you need is NAD(+)? *Pharmacol. Rev.* 64, 166–187. doi: 10.1124/pr.110.003905

Carino, A., Cipriani, S., Marchianò, S., Biagioli, M., Santorelli, C., Donini, A., et al. (2017). BAR502, a dual FXR and GPBAR1 agonist, promotes browning of white adipose tissue and reverses liver steatosis and fibrosis. *Sci. Rep.* 7:42801. doi: 10.1038/srep42801

Cesari, M., Pahor, M., and Incalzi, R. A. (2010). Plasminogen activator inhibitor-1 (PAI-1): a key factor linking fibrinolysis and age-related subclinical and clinical conditions. *Cardiovasc. Ther.* 28, e72–91. doi: 10.1111/j.1755-5922.2010.00171.x

Chávez-Talavera, O., Tailleux, A., Lefebvre, P., and Staels, B. (2017). Bile acid control of metabolism and inflammation in obesity, type 2 diabetes, dyslipidemia, and nonalcoholic fatty liver disease. *Gastroenterology* 152, 1679–1694.e3. doi: 10.1053/j.gastro.2017.01.055

Chen, W., Kang, C., Wang, S., and Lee, H. (2012). α-Lipoic acid regulates lipid metabolism through induction of sirtuin 1 (SIRT1) and activation of AMP-activated protein kinase. *Diabetologia* 55, 1824–1835. doi: 10.1007/s00125-012-2530-4

Chirala, S. S., Jayakumar, A., Gu, Z. W., and Wakil, S. J. (2001). Human fatty acid synthase: role of interdomain in the formation of catalytically active synthase dimer. *Proc. Natl. Acad. Sci. U.S.A.* 98, 3104–3108. doi: 10.1073/pnas.051635998

Chu, H., Duan, Y., Yang, L., and Schnabl, B. (2018). Small metabolites, possible big changes: a microbiota-centered view of non-alcoholic fatty liver disease. *Gut* 68, 359–370. doi: 10.1136/gutjnl-2018-316307

Collins, L., and Costello, R. A. (2020). *Glucagon-Like Peptide-1 Receptor Agonists.* Treasure Island, FL: StatPearls Publishing.

Cui, Y., Jiang, L., Shao, Y., Mei, L., and Tao, Y. (2019). Anti-alcohol liver disease effect of Gentianae macrophyllae extract through MAPK/JNK/p38 pathway. *J. Pharm. Pharmacol.* 71, 240–250. doi: 10.1111/jphp.13027

Diniz, T. A., de Lima Junior, E. A., Teixeira, A. A., Biondo, L. A., da Rocha, L. A. F., Valadão, I. C., et al. (2020). Aerobic training improves NAFLD markers and insulin resistance through AMPK-PPAR-α signaling in obese mice. *Life Sci.* 266:118868. doi: 10.1016/j.lfs.2020.118868

Dodson, M., de la Vega, M. R., Cholanians, A. B., Schmidlin, C. J., Chapman, E., and Zhang, D. (2019). Modulating NRF2 in disease: timing is everything. *Annu. Rev. Pharmacol. Toxicol.* 59, 555–575. doi: 10.1146/annurev-pharmtox-010818-021856

Engstler, A. J., Aumiller, T., Degen, C., Dürr, M., Weiss, E., Maier, I. B., et al. (2016). Insulin resistance alters hepatic ethanol metabolism: studies in mice and children with non-alcoholic fatty liver disease. *Gut* 65, 1564–1571. doi: 10.1136/gutjnl-2014-308379

Eslam, M., Valenti, L., and Romeo, S. (2018). Genetics and epigenetics of NAFLD and NASH: clinical impact. *J. Hepatol.* 68, 268–279. doi: 10.1016/j.jhep.2017.09.003

Estes, C., Anstee, Q. M., Arias-Loste, M. T., Bantel, H., Bellentani, S., Caballeria, J., et al. (2018). Modeling NAFLD disease burden in China, France, Germany, Italy, Japan, Spain, United Kingdom, and United States for the period 2016-2030. *J. Hepatol.* 69, 896–904. doi: 10.1016/j.jhep.2018.05.036

Estes, C., Razavi, H., Loomba, R., Younossi, Z., and Sanyal, A. J. (2017). Modeling the epidemic of nonalcoholic fatty liver disease demonstrates an exponential increase in burden of disease. *Hepatology* 67, 123–133. doi: 10.1002/hep.29466

Fan, L., Lai, R., Ma, N., Dong, Y., Li, Y., Wu, Q., et al. (2021). miR-552-3p modulates transcriptional activities of FXR and LXR to ameliorate hepatic glycolipid metabolism disorder. *J. Hepatol.* 74, 8–19. doi: 10.1016/j.jhep.2020.07.048

Fang, S., Suh, J. M., Reilly, S. M., Yu, E., Osborn, O., Lackey, D., et al. (2015). Intestinal FXR agonism promotes adipose tissue browning and reduces obesity and insulin resistance. *Nat. Med.* 21, 159–165. doi: 10.1038/nm.3760

Feng, X., Yu, W., Li, X., Zhou, F., Zhang, W., Shen, Q., et al. (2017). Apigenin, a modulator of PPARγ, attenuates HFD-induced NAFLD by regulating hepatocyte lipid metabolism and oxidative stress via Nrf2 activation. *Biochem. Pharmacol.* 136, 136–149. doi: 10.1016/j.bcp.2017.04.014

Ferré, P., and Foufelle, F. (2010). Hepatic steatosis: a role for de novo lipogenesis and the transcription factor SREBP-1c. *Diabetes Obes. Metab.* 12, 83–92. doi: 10.1111/j.1463-1326.2010.01275.x

Fischer, M., You, M., Matsumoto, M., and Crabb, D. W. (2003). Peroxisome proliferator-activated receptor alpha (PPARalpha) agonist treatment reverses PPARalpha dysfunction and abnormalities in hepatic lipid metabolism in ethanol-fed mice. *J. Biol. Chem.* 278, 27997–28004. doi: 10.1074/jbc.M302140200

Fortin, É., Blouin, R., Lapointe, J., Petit, H. V., and Palin, M. F. (2017). Linoleic acid, α-linolenic acid and enterolactone affect lipid oxidation and expression of lipid metabolism and antioxidant-related genes in hepatic tissue of dairy cows. *Br. J. Nutr.* 117, 1199–1211. doi: 10.1017/S0007114517000976

Foster, F. M., Traer, C. J., Abraham, S. M., and Fry, M. J. (2003). The phosphoinositide (PI) 3-kinase family. *J. Cell Sci.* 116, 3037–3040. doi: 10.1242/jcs.00609

French, S. W. (2013). The importance of CYP2E1 in the pathogenesis of alcoholic liver disease and drug toxicity and the role of the proteasome. *Subcell. Biochem.* 67, 145–164. doi: 10.1007/978-94-007-5881-0_4

Friedman, S. L., Neuschwander-Tetri, B. A., Rinella, M., and Sanyal, A. J. (2018). Mechanisms of NAFLD development and therapeutic strategies. *Nat. Med.* 24, 908–922. doi: 10.1038/s41591-018-0104-9

Fu, R., Zhou, J., Wang, R., Sun, R., Feng, D., Wang, Z., et al. (2019). Protocatechuic acid-mediated miR-219a-5p activation inhibits the p66shc oxidant pathway to alleviate alcoholic liver injury. *Oxid. Med. Cell Longev.* 2019:3527809. doi: 10.1155/2019/3527809

Gai, Z., Visentin, M., Gui, T., Zhao, L., Thasler, W. E., Häusler, S., et al. (2018). Effects of farnesoid X receptor activation on arachidonic acid metabolism, NF-kB signaling, and hepatic inflammation. *Mol. Pharmacol.* 94, 802–811. doi: 10.1124/mol.117.111047

Gao, X., Nan, Y., Zhao, Y., Yuan, Y., Ren, B., Sun, C., et al. (2017). Atorvastatin reduces lipid accumulation in the liver by activating protein kinase A-mediated phosphorylation of perilipin 5. *Biochim. Biophys. Acta Mol. Cell Biol. Lipids* 1862, 1512–1519. doi: 10.1016/j.bbalip.2017.09.007

Ge, M., Yao, W., Yuan, D., Zhou, S., Chen, X., Zhang, Y., et al. (2017). Brg1-mediated Nrf2/HO-1 pathway activation alleviates hepatic ischemia-reperfusion injury. *Cell Death Dis.* 8:e2841. doi: 10.1038/cddis.2017.236

Giorgio, M., Migliaccio, E., Orsini, F., Paolucci, D., Moroni, M., Contursi, C., et al. (2005). Electron transfer between cytochrome c and p66Shc generates reactive oxygen species that trigger mitochondrial apoptosis. *Cell* 122, 221–233. doi: 10.1016/j.cell.2005.05.011

Go, G. W. (2015). Low-density lipoprotein receptor-related protein 6 (LRP6) is a novel nutritional therapeutic target for hyperlipidemia, non-alcoholic fatty liver disease, and atherosclerosis. *Nutrients* 7, 4453–4464. doi: 10.3390/nu7064453

Grander, C., Adolph, T. E., Wieser, V., Lowe, P., Wrzosek, L., Gyongyosi, B., et al. (2018). Recovery of ethanol-induced Akkermansia muciniphila depletion ameliorates alcoholic liver disease. *Gut* 67, 891–901. doi: 10.1136/gutjnl-2016-313432

Gutiérrez-Juárez, R., Pocai, A., Mulas, C., Ono, H., Bhanot, S., Monia, B. P., et al. (2017). Critical role of stearoyl-CoA desaturase-1 (SCD1) in the onset of diet-induced hepatic insulin resistance. *J. Clin. Invest.* 116, 1686–1695. doi: 10.1172/JCI26991

Gyamfi, M. A., and Wan, Y. J. (2010). Pathogenesis of alcoholic liver disease: the role of nuclear receptors. *Exp. Biol. Med.* 235, 547–560. doi: 10.1258/ebm.2009.009249

Han, C. Y., Rho, H. S., Kim, A., Kim, T. H., Jang, K., Jun, D. W., et al. (2018). FXR inhibits endoplasmic reticulum stress-induced nlrp3 inflammasome in hepatocytes and ameliorates liver injury. *Cell Rep.* 24, 2985–2999. doi: 10.1016/j.celrep.2018.07.068

Han, Y. M., Lee, Y. J., Jang, Y. N., Kim, H. M., Seo, H. S., Jung, T. W., et al. (2020). Aspirin improves nonalcoholic fatty liver disease and atherosclerosis through regulation of the PPARδ-AMPK-PGC-1α pathway in dyslipidemic conditions. *Biomed. Res. Int.* 2020:7806860. doi: 10.1155/2020/7806860

Haneklaus, M., and O'Neill, L. A. (2015). NLRP3 at the interface of metabolism and inflammation. *Immunol. Rev.* 265, 53–62. doi: 10.1111/imr.12285

Hao, T., Chen, H., Wu, S., and Tian, H. (2019). LRG ameliorates steatohepatitis by activating the AMPK/mTOR/SREBP1 signaling pathway in C57BL/6J mice fed a high-fat diet. *Mol. Med. Rep.* 20, 701–708. doi: 10.3892/mmr.2019.10304

Hardy, T., and Mann, D. A. (2016). Epigenetics in liver disease: from biology to therapeutics. *Gut* 65,1895–1905. doi: 10.1136/gutjnl-2015-311292

He, Q., Sha, S., Sun, L., Zhang, J., and Dong, M. (2016). GLP-1 analogue improves hepatic lipid accumulation by inducing autophagy via AMPK/mTOR pathway. *Biochem. Biophys. Res. Commun.* 476, 196–203. doi: 10.1016/j.bbrc.2016.05.086

Henao-Mejia, J., Elinav, E., Jin, C., Hao, L., Mehal, W. Z., Strowig, T., et al. (2012). Inflammasome-mediated dysbiosis regulates progression of NAFLD and obesity. *Nature* 482, 179–185. doi: 10.1038/nature10809

Hiebl, V., Ladurner, A., Latkolik, S., and Dirsch, V. M. (2018). Natural products as modulators of the nuclear receptors and metabolic sensors LXR, FXR and RXR. *Biotechnol. Adv.* 36, 1657–1698. doi: 10.1016/j.biotechadv.2018.03.003

Huang, C., Shiu, S. M., Wu, M., Chen, W., Wang, S., and Lee, H. (2013). Monacolin K affects lipid metabolism through SIRT1/AMPK pathway in HepG2 cells. *Arch. Pharm. Res.* 36, 1541–1551. doi: 10.1007/s12272-013-0150-2

Huang, D., Li, T., Li, X., Zhang, L., Sun, L., He, X., et al. (2014). HIF-1-mediated suppression of acyl-CoA dehydrogenases and fatty acid oxidation is critical for cancer progression. *Cell Rep.* 8, 1930–1942. doi: 10.1016/j.celrep.2014.08.028

Huang, M., Kong, B., Zhang, M., Rizzolo, D., Armstrong, L. E., Schumacher, J. D., et al. (2020). Enhanced alcoholic liver disease in mice with intestine-specific farnesoid X receptor deficiency. *Lab. Invest.* 100, 1158–1168. doi: 10.1038/s41374-020-0439-y

Huang, R., Hu, W., Hou, S., Zhao, H., Wang, X., and Chen, G. (2020). The chemical constituents of *Gentiana macrophylla* pall. under acidic condition using gentiopicroside-rich secoiridoids extract. *Phytochemistry Lett.* 39, 30–34. doi: 10.1016/j.phytol.2020.07.004

Hughes, M. M., and O'Neill, L. A. J. (2018). Metabolic regulation of NLRP3. *Immunol. Rev.* 281, 88–98. doi: 10.1111/imr.12608

Ishikawa, H., and Barber, G. N. (2008). STING is an endoplasmic reticulum adaptor that facilitates innate immune signalling. *Nature* 455, 674–678. doi: 10.1038/nature07317

Jain, A., Lamark, T., Sjøttem, E., Larsen, K. B., Awuh, J. A., Øvervatn, A., et al. (2010). p62/SQSTM1 is a target gene for transcription factor NRF2 and creates a positive feedback loop by inducing antioxidant response element-driven gene transcription. *J. Biol. Chem.* 285, 22576–22591. doi: 10.1074/jbc.M110.118976

Jiang, B., Le, L., Pan, H., Hu, K., Xu, L., and Xiao, P. (2014). Dihydromyricetin ameliorates the oxidative stress response induced by methylglyoxal via the AMPK/GLUT4 signaling pathway in PC12 cells. *Brain Res. Bull.* 109, 117–126. doi: 10.1016/j.brainresbull.2014.10.010

Jiang, H., He, H., Chen, Y., Huang, W., Cheng, J., and Ye, J. (2017). Identification of a selective and direct NLRP3 inhibitor to treat inflammatory disorders. *J. Exp. Med.* 214, 3219–3238. doi: 10.1084/jem.20171419

Jiang, L., Zhang, S., Li, C., Tang, J., Che, F., and Lu, Y. (2017). Roles of the Nrf2/HO-1 pathway in the anti-oxidative stress response to ischemia-reperfusion brain injury in rats. *Eur. Rev. Med. Pharmacol. Sci.* 21, 1532–1540.

Jin, R., Krasinskas, A., Le, N. A., Konomi, J. V., Holzberg, J., and Romero, R. (2018). Association between plasminogen activator inhibitor-1 and severity of liver injury and cardiovascular risk in children with non-alcoholic fatty liver disease. *Pediatr. Obes.* 13, 23–29. doi: 10.1111/ijpo.12183

Johnston, M. P., Patel, J., and Byrne, C. D. (2020). Causes of mortality in non-alcoholic fatty liver disease (NAFLD) and alcohol related fatty liver disease (AFLD). *Curr. Pharm. Des.* 26, 1079–1092. doi: 10.2174/1381612826666200128094231

Jung, T. W., Kim, H. C., Abd El-Aty, A. M., and Jeong, J. H. (2018). Maresin 1 attenuates NAFLD by suppression of endoplasmic reticulum stress via AMPK-SERCA2b pathway. *J. Biol. Chem.* 293, 3981–3988. doi: 10.1074/jbc.RA117.000885

Kanda, T., Goto, T., Hirotsu, Y., Masuzaki, R., Moriyama, M., and Omata, M. (2020). Molecular mechanisms: connections between nonalcoholic fatty liver disease, steatohepatitis and hepatocellular carcinoma. *Int. J. Mol. Sci.* 21:1525. doi: 10.3390/ijms21041525

Kato, H., Sakaki, K., and Mihara, K. (2006). Ubiquitin-proteasome-dependent degradation of mammalian ER stearoyl-CoA desaturase. *J. Cell Sci.* 119, 2342–2353. doi: 10.1242/jcs.02951

Katz, H. R. (2007). Inhibition of pathologic inflammation by leukocyte Ig-like receptor B4 and related inhibitory receptors. *Immunol. Rev.* 217, 222–230. doi: 10.1111/j.1600-065X.2007.00522.x

Kay, H. Y., Kim, W. D., Hwang, S. J., Choi, H. S., Gilroy, R. K., Wan, Y. J., et al. (2011). Nrf2 inhibits LXRα-dependent hepatic lipogenesis by competing with FXR for acetylase binding. *Antioxid. Redox Signal.* 15, 2135–2146. doi: 10.1089/ars.2010.3834

Kohjima, M., Higuchi, N., Kato, M., Kotoh, K., Yoshimoto, T., and Fujino, T. (2008). SREBP-1c, regulated by the insulin and AMPK signaling pathways, plays a role in nonalcoholic fatty liver disease. *Int. J. Mol. Med.* 21, 507–511. doi: 10.3892/ijmm.21.4.507

Kraus, W. L., and Hottiger, M. O. (2013). PARP-1 and gene regulation: progress and puzzles. *Mol. Aspects Med.* 34, 1109–1123. doi: 10.1016/j.mam.2013.01.005

Lackner, C., Spindelboeck, W., Haybaeck, J., Douschan, P., Rainer, F., and Terracciano, L. (2016). Histological parameters and alcohol abstinence determine long-term prognosis in patients with alcoholic liver disease. *J. Hepatol.* 66, 610–618. doi: 10.1016/j.jhep.2016.11.011

Lee, C. (2017). Collaborative power of Nrf2 and PPARγ activators against metabolic and drug-induced oxidative injury. *Oxid. Med. Cell. Longev.* 2017:1378175. doi: 10.1155/2017/1378175

Lee, N. Y., Yoon, S. J., Han, D. H., Gupta, H., Youn, G. S., and Shin, M. J. (2020). Lactobacillus and Pediococcus ameliorate progression of non-alcoholic fatty liver disease through modulation of the gut microbiome. *Gut Microbes* 11, 882–899. doi: 10.1080/19490976.2020.1712984

Li, D., Cui, Y., Wang, X., Liu, F., and Li, X. (2021). Apple polyphenol extract alleviates lipid accumulation in free-fatty-acid-exposed HepG2 cells via activating autophagy mediated by SIRT1/AMPK signaling. *Phytother. Res.* 35, 1416–1431. doi: 10.1002/ptr.6902

Li, S., Tan, H., Wang, N., Zhang, Z., Lao, L., Wong, C. W., et al. (2015). The role of oxidative stress and antioxidants in liver diseases. *Int. J. Mol. Sci.* 16, 26087–26124. doi: 10.3390/ijms161125942

Li, X., Monks, B., Ge, Q., and Birnbaum, M. J. (2007). Akt/PKB regulates hepatic metabolism by directly inhibiting PGC-1alpha transcription coactivator. *Nature* 447, 1012–1016. doi: 10.1038/nature05861

Liao, X., Song, L., Zhang, L., Wang, H., Tong, Q., Xu, J., et al. (2018). LAMP3 regulates hepatic lipid metabolism through activating PI3K/Akt pathway. *Mol. Cell. Endocrinol.* 470, 160–167. doi: 10.1016/j.mce.2017.10.010

Liou, C. J., Wei, C. H., Chen, Y. L., Cheng, C. Y., Wang, C. L., and Huang, W. C. (2018). Fisetin protects against hepatic steatosis through regulation of the Sirt1/AMPK and fatty acid β-oxidation signaling pathway in high-fat diet-induced obese mice. *Cell. Physiol. Biochem.* 49, 1870–1884. doi: 10.1159/000493650

Liu, X., Wang, Y., Wu, D., Li, S., Wang, C., and Han, Z. (2019). Magnolol prevents acute alcoholic liver damage by activating PI3K/Nrf2/PPARγ and inhibiting NLRP3 signaling pathway. *Front. Pharmacol.* 10:1459. doi: 10.3389/fphar.2019.01459

Liu, Y., Han, X., Bian, Z., Peng, Y., You, Z., and Wang, Q. (2012). Activation of liver X receptors attenuates endotoxin-induced liver injury in mice with nonalcoholic fatty liver disease. *Dig. Dis. Sci.* 57, 390–398. doi: 10.1007/s10620-011-1902-9

Loomba, R., Friedman, S. L., and Shulman, G. I. (2021). Mechanisms and disease consequences of nonalcoholic fatty liver disease. *Cell* 184, 2537–2564. doi: 10.1016/j.cell.2021.04.015

Lu, Y., Jiang, Z., Dai, H., Miao, R., Shu, J., and Gu, H. (2018). Hepatic leukocyte immunoglobulin-like receptor B4 (LILRB4) attenuates nonalcoholic fatty liver disease via SHP1-TRAF6 pathway. *Hepatology* 67, 1303–1319. doi: 10.1002/hep.29633

Luo, C., Sun, H., Peng, J., Gao, C., Bao, L., Ji, R., et al. (2021). Rosmarinic acid exerts an antagonistic effect on nonalcoholic fatty liver disease by regulating the YAP1/TAZ-PPARγ/PGC-1α signaling pathway. *Phytother. Res.* 35, 1010–1022. doi: 10.1002/ptr.6865

Makariou, S. E., Elisaf, M., Challa, A., Tentolouris, N., and Liberopoulos, E. N. (2017). No effect of vitamin D supplementation on cardiovascular risk factors in subjects with metabolic syndrome: a pilot randomised study. *Arch. Med. Sci. Atheroscler. Dis.* 2, e52–e60. doi: 10.5114/amsad.2017.70504

Matsuda, S., Kobayashi, M., and Kitagishi, Y. (2013). Roles for PI3K/AKT/PTEN pathway in cell signaling of nonalcoholic fatty liver disease. *ISRN Endocrinol.* 2013:472432. doi: 10.1155/2013/472432

McIlvride, S., Nikolova, V., Fan, H. M., McDonald, J. A. K., Wahlström, A., Bellafante, E., et al. (2019). Obeticholic acid ameliorates dyslipidemia but not glucose tolerance in mouse model of gestational diabetes. *Am. J. Physiol. Endocrinol. Metab.* 317, E399–E410. doi: 10.1152/ajpendo.00407.2018

Meng, Q., Feng, Z., Zhang, X., Hu, L., Wang, M., Zhang, H., et al. (2019). PPAR-γ activation exerts an anti-inflammatory effect by suppressing the NLRP3 inflammasome in spinal cord-derived neurons. *Mediators Inflamm.* 2019:6386729. doi: 10.1155/2019/6386729

Mirhafez, S. R., Rezai, A., Dehabeh, M., Nobakht, M., Gh,. B. F., Bidkhori, M., Sahebkar, A., et al. (2021). Efficacy of phytosomal curcumin among patients with non-alcoholic fatty liver disease. *Int. J. Vitam. Nutr. Res.* 91, 278–286. doi: 10.1024/0300-9831/a000629

Mitrovic, B., Gluvic, Z., Macut, D., Obradovic, M., Sudar-Milovanovic, E., Soskic, S., et al. (2021). Effects of metformin-single therapy on the level of inflammatory markers in serum of non-obese T2DM patients with NAFLD. *Endocr. Metab. Immune Disord. Drug Targets.* doi: 10.2174/1871530321666210225110140. [Epub ahead of print].

Muñoz-Garach, A., Cornejo-Pareja, I., and Tinahones, F. J. (2016). Does metabolically healthy obesity exist? *Nutrients* 8:320. doi: 10.3390/nu8060320

Nakajima, T., Kamijo, Y., Tanaka, N., Sugiyama, E., Tanaka, E., and Kiyosawa, K. (2004). Peroxisome proliferator-activated receptor alpha protects against alcohol-induced liver damage. *Hepatology* 40, 972–980. doi: 10.1002/hep.20399

Newsome, P. N., Buchholtz, K., Cusi, K., Linder, M., Okanoue, T., Ratziu, V., et al. (2021). A placebo-controlled trial of subcutaneous semaglutide in nonalcoholic steatohepatitis. *N. Engl. J. Med.* 384, 1113–1124. doi: 10.1056/NEJMoa2028395

Ntambi, J. M., Miyazaki, M., Stoehr, J. P., Lan, H., Kendziorski, C. M., Yandell, B. S., et al. (2002). Loss of stearoyl-CoA desaturase-1 function protects mice against adiposity. Proc. *Natl. Acad. Sci. U.S.A.* 99, 11482–11486. doi: 10.1073/pnas.132384699

Ozols, J. (1997). Degradation of hepatic stearyl CoA delta 9-desaturase. *Mol. Biol. Cell* 8, 2281–2290. doi: 10.1091/mbc.8.11.2281

Palian, B. M., Rohira, A. D., Johnson, S. A., He, L., Zheng, N., Dubeau, L., et al. (2014). Mafl is a novel target of PTEN and PI3K signaling that negatively regulates oncogenesis and lipid metabolism. *PLoS Genet.* 10:e1004789. doi: 10.1371/journal.pgen.1004789

Pan, Y., Wang, N., Xia, P., Wang, E., Guo, Q., and Ye, Z. (2018). Inhibition of Rac1 ameliorates neuronal oxidative stress damage via reducing Bcl-2/Rac1 complex formation in mitochondria through PI3K/Akt/mTOR pathway. *Exp. Neurol.* 300,149–166. doi: 10.1016/j.expneurol.2017.10.030

Panda, S., and Kar, A. (2007). Apigenin (4',5,7-trihydroxyflavone) regulates hyperglycaemia, thyroid dysfunction and lipid peroxidation in alloxan-induced diabetic mice. *J. Pharm. Pharmacol.* 59, 1543–1548. doi: 10.1211/jpp.59.11.0012

Pár, A., and Pár, G. (2019). Alcoholic liver disease: the roles of genetic-epigenetic factors and the effect of abstinence. *Orvosi. Hetilap.* 160, 524–532. doi: 10.1556/650.2019.31352

Park, E. J., Kim, Y. M., Kim, H. J., Jang, S. Y., Oh, M. H., Lee, D. H., et al. (2016). (S)YS-51, a novel isoquinoline alkaloid, attenuates obesity-associated non-alcoholic fatty liver disease in mice by suppressing lipogenesis, inflammation and coagulation. *Eur. J. Pharmacol.* 788, 200–209. doi: 10.1016/j.ejphar.2016.06.040

Peterson, T. R., Sengupta, S. S., Harris, T. E., Carmack, A. E., Kang, S. A., and Balderas, E. (2011). mTOR complex 1 regulates lipin 1 localization to control the SREBP pathway. *Cell* 146, 408–420. doi: 10.1016/j.cell.2011.06.034

Petrasek, J., Iracheta-Vellve, A., Csak, T., Satishchandran, A., Kodys, K., Kurt-Jones, E. A., et al. (2013). STING-IRF3 pathway links endoplasmic reticulum stress with hepatocyte apoptosis in early alcoholic liver disease. *Proc. Natl. Acad. Sci. U.S.A.* 110, 16544–16549. doi: 10.1073/pnas.1308331110

Petroni, M. L., Brodosi, L., Marchignoli, F., Musio, A., and Marchesini, G. (2019). Moderate alcohol intake in non-alcoholic fatty liver disease: to drink or not to drink? *Nutrients* 11:3048. doi: 10.3390/nu11123048

Porcu, C., Sideri, S., Martini, M., Cocomazzi, A., Galli, A., Tarantino, G., et al. (2018). Oleuropein induces AMPK-dependent autophagy in NAFLD mice, regardless of the gender. *Int. J. Mol. Sci.* 19:3948. doi: 10.3390/ijms19123948

Qiu, P., Dong, Y., Li, B., Kang, X., Gu, C., Zhu, T., et al. (2017). Dihydromyricetin modulates p62 and autophagy crosstalk with the Keap-1/Nrf2 pathway to alleviate ethanol-induced hepatic injury. *Toxicol. Lett.* 274, 31–41. doi: 10.1016/j.toxlet.2017.04.009

Quan, H. Y., Kim, D. Y., Kim, S. J., Jo, H. K., Kim, G. W., and Chung, S. H. (2013). Betulinic acid alleviates non-alcoholic fatty liver by inhibiting SREBP1 activity via the AMPK-mTOR-SREBP signaling pathway. *Biochem. Pharmacol.* 85, 1330–1340. doi: 10.1016/j.bcp.2013.02.007

Reddy, R. C., and Standiford, T. J. (2010). Nrf2 and PPAR{gamma}: PPARtnering against oxidant-induced lung injury. *Am. J. Respir. Crit. Care Med.* 182,

134–135. doi: 10.1164/rccm.201004-0457ED

Rehm, J., Samokhvalov, A. V., and Shield, K. D. (2013). Global burden of alcoholic liver diseases. *J. Hepatol.* 59, 160–168. doi: 10.1016/j.jhep.2013.03.007

Sampath, H., and Ntambi, J. M. (2014). Role of stearoyl-CoA desaturase-1 in skin integrity and whole body energy balance. *J. Biol. Chem.* 89, 2482–2488. doi: 10.1074/jbc.R113.516716

Saravanan, S., Islam, V. I., Thirugnanasambantham, K., Pazhanivel, N., Raghuraman, N., and Paulraj, M. G. (2014). Swertiamarin ameliorates inflammation and osteoclastogenesis intermediates in IL-1β induced rat fibroblast-like synoviocytes. *Inflamm. Res.* 63, 451–462. doi: 10.1007/s00011-014-0717-5

Sarin, S. K., Kumar, M., Eslam, M., George, J., Mahtab, M. A., Akbar, S. M. F., et al. (2020). Liver diseases in the asia-pacific region: a lancet gastroenterology & hepatology commission. *Lancet Gastroenterol. Hepatol.* 5, 167–228. doi: 10.1016/S2468-1253(19)30342-5

Schwimmer, J. B. (2007). Definitive diagnosis and assessment of risk for nonalcoholic fatty liver disease in children and adolescents. *Semin. Liver Dis.* 27, 312–318. doi: 10.1055/s-2007-985075

Sharifi, N., and Amani, R. (2019). Vitamin D supplementation and non-alcoholic fatty liver disease: a critical and systematic review of clinical trials. *Crit. Rev. Food Sci. Nutr.* 59, 693–703. doi: 10.1080/10408398.2017.1389693

Shellito, J. E., Zheng, M. Q., Ye, P., Ruan, S., Shean, M. K., and Kolls, J. (2001). Effect of alcohol consumption on host release of interleukin-17 during pulmonary infection with *Klebsiella pneumoniae. Alcohol. Clin. Exp. Res.* 25, 872–881. doi: 10.1111/j.1530-0277.2001.tb02293.x

Shen, Y., Lindemeyer, A. K., Gonzalez, C., Shao, X. M., Spigelman, I., Olsen, R. W., et al. (2012). Dihydromyricetin as a novel anti-alcohol intoxication medication. *J. Neurosci.* 32, 390–401. doi: 10.1523/JNEUROSCI.4639-11.2012

Shi, L., Zhang, T., Liang, X., Hu, Q., Huang, J., Zhou, Y., et al. (2015). Dihydromyricetin improves skeletal muscle insulin resistance by inducing autophagy via the AMPK signaling pathway. *Mol. Cell. Endocrinol.* 409, 92–102. doi: 10.1016/j.mce.2015.03.009

Tarantino, G., and Balsano, C. (2020). Gastrointestinal peptides and nonalcoholic fatty liver disease. *Curr. Opin. Endocrinol. Diabetes Obes.* 27, 11–15. doi: 10.1097/MED.0000000000000514

Tarantino, G., Citro, V., and Capone, D. (2019). Nonalcoholic fatty liver disease: a challenge from mechanisms to therapy. *J. Clin. Med.* 9, 15. doi: 10.3390/jcm9010015

Tilg, H., and Mathurin, P. (2016). Altered intestinal microbiota as a major driving force in alcoholic steatohepatitis. *Gut* 65, 728–729. doi: 10.1136/gutjnl-2015-311014

Tong, X., and Pelling, J. C. (2013). Targeting the PI3K/Akt/mTOR axis by apigenin for cancer prevention. *Anticancer Agents Med. Chem.* 13, 971–978. doi: 10.2174/18715206113139990119

Traussnigg, S., Halilbasic, E., Hofer, H., Munda, P., Stojakovic, T., Fauler, G., et al. (2021). Open-label phase II study evaluating safety and efficacy of the non-steroidal farnesoid X receptor agonist PX-104 in non-alcoholic fatty liver disease. *Wien. Klin. Wochenschr.* 133, 441–451. doi: 10.1007/s00508-020-01735-5

Um, M. Y., Hwang, K. H., Ahn, J., and Ha, T. Y. (2013). Curcumin attenuates diet-induced hepatic steatosis by activating AMP-activated protein kinase. *Basic Clin. Pharmacol. Toxicol.* 113, 152–157. doi: 10.1111/bcpt.12076

Wang, L., Zhang, B., Huang, F., Liu, B., and Xie, Y. (2016). Curcumin inhibits lipolysis via suppression of ER stress in adipose tissue and prevents hepatic insulin resistance. *J. Lipid. Res.* 57, 1243–1255. doi: 10.1194/jlr.M067397

Wang, S., Shi, X., Feng, M., Wang, X., Zhang, Z., Zhao, X., et al. (2016). Puerarin protects against CCl4-induced liver fibrosis in mice: possible role of PARP-1 inhibition. *Int. Immunopharmacol.* 38, 238–245. doi: 10.1016/j.intimp.2016.06.008

Wang, S., Yang, F., Shang, L., Zhang, Y., Zhou, Y., and Shi, X. (2019). Puerarin protects against high-fat high-sucrose diet-induced non-alcoholic fatty liver disease by modulating PARP-1/PI3K/AKT signaling pathway and facilitating mitochondrial homeostasis. *Phytother. Res.* 33, 2347–2359. doi: 10.1002/ptr.6417

Wang, X., Zheng, Z., Caviglia, J. M., Corey, K. E., Herfel, T. M., Cai, B., et al. (2016). Hepatocyte TAZ/WWTR1 promotes inflammation and fibrosis in nonalcoholic steatohepatitis. *Cell Metab.* 24, 848–862. doi: 10.1016/j.cmet.2016.09.016

Wang, Z., Li, B., Jiang, H., Ma, Y., Bao, Y., Zhu, X., et al. (2021). IL-8 exacerbates alcohol-induced fatty liver disease via the Akt/HIF-1α pathway in human IL-8-expressing mice. *Cytokine* 138, 155402. doi: 10.1016/j.cyto.2020.155402

Wilding, J. P. H., Batterham, R. L., Calanna, S., Davies, M., Van Gaal, L. F., Lingvay, I., et al. (2021). STEP 1 study group. once-weekly semaglutide in adults with overweight or obesity. *N. Engl. J. Med.* 384:989. doi: 10.1056/NEJMoa2032183

Xiao, J., Liu, Y., Xing, F., Leung, T. M., Liong, E. C., and Tipoe, G. L. (2016). Bee's honey attenuates non-alcoholic steatohepatitis-induced hepatic injury through the regulation of thioredoxin-interacting protein-NLRP3 inflammasome pathway. *Eur. J. Nutr.* 55, 1465–1477. doi: 10.1007/s00394-015-0964-4

Xiao, J., Wang, F., Wong, N., He, J., Zhang, R., and Sun, R. (2019). Global liver disease burdens and research trends: analysis from a Chinese perspective. *J. Hepatol.* 71, 212–221. doi: 10.1016/j.jhep.2019.03.004

Xie, K., He, X., Chen, K., Sakao, K., and Hou, D. (2020). Ameliorative effects and molecular mechanisms of vine tea on western diet-induced NAFLD. *Food Funct.* 11, 5976–5991. doi: 10.1039/D0FO00795A

Xu, M., Zhou, Z., Parker, R., and Gao, B. (2017). Targeting inflammation for the treatment of alcoholic liver disease. *Pharmacol. Ther.* 180, 77–89. doi: 10.1016/j.pharmthera.2017.06.007

Xu, Y., Chen, D., Lin, X., Zhao, Q., Guo, J., Chen, L., et al. (2019). The LRP6 functional mutation rs2302685 contributes to individual susceptibility to alcoholic liver injury related to the Wnt/β-catenin-TCF1-CYP2E1 signaling pathway. *Arch. Toxicol.* 93, 1679–1695. doi: 10.1007/s00204-019-02447-0

Yan, C., Tian, X., Li, J., Liu, D., Ye, D., Xie, Z., et al. (2021). A high-fat diet attenuates AMPK α1 in adipocytes to induce exosome shedding and nonalcoholic fatty liver development *in vivo. Diabetes* 70, 577–588. doi: 10.2337/db20-0146

Yan, C., Zhang, Y., Zhang, X., Aa, J., Wang, G., and Xie, Y. (2018). Curcumin regulates endogenous and exogenous metabolism via Nrf2-FXR-LXR pathway in NAFLD mice. *Biomed. Pharmacother.* 105, 274–281. doi: 10.1016/j.biopha.2018.05.135

Yang, J., Mowry, L. E., Nejak-Bowen, K. N., Okabe, H., Diegel, C. R., Lang, R. A., et al. (2014). β-catenin signaling in murine liver zonation and regeneration: a Wnt-Wnt situation! *Hepatology* 60, 964–976. doi: 10.1002/hep.27082

Yang, X., Sheng, S., Du, X., Su, W., Tian, J., and Zhao, X. (2021). Hepatocyte-specific TAZ deletion downregulates p62/Sqstml expression in nonalcoholic steatohepatitis. *Biochem. Biophys. Res. Commun.* 535, 60–65. doi: 10.1016/j.bbrc.2020.12.038

You, M., Jogasuria, A., Lee, K., Wu, J., Zhang, Y., Lee, Y. K., Sadana, P., et al. (2017). Signal transduction mechanisms of alcoholic fatty liver disease:emer ging role of lipin-1. *Curr. Mol. Pharmacol.* 10, 226–236. doi: 10.2174/1874467208666150817112109

You, M., Matsumoto, M., Pacold, C. M., Cho, W. K., and Crabb, D. W. (2004). The role of AMP-activated protein kinase in the action of ethanol in the liver. *Gastroenterology* 127, 1798–1808. doi: 10.1053/j.gastro.2004.09.049

You, M., and Rogers, C. Q. (2009). Adiponectin: a key adipokine in alcoholic fatty liver. *Exp. Biol. Med.* 234, 850–859. doi: 10.3181/0902-MR-61

Younossi, Z., Anstee, Q. M., Marietti, M., Hardy, T., Henry, L., Eslam, M., et al. (2018). Global burden of NAFLD and NASH: trends, predictions, risk factors and prevention. *Nat. Rev. Gastroenterol. Hepatol.* 15, 11–20. doi: 10.1038/nrgastro.2017.109

Younossi, Z., and Henry, L. (2016). Contribution of alcoholic and nonalcoholic fatty liver disease to the burden of liver-related morbidity and mortality. *Gastroenterology* 150, 1778–1785. doi: 10.1053/j.gastro.2016.03.005

Younossi, Z., Tacke, F., Arrese, M., Chander Sharma, B., Mostafa, I., and Bugianesi, E. (2019). Global perspectives on nonalcoholic fatty liver disease and nonalcoholic steatohepatitis. *Hepatology* 69, 2672–2682. doi: 10.1002/hep.30251

Zeng, L., Tang, W., Yin, J., Feng, L., Li, Y., Yao, X., et al. (2016). Alisol A 24-acetate prevents hepatic steatosis and metabolic disorders in HepG2 cells. *Cell. Physiol. Biochem.* 40, 453–464. doi: 10.1159/000452560

Zhan, Z., Wu, M., Shang, Y., Jiang, M., Liu, J., Qiao, C., et al. (2021). Taxifolin ameliorate high-fat-diet feeding plus acute ethanol binge-induced steatohepatitis through inhibiting inflammatory caspase-1-dependent pyroptosis. *Food Funct.* 12, 362–372. doi: 10.1039/D0FO02653K

Zhang, P., Meng, X., Li, D., Calderone, R., Mao, D., and Sui, B. (2018). Commensal homeostasis of gut microbiota-host for the impact of obesity. *Front. Physiol.* 8:1122. doi: 10.3389/fphys.2017.01122

Zhang, S., Zheng, L., Dong, D., Xu, L., Yin, L., Qi, Y., et al. (2013). Effects of flavonoids from Rosa laevigata Michx fruit against high-fat diet-induced non-alcoholic fatty liver disease in rats. *Food Chem.* 141, 2108–2116. doi: 10.1016/j.foodchem.2013.05.019

Zhang, X., Ji, X., Wang, Q., and Li, J. (2018). New insight into inter-organ crosstalk contributing to the pathogenesis of non-alcoholic fatty liver disease (NAFLD). *Protein Cell* 9, 164–177. doi: 10.1007/s13238-017-0436-0

Zhang, Z., Mocanu, V., Cai, C., Dang, J., Slater, L., Deehan, E. C., et al. (2019). Impact of fecal microbiota transplantation on obesity and metabolic syndrome-a systematic review. *Nutrients* 11:2291. doi: 10.3390/nu11 102291

Zhao, L., Ye, J., Wu, G., Peng, X., Xia, P., and Ren, Y. (2015). Gentiopicroside prevents interleukin-1 beta induced inflammation response in rat articular chondrocyte. *J. Ethnopharmacol.* 172, 100–107. doi: 10.1016/j.jep.2015.06.031

Zhao, X., Gong, L., Wang, C., Liu, M., Hu, N., Dai, X., et al. (2021). Quercetin mitigates ethanol-induced hepatic steatosis in zebrafish via P2X7R-mediated PI3K/Keap1/Nrf2 signaling pathway. *J. Ethnopharmacol.* 268:113569. doi: 10.1016/j.jep.2020.113569

Zhong, F., Hu, Z., Jiang, K., Lei, B., Wu, Z., Yuan, G., et al. (2019). Complement C3 activation regulates the production of tRNA-derived fragments Gly-tRFs and promotes alcohol-induced liver injury and steatosis. *Cell Res.* 29, 548–561. doi: 10.1038/s41422-019-0175-2

Zhong, Q., Wu, Y., Xiong, F., Liu, M., Liu, Y., Wang, C., et al. (2021). Higher flavonoid intake is associated with a lower progression risk of non-alcoholic fatty liver disease in adults: a prospective study. *Br. J. Nutr.* 125, 460–470. doi: 10.1017/S0007114520002846

Zhou, G., Myers, R., Li, Y., Chen, Y., Shen, X., and Fenyk-Melody, J. (2001). Role of AMP-activated protein kinase in mechanism of metformin action. *J. Clin. Invest.* 108, 1167–1174. doi: 10.1172/JCI13505

Zhou, J., and Chng, W. J. (2013). Roles of thioredoxin binding protein (TXNIP) in oxidative stress, apoptosis and cancer. *Mitochondrion* 13, 163–169. doi: 10.1016/j.mito.2012.06.004

Zhuge, Q., Zhang, Y., Liu, B., and Wu, M. (2020). Blueberry polyphenols play a preventive effect on alcoholic fatty liver disease C57BL/6 J mice by promoting autophagy to accelerate lipolysis to eliminate excessive TG accumulation in hepatocytes. *Ann. Palliat. Med.* 9, 1045–1054. doi: 10.21037/apm.2020.03.38

11

Liver Metabolomics Reveals the Effect of *Lactobacillus reuteri* on Alcoholic Liver Disease

Tian-xiang Zheng[1†], Shi-lin Pu[1†], Peng Tan[2], Yi-chao Du[2], Bao-lin Qian[1], Hao Chen[1], Wen-guang Fu[1,2] and Mei-zhou Huang[2*]*

[1] Department of Hepatobiliary Surgery, The Affiliated Hospital of Southwest Medical University, Luzhou, China, [2] Academician (Expert) Workstation of Sichuan Province, The Affiliated Hospital of Southwest Medical University, Luzhou, China

Correspondence:
Wen-guang Fu
fuwg@swmu.edu.cn
Mei-zhou Huang
13141254071@163.com

[†] These authors have contributed equally to this work

Alcoholic liver disease (ALD), a type of chronic liver disease that is prevalent worldwide, is still identified to have a poor prognosis despite many medical treatment protocols. Thus, it is urgent to develop and test new treatment protocols for ALD. *Lactobacillus reuteri* (*L. reuteri*) has been widely used in the clinical treatment of digestive system diseases, but studies on the protective effect of *L. reuteri* on ALD are considered to be rare. Therefore, in the present study, we examined the effect of *L. reuteri* on ALD and provide data that are significant in the development of new treatment protocols for ALD. An ALD model has been established in C57BL/6J mice treated according to the Gao-binge modeling method. Mice in the treatment group were administered with *L. reuteri*˙ Hematoxylin and eosin (H&E) staining, oil red O staining, immunohistochemistry, and biochemical analyses were performed to detect the phenotypic changes in the liver among mice in the different treatment groups. *L. reuteri* treatment reversed inflammatory cell infiltration and lipid accumulation. Moreover, AST, ALT, TG, and TCH levels were also reduced in the probiotics-treatment group. Five candidate biomarkers were found in the liver metabolites of different treatment groups by UPLC/QTOF-MS and a multivariate analysis. Several fatty acid metabolic pathways such as linoleic acid metabolism and glycerolipid metabolism were involved. All these findings suggested that *L. reuteri* treatment reversed the phenotype of ethanol-induced hepatitis and metabolic disorders. These findings provide evidence that *L. reuteri* might serve as a new therapeutic strategy for ALD.

Keywords: alcoholic liver disease, alcoholic hepatitis, *Lactobacillus reuteri*, metabolomics analysis, fatty acid metabolism

INTRODUCTION

Alcoholic liver disease (ALD) has been identified as one of the most common liver diseases worldwide. According to the latest World Health Organization estimates, 3,000,000 alcohol-related deaths, were reported in 2016, which accounted for 5.1% of the global disease burden (World Health Organization, 2018). Alcohol can reportedly inhibit mitochondrial β-oxidation, increase fatty acid synthesis, and accumulate fatty acids in the liver, which results in the perturbation of lipid metabolism homeostasis. ALD is also underlying cause of many liver diseases, including alcoholic steatohepatitis (ASH) and hepatocellular carcinoma (HCC). ASH is an advanced stage of ALD, characterized by chronic liver injury, inflammation, and fibrosis and can ultimately progress to

HCC (Seitz et al., 2018). Corticosteroids and pentoxifylline (TNF-α inhibitor) are commonly used to treat ASH, but they fail to decrease the risk of 6-month mortality (Singh et al., 2015; Thursz et al., 2015). Therefore, the discovery of a new feasible approach for the treatment of ALD is urgently needed.

In recent years, the gut microbiome has attracted increased attention in the field of metabolic diseases. *Lactobacillus reuteri*, a type of probiotic, has been demonstrated to be beneficial in many diseases, including diarrhea and infant colic (Jimenez-Gutierrez et al., 2014; Chau et al., 2015). *L. reuteri* has been reported to inhibit Gram-negative bacteria by secreting reuterin, a well-known antimicrobial compound, and several other antimicrobial substances, such as reutericyclin, lactic acid, and acetic acid (Yang et al., 2015; Greifova et al., 2017). It has been demonstrated that *L. reuteri* can attenuate multi-organ inflammation while remodeling the gut microbiome of *foxp3*-mutant mice with gut microbial dysbiosis (He et al., 2017). Many studies on obesity, type 2 diabetes, and fatty liver disease have shown that *L. reuteri* treatment reversed insulin resistance, hepatic steatosis, and inflammation (Hsieh et al., 2013; Marie-Christine et al., 2015; Dahiya et al., 2017).

Alcoholic liver disease is also a type of metabolic disease. The commonly used methods of histological analysis and the detection of several biochemical biomarkers lack the comprehensive recognition of metabolic changes. Metabolomics analysis is an indispensable and readily used method that can detect changes in metabolism in response to various stimuli by analyzing alterations in endogenous small molecule metabolites (Noorbakhsh et al., 2019). Therefore, metabolomics analysis is determined to be superior in the detection of liver metabolites, guiding clinical diagnosis and determination of prognosis. Few studies have focused on the metabolic effect of *L. reuteri* on ALD. Thus, a metabolomics analysis was performed in this study. We also hypothesize that *L. reuteri* treatment can reverse the progression of ALD by ameliorating disorders of liver metabolism.

MATERIALS AND METHODS

Animals

Male C57BL/6 mice (8–10 weeks of age) were obtained from Chengdu Dashuo Biotechnological Company. A Lieber-DeCarli liquid ethanol diet and a control diet were purchased from TROPHIC Animal Feed High-tech Co., Ltd., China. Edible alcohol (95%) was purchased from Henan Xinheyang Alcohol Co., Ltd. *L. reuteri* DSM17938 was purchased from BioGaia. All mice were housed in a specific pathogen-free environment (temperature 23°C ± 2°C, humidity 55% ± 5%, and a 12-h light/dark cycle) with free access to water and the liquid ethanol diet or the control diet.

Eighteen male mice were randomly assigned to three groups. The control group was fed a control diet (TROPHIC Animal Feed High-tech Co., Ltd., Nantong, China); meanwhile, the model and probiotics-treatment groups were fed an ethanol diet (TROPHIC Animal Feed High-tech Co., Ltd., Nantong, China). Moreover, the model and probiotics-treatment groups were administered edible alcohol by oral gavage (0.25 g/ml ethanol, 5 g/kg of body weight) weekly. In addition, probiotics-treatment group was, respectively, treated with *L. reuteri* (2×10^7 CFU, daily). After 8 weeks, the mice were sacrificed by isoflurane inhalation (3–4%). Another group of five mice was treated by control diet and *L. reuteri* (2×10^7 CFU, daily) for 8 weeks to access the safety of *L. reuteri*. Different groups were given equal amounts of ethanol diet precisely daily, and the residual was recorded the next day and the amount of food was adjusted to make sure they ingested a similar amount of alcohol. All experiments were approved by the Animal Care and Use Committee of Southwest Medical University (approval No. XNYKDX202005) and were performed in accordance with the Guidelines for the Care and Use of Laboratory Animals issued by the United States National Institutes of Health.

Sample Collection and Preparation

Plasma samples were collected and centrifuged at 10,000 rpm for 10 min at 4°C, and the resultant supernatants were stored at −80°C for biochemical analysis. Liver and intestinal tissues were removed immediately and later placed in phosphate-buffered saline solution for cleaning. Then, the samples were stored at −80°C for histologic analyses. To perform the metabolomics analysis, 0.2 g of each liver sample was added to 2 ml of a methanol and water (4:1) mixture, homogenized for 1 min, extracted by ultrasonication on an ice water bath for 8 min (80 Hz), and filtered through a 0.22-μm nylon filter in order to obtain 1.6 ml of supernatant.

Detection of Biochemical Biomarkers in Serum

The levels of serum aspartate aminotransferase (AST), alanine aminotransferase (ALT), alkaline phosphatase (ALP), triglycerides (TG), and total cholesterol (TCH) were detected using an automatic biochemical analyzer (Erba XL-640, Germany).

ELISA of Lipopolysaccharide (LPS) and TNF-α in Serum

The ELISA kits of Lipopolysaccharide (LPS) and TNF-α in serum were purchased from Bioswamp (Wuhan, China).

Liver Morphology and Intestinal Tight Junctions

Liver and intestinal samples were fixed in 4% paraformaldehyde for 24 h, embedded in paraffin, and cut into sections. The sections were examined by light microscopy (100 ×, 400 ×) after hematoxylin and eosin (H&E) staining, oil red O staining, and immunohistochemical staining for ZO-1 and occludin according to the manufacturer's protocols.

Metabolomics Analysis

Chromatographic Conditions

The liver metabolomics analysis was performed using an Agilent 1290 ultrahigh-pressure liquid chromatography machine (Agilent Technologies, Palo Alto, CA, United States). ZORBAX Eclipse Plus C18 RRHD columns (2.1 × 150 mm, 1.8 μm) with a temperature that was maintained at 35°C were used in this analysis. The mobile phase was composed of A (0.1% formic acid in water) and B (0.1% formic acid in acetonitrile). The flow rate of the mobile phase was set at 0.4 ml/min. The linear gradient elution program was set as follows: at 0–2 min, 98% A and 2% B; 2–9 min, 98% A and 2% B; 9–15 min, 55% A and 45% B; 15–22 min, 30% A and 70% B; 22–24 min, 2% A and 98% B; and 24–26 min, 98% A and 2% B.

Mass Spectrometry Conditions

The metabolomics analysis was performed using an Agilent 6530 quadrupole time-of-flight Mass Spectrometer (Agilent Technologies, Palo Alto, CA, United States), which was equipped with an electrospray ionization (ESI) source. The positive and negative modes were used to collect the data from 50 to 1000 m/z at a rate of 1 spectra/s. The optimal conditions were set as follows: fragmentation voltage: 135 V; the skimmer voltage: 65 V; capillary voltage: ESI + : 4.0 kv, ESI-: 3.5 kv; desolvation gas flow: nitrogen, 10 L/min, 350°C, atomizer pressure: 45 psig.

Multivariate Statistical Analysis of the Serum Metabolite Data

MassHunter Qualitative Analysis (Agilent Technologies, United States) was applied to transform the original mass spectrometry data into the general mzData format, which was obtained from the LC-MS analysis. In order to obtain the generated data matrix, which consisted of m = z, retention time, and peak area, XCMS was employed for data processing such as peak recognition, filtering, and alignment. The generated data matrix was then imported to SIMCA (version 13.0, Umetrics AB, Sweden) to perform the multivariate statistical analysis by principal component analysis (PCA) and orthogonal partial least squares discriminant analysis (OPLS-DA); then, the result was obtained in the form of a score spot. The R^2X, R^2Y, and Q^2 parameters were introduced to describe the result of OPLS-DA to obtain Variable Importance in Projection (VIP) using the permutation test in case of model overfitting and a *t*-test in order to evaluate statistical significance. The biomarkers were further screened in accordance with a VIP value >1, $p < 0.05$, and fold changes >1.5 or < 0.5.

Biomarker Identification and Metabolic Pathway Analysis

Human Metabolome Database (HMDB) was used to infer the possible molecular formula of compounds according to m = z and the relative isotopic abundance of the molecular ion peak. The molecular ion peaks were analyzed by secondary mass spectrometry under a different collision energy to obtain accurate fragment information. The final compounds were determined according to their accurate molecular ion mass, fragment information, and isotope abundance by interpreting the data according to databases such as the Human Metabolome Database (HMDB) and the Kyoto Encyclopedia of Genes and Genomes (KEGG).

Statistical Analysis

Statistical analysis was performed using SPSS 17.0. *T*-test was used in the OPLS-DA model to ensure the reliability of the results. Differences of the body weight, liver weight, liver/body weight ratio, biochemical biomarkers, LPS and TNF-α in serum among three groups were compared using one-way analysis of variance with Tukey's test. Data are expressed as the mean ± SD. All differences were considered statistically significant when $p < 0.05$.

RESULTS

Establishment of the Mouse Model

To determine whether *L. reuteri* exerts protective effects on ALD, 18 male C57BL/6 mice were divided into 3 groups (**Figure 1A**). The control group was fed a control diet, while the ethanol group and the probiotics-treatment group were both fed a liquid ethanol diet and were administered edible alcohol via oral gavage (0.25 g/ml ethanol, 5 g/kg of body weight) weekly. *L. reuteri* was added to the drinking water in the probiotics-treatment group (2×10^7 CFU, daily). Compared with the control group, mice, which were fed an ethanol diet, showed a significant increase in liver/body weight ratio, body weight and liver weight, while these increases were significantly reversed by *L. reuteri* treatment (**Figures 1B–D**).

L. reuteri Treatment Ameliorated the Steatohepatitis Phenotype and the Expression of Intestinal ZO-1

To further detect the effects of *L. reuteri* on ALD, H&E staining and oil red O staining were performed to detect the histomorphological changes of steatohepatitis induced by an ethanol diet. Inflammatory cell infiltration and lipid vacuolation were observed in the livers of mice fed an ethanol diet (**Figure 2A**), and the levels were significantly determined to be different from those in mice in the control group. Oil red O staining also revealed accumulation of lipid droplets (**Figure 2B**). We then performed a serum biochemical analysis to explore the effects of *L. reuteri*. Compared with mice fed an ethanol diet, probiotics-treated mice showed an amelioration of liver injury, which manifested as a decrease in AST and ALT levels (**Figures 2C,D**). In addition, the biochemical analysis showed an accumulation of TG and TCH, which was consistent with the histologic analyses (**Figures 2E,F**). Serum LPS and TNF-α ELISA were performed to further detect the protective effect of *L. reuteri* treatment on liver (**Figures 2G,H**). To confirm the safety of *L. reuteri*, a group of mice was treated by control diet and *L. reuteri* in drinking water. The body weight, liver weight, liver/body weight ratio, HE and oil red o staining and other biochemical biomarkers in serum were compared with control group and the results showed no significant difference between these two groups (**Supplementary Materials**). The results indicated that *L. reuteri* treatment reversed the endotoxemia and inflammation induced by ethanol. These findings clearly indicated that the phenotype of steatohepatitis induced by ethanol was ameliorated using *L. reuteri* treatment.

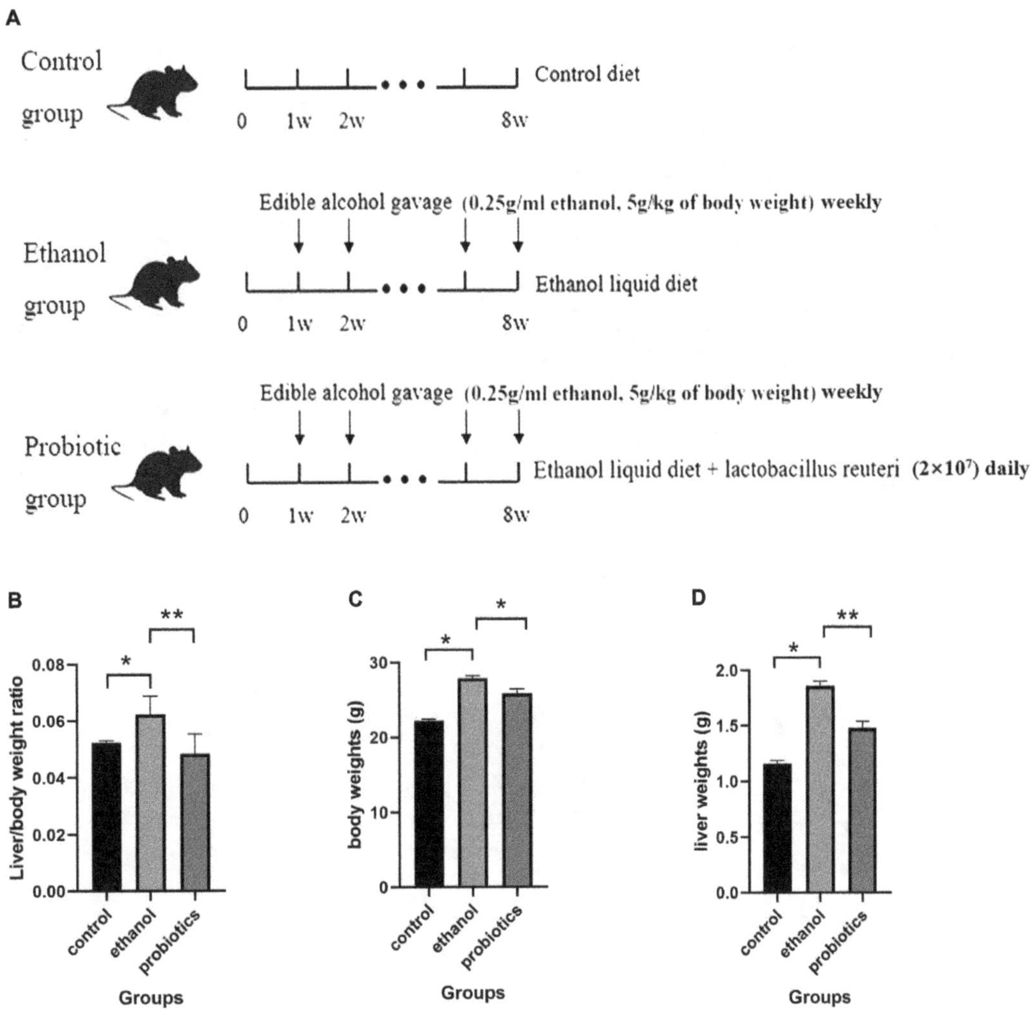

FIGURE 1 | (A) Diagram of the mouse model. Mice were divided into three groups: control group, the ethanol group, and the probiotics group. The control group was fed a control diet. The ethanol group and probiotics group were fed a liquid ethanol diet and were administered edible alcohol via oral gavage (0.25 g/ml ethanol, 5 g/kg of body weight) weekly. Moreover, mice in the probiotics group were also treated with *L. reuteri* (2 × 107 CFU, daily). **(B)** Liver to body weight ratio of the three groups. **(C)** Body weight of three groups. **(D)** Liver weight of three groups. $^{*}p < 0.05$, $^{**}p < 0.01$.

Lactobacillus reuteri has been reported to be beneficial for the expression of intestinal tight junction (TJ) proteins in colitis, which improves gut barrier function and might affect ethanol-induced hepatitis (Ahl et al., 2016). Therefore, TJ protein expression was detected in the three groups using immunohistochemical staining. ZO-1 expression was significantly suppressed in mice fed an ethanol diet, which was reversed by *L. reuteri* treatment, while occludin expression was not significantly different among the three groups (**Figures 3A,B**).

L. reuteri Reversed Polyunsaturated Fatty Acid Metabolism Disorder

To further explore the way in which *L. reuteri* reversed the progression of ALD, especially the metabolic changes, we performed a metabolomics analysis of mouse liver samples. UPLC Q-TOF/MS was used to elute and acquire data. Representative total ion chromatograms of the cells and cell culture supernatants showed good separation and strong sensitivity of the established method (**Supplementary Figure S1**). PCA, which is an unsupervised pattern recognition analytical method based on the LC-MS data, was then used to visualize the trends among the groups. In the positive and negative ion mode, the PCA score plots of the liver samples showed a clear separation, which implied the perturbation of liver metabolic profiles among the three groups (**Figures 4A,B**). The model R2X parameters, which represent the model's ability to interpret variables, were determined to be at 0.545 and 0.649 in the positive and negative ion mode, respectively, which indicates that 54.5 and 64.9% of the variables are used in building the analysis model in the positive and negative mode, respectively.

To improve the classification, OPLS-DA was introduced. The OPLS-DA score plots have been determined to show that

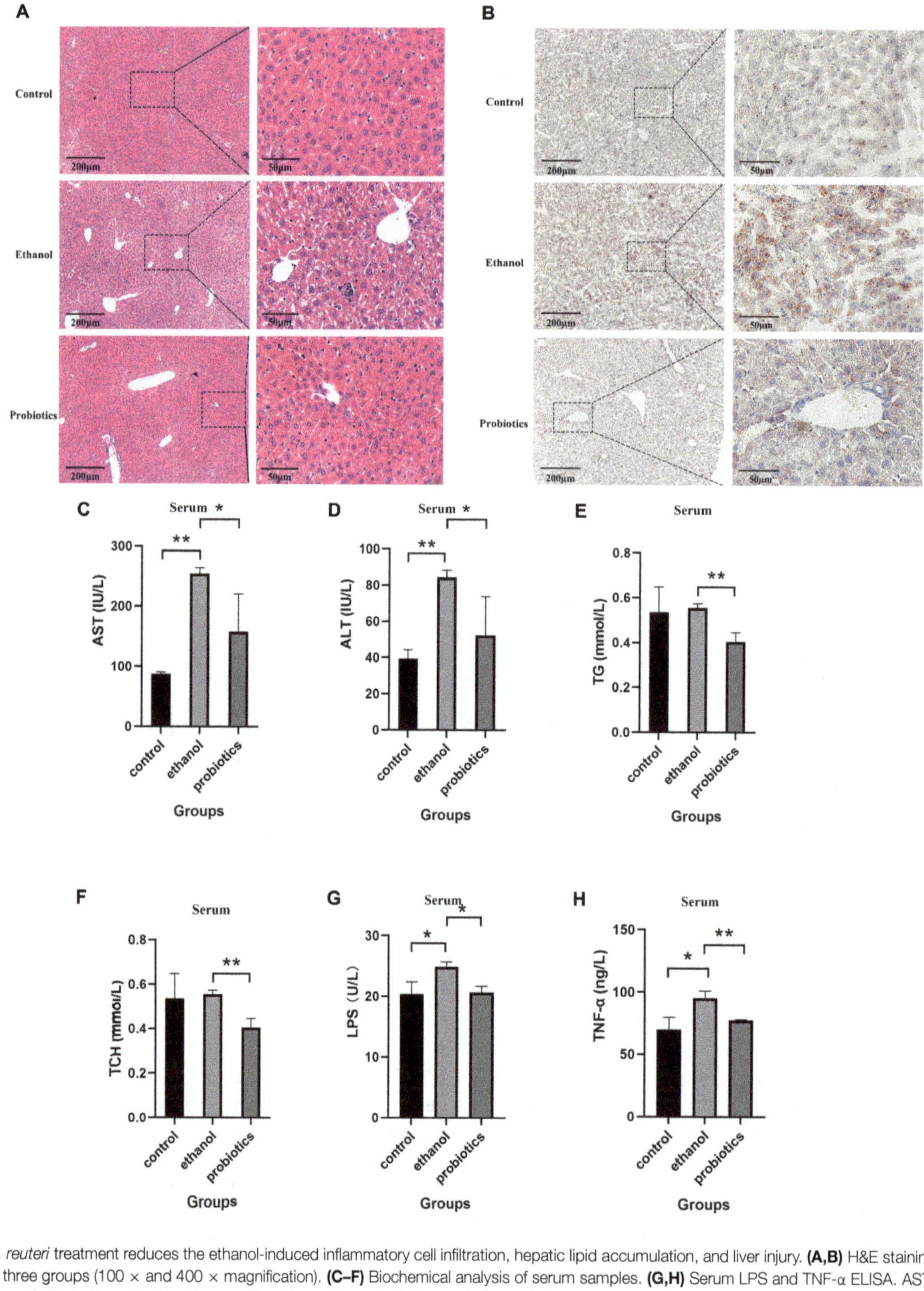

FIGURE 2 | *L. reuteri* treatment reduces the ethanol-induced inflammatory cell infiltration, hepatic lipid accumulation, and liver injury. **(A,B)** H&E staining and oil red O staining in the three groups (100 × and 400 × magnification). **(C–F)** Biochemical analysis of serum samples. **(G,H)** Serum LPS and TNF-α ELISA. AST: aspartate aminotransferase, ALT: alanine aminotransferase, TG: triglycerides and TCH: total cholesterol. $^{*}p < 0.05$, $^{**}p < 0.01$.

the three groups were clearly separated, which suggested that significant metabolic changes were induced by an ethanol diet and were reversed by *L. reuteri* treatment (**Figures 4C,D**). This finding is consistent with the PCA result. To ensure the reliability of the results, permutation test is widely used in the OPLS-DA model of metabolomics analysis. The intercept of the R2 and Q2 parameters reached 0.699 and −0.767 in the positive ion mode, respectively, and 0.821 and −0.553 in the negative ion mode, respectively, which further indicated that overfitting did not occur (**Figures 4E,F**). The VIP value, which was obtained from the OPLS-DA model, was then used to identify metabolites using Student's *t*-test to ensure that the metabolites selected

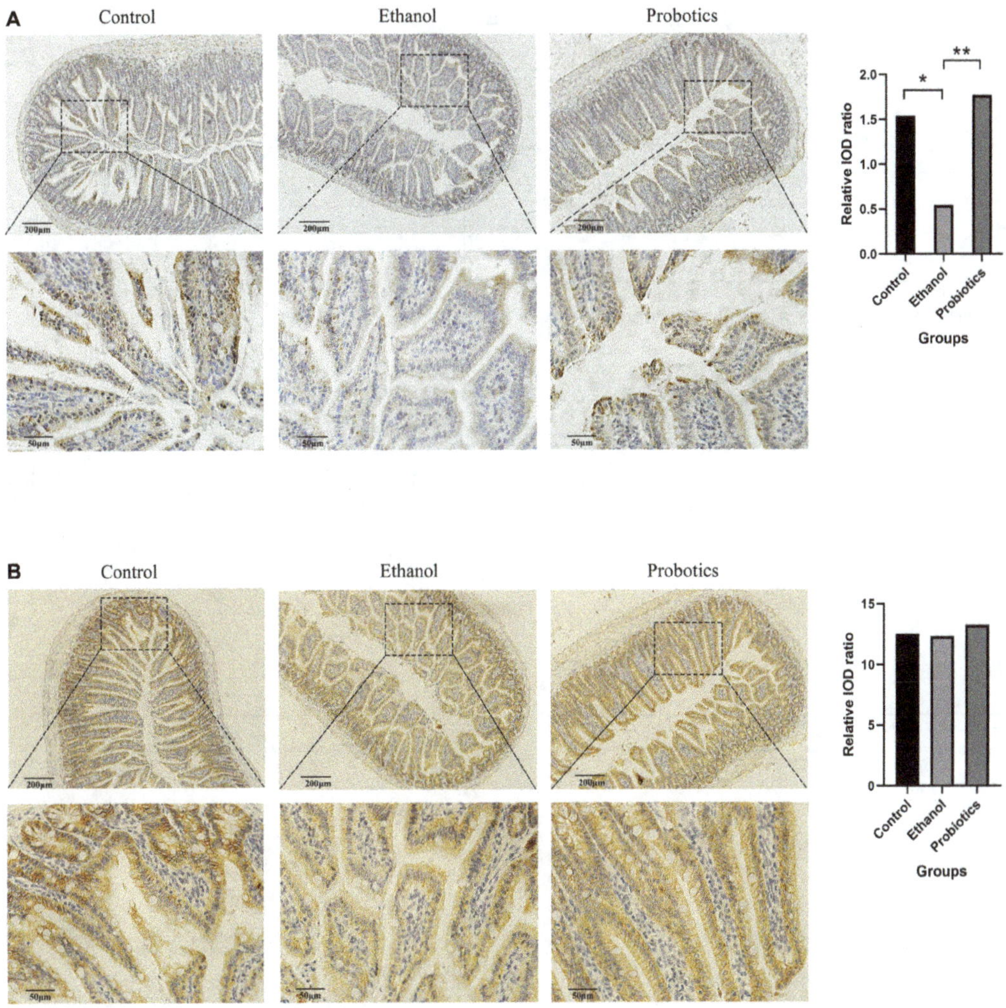

FIGURE 3 | Immunohistochemical staining of intestinal tight junctions. **(A)** ZO-1 expression was significantly repressed in mice fed an ethanol diet and was reversed by *L. reuteri* treatment. **(B)** Occludin expression was not significantly different among the three groups (100 × and 400 × magnification). $^{*}p < 0.05$, $^{**}p < 0.01$.

were statistically significant. The compounds for which the VIP value was >1 and $p < 0.05$ were screened. In the positive and negative ion modes, 15 and 8 potential biomarkers were screened, respectively.

Twenty-three potential biomarkers were then identified in the search for MS/MS fragmentation patterns in HMDB and consisted of the following: 7 fatty acids and their metabolites and 11 lysophosphatidylethanolamine (LysoPE). In addition, five candidate biomarkers were observed that can be identified in the KEGG database with a fold change >1.5 or < 0.5; these included xanthosine, palmitic acid (PA, 16:0), and n-3 polyunsaturated fatty acids, such as linoleic acid (LA, 18:2), arachidonic acid (AA, 20:4), and docosapentaenoic acid (DPA, 22:5) (**Table 1**). Interestingly, all candidate biomarkers were found in the negative ion mode.

To examine the effects of the candidate biomarkers on metabolic pathways, enrichment analysis of KEGG pathways was performed for the nine potential biomarkers that could be identified in the KEGG database. As shown in **Figures 5A,B**, alpha-linolenic acid and LA metabolism, glycerolipid metabolism, fatty acid elongation in mitochondria, fatty acid biosynthesis, fatty acid metabolism, mitochondrial beta-oxidation of long-chain saturated fatty acids, phospholipid biosynthesis, sphingolipid metabolism, steroid biosynthesis, bile acid biosynthesis, AA metabolism, and the purine metabolism pathways were found to be involved in the metabolic change between ethanol diet group and probiotics treatment group. The alpha-linolenic acid and linoleic acid metabolism pathways had the highest enrichment degree and involved linoleic acid (LA), arachidonic acid (AA), and 12(13)-EpOME. These findings suggested that fatty acid metabolism was disturbed by an ethanol diet and that this disturbance was reversed via *L. reuteri* treatment.

DISCUSSION

Alcoholic liver disease has been identified as the most common type of chronic liver disease and is the main cause of liver-related mortality worldwide, which results in a significant burden

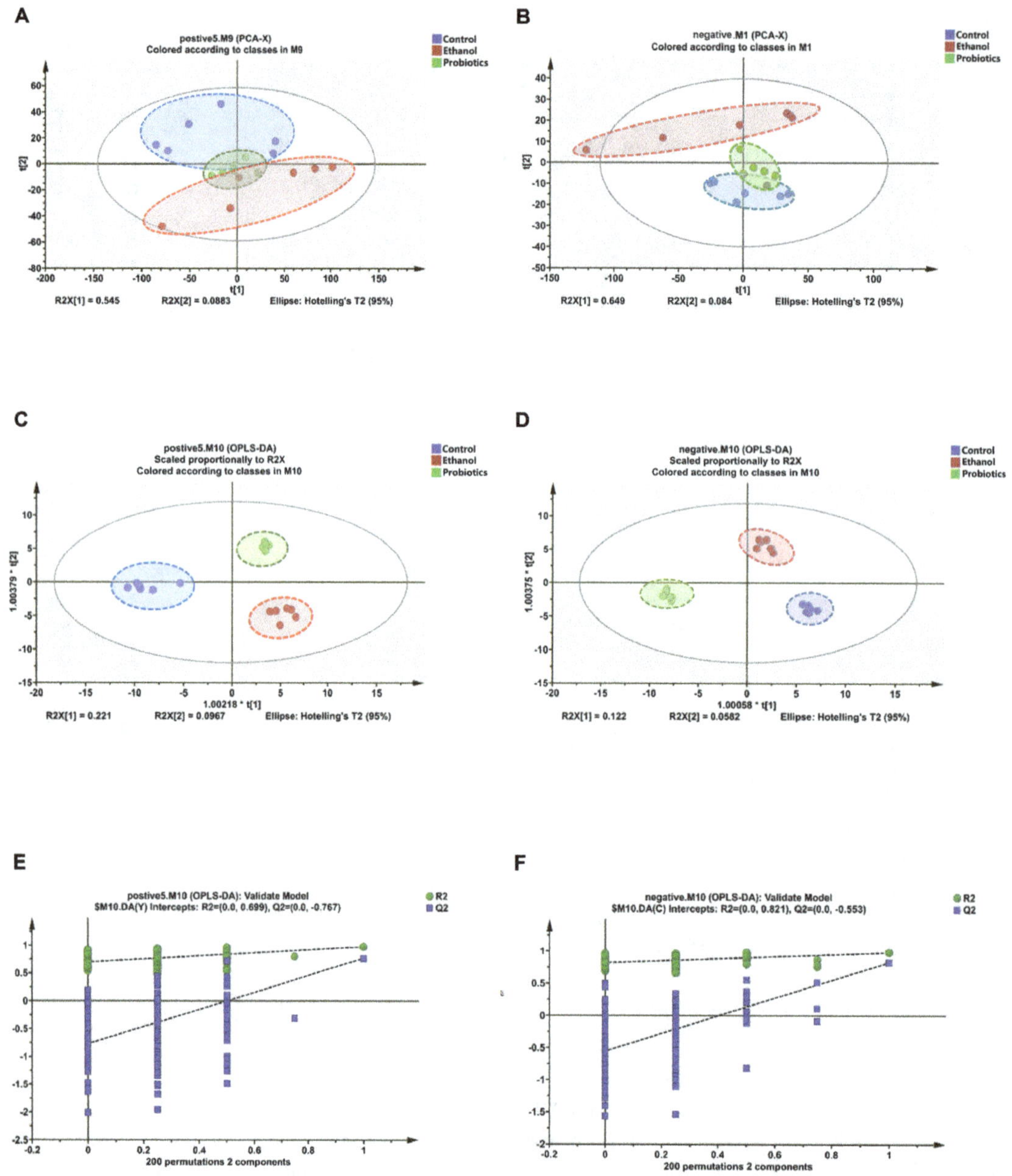

FIGURE 4 | Differentiation of the liver metabolic profiles of the control group, ethanol group, and the probiotics group. **(A,B)** PCA score plots based on the liver metabolic profiles of the three groups in the positive and negative modes: ESI + : R2 = 0.545, ESI-: R2 = 0.649. **(C,D)** OPLS-DA score plots of the three groups in the positive and negative modes: ESI + : R2X = 0.735, R2Y = 0.995, Q2 = 0.728; ESI-: R2X = 0.711, R2Y = 0.974, Q2 = 0.792. **(E,F)** Permutation test of the OPLS-DA model: ESI + : the intercepts of R2 = 0.699 and Q2 = -0.767, ESI-: the intercepts of R2 = 0.821 and Q2 = −0.553.

to society and a threat to human health (Rehm et al., 2013). Given that the currently used drugs provide a limited survival benefit, there is an urgent demand to discover a new potential therapy (Seitz et al., 2018). In recent years, the protective effects of probiotics on metabolic diseases have been widely examined. *L. reuteri* has been demonstrated to be beneficial in many digestive system diseases and metabolic diseases, such as colitis and type 2 diabetes (Gao et al., 2015; Dahiya et al., 2017). Thus, we performed a metabolomics analysis to examine the metabolic protective effects of *L. reuteri* on ALD.

To investigate whether *L. reuteri* exerts a protective effect on ALD, it was administered to C57BL/6 mice together with ethanol. H&E staining showed an amelioration of steatosis and inflammatory cell infiltration under *L. reuteri* treatment; meanwhile, oil red O staining showed less lipid droplet accumulation. Consistent with the histomorphology analysis, the levels of AST, ALT, TG, TCH, LPS, and TNF-α were reduced under *L. reuteri* treatment. Besides, ZO-1 and occludin IHC were performed and the results showed ZO-1 was suppressed by alcohol and reversed after treated by *L. reuteri* while occludin

TABLE 1 | The result of candidate biomarkers.

Metabolite	VIP	*p*-value	Fold Change(P/E)	RT (min)	SM
Linoleic acid (18:2)	6.328	0.009	1.68	13.26	–
Arachidonic acid (20:4)	4.590	0.015	2.20	15.72	–
Docosapentaenoic acid (DPA, 22:5)	3.434	0.038	2.28	22.06	–
Xanthosine	1.779	0.001	2.01	5.08	–
Palmitic acid (16:0)	2.962	0.028	1.72	23.35	–

RT, retention time; VIP, variable importance in projection; SM, scan mode; +, metabolites identified in the positive (ESI +) electrospray ionization mode; –, metabolites identified in the negative (ESI-) electrospray ionization mode. P/E, the probiotics group compared with the ethanol group.

was not affected by ethanol diet. However, occludin was indicated decreased in the colon of ethanol fed mice (Mir et al., 2016). The mechanism needs to be explored in our next research. Studies of liver and intestinal inflammation suggested that *L. reuteri* treatment reduced the expression levels of hepatic IL-1β, IL-6, and TNF-α and promoted the expression of the anti-inflammatory cytokine IL-10 by suppressing the mitogen-activated protein kinase and NF-κB signaling pathways (Liu et al., 2012; Hsu et al., 2017). Hypercholesterolemic rats treated with a probiotics mixture containing *L. reuteri* have exhibited decreased lipid accumulation and reduced expression levels of cholesterol synthesis-related proteins, such as sterol regulatory element-binding protein 1 (SREBP1), fatty acid synthase, and acetyl-CoA carboxylase in the liver (Kim et al., 2017). These findings might explain the mechanism by which *L. reuteri* reverses liver injury and lipid accumulation.

To further examine the metabolic changes, metabolomics was introduced to comprehensively detect changes in the liver samples. PCA and OPLS-DA scores showed a significant difference in the metabolic characteristics among the control group, model group, and treatment group. Twenty-three potential biomarkers were then screened, including 7 fatty acids and their metabolites as well as 11 LysoPE; xanthosine, PA, LA, AA, and DPA were also identified as 5 candidate biomarkers with fold changes >1.5, which indicates a significant change in fatty acid metabolism. Their biological functions and related metabolic pathways can explain the protective effects of *L. reuteri*. Nine biomarkers that could be found in the KEGG database were detected by KEGG enrichment analysis in order to identify the possible pathways involved. The enrichment of PA and three polyunsaturated fatty acids (PUFA), LA, AA, and DPA was worthy of further attention.

Palmitic acid is a type of saturated long-chain fatty acids (LCFA). Chronic alcohol abuse reduces the production of LCFA via suppressing the bacterial genes involved in the biosynthesis of saturated fatty acids, including malonyl CoA:ACP acyltransferase (FabD; [EC:2.3.1.39]), 3-oxoacyl-[acyl-carrier-protein] synthase II (FabF; [EC:2.3.1.179]) and 3-oxoacyl-[acyl-carrier protein] reductase (FabG; [EC:1.1.1.100]), leading to the limit the proliferation of lactobacilli which metabolizes saturated LCFA (Chen et al., 2015). Meanwhile, alcohol-induced liver injury and steatosis were reversed after the supplementation of saturated LCFA via preventing gut leakiness and restoring the eubiosis.

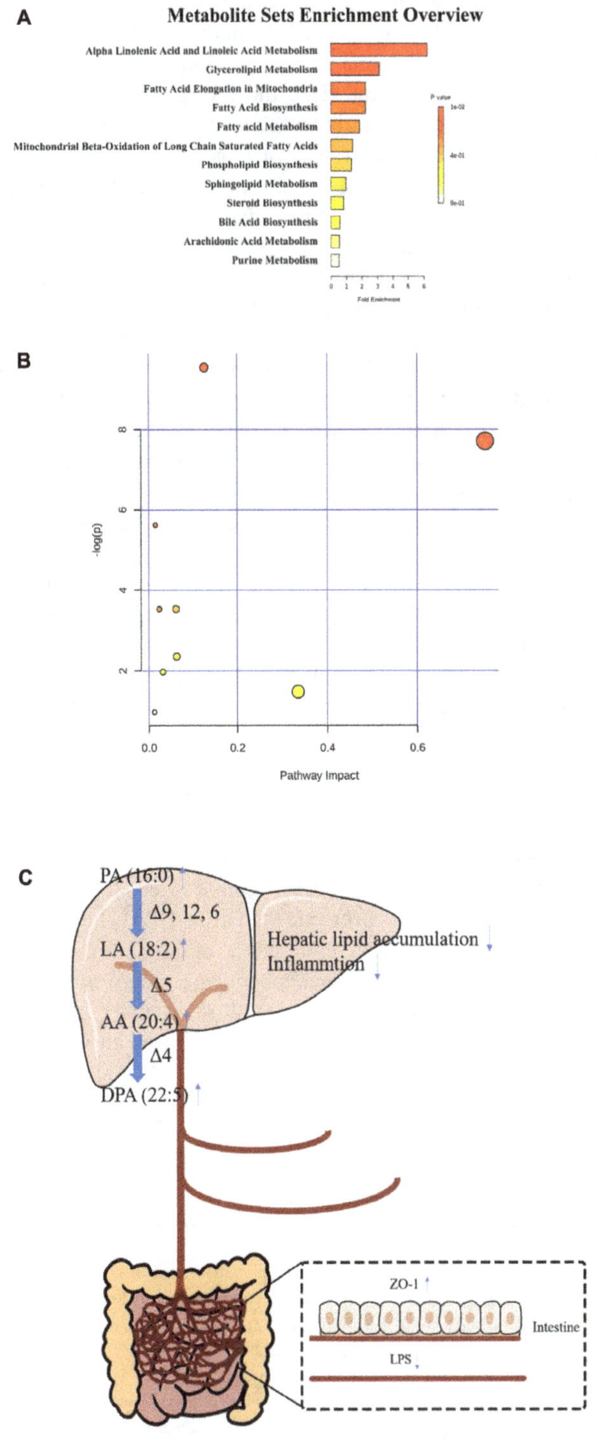

FIGURE 5 | The enriched KEGG pathways **(A,B)** and the diagram of the protective effect of *L. reuteri* on ALD **(C)**.

Linoleic acid is an n-6 PUFA that can be metabolized to AA. Several meta-analyses and prospective cohort studies have shown that a higher level of LA was associated with a decreased risk of coronary heart disease, while another study on hyperlipidemia showed a hypolipidemic effect on mice fed a high-fat diet, which suggests its potential use for ameliorating fatty acid metabolism (Jang et al., 2008; Farvid et al., 2014; Marklund et al., 2019). Jina et al. examined associations among LA, AA, and the lipoprotein subclasses VLDL, LDL, and HDL and showed that high levels of LA and AA were significantly associated with a low level of large VLDL particles and a high level of large HDL particles (Choo et al., 2010). These findings might explain why the increased levels of LA and AA exerted protective effects on liver steatosis under *L. reuteri* treatment.

Chronic alcohol consumption can lead to a decrease in Δ-6, Δ-5, and Δ-9 desaturase activity, which is essential for the formation of AA (Risti-Medi et al., 2013). Despite the traditional view that AA is a substrate for pro-inflammatory eicosanoids, substantial evidence supports the concept that AA also serves as a precursor for a group of potent anti-inflammatory mediators. In addition to its ability to be transformed into the pro-inflammatory prostaglandin E2 and leukotrienes by cyclooxygenase (COX) and 5-lipoxygenase (LO), AA can also be transformed into lipoxins, resolvins, protectins, maresins, PGE1, and PGI2, which are found to represent a series of potent bioactive compounds that have been reported to have anti-inflammatory effects in chronic liver diseases, such as ALD, NAFLD, and cirrhosis (Das, 2019). Lactobacillus rhamnosus GG has been reported beneficial to ameliorating the reduction of AA induced by ethanol diet (Shi et al., 2015).

Docosapentaenoic acid is an n-3 PUFA that has been demonstrated to inhibit the expression of pro-inflammatory cytokines, such as TNF-α, IL-1β, and IL-6, and to improve the expression of the anti-inflammatory cytokine IL-10 (Tian et al., 2017; Zheng et al., 2019). Kimberly et al. found that the n-3 DPA-derived protectin (PDn-3 DPA) biosynthetic pathway regulated the differentiation of human monocytes, which altered the macrophage phenotype, efferocytosis, and bacterial phagocytosis (Pistorius et al., 2018). Remarkably, Zheng et al. (2019) demonstrated that DPA could lead to a decrease in the substrate needed for the synthesis of pro-inflammatory eicosanoids (PGE2 and LTB4) in a dextran sulfate sodium (DSS)-induced colitis model. This finding might explain why an increased level of AA did not lead to an increased level of pro-inflammatory eicosanoids in our study.

Increased levels of PUFAs prevent liver inflammation and lipid accumulation, which indicates that fatty acid metabolism is a therapeutic target for the management of ALD. An eradication of bacteria group was established via antibiotics (ampicillin, vancomycin, neomycin, and metronidazole) in our initially. However, the morality of mice is uncontrollable when gavaged with ethanol and we failed to collect the samples of this group. The effect of eradicating gut bacteria on ALD needs to be further explored. Besides, further studies on fatty acid metabolism in ALD are therefore needed.

In conclusion, all these findings suggested that *L. reuteri* treatment reversed the phenotype of ethanol-induced hepatitis and disorders of fatty acid metabolism (**Figure 5C**). We speculate that *L. reuteri* might exert a protective effect on ALD by ameliorating fatty acid metabolism. These findings provide evidence that *L. reuteri* may serve as a new therapeutic strategy for ALD.

AUTHOR CONTRIBUTIONS

S-P and T-Z designed and established the mouse model. T-Z finished manuscript-writing and performed data analysis. PT and Y-D performed histomorphological analysis. B-Q and HC collected tissue samples. W-F and M-H supervised the study and revised the manuscript. All authors contributed to the article and approved the submitted version.

REFERENCES

Ahl, D., Liu, H., Schreiber, O., Roos, S., Phillipson, M., and Holm, L. (2016). *Lactobacillus reuteri* increases mucus thickness and ameliorates dextran sulphate sodium-induced colitis in mice. *Acta Physiol.* 217, 300–310. doi: 10.1111/apha.12695

Chau, K., Lau, E., Greenberg, S., Jacobson, S., Yazdani-Brojeni, P., Verma, N., et al. (2015). Probiotics for infantile colic: a randomized, double-blind, placebo-controlled trial investigating *Lactobacillus reuteri* DSM 17938. *J. Pediatr.* 166, 74–78. doi: 10.1016/j.jpeds.2014.09.020

Chen, P., Torralba, M., Tan, J., Embree, M., Zengler, K., Starkel, P., et al. (2015). Supplementation of saturated long-chain fatty acids maintains intestinal eubiosis and reduces ethanol-induced liver injury in mice. *Gastroenterology* 148, 203–214.e16. doi: 10.1053/j.gastro.2014.09.014

Choo, J., Ueshima, H., Curb, J. D., Shin, C., Evans, R. W., El-Saed, A., et al. (2010). Serum n-6 fatty acids and lipoprotein subclasses in middle-aged men: the population-based cross-sectional ERA-JUMP study. *Am. J. Clin. Nutr.* 91, 1195–1203. doi: 10.3945/ajcn.2009.28500

Dahiya, D. K., Renuka, Puniya, M., Shandilya, U. K., Dhewa, T., Kumar, N., et al. (2017). Gut microbiota modulation and its relationship with obesity using prebiotic fibers and probiotics: a review. *Front. Microbiol.* 8:563. doi: 10.3389/fmicb.2017.00563

Das, U. N. (2019). Beneficial role of bioactive lipids in the pathobiology, prevention, and management of HBV, HCV and alcoholic hepatitis, NAFLD, and liver cirrhosis: a review. *J. Adv. Res.* 17, 17–29. doi: 10.1016/j.jare.2018.12.006

Farvid, M. S., Ding, M., Pan, A., Sun, Q., Chiuve, S. E., Steffen, L. M., et al. (2014). Dietary linoleic acid and risk of coronary heart disease: a systematic review and meta-analysis of prospective cohort studies. *Circulation* 130, 1568–1578. doi: 10.1161/circulationaha.114.010236

Gao, C., Major, A., Rendon, D., Lugo, M., Jackson, V., Shi, Z., et al. (2015). Histamine H2 receptor-mediated suppression of intestinal inflammation by probiotic *Lactobacillus reuteri*. *mBio* 6:e01358-15. doi: 10.1128/mBio.01358-15

Greifova, G., Majekova, H., Greif, G., Body, P., Greifova, M., and Dubnickova, M. (2017). Analysis of antimicrobial and immunomodulatory substances produced by heterofermentative *Lactobacillus reuteri*. *Folia Microbiol.* 62, 515–524. doi: 10.1007/s12223-017-0524-9

He, B., Hoang, T. K., Wang, T., Ferris, M., Taylor, C. M., Tian, X., et al. (2017). Resetting microbiota by *Lactobacillus reuteri* inhibits T reg deficiency-induced autoimmunity via adenosine A2A receptors. *J. Exp. Med.* 214, 107–123. doi: 10.1084/jem.20160961

Hsieh, F.-C., Lee, C.-L., Chai, C.-Y., Chen, W. T., Lu, Y. C., and Wu, C. S. (2013). Oral administration of *Lactobacillus reuteri* GMNL-263 improves insulin resistance and ameliorates hepatic steatosis in high fructose-fed rats. *Nutr. Metab.* 10:35. doi: 10.1186/1743-7075-10-35

Hsu, T. C., Huang, C. Y., Liu, C. H., Hsu, K. C., Chen, Y. H., and Tzang, B. S. (2017). *Lactobacillus paracasei* GMNL-32, *Lactobacillus reuteri* GMNL-89 and *L. reuteri* GMNL-263 ameliorate hepatic injuries in lupus-prone mice. *Br. J. Nutr.* 117, 1066–1074. doi: 10.1017/s0007114517001039

Jang, A., Srinivasan, P., Lee, N. Y., Song, H. P., Lee, J. W., Lee, M., et al. (2008). Comparison of hypolipidemic activity of synthetic gallic acid-linoleic acid ester with mixture of gallic acid and linoleic acid, gallic acid, and linoleic acid on high-fat diet induced obesity in C57BL/6 Cr Slc mice. *Chem. Biol. Interact.* 174, 109–117. doi: 10.1016/j.cbi.2008.05.018

Jimenez-Gutierrez, P., Lopez-Velazquez, G., Jimenez-Gutierrez, C., Mancilla-Ramirez, J., Estevez-Jimenez, J., and Parra, M. (2014). Diarrhea in preschool children and *Lactobacillus reuteri*: a randomized controlled trial. *Pediatrics* 133, e904–e909. doi: 10.1542/peds.2013-0652

Kim, S. J., Park, S. H., Sin, H. S., Jang, S. H., Lee, S. W., Kim, S. Y., et al. (2017). Hypocholesterolemic effects of probiotic mixture on diet-induced hypercholesterolemic rats. *Nutrients* 9:293. doi: 10.3390/nu9030293

Liu, Y., Fatheree, N. Y., Mangalat, N., and Rhoads, J. M. (2012). *Lactobacillus reuteri* strains reduce incidence and severity of experimental necrotizing enterocolitis via modulation of TLR4 and NF-kappaB signaling in the intestine. *Am. J. Physiol. Gastrointest. Liver Physiol.* 302, G608–G617. doi: 10.1152/ajpgi.00266.2011

Marie-Christine, S., Strassburger, K., Bettina, N., Hubert, K., Peter, N., Volker, B., et al. (2015). Intake of *Lactobacillus reuteri* improves incretin and insulin secretion in glucose-tolerant humans: a proof of concept. *Diabetes Care* 38, 1827–1834. doi: 10.2337/dc14-2690

Marklund, M., Wu, J. H. Y., Imamura, F., Del Gobbo, L. C., Fretts, A., de Goede, J., et al. (2019). Biomarkers of dietary omega-6 fatty acids and incident cardiovascular disease and mortality. *Circulation* 139, 2422–2436. doi: 10.1161/CIRCULATIONAHA.118.038908

Mir, H., Meena, A. S., Chaudhry, K. K., Shukla, P. K., Gangwar, R., Manda, B., et al. (2016). Occludin deficiency promotes ethanol-induced disruption of colonic epithelial junctions, gut barrier dysfunction and liver damage in mice. *Biochim. Biophys. Acta* 1860, 765–774. doi: 10.1016/j.bbagen.2015.12.013

Noorbakhsh, H., Yavarmanesh, M., Mortazavi, S. A., Adibi, P., and Moazzami, A. A. (2019). Metabolomics analysis revealed metabolic changes in patients with diarrhea-predominant irritable bowel syndrome and metabolic responses to a synbiotic yogurt intervention. *Eur. J. Nutr.* 58, 3109–3119. doi: 10.1007/s00394-018-1855-2

Pistorius, K., Souza, P. R., De Matteis, R., Austin-Williams, S., Primdahl, K. G., Vik, A., et al. (2018). PDn-3 DPA pathway regulates human monocyte differentiation and macrophage function. *Cell Chem. Biol.* 25, 749–760.e9. doi: 10.1016/j.chembiol.2018.04.017

Rehm, J., Samokhvalov, A. V., and Shield, K. D. (2013). Global burden of alcoholic liver diseases. *J. Hepatol.* 59, 160–168. doi: 10.1016/j.jhep.2013.03.007

Risti-Medi, D., Takiæ, M., Vuèiæ, V., Kandi, D., Kosti, N., and Glibeti, M. (2013). Abnormalities in the serum phospholipids fatty acid profile in patients with alcoholic liver cirrhosis a pilot study. *J. Clin. Biochem. Nutr.* 53, 49–54. doi: 10.3164/jcbn.12-79

Seitz, H. K., Bataller, R., Cortez-Pinto, H., Gao, B., Gual, A., Lackner, C., et al. (2018). Alcoholic liver disease. *Nat. Rev. Dis. Primers.* 4:16. doi: 10.1038/s41572-018-0014-7

Shi, X., Wei, X., Yin, X., Wang, Y., Zhang, M., Zhao, C., et al. (2015). Hepatic and fecal metabolomic analysis of the effects of *Lactobacillus rhamnosus* GG on alcoholic fatty liver disease in mice. *J. Proteome Res.* 14, 1174–1182. doi: 10.1021/pr501121c

Singh, S., Murad, M. H., Chandar, A. K., Bongiorno, C. M., Singal, A. K., Atkinson, S. R., et al. (2015). Comparative effectiveness of pharmacological interventions for severe alcoholic hepatitis: a systematic review and network meta-analysis. *Gastroenterology* 149, 958–970.e12. doi: 10.1053/j.gastro.2015.06.006

Thursz, M. R., Richardson, P., Allison, M., Austin, A., Bowers, M., Day, C. P., et al. (2015). Prednisolone or pentoxifylline for alcoholic hepatitis. *N. Engl. J. Med.* 372, 1619–1628. doi: 10.1056/NEJMoa1412278

Tian, Y., Katsuki, A., Romanazzi, D., Miller, M. R., Adams, S. L., Miyashita, K., et al. (2017). Docosapentaenoic Acid (22:5n-3) downregulates mRNA expression of pro-inflammatory factors in LPS-activated murine macrophage like RAW264.7 Cells. *J. Oleo Sci.* 66, 1149–1156. doi: 10.5650/jos.ess17111

World Health Organization (2018). *Global Status Report on Alcohol and Health 2018*. Geneva: World Health Organization.

Yang, Y., Zhao, X., Le, M. H., Zijlstra, R. T., and Ganzle, M. G. (2015). Reutericyclin producing *Lactobacillus reuteri* modulates development of fecal microbiota in weanling pigs. *Front. Microbiol.* 6:762. doi: 10.3389/fmicb.2015.00762

Zheng, Z., Dai, Z., Cao, Y., Shen, Q., and Zhang, Y. (2019). Docosapentaenoic acid (DPA, 22:5n-3) ameliorates inflammation in an ulcerative colitis model. *Food Funct.* 10, 4199–4209. doi: 10.1039/C8FO02338G

12

miR-378b Regulates Insulin Sensitivity by Targeting Insulin Receptor and p110α in Alcohol-Induced Hepatic Steatosis

Yuan-yuan Li[1†], Yu-juan Zhong[1†], Qi Cheng[1], Ying-zhao Wang[1], Yuan-yuan Fan[1], Cheng-fang Yang[1], Zuheng Ma[2], Yong-wen Li[1,3] and Li Li[1*]*

[1] College of Pharmacy, Guilin Medical University, Guilin, China, [2] Department of Molecular Medicine and Surgery, Karolinska Institutet, Stockholm, Sweden, [3] Center for Diabetic Systems Medicine, Guangxi Key Laboratory of Excellence, Guilin, China

***Correspondence:**
Yong-wen Li
liyongwen99@163.com
Li Li
liyongwen168@163.com

[†]These authors have contributed equally to this work

Insulin resistance has been implicated in alcoholic liver disease. A previous study has shown that microRNAs (miRNAs) play a major role in the production, secretion, and function of insulin. MiRNAs are capable of repressing multiple target genes that in turn negatively regulate various physiological and pathological activities. However, current information on the biological function of miRNAs in insulin resistance is limited. The goal of the present study was to elucidate the role of miR-378b in alcohol-induced hepatic insulin resistance and its underlying mechanism. This study has observed that miR-378b is up-regulated in National Institute on Alcohol Abuse and Alcoholism (NIAAA) alcoholic mouse models as well as in ethanol-induced L-02 cells *in vitro*. Furthermore, miR-378b overexpression impaired the insulin signaling pathway, and inhibition of miR-378b improved insulin sensitivity *in vivo* and *in vitro*. A mechanistic study revealed that IR and p110α are direct targets of miR-378b. Together, these results suggest that miR-378b controls insulin sensitivity by targeting the insulin receptor (IR) as well as p110α and possibly play an inhibitory role in the development of insulin resistance, thereby providing insights into the development of novel diagnostic and treatment methods.

Keywords: MiR-378b, insulin resistance, insulin receptor, p110α, alcoholic hepatic steatosis

INTRODUCTION

Alcoholic liver disease (ALD) is a common liver disorder with high global morbidity and mortality rates (Ramaiah et al., 2004). ALD pathogenesis consists of stages including steatosis, steatohepatitis, and fibrosis/cirrhosis (Chacko and Reinus, 2016). One of the most important organs for insulin action is the liver. Insulin resistance plays a pivotal role in the formation of ALD (Magdaleno et al., 2017; Chen et al., 2018). However, excessive alcohol uptake also increases the risk for insulin resistance, which is characterized by the inability of insulin-sensitive tissues to respond to insulin, resulting in various metabolic syndromes (Aberg et al., 2018; Tatsumi et al., 2018). Alcohol overconsumption may promote the pathogenesis of hepatic insulin resistance by inhibiting insulin signaling (Carr and Correnti, 2015). In addition, hepatic steatosis induced by alcohol leads to intracellular metabolic imbalance, can promote insulin resistance in liver cells (Samuel and

Shulman, 2012; Perry et al., 2014). Thus, ALD and insulin resistance are intertwined in liver diseases.

Insulin receptor/insulin-receptor substrate (IR/IRS), combined with phosphoinositide 3-kinase (PI3K) heterodimers and serine-threonine protein kinase (Akt/PKB), are three well-defined and major nodes of the insulin signaling pathway (Taniguchi et al., 2006). PI3K comprises a regulatory subunit (p85) as well as a catalytic subunit (p110). In addition, p110α plays a central role in hepatic insulin/PI3K signaling and regulates glucose and lipid homeostasis (Liu et al., 2014). In normal physiological conditions, insulin binds to insulin receptors (IRs) on target tissues that in turn stimulates receptor autophosphorylation and internalization, thereby recruiting and activating insulin receptor substrate proteins 1 and 2 (IRS1/2). Then, IRS1/2 activates PI3K that converts phosphatidylinositol 4,5-bisphosphate (PIP2) into phosphatidylinositol (3,4,5)-trisphosphate (PIP3), which is situated on the cell membrane. Akt then binds to PIP3 at its pleckstrin homology domain, followed by its phosphorylation and activation (He et al., 2007; Samuel and Shulman, 2016; Parker et al., 2018). Elevated blood glucose stimulates islet β cells to secrete insulin and activates the PI3K/AKT signaling pathway in the liver, which play the following roles: 1) Inhibition of glycogen synthase kinase 3 (GSK3) increase glycogen synthase (GS) activity and thereby promote liver glycogen synthesis; 2) promote phosphorylation of forkhead box factor 1 (FoxO1) and reduces gluconeogenesis; 3) activate sterol regulatory element binding protein 1 (SREBP-1) and promote the synthesis of endogenous fatty acids (Perry et al., 2014; Carr and Correnti, 2015). Chronic ethanol consumption can disrupt IR, IRS1/2, PI3K, PIP3, and Akt expression or phosphorylation, which in turn decreases hepatocyte sensitivity to insulin and blocks the PI3K-Akt pathway, resulting in the decrease of glycogen synthesis, the increase of gluconeogenesis, the increase of fatty acid *de novo* synthesis, the increase of blood lipid. However, the body can only compensate for insulin resistance by increasing insulin secretion. A growing body of evidence shows that the decline of IR also contributes to the cause and development of IR and type 2 diabetes mellitus (T2DM). Knocking out IR leads to severe insulin resistance and impaired glucose homeostasis (Yang et al., 2015). Therefore, the expression levels of hepatic IR and p110α play an important role in insulin sensitivity of the whole body. However, the underlying mechanism of ethanol-induced downregulation of IR and p110α is still not fully understood.

MicroRNAs (miRNAs) pertain to endogenous non-coding RNAs that are 19–25 nucleotides in length and are conserved across species (Kim, 2005). Mature miRNAs have 2–8 relatively conserved nucleotides at its 5'-termini that are called "seed sequences" that interact with its target messenger RNA (mRNA) *via* specific base pairing. This miRNA interaction induces the degradation and/or disrupts the translation of its target gene mRNA, which is considered as a post-transcriptional regulatory mechanism of target gene expression (Bartel, 2004; Bartel, 2005). Although the specific target genes and biological functions of various miRNAs remain unclear, miRNAs are thought to play a central role in maintaining normal and pathological states. Growing evidence has shown that miRNAs are largely involved in the control of insulin signaling. For example, let-7 and miR-103/107 are mainly involved in controlling insulin signaling in peripheral tissues by targeting caveolin-1 and IR/IRS2, respectively (Frost and Olson, 2011; Trajkovski et al., 2011). Obesity caused by consumption of a high-fat diet induces insulin resistance in mice, which is associated with the upregulation of specific miRNAs, including miR-802, miR-29a, and miR-195 (Kornfeld et al., 2013; Yang et al., 2014a; Yang et al., 2014b). Human miR-378b, which has been localized to chromosome 3, belongs to the miR-378 family, and its seed sequence similar to miR-378a. An earlier study has revealed that miR-378b is upregulated during keratinocyte differentiation as well as promotes cell differentiation *via* NKX3.1 (Wang et al., 2015). In addition, the upregulation of miR-378b leads to the obstruction of the insulin signaling pathway and glucose metabolism (Liu et al., 2014). Unfortunately, the role of miR-378b in ethanol-induced liver insulin sensitivity remains unclear.

Numerous studies have shown that alcohol can cause alcoholic liver damage by activating oxidative stress, inhibiting liver fat-acid metabolism, and increasing liver lipid synthesis (Li et al., 2017; Li et al., 2018; Yang C. et al., 2018; Yang C. F. et al., 2018). Studies have also revealed that alcohol reduces hepatic glycogen synthesis and increases gluconeogenesis by regulating the liver insulin signaling pathway (Pang et al., 2009; Magdaleno et al., 2017). However, the exact mechanism remains unclear. Earlier, we found that miR-378b is upregulated in the liver tissues of ALD rats compared to ALD rats treated with methyl ferulic acid through high-throughput sequencing. Therefore, this study focused on the role and regulation of miR-378b in alcohol-induced liver insulin resistance. In this study, we show that the level of miR-378b is upregulated in the hepatic tissue ethyl alcohol (EtOH)-fed mice and EtOH-induced L-02 cells. This study shows that miR-378b directly targets the three prime untranslated region (3'UTR) of the IR and p110α genes to downregulate their protein expression, thereby disrupting insulin signaling. Hence, miR-378b upregulation in ALD is implicated in the pathogenesis of hepatic insulin resistance.

MATERIALS AND METHODS

Animals and Protocols

Weight 20–25g male C57BL/6 mice, purchased by Hunan Sja Laboratory Animal Co., Ltd. (Hunan, China). The animal experiments have been approved by the Institutional Ethical Committee of Guilin Medical University. All experimental procedures were performed following the Health Guideline of Animal Use and Care Committee of Guilin Medical University. The mice were randomly assigned to either the control diet (CD)-fed group or EtOH-fed group. An National Institute on Alcohol Abuse and Alcoholism (NIAAA) model was constructed as earlier described with minor modifications (Bertola et al., 2013). Briefly, following a one-week period of acclimation using a control liquid diet, the mice of the EtOH-fed group were fed ethanol (5% v/v) liquid diets (LD) (Trophic Animal Feed High-Tech Co., Ltd., Nantong, China), whereas the mice in the CD-fed group received LD. All mice were pair-fed for four weeks. Mice were euthanized and we collected blood and liver tissues for further analysis.

Adeno-Associated Virus Administration

The full mouse miR-378b sequences were amplified by PCR from mouse genomic DNA and cloned into pAAV-MCS digested by *BamHI* and *HindIII*. The adeno-associated virus (AAV, serotype 9, a gift from GeneChem, Shanghai, China), which has higher infection efficiency and induces long-lasting expression, was used in packaging recombinant AAV (Mingozzi and High, 2011). The packaged adeno-associated virus was named AAV-miR-378b. The empty (untransformed) adeno-associated virus vector named AAV-NC and served as control. Then, AAV-miR-378b, AAV-NC were given at a dose of 1×10^{11} vg per animal *via* tail vein injection using a 1-ml sterile syringe prior to ALD model construction.

Tolerance Tests

Glucose-tolerance test (GTT) and Insulin-tolerance test (ITT) were carried out as previously described with minor modification (Qu et al., 2019). Glucose-tolerance test (GTT) was conducted on mice that were fasted overnight (12 h). After measuring fasted blood glucose (FBG) levels, each mouse received an intraperitoneal (i.p.) glucose injection at a dose of 2 g/kg body weight. Blood glucose levels in the tail vein were assessed after 15, 30, 60, and 120 min, respectively. Insulin-tolerance test (ITT) was performed using mice that were fasted for 6 h. After measuring FBG levels, every mouse was treated with insulin at a dose of 0.75 U/kg body weight as shown in the figures. Blood glucose levels were taken at indicated time points.

Histopathological Analysis

Histopathological analysis was carried out as previously described with minor modification (Li et al., 2017). Liver tissues were fixed for 24 h in 10% phosphate-buffered formalin and buried in paraffin blocks, followed by staining for routine histological analysis. H&E staining was performed using standard protocols. Pathological changes were evaluated and photomicrographs were collected using an optical microscope (OLYMPUS BX41, OLYMPUS, Tokyo, Japan).

Serum and Liver Biochemical Analysis

Hepatic lipids were extracted using a previously reported method (Cheng et al., 2018). Total triglycerides (TGs) in sera and livers were assessed using an Erba XL-600 automatic biochemical analyzer with TG determination kits (U82811020, Guilin Unitech Medical Electronics Co., Ltd., Guilin, China). The levels of alanine aminotransferase (ALT) and aspartate aminotransferase (AST) were measured using commercially available diagnostic kits (Guilin Elite Medical Electronics Co., Ltd., Guilin, China) by the Erba XL-600 automatic biochemistry analyzer. The levels of glucose and insulin were measured using biochemical (U83730050, Guilin Unitech Medical Electronics Co., Ltd., Guilin, China) and ultra-sensitive mouse insulin immunoassay kit (Li Ka Shing Faculty of Medicine, The University of Hong Kong) according to the supplier's protocol, respectively. Homeostasis model assessment of insulin resistance (HOMA-IR) index was calculated according to the formula: [fasting glucose level (mM)] × [fasting serum insulin (mU/L)]/ 22.5 (Du et al., 2018).

Cell Culture

Human hepatocyte L-02 cells (no GDC079) were obtained from the China Center for Type Culture Collection of Wuhan University (Wuhan, China). The L-02 cells were cultured in Dulbecco's modified Eagle medium (DMEM) (817147, Thermo Fisher, MA, USA) medium containing 10% fetal bovine serum (FBS) (E600001-0100, Sangon Biotech, Inc., Shanghai, China) as well as 5% penicillin-streptomycin mixture (1212018, Sangon Biotech Inc., Shanghai, China). The cells were grown at 37°C in 5% CO_2 air. In addition, our previous study found that 200 mM ethanol successfully induced insulin resistance in L-02 cells (Cheng et al., 2019), so we performed a subsequent experiment with an ethanol concentration of 200 mM.

Measurement of Hepatocyte Glycogen Content

The glycogen content of L-02 cells and liver were assessed using glycogen kits (A043-1-1, Nanjing Jiancheng Bioengineering Institute, Nanjing, China) using the anthrone reagent method. Glycogen levels were normalized to the observed total protein contents. Total protein concentration was measured using the bicinchoninic acid assay (BCA) kit (P0010S, Beyotime Biotechnology, Beijing, China) and conducted following the supplier's protocols.

Plasmid Construction and Transfection

The synthetic miR-378b mimic, inhibitor, and negative control RNA were obtained from GeneChem (Shanghai, China). Transfection was conducted using Gene Pulser Xcell™ Electroporation system (Bio-Rad Laboratories, Inc., Hercules, CA, USA) following the supplier's protocols. After 12 h transfection, the medium was changed to DMEM containing 200 mM ethanol. The treated cells were harvested after 48 h for the further analysis.

RNA Isolation and Quantitative Real-Time PCR

Total RNA of liver tissues or L-02 cells were extracted using TRIzol reagent (DP419, Tiangen Biotech Co., Ltd., Beijing, China), following the supplier's protocol. Before reverse transcription using FastQuant RT Kit (KR106, Tiangen Biotech Co., Ltd., Beijing, China), total RNA was quantified in a NanoDrop One Ultra Micro Nucleic Acid Protein Analyzer (Gene Company Ltd., Kunming, China). Target genes were amplified using the MJ PTC-200 PCR system (Bio-Rad, Hercules, CA, USA) and the RT PCR kit (2× Taq PCR Master Mix, Aidlab Biotech Co., Ltd., Beijing, China). The PCR products were identified using 1.5% agarose gel electrophoresis. The mRNA level of β-actin was used as an internal control. For miRNA detection, total RNA was reverse-transcribed using All-in-One™ miRNA First-Strand cDNA Synthesis kit (QP103, GeneCopoeia™, Guangzhou, China) and subsequently measured by quantitative real-time (qRT)-PCR using miR-378b specific primer (GeneCopoeia™, Guangzhou, China). The U6 was used as the reference gene on the expression levels of miR-378b. Primer sequences were listed as following: p110α (forward 5'-CCACGACCATCATCAGGTGAA-3'; reverse 5'-CCTCACGGAGGC ATTCTAAAGT -3'), IR (forward 5'-AAAACGAGGCCCGAAGATTTC-3'; reverse 5'-GAGCCCATAGACCCGGAAG-3').

Western Blotting and Antibodies

L-02 cells or liver tissues were lysed with RIPA lysis buffer (P0013B, Beyotime Institute of Biotechnology, Shanghai, China) supplemented with protease inhibitor (100×) and phosphatase inhibitor (C900369-0260, Sangon Biotech Inc., Shanghai, China). Protein concentrations were assessed using a modified form BCA protein concentration assay kit (Beyotime Bio Co., Nanjing, China). Proteins were separated by sodium dodecyl sulfate-polyacrylamide gel electrophoresis (SDS-PAGE) and then transferred onto the nitrocellulose membrane (Pall Co., NY, USA). Then, the membranes were incubated with the appropriate antibodies. The antigen-antibody complex on the membrane was detected with enhanced chemiluminescence (ECL) reagent (E002-100, 7sea Biotech Co., Shanghai, China). ImageJ was used for blotting and quantitative analysis. The intensity values were normalized to that of β-actin. The p110α antibody (#4249) was obtained from Cell Signaling Technology (Cell Signaling, Danvers, MA, USA). The phosphorylated AKT1 (D155022) and AKT1 (D151621) antibodies were purchased from Sangon Biotech Co., Ltd. (Shanghai, China). Primary antibodies against for p-IR Anti-Insulin Receptor (phospho Y1185) (ab62321), IR (ab131238), p85α (ab191606), AKT1 (ab227385), p-AKT1 (ab81283) were purchased from Abcam Technology (Cambridge, UK). The β-actin (TA-09), mouse anti-goat (EM3511-01) and goat anti-rabbit secondary antibodies (EM35110-01) were supplied by ZSGB Biotech Co., Ltd. (Beijing, China).

Co-Immunoprecipitation Assay

To study the relationship between p85α and p110α, an immunoprecipitation assay was performed in accordance with the manufacturer's approach. After homogenized as described above, liver tissues or cell lysates were incubated overnight with specific antibodies at 4°C. Then, the mixture with the pre-formed antibody-antigen complex was added to the protein A-coupled beads (C600688-A, Sangon Biotech Inc., Shanghai, China). After incubating for 2 h at 4°C, discarded the supernatant, and the beads were washed seven times using cold phosphate-buffered saline (PBS). After the final wash, 50 μl of the sample buffer were added and boiled for western blotting.

Luciferase Reporter Assays

To validate that IR/p110α gene is indeed the target of miR-378b, we purchased a plasmid harboring luciferase with the 3' UTR sequence of IR/p110α mRNA. Then, the mutant or wild-type of 3' UTR sequences of IR/p110α were inserted into the XbaI restriction sites of the pGL3 vector (GeneChem, Shanghai, China). 293T cells (Cell Bank of Chinese Academy of Sciences, Shanghai, China) infected with miR-378 mimics or ctrl RNA were seeded into 24-well plates. 0.6 μg pGL3 vector with above sequence was cotransfected with 0.05 μg pRL-TK vector into the cells by Lipofectamine 2000 (11668-019, Invitrogen, Carlsbad, CA, USA). At 48 h after transfection, 293T cells were harvested. The Dual-Luciferase Reporter Assay System (E2920, Promega, Madison, WI, USA) was used to measure luciferase activity.

Statistical Analysis

All the experiments were conducted at least thrice independently, and the results were expressed as the means ± SD. A p value <0.05 was deemed statistically significant. Statistical significance was evaluated using an analysis of variance (ANOVA) and the student's t-test. The software used for data analysis and drawing were GraphPad Prism 7.0 and Excel. No data, samples, or animals were excluded or omitted from reporting.

RESULTS

Expression Level of mir-378b Increased in Ethyl Alcohol Fed Mice

To evaluate the liver damage in EtOH-fed and CD-fed mice, HE staining was performed. Histopathological analysis revealed that the liver tissues of EtOH-fed mice had numerous fat vacuoles of variable size, the liver cell cord was irregularly structured, and the hepatic cells disorganized, whereas the liver tissues in CD-fed mice exhibited normal lobular structure with radiating hepatic cords, without signs of fatty tissue degeneration (**Figure 1A**). Furthermore, there was no remarkable difference in the weights between EtOH-fed and CD-fed mice (**Figure 1B**). However, the liver index of the EtOH-fed group increased by 43.4% compared with the CD-fed group (**Figure 1C**). Compared with the control group, liver TG and serum TG levels in the EtOH-fed mice significantly increased by 44.7 and 59.2%, respectively (**Figures 1D, E**).

The EtOH-fed mice showed higher FBG levels and impaired glucose processing throughout the body by GTT and ITT (**Figures 1F, G**). The HOMA-IR index in EtOH-fed mice also significantly increased by 339.7% compared with the controls. The results clearly showed that glucose tolerance and insulin tolerance were impaired, and hyperglycemia developed in EtOH-fed mice, which are the characteristics of insulin resistance (**Figures 1H–J**). Because this study was centered on miRNAs that are related to ethanol-induced insulin resistance, we employed EtOH-fed mice in identifying miRNAs that are modulated by alcohol. qRT-PCR analysis showed that miR-378b expression in the model mice was over three-fold greater than that in CD-fed mice (**Figure 1K**). These results suggest that liver miR-378b high expression level is related to liver insulin resistance.

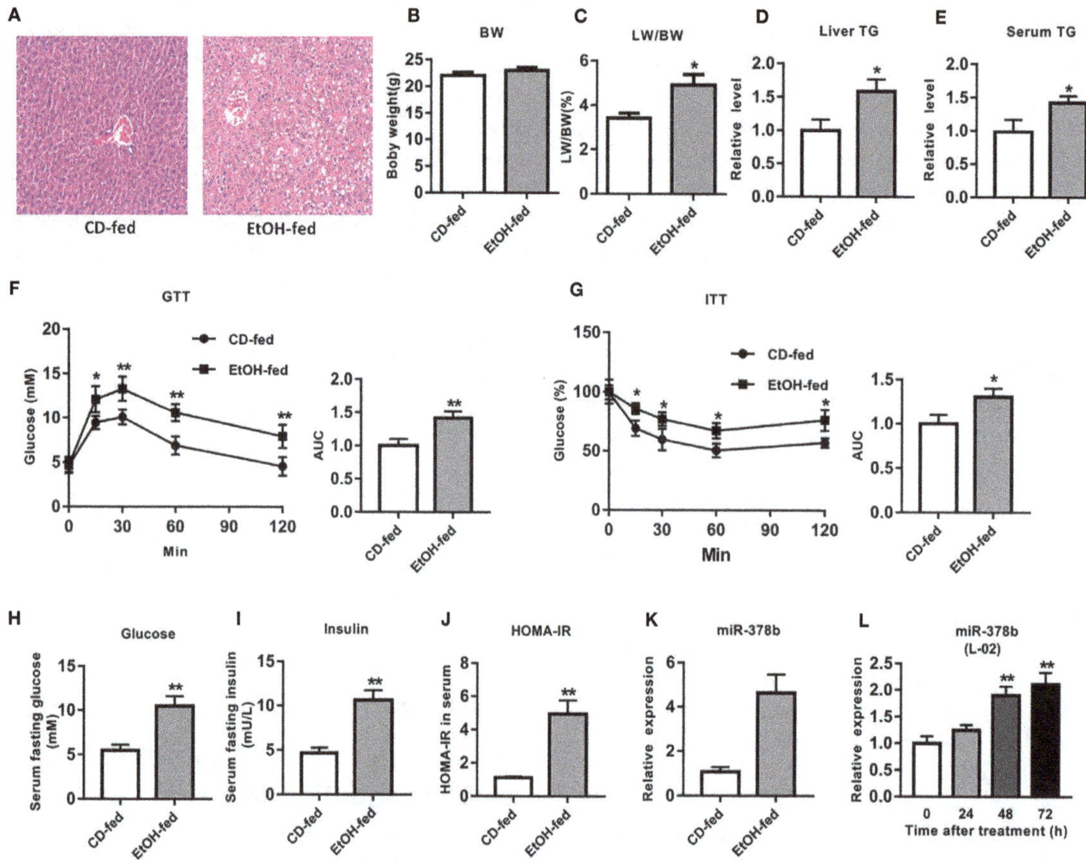

FIGURE 1 | miR-378b is upregulated in EtOH-fed mice and EtOH-induced L-02 cells. **(A)** Representative images of H&E staining of liver sections from control diet (CD)-fed mice (left) or EtOH-fed mice (right). **(B)** Body weights of the mice before the experiment and before being killed. **(C)** The liver index. **(D)** Liver triglyceride (TG) levels. **(E)** Serum TG levels. **(F)** Glucose-tolerance test (GTT) and area under the curve (AUC) data. **(G)** Insulin-tolerance test (ITT) and area under the curve (AUC) data. **(H)** Fasting serum glucose levels. **(I)** Fasting serum insulin concentrations. **(J)** Homeostasis model assessment of insulin resistance (HOMA-IR) index. **(K)** The expression level of miR-378b in liver tissues. **(L)** The expression level of miR-378b in L-02 cells. All data are expressed as the mean ± SD of at least three separate experiments (n=6). $^{*}p < 0.05$ *vs.* control; $^{**}p < 0.01$ *versus* control.

miR-378b Is Upregulated in EtOH-Induced L-02 Cells

To study the function of mir-378b in the control of insulin sensitivity, the levels of miR-378b in L-02 cells was examined under normal and ethanol-induced conditions. Subsequently, L-02 cells were treated with ethanol for different durations, then the levels of miR-378b were assessed by qRT-PCR. Interestingly, the expression levels of miR-378b significantly increased in time dependent manner after ethanol treatment, and the levels of miR-378b in L-02 cells induced by ethanol for 48 and 72 h significantly increased by 65.2 and 111.7%, respectively, when compared with the control group (**Figure 1L**). Together, these results indicate that miR-378b is upregulated in the EtOH-treated L-02 cells, thereby implicating miR-378b in insulin resistance.

Upregulation of miR-378b Disrupts Insulin Sensitivity in L-02 Cells

To research the impact of miR-378b on the insulin signaling pathway, L-02 cells were transfected with miR-378b mimic and incubated in the presence of ethanol. qRT-PCR analysis indicated that miR-378b level marked rise by 1.83-fold compared with the control group after miR-378b mimic transfection (**Figure 2A**). Moreover, the glucose levels of the medium in the miR-378b overexpression group and EtOH-induced group were significantly increased by 90.1 and 53.5%, respectively, when compared with the control group (**Figure 2B**). The miR-378b mimic also remarkable reduced glycogen levels by 26.7% in L-02 cells (**Figure 2C**). Furthermore, we analyzed the expression of the insulin signaling pathway in L-02 cells transfected with miR-378b mimic and found that the levels of IR and p-IR significantly decreased by 54.3 and 38.2%, respectively, after stimulation with EtOH relative to the control group (**Figure 2D**). In addition, the influence of p85α and p110α on the PI3K-AKT signaling pathway in hepatocytes were examined by immunoprecipitation. The results showed that the protein expression levels of p110α combined with p85α significantly decreased by 47.7% when transfected with miR-378b mimics and incubated in the presence of ethanol (**Figure

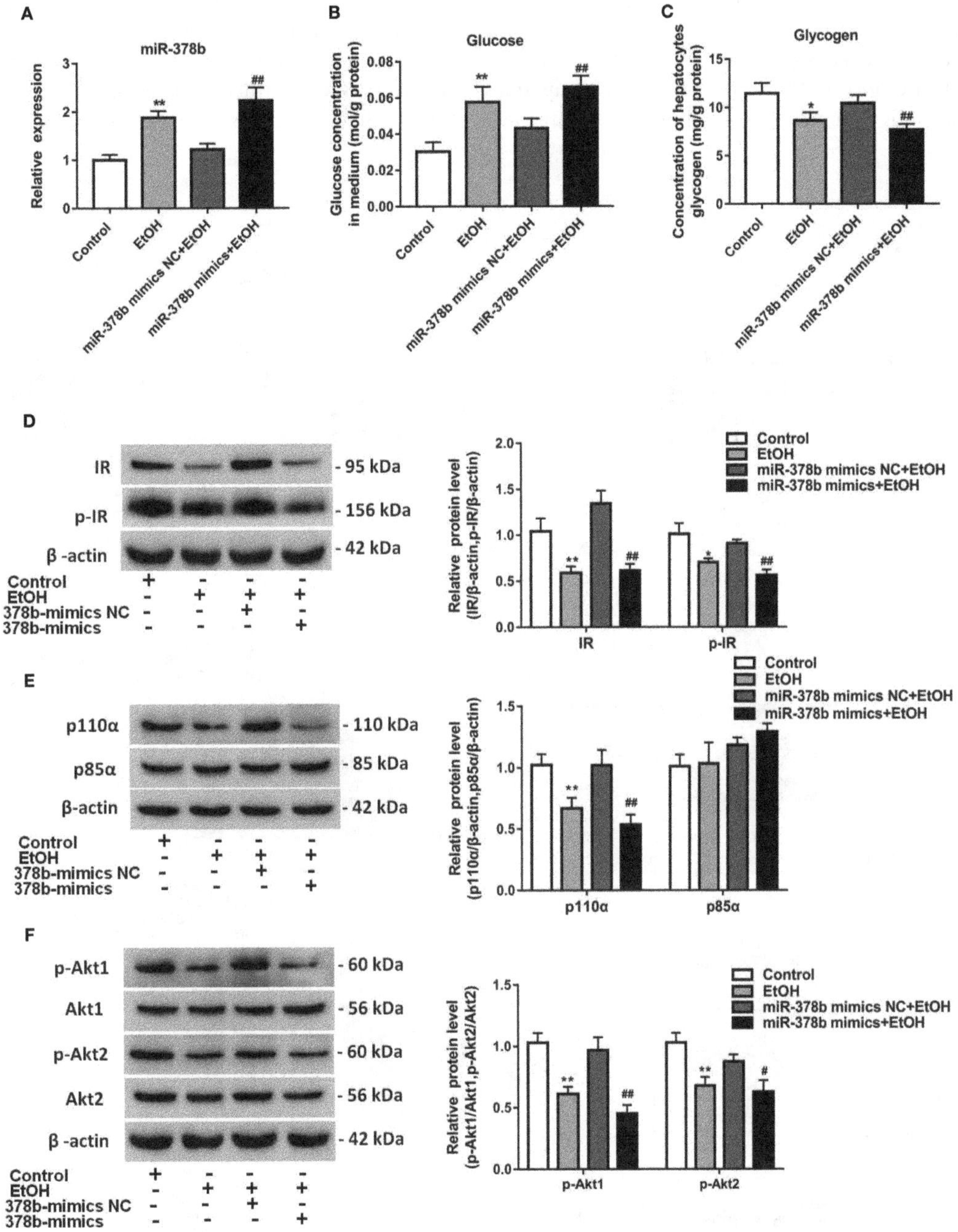

FIGURE 2 | miR-378b overexpression suppresses insulin sensitivity in L-02 cells. **(A)** The expression level of miR-378b in L-02 cells. **(B)** The glucose levels in medium. **(C)** The glycogen content in L-02 cells. **(D)** Western blot analysis for protein expression of insulin receptor (IR) and p-IR. **(E)** Western blot analysis for protein expression of p85α and p110α. **(F)** Western blot analysis for protein expression of Akt1, Akt 2, p-Akt1, p-Akt2. All data are expressed as the mean ± SD of at least three separate experiments. $^{*}p < 0.05$, $^{**}p < 0.01$ *vs*. control. $^{\#}p < 0.05$, $^{\#\#}p < 0.01$ *vs*. miR-378b-mimics NC.

2E). In addition, the protein expression levels of p-Akt1 and p-Akt2 markedly decreased by 53.4 and 28.2%, respectively, in the miR-378b overexpression group compared with the control groups (**Figure 2F**). In a word, these findings suggest that the over expressed miR-378b aggravates insulin resistance in L-02 cells.

Suppression of miR-378b Alleviates EtOH-Induced Insulin Resistance *In Vitro*

The expression of miR-378b increased in EtOH-induced insulin resistant L-02 cells. Insulin sensitivity impaired by miR-378b overexpression was also observed in L-02 cells. Based on the results earlier described, we postulated that miR-378b inhibition also enhances insulin sensitivity in conditions of EtOH-induced insulin resistance. To verify our hypothesis, we transfected L-02 cells with miR-378b inhibitor and incubated these in the presence of ethanol. **Figure 3A** shows that the level of miR-378b significantly ascended by 83.2% in the ethanol group and transfection of the miR-378b inhibitor significantly decreased its level by 28.4% in L-02 cells. In addition, compared with the control group, the glucose levels in the medium significantly decreased by 37.1%, and glycogen levels significantly increased by 27.6% with transfection of miR-378b inhibitor in L-02 cells (**Figures 3B, C**). Furthermore, we analyzed the expression of the insulin signaling pathway in L-02 cells transfected with miR-

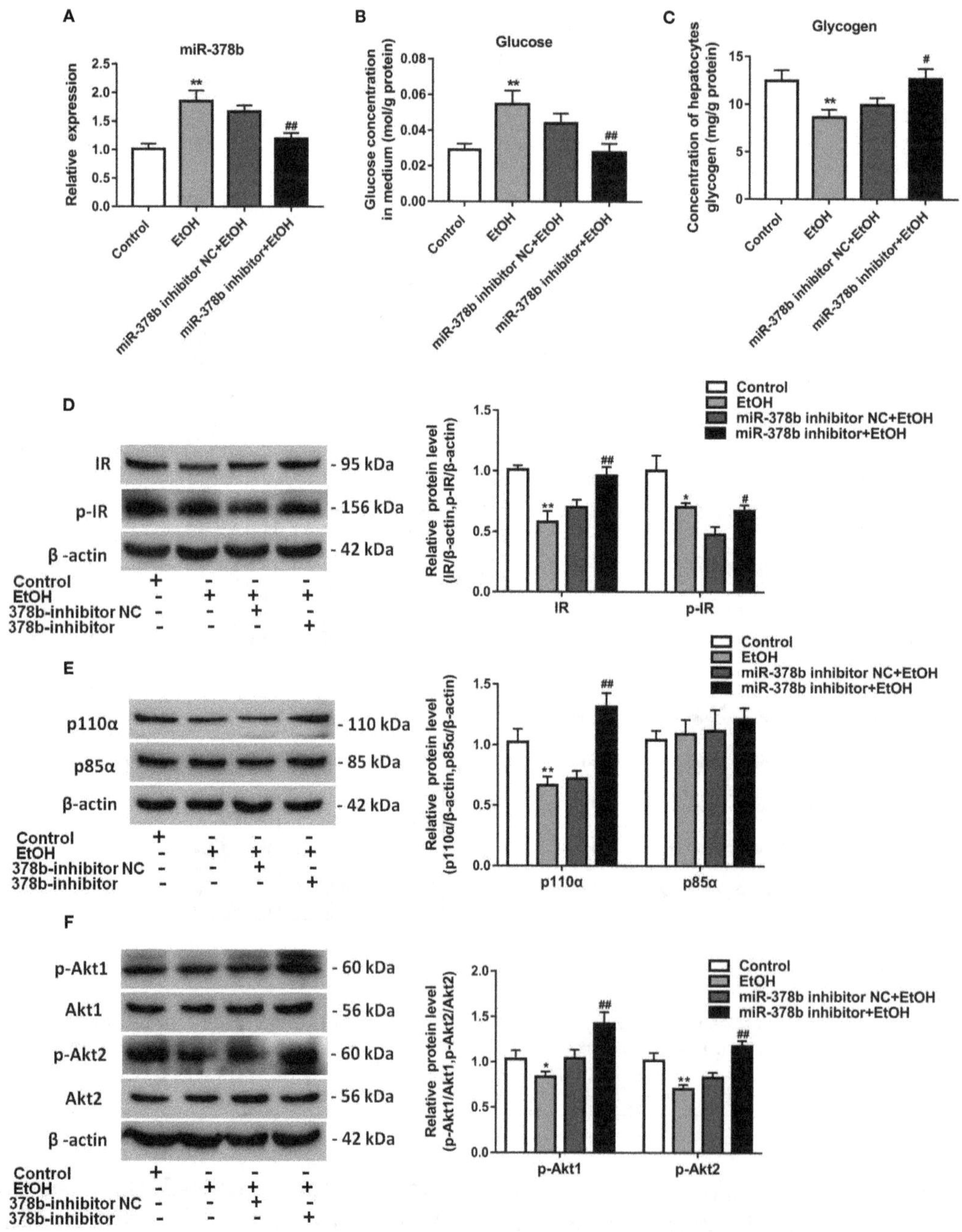

FIGURE 3 | Suppression of miR-378b alleviates EtOH-induced insulin resistance *in vitro*. **(A)** The expression level of miR-378b in L-02 cells. **(B)** The glucose levels in medium. **(C)** The glycogen content in L-02 cells. **(D)** Western blot analysis for protein expression of insulin receptor (IR) and p-IR. **(E)** Western blot analysis for protein expression of p85α and p110α. **(F)** Western blot analysis for protein expression of Akt1, Akt 2, p-Akt1, p-Akt2. All data were expressed as the mean ± SD of at least three separate experiments. $^{*}p < 0.05$, $^{**}p < 0.01$ *vs*. control. $^{\#}p < 0.05$, $^{\#\#}p < 0.01$ *vs*. miR-378b-inhibitor NC.

378b inhibitor and found that the levels of IR and p-IR, significantly increased by 37.1 and 41.2%, respectively, in the L-02 cells transfected with miR-378b compared with the negative control groups (**Figure 2D**). Furthermore, immunoprecipitation showed that the protein levels of p110α and p85α significantly increased by 82.4% after transfection with the miR-378b inhibitor and incubated in the presence of ethanol (**Figure 3E**). In addition, the protein levels of p-Akt1 and p-Akt2 expressed in liver tissue significantly increased by 36.9 and 42.3%, respectively, in the miR-378b inhibitor group compared with the negative control groups (**Figure 2F**). As expected, these effects of ethanol were reversed after transfecting with the miR-378b inhibitor, indicating that inhibition of miR-378b increased insulin sensitivity in L-02 cells (**Figures 3D–F**).

miR-378b Directly Targets IR and p110α

To elucidate the molecular mechanism underlying the miR-378b-mediated insulin signaling pathway, using TargetScan bioinformatics tools, we hypothesized that IR and p110α are two potential targets of miR-378b, with their 3′ UTRs as miRNA-binding sites (**Figures 4A, B**). Bioinformatics analysis showed that IR and p110α are key components of insulin signaling. To further investigate whether these observed suppressive effects are direct actions, specific fragments of the wild-type and mutated IR and p110α 3′ UTRs were ligated to a luciferase reporter vector. The results showed that miR-378b mimics reduced luciferase activity by 26.2 and 129.8% of the reporter containing human IR and p110α-3′ UTRs, respectively, in 293T cells but had no effect on the reporters with mutated IR and p110α-3′ UTRs (**Figures 4C, D**), suggesting that IR and p110α are indeed miR-378b targets. To further determine whether p110α and IR are regulated by miR-378b, we transfected L-02 cells with either miR-378b mimics or inhibitor. IR and p110α proteins in the L-02 cells were respectively downregulated by 42 and 36.6% after transfection with the miR-378b mimics (**Figures 4E, G**). In contrast, L-02 cells transfected with miR-378b inhibitor resulted in the upregulation of IR and p110α by 54.2 and 142.8%, respectively (**Figures 4F, H**). No significant change in the mRNA level of IR and p110α (**Figures 4I–L**). On the basis of those study results, we suggested that the possible mechanism of miR-378b targeting IR and p110α is that miR-378b partially binds to the mRNA of IR and regulates the translation process of IR and p110α, but has no effect on the transcription process of IR and p110α.

miR-378b Overexpression Aggravates Insulin Signaling *In Vivo*

To study the influence of miR-378b overexpression on EtOH-induced insulin resistance *in vivo*, we injected EtOH-fed mice with adeno-associated virus particles containing AAV-miR-378b-up or AAV-miR-378b-up-NC *via* tail vein. **Figure 5A** shows that the transfer effect of AAV-miR-378b-up or AAV-miR-378b-up-NC was almost the same in the tissue of EtOH-fed mice liver. MiR-378b expression in the liver of AAV-miR-378b-up-treated mice was 3.54-fold higher than that in the liver of the negative control mice (**Figure 5D**). Moreover, the TG levels in both serum and liver significantly increased by 34.1 and 39.8% in EtOH-fed mice after AAV-miR-378b-up injection (**Figure 5B**). The increase in lipid accumulation in EtOH-fed mice overexpressing miR-378b was further confirmed by H&E staining (**Figure 5C**). Moreover, the results showed that the ALT and AST levels were significantly increased by AAV-miR-378b-up-treated (**Figures 5E, F**). In addition, compared with the AAV-miR-378b-up-NC group, the glycogen levels significantly decreased by AAV-miR-378b-up-treated (**Figures 5G**). Furthermore, miR-378b overexpression resulted in impaired glucose tolerance and insulin tolerance (**Figures 5H, I**). These results show that miR-378b overexpression influences insulin signaling.

The above findings prompted us to investigate the effect of miR-378b on the insulin signaling pathway. Therefore, to assess whether the upregulation of miR-378b induces insulin resistance in EtOH-fed mice, we injected miR-378b into EtOH-fed mice and assessed the phosphorylation of various insulin signaling intermediates. MiR-378b overexpression significantly reduced IR phosphorylation and IR expression by 49.2 and 26.9%, respectively, in EtOH-fed mice (**Figure 5J**). In addition, phosphorylation of the downstream molecules of IR such as Akt1, and Akt2 were significantly reduced by 41.9%, and 40.8%, respectively (**Figures 5J, L**). Furthermore, the protein expression of p110α bound to p85α was also significantly reduced by 37.1% in EtOH-fed mice injected with AAV-miR-378b-up (**Figure 5K**). Based on these results, we proposed that the over expressed miR-378b aggravates insulin resistance *in vivo*.

Loss of miR-378b Improves Insulin Resistance in EtOH-Fed Mice

Suppression of miR-378b protected hepatocytes from EtOH-induced insulin resistance. Next, the results observed in L-02 cells were extended to mouse models of EtOH-fed insulin resistance. Adeno-associated virus expressing a miR-378b-inhibitor (AAV-miR-378b-down) or a negative control adeno-associated virus vector containing GFP (AAV-miR-378b-down-NC) were injected from the tail vein into the liver of mice. The adeno-associated virus showed fluorescence, and the transfection efficiency of AAV-miR-378b-down or AAV-miR-378b-down-NC was almost the same by fluorescence microscopy (**Figure 6A**). Transfection of AAV-miR-378b-down reduced the expression of miR-378b by 30.3% compared with the AAV-miR-378b-down-NC group (**Figure 6D**). Moreover, AAV-miR-378b-down infection resulted in a marked reduction in hepatic TG content by 17.2%, as well as serum TG levels by 24.7% in EtOH-fed mice (**Figure 6B**). The H&E staining revealed that the hepatic lipid accumulation levels were significantly elevated compared with the controls in both chronic alcohol diet-fed mice as well as AAV-miR-378b-down-NC infected mice (**Figure 6C**). Moreover, the results showed that the increased levels of ALT and AST induced by ethanol in serum were significantly attenuated by AAV-miR-378b-down- treated (**Figures 6E, F**). In addition, compared with the AAV-miR-378b-down-NC group, the glycogen levels were significantly increased by AAV-miR-378b-down-treated (**Figures 6G**). In contrast, administration of

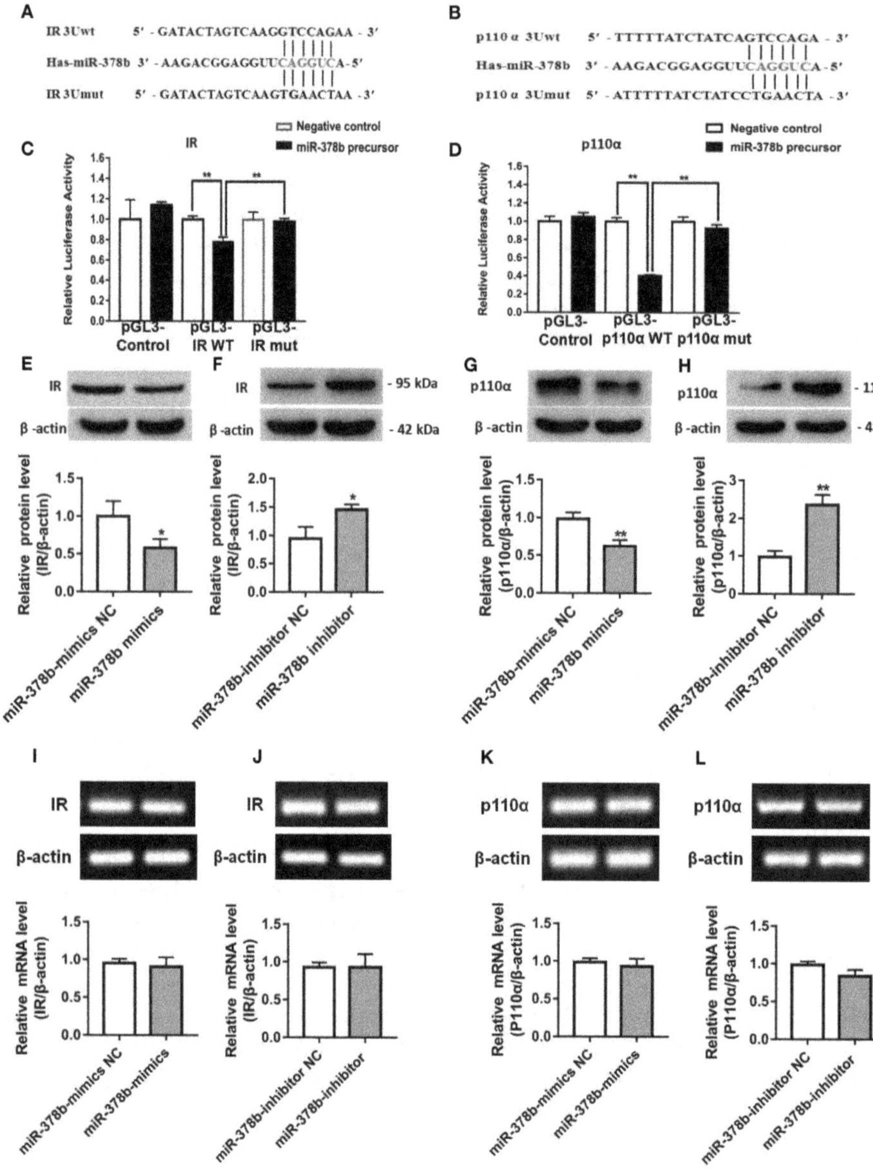

FIGURE 4 | miR-378b directly targets IR and p110α. **(A, B)** Predicted duplex formation between miR-378b and human wild-type/mutant IR-3'-UTR (IR-3U-wt/mut) or human wild-type/mutant p110α-3'-UTR (p110α-3U-wt/mut). **(C, D)** Luciferase reporter assay for the interaction between wild-type 3'-UTR of insulin receptor (IR) or of p110α and miR-378b, as well as mutant 3'-UTR of IR or of p110α and miR-378b in the 293T cells. **(E–H)** Western blot analysis for protein expression of IR or p110α in L-02 cells. **(I–L)** Messenger RNA (mRNA) expression levels of IR or p110α in L-02 cells. All data were expressed as the mean ± SD of at least three separate experiments. *$p < 0.05$, **$p < 0.01$ *vs*. control.

AAV-miR-378b-down significantly reduced the development of alcoholic insulin resistance. GTT showed that exogenous glucose was cleared faster in AAV-miR-378b-down-treated mice than in AAV-miR-378b-down-NC-treated mice. Meanwhile, ITT revealed that injection of miR-378b increased insulin sensitivity in EtOH-fed mice (**Figures 6H, I**).

To address the mechanisms underlying EtOH-induced insulin resistance regulation by miR-378b, we tested the action of miR-378b on the expression of insulin signaling intermediates by adeno-associated virus-mediated inhibition of miR-378b. As expected, western blot analysis showed that inhibition of miR-378b significantly increased IR levels by 67% and IR, Akt1, and Akt2 phosphorylation levels by 68.1, 41.6, and 28.4%, respectively, in EtOH-fed mice (**Figures 6J, L**). Moreover, we assessed the effects of p85α and p110α on liver PI3K-AKT signaling pathway using immunoprecipitation. p85α protein expression levels in mice did not change with injection of AAV-miR-378b-down. However, the protein expression of p110α bound to p85α was significantly increased by 69.3% in EtOH-fed mice injected with AAV-miR-378b-down (**Figure**

6K). Collectively, these findings indicate that inhibition of miR-378b in EtOH-fed mice improves insulin resistance.

DISCUSSION

Growing evidence suggests that miRNAs play central roles in various aspects of insulin resistance. Furthermore, the development of insulin resistance controls the progression from simple steatosis toward cirrhosis in ALD (Carr and Correnti, 2015). Thus, elucidating the mechanistic processes underlying insulin signaling may improve our understanding of the development of alcohol-induced insulin resistance. In the present study, we found that miR-378b expression boosted in the EtOH-fed mice and EtOH-trigger L-02 cells and at the same time, it was accompanied with insulin signal pathway dysfunction. Further investigation show that the over expressed miR-378b reduced PI3K/AKT activation, whereas inhibition of miR-378b improved insulin resistance *in vivo and in vitro*. Our findings demonstrate for the first time that miR-378b has a key role in alcohol-induced hepatic insulin resistance.

MiRNA can directly or indirectly regulate insulin sensitivity through epigenetic mechanisms (Yang et al., 2012). The possible targets of differentially expressed miRNAs have central roles in insulin secretion, lipid metabolism, glucose metabolism, and inflammation, which are the main process involved in the occurrence and development of alcoholic liver disease (Hartmann and Tacke, 2016; Satishchandran et al., 2018). A previous study has shown that mice with liver fibrosis have downregulated miR-378b levels in the liver (Hyun et al., 2016). However, our results suggested that miR-378b expression in the livers of NIAAA mice (EtOH-fed) were significantly increased. Some factors such as feeding periods, different diet compositions, and degree of liver damage may explain the observed contradiction. Previous reports have display that the expression patterns of circulatory and hepatic miRNA shows a

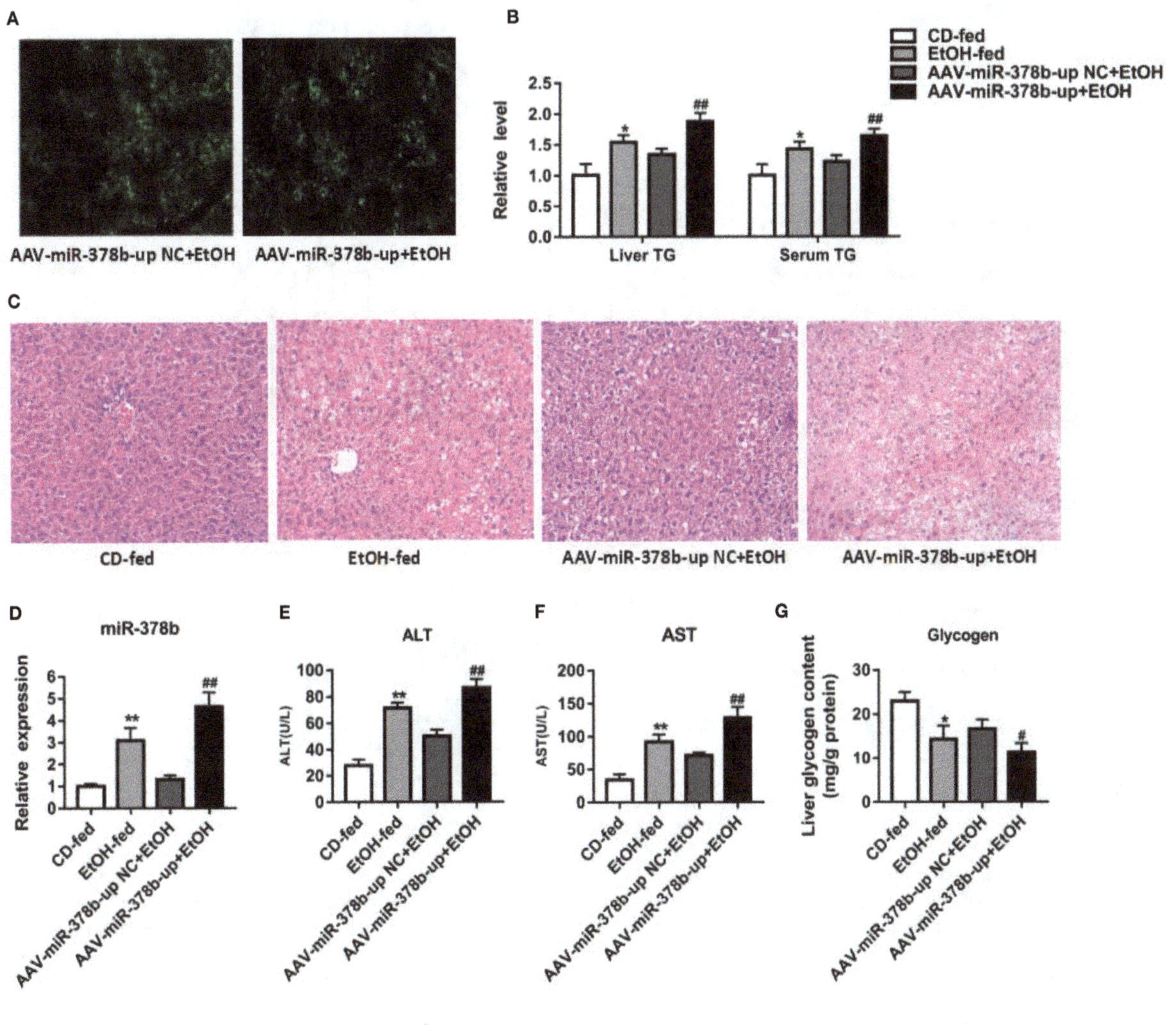

FIGURE 5 | Continued

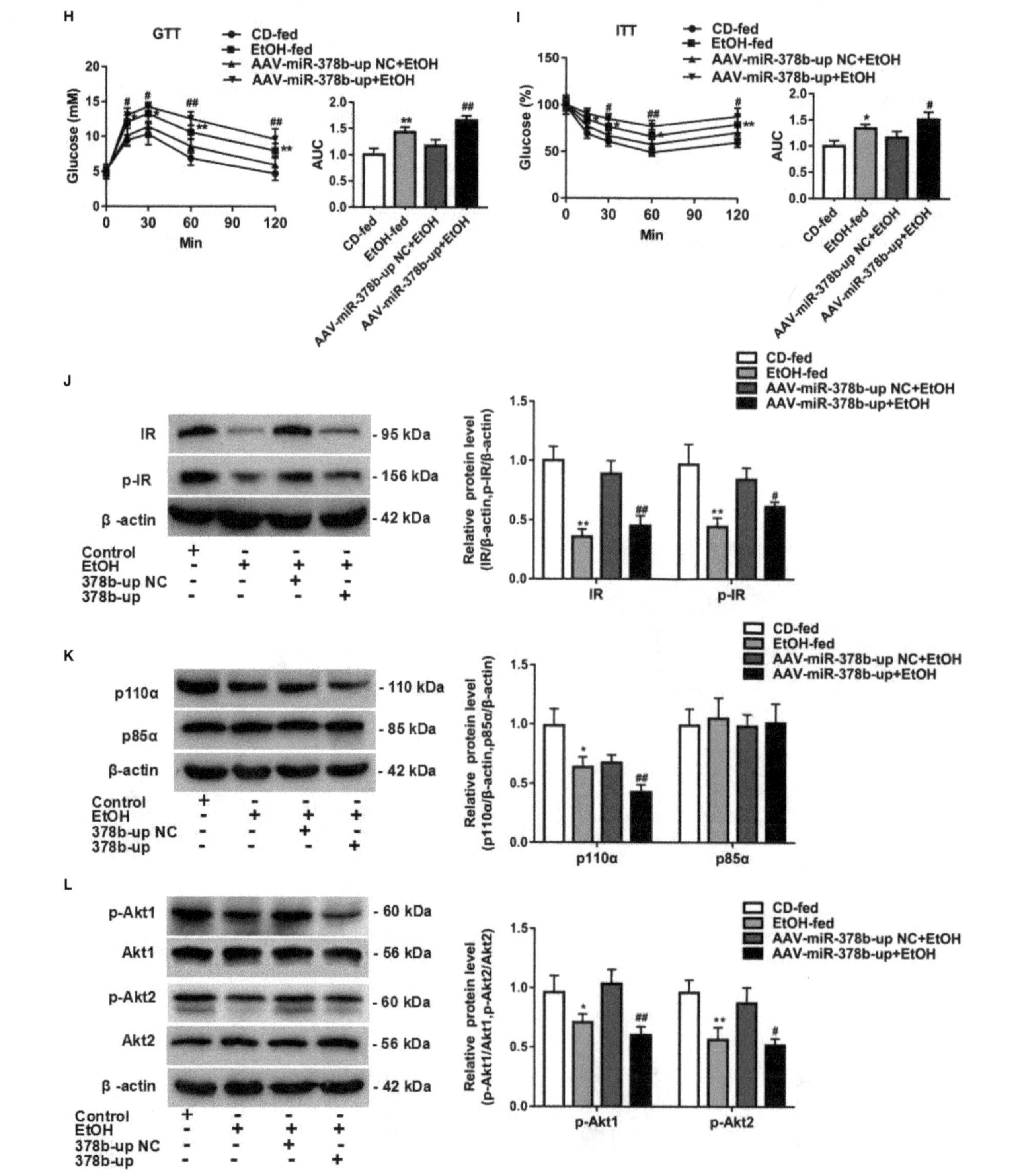

FIGURE 5 | miR-378b overexpression aggravates insulin signaling *in vivo.* **(A)** The infection efficiency of AAV-miR-378b-up NC and AAV-miR-378b-up in liver tissue. **(B)** Liver and serum triglyceride (TG) levels. **(C)** Representative images of H&E staining of liver sections. **(D)** The expression of miR-378b in liver tissue. **(E)** Serum alanine aminotransferase (ALT) levels. **(F)** Serum aspartate aminotransferase (AST) levels. **(G)** Liver glycogen content. **(E)** Serum TG levels. **(H)** Glucose-tolerance test (GTT). **(I)** Insulin-tolerance test (ITT). **(J)** Western blot analysis for protein expression of insulin receptor (IR) and p-IR. **(K)** Western blot analysis for protein expression of p85α and p110α. **(L)** Western blot analysis for protein expression of Akt1, Akt 2, p-Akt1, p-Akt2. All data were expressed as the mean ± SD of at least three separate experiments (n=6). $^{*}p < 0.05$, $^{**}p < 0.01$ compared with the CD-fed group. $^{\#}p < 0.05$, $^{\#\#}p < 0.01$ compared with the AAV-miR-378b-up NC group.

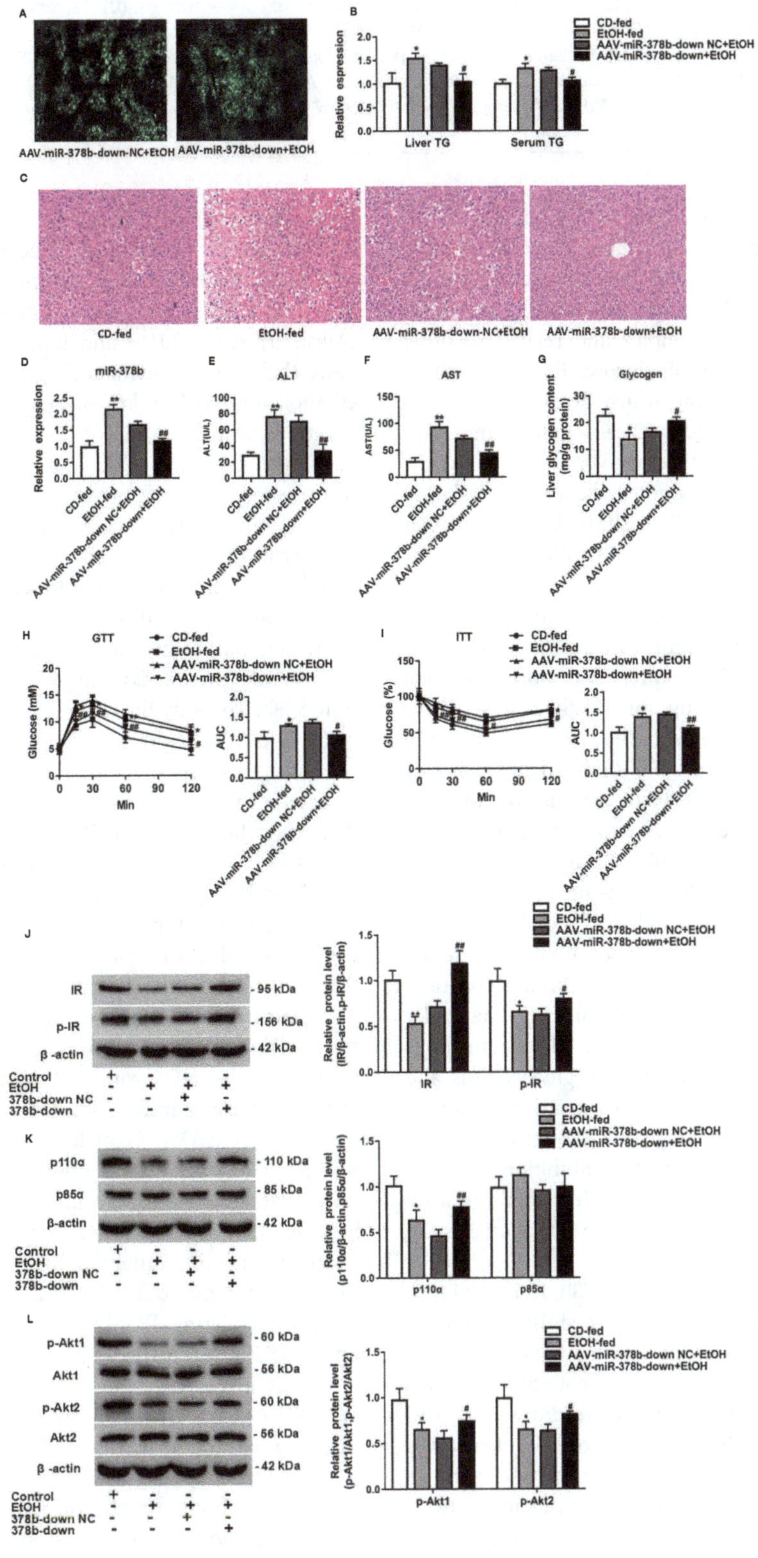

FIGURE 6 | Continued

FIGURE 6 | Loss of miR-378b improves insulin resistance in EtOH-fed mice. **(A)** The infection efficiency of AAV-miR-378b-down NC and AAV-miR-378b-down in liver tissue. **(B)** Liver and serum triglyceride (TG) levels. **(C)** Representative images of H&E staining of liver sections. **(D)** The expression of miR-378b in liver tissue. **(E)** Serum alanine aminotransferase (ALT) levels. **(F)** Serum aspartate aminotransferase (AST) levels. **(G)** Liver glycogen content. **(E)** Serum TG levels. **(H)** Glucose-tolerance test (GTT). **(I)** Insulin-tolerance test (ITT). **(J)** Western blot analysis for protein expression of insulin receptor (IR) and p-IR. **(K)** Western blot analysis for protein expression of p85α and p110α. **(L)** Western blot analysis for protein expression of Akt1, Akt 2, p-Akt1, p-Akt2. All data were expressed as the mean ± SD of at least three separate experiments (n=6). *$p < 0.05$, **$p < 0.01$ compared with the control diet (CD)-fed group. #$p < 0.05$, ##$p < 0.01$ compared with the AAV-miR-378b-down NC group.

reverse trend (Coulouarn et al., 2009; Choi et al., 2013). Furthermore, a study suggested that alcohol overconsumption and overnutrition could promote the development of insulin resistance (Carr and Correnti, 2015). Furthermore, the metabolic disorders of rodent species are complex and related to other factors, including elevated levels of glucose, lipid, as well as hormones. Therefore, to determine which factor controls the expression of miR-378b, we treated L-02 cells with ethanol. Our results showed that treatment with ethanol notably raised the miR-378b expression level and disrupted the phosphorylation levels of insulin signaling pathway. This study data suggest that ethanol controls miR-378b expression, and miR-378b may be involved in hepatic insulin resistance.

miR-378b, a member of the miR-378 family, is highly conserved across species, from chimp to humans. A previous study has shown that miR-378b is expressed in normal human dermal fibroblasts, and circulating miR-378b is a sensitive biomarker for photo-aging (Joo et al., 2017). It was also found to protect dermal fibroblasts from UVB-inhibited collagen I by targeting SIRT6 (Kim et al., 2017). However, the role of miR-378b in the pathogenesis of hepatic insulin resistance remains elusive. To determine the role of miR-378b in hepatic insulin resistance, we transfected miR-378b mimics or inhibitor or NC into L-02 cells. As expected, our research data indicated that the over expressed miR-378b lowered insulin sensitivity and caused the insulin signaling pathway dysfunction. On the contrary, further study indicated that miR-378b blocker markedly improved insulin sensitivity in L-02 cells. These findings suggest that the liver plays a central role in glucogenesis and lipogenesis (Baranowski et al., 2014). In this study, we observed that the overexpression of miR-378b in L-02 cells markedly decreased glycogen content, whereas the inhibition of miR-378b enhanced glycogen content. In brief, our research demonstrated that miR-378b has a negative effect on insulin signaling pathway *in vitro*.

In the current study, two targets of miR-378b, IR and p110α, have been identified and experimentally verified. IR is a ligand-activated receptor and member of the tyrosine kinase family of transmembrane signaling proteins, which are collectively known as major regulators of cell growth, differentiation, and metabolism (Lee and Pilch, 1994). Furthermore, IR also serves as an important center of Insulin signal transduction, with its activation tightly regulated. During insulin stimulation, IR is activated *via* autophosphorylation, which consequently phosphorylates numerous IRS proteins. PI3K, which is composed of a catalytic subunit p85 and regulatory subunit p110, functions in various pathological and physiological conditions, including metabolic regulation, immune responses, and cancer (Pentassuglia et al., 2016). p110α, a subunit of Pi3k that is known to be highly expressed in mammalian tissues. Previous studies on p110α have focused on breast (Bhat-Nakshatri et al., 2016) and lung cancer (Bonelli et al., 2015). Nevertheless, our understanding of biological effect of p110α in ethanol-induced insulin resistance is limited. A previous study suggested that inhibition of IR or p110α significantly decreases AKT phosphorylation (Liu et al., 2014; Srivastava et al., 2018). In this research, our data indicated that the levels of IR and p110α were significantly lowered in the liver of NIAAA mice. Furthermore, In L-02 cells, miR-378b is usually negatively correlated with IR or P110. In addition, using TargetScan, IR and p110α were identified as miR-378b target genes. Luciferase constructs harboring the 3'-UTRs of IR or p110α resulted in significantly lower activity in 293T cells that were overexpressing miR-378b. To verify the role of miR-378b in the downregulation of IR or p110α, we transfected miR-378b mimics, inhibitor, or NC into L-02 cells. MiR-378b overexpression resulted in a decrease in IR or p110α expression, whereas the downregulation of miR-378b improved IR or p110α expression. These findings further support the contribution of miR-378b in hepatic insulin resistance.

We also established an NIAAA mice model using Lieber-DeCarli liquid diet supplemented with 5% ethanol. We observed that miR-378b expression increased in the livers of EtOH-fed mice. Furthermore, our research also verified the impairment of the insulin signaling pathway in the liver of EtOH-fed mice relative to the NC group. We conducted a gain-of-function experiment using miR-378b. After tail vein injection of AAV-miR-378b or AAV-NC, at least a two-fold increase in hepatic miR-378b expression was observed in the livers of EtOH-fed mice relative to the NC group. Remarkably, the over expressed hepatic miR-378b pronouncedly increased TG levels and disrupted insulin signaling, whereas inhibition of miR-378b significantly reduced TG levels and enhanced insulin signaling by downregulating IR/p110α. Our findings indicate that the upregulation of miR-378b contributes to hepatic insulin resistance in EtOH-fed mice. In sum, Our research show that miR-378b has a negative effect on activation of the insulin signaling pathway *in vitro*.

In conclusion, our researches show that excessive drinking can induce high expression of miR-378b. miR-378b has incomplete binding to IR and p110α mRNA 3-UTRs, so it does not affect the stability of IR and p110α mRNA and does not affect the transcription process. Instead, it can affect the protein translation process of IR and p110α mRNA, so that IR and p110α proteins are down-regulated in the liver, and AKT phosphorylation is reduced, affecting the insulin signaling cascade in the liver. Due to the inhibition of the PI3K/AKT pathway, glycogen synthesis in the liver is reduced and blood glucose is increased, which promote the *de novo* synthesis of liver fatty acids and increase adrenoleukodystrophy (VLDL) secretion, leading to fatty liver and hyperlipidemia. High expression of miR-378b in the liver is closely related to ALD formation, and miR-378b is a promising new target for ALD drug therapy.

AUTHOR CONTRIBUTIONS

Y-YL and Y-JZ conducted experiments, analyzed data, and wrote manuscript. Y-ZW, Y-YF, C-FY, and ZM conducted experiments and analyzed data. LL, Y-WL, and QC analyzed data and revised manuscript. LL and Y-WL served as the guarantors of this work and as such, received full access to all the results in the study and take full responsibility for data integrity and analytical accuracy.

REFERENCES

Aberg, F., Helenius-Hietala, J., Puukka, P., Farkkila, M., and Jula, A. (2018). Interaction between alcohol consumption and metabolic syndrome in predicting severe liver disease in the general population. *Hepatol. (Baltimore Md.)* 67, 2141–2149. doi: 10.1002/hep.29631

Baranowski, M., Zabielski, P., Blachnio-Zabielska, A. U., Harasim, E., Chabowski, A., Górski, J., et al. (2014). Insulin-sensitizing effect of LXR agonist T0901317 in high-fat fed rats is associated with restored muscle GLUT4 expression and insulin-stimulated AS160 phosphorylation. *Cell. Physiol. Biochem. : Int. J. Exp. Cell. Physiol. Biochem. Pharmacol.* 33, 1047–1057. doi: 10.1159/000358675

Bartel, D. P. (2004). MicroRNAs: genomics, biogenesis, mechanism, and function. *Cell* 116, 281–297. doi: 10.1016/S0092-8674(04)00045-5

Bartel, B. (2005). MicroRNAs directing siRNA biogenesis. *Nat. Struct. Mol. Biol.* 12, 569–571. doi: 10.1038/nsmb0705-569

Bertola, A., Mathews, S., Ki, S. H., Wang, H., and Gao, B. (2013). Mouse model of chronic and binge ethanol feeding (the NIAAA model). *Nat. Protoc.* 8, 627–637. doi: 10.1038/nprot.2013.032

Bhat-Nakshatri, P., Goswami, C. P., Badve, S., Magnani, L., Lupien, M., and Nakshatri, H. (2016). Molecular Insights of Pathways Resulting from Two Common PIK3CA Mutations in Breast Cancer. *Cancer Res.* 76, 3989–4001. doi: 10.1158/0008-5472.CAN-15-3174

Bonelli, M. A., Cavazzoni, A., Saccani, F., Alfieri, R. R., Quaini, F., La Monica, S., et al. (2015). Inhibition of PI3K Pathway Reduces Invasiveness and Epithelial-to-Mesenchymal Transition in Squamous Lung Cancer Cell Lines Harboring PIK3CA Gene Alterations. *Mol. Cancer Ther.* 14 (8), 1916–1927. doi: 10.1158/1535-7163.MCT-14-0892

Carr, R. M., and Correnti, J. (2015). Insulin resistance in clinical and experimental alcoholic liver disease. *Ann. New York Acad. Sci.* 1353, 1–20. doi: 10.1111/nyas.12787

Chacko, K. R., and Reinus, J. (2016). Spectrum of Alcoholic Liver Disease. *Clinics Liver Dis.* 20, 419–427. doi: 10.1016/j.cld.2016.02.002

Chen, H., Shen, F., Sherban, A., Nocon, A., Li, Y., Wang, H., et al. (2018). DEP domain-containing mTOR-interacting protein suppresses lipogenesis and ameliorates hepatic steatosis and acute-on-chronic liver injury in alcoholic liver disease. *Hepatol. (Baltimore Md.)* 68, 496–514. doi: 10.1002/hep.29849

Cheng, Q., Li, Y. W., Yang, C. F., Zhong, Y. J., He, H., Zhu, F.-c., et al. (2018). Methyl ferulic acid attenuates ethanol-induced hepatic steatosis by regulating AMPK *and* FoxO1 Pathways in Rats and L-02 cells. *Chemico-Biol. Interact.* 291, 180–189. doi: 10.1016/j.cbi.2018.06.028

Cheng, Q., Li, Y. W., Yang, C. F., Zhong, Y. J., and Li, L. (2019). Ethanol-Induced Hepatic Insulin Resistance is Ameliorated by Methyl Ferulic Acid Through the PI3K/AKT Signaling Pathway. *Front. Pharmacol.* 10, 949. doi: 10.3389/fphar.2019.00949

Choi, Y., Dienes, H. P., and Krawczynski, K. (2013). Kinetics of miR-122 expression in the liver during acute HCV infection. *PloS One* 8, e76501. doi: 10.1371/journal.pone.0076501

Coulouarn, C., Factor, V. M., Andersen, J. B., Durkin, M. E., and Thorgeirsson, S. S. (2009). Loss of miR-122 expression in liver cancer correlates with suppression of the hepatic phenotype and gain of metastatic properties. *Oncogene* 28, 3526–3536. doi: 10.1038/onc.2009.211

Du, X., Li, X., Chen, L., Zhang, M., Lei, L., Gao, W., et al. (2018). Hepatic miR-125b inhibits insulin signaling pathway by targeting PIK3CD. *J. Cell Physiol.* 233 (8), 6052–6066. doi: 10.1002/jcp.26442

Frost, R. J., and Olson, E. N. (2011). Control of glucose homeostasis and insulin sensitivity by the Let-7 family of microRNAs. *Proc. Natl. Acad. Sci. United States America* 108, 21075–21080. doi: 10.1073/pnas.1118922109

Hartmann, P., and Tacke, F. (2016). Tiny RNA with great effects: miR-155 in alcoholic liver disease. *J. Hepatol.* 64 (6), 1214–1216. doi: 10.1016/j.jhep.2016.02.039

He, J., de la Monte, S., and Wands, J. R. (2007). Acute ethanol exposure inhibits insulin signaling in the liver. *Hepatol. (Baltimore Md.)* 46, 1791–1800. doi: 10.1002/hep.21904

Hyun, J., Wang, S., Kim, J., Rao, K. M., Park, S. Y., Chung, I., et al. (2016). MicroRNA-378 limits activation of hepatic stellate cells and liver fibrosis by suppressing Gli3 expression. *Nat. Commun.* 7, 10993. doi: 10.1038/ncomms10993

Joo, D., An, S., Choi, B. G., Kim, K., Choi, Y. M., Ahn, K. J., et al. (2017). MicroRNA378b regulates alpha1type 1 collagen expression via sirtuin 6 interference. *Mol. Med. Rep.* 16, 8520–8524. doi: 10.3892/mmr.2017.7657

Kim, K., An, S., Choi, B. G., Choi, Y. M., and Ahn, K. J. (2017). Arctiin regulates collagen type 1alpha chain 1 mRNA expression in human dermal fibroblasts via the miR378bSIRT6 axis. *Mol. Med. Rep.* 16, 9120–9124. doi: 10.3892/mmr.2017.7679

Kim, V. N. (2005). MicroRNA biogenesis: coordinated cropping and dicing. *Nat. Rev. Mol. Cell Biol.* 6, 376–385. doi: 10.1038/nrm1644

Kornfeld, J. W., Baitzel, C., Konner, A. C., Nicholls, H. T., Vogt, M. C., Herrmanns, K., et al. (2013). Obesity-induced overexpression of miR-802 impairs glucose metabolism through silencing of Hnf1b. *Nature* 494, 111–115. doi: 10.1038/nature11793

Lee, J., and Pilch, P. F. (1994). The insulin receptor: structure, function, and signaling. *Am. J. Physiol.* 266, C319–C334. doi: 10.1152/ajpcell.1994.266.2.C319

Li, C., Li, L., Yang, C. F., Zhong, Y. J., Zhong, Y.-j., Wu, D., et al. (2017). Hepatoprotective effects of Methyl ferulic acid on alcohol-induced liver oxidative injury in mice by inhibiting the NOX4/ROS-MAPK pathway. *Biochem. Biophys. Res. Commun.* 493, 277–285. doi: 10.1016/j.bbrc.2017.09.030

Li, L., Zhong, Y., Ma, Z., Yang, C., Wei, H., Chen, L., et al. (2018). Methyl ferulic acid exerts anti-apoptotic effects on L-02 cells via the ROS-mediated signaling pathway. *Int. J. Oncol.* 53, 225–236. doi: 10.3892/ijo.2018.4379

Liu, W., Cao, H., Ye, C., Chang, C., Lu, M., Jing, Y., et al. (2014). Hepatic miR-378 targets p110alpha and controls glucose and lipid homeostasis by modulating hepatic insulin signalling. *Nat. Commun.* 5, 5684. doi: 10.1038/ncomms6684

Magdaleno, F., Blajszczak, C. C., and Nieto, N. (2017). Key Events Participating in the Pathogenesis of Alcoholic Liver Disease. *Biomolecules* 7, E9. doi: 10.3390/biom7010009

Mingozzi, F., and High, K. A. (2011). Therapeutic in vivo gene transfer for genetic disease using AAV: progress and challenges. *Nat. Rev. Genet.* 12, 341–355. doi: 10.1038/nrg2988

Pang, M., de la Monte, S. M., Longato, L., Tong, M., He, J., Chaudhry, R., et al. (2009). PPARdelta agonist attenuates alcohol-induced hepatic insulin resistance and improves liver injury and repair. *J. Hepatol.* 50, 1192–1201. doi: 10.1016/j.jhep.2009.01.021

Parker, R., Kim, S. J., and Gao, B. (2018). Alcohol, adipose tissue and liver disease: mechanistic links and clinical considerations. *Nat. Rev. Gastroenterol. Hepatol.* 15, 50–59. doi: 10.1038/nrgastro.2017.116

Pentassuglia, L., Heim, P., Lebboukh, S., Morandi, C., Xu, L., and Brink, M. (2016). Neuregulin-1beta promotes glucose uptake via PI3K/Akt in neonatal rat cardiomyocytes. *Am. J. Physiol. Endocrinol. Metab.* 310, E782–E794. doi: 10.1152/ajpendo.00259.2015

Perry, R. J., Samuel, V. T., Petersen, K. F., and Shulman, G. I. (2014). The role of hepatic lipids in hepatic insulin resistance and type 2 diabetes. *Nature* 510, 84–91. doi: 10.1038/nature13478

Qu, Y. L., Deng, C. H., Luo, Q., Shang, X.-Y., Wu, J.-X., Shi, Y., et al. (2019). Arid1a regulates insulin sensitivity and lipid metabolism. *EBioMedicine* 42, 481–493. doi: 10.1016/j.ebiom.2019.03.021

Ramaiah, S., Rivera, C., and Arteel, G. (2004). Early-phase alcoholic liver disease: an update on animal models, pathology, and pathogenesis. *Int. J. Toxicol.* 23, 217–231. doi: 10.1080/10915810490502069

Samuel, V. T., and Shulman, G. I. (2012). Mechanisms for insulin resistance: common threads and missing links. *Cell* 148, 852–871. doi: 10.1016/j.cell.2012.02.017

Samuel, V. T., and Shulman, G. I. (2016). The pathogenesis of insulin resistance: integrating signaling pathways and substrate flux. *J. Clin. Invest.* 126, 12–22. doi: 10.1172/JCI77812

Satishchandran, A., Ambade, A., Rao, S., Hsueh, Y.-C., Iracheta-Vellve, A., Tornai, D., et al. (2018). MicroRNA 122, Regulated by GRLH2, Protects Livers of Mice and Patients From Ethanol- Induced Liver Disease. *Gastroenterology* 154 (1), 238–252.e7. doi: 10.1053/j.gastro.2017.09.022

Srivastava, A., Shankar, K., Beg, M., Rajan, S., Gupta, A., Varshney, S., et al. (2018). Chronic hyperinsulinemia induced miR-27b is linked to adipocyte insulin resistance by targeting insulin receptor. *J. Mol. Med. (Berlin Germany)* 96, 315–331. doi: 10.1007/s00109-018-1623-z

Taniguchi, C. M., Emanuelli, B., and Kahn, C. R. (2006). Critical nodes in signalling pathways: insights into insulin action. *Nat. Rev. Mol. Cell Biol.* 7, 85–96. doi: 10.1038/nrm1837

Tatsumi, Y., Morimoto, A., Asayama, K., Sonoda, N., Miyamatsu, N., Ohno, Y., et al. (2018). Association between alcohol consumption and incidence of impaired insulin secretion and insulin resistance in Japanese: The Saku study. *Diabetes Res. Clin. Pract.* 135, 11–17. doi: 10.1016/j.diabres.2017.10.021

Trajkovski, M., Hausser, J., Soutschek, J., Bhat, B., Akin, A., Zavolan, M., et al. (2011). MicroRNAs 103 and 107 regulate insulin sensitivity. *Nature* 474, 649–653. doi: 10.1038/nature10112

Wang, X. L., Zhang, T., Wang, J., Zhang, D. B., Zhao, F., Lin, X.-w., et al. (2015). MiR-378b Promotes Differentiation of Keratinocytes through NKX3.1. *PloS One* 10, e0136049. doi: 10.1371/journal.pone.0136049

Yang, Y. M., Seo, S. Y., Kim, T. H., and Kim, S. G. (2012). Decrease of microRNA-122 causes hepatic insulin resistance by inducing protein tyrosine phosphatase 1B, which is reversed by licorice flavonoid. *Hepatol. (Baltimore Md.)* 56, 2209–2220. doi: 10.1002/hep.25912

Yang, W. M., Jeong, H. J., Park, S. Y., and Lee, W. (2014a). Induction of miR-29a by saturated fatty acids impairs insulin signaling and glucose uptake through translational repression of IRS-1 in myocytes. *FEBS Lett.* 588, 2170–2176. doi: 10.1016/j.febslet.2014.05.011

Yang, W. M., Jeong, H. J., Park, S. Y., and Lee, W. (2014b). Saturated fatty acid-induced miR-195 impairs insulin signaling and glycogen metabolism in HepG2 cells. *FEBS Lett.* 588, 3939–3946. doi: 10.1016/j.febslet.2014.09.006

Yang, W. M., Jeong, H. J., Park, S. W., and Lee, W. (2015). Obesity-induced miR-15b is linked causally to the development of insulin resistance through the repression of the insulin receptor in hepatocytes. *Mol. Nutr. Food Res.* 59, 2303–2314. doi: 10.1002/mnfr.201500107

Yang, C., Li, L., Ma, Z., Zhong, Y., Pang, W., Xiong, M., et al. (2018). Hepatoprotective effect of methyl ferulic acid against carbon tetrachloride-induced acute liver injury in rats. *Exp. Ther. Med.* 15, 2228–2238. doi: 10.3892/etm.2017.5678

Yang, C. F., Zhong, Y. J., Ma, Z., Li, L., Shi, L., Chen, L., et al. (2018). NOX4/ROS mediate ethanolinduced apoptosis via MAPK signal pathway in L02 cells. *Int. J. Mol. Med.* 41, 2306–2316. doi: 10.3892/ijmm.2018.3390

13

Qinggan Huoxue Recipe Alleviates Alcoholic Liver Injury by Suppressing Endoplasmic Reticulum Stress Through LXR-LPCAT3

Yifei Lu[1,2]*, Mingmei Shao*[1,3]*, Hongjiao Xiang*[1]*, Junmin Wang*[1]*, Guang Ji*[4]** and Tao Wu*[1,4]*

[1]Institute of Interdisciplinary Integrative Medicine Research, Shanghai University of Traditional Chinese Medicine, Shanghai, China, [2]Yueyang Hospital of Integrated Traditional Chinese and Western Medicine, Shanghai University of Traditional Chinese Medicine, Shanghai, China, [3]Teaching Department, Baoshan District Hospital of Intergrated Traditional Chinese and Western Medicine, Shanghai, China, [4]Institute of Digestive Disease, Longhua Hospital, Shanghai University of Traditional Chinese Medicine, Shanghai, China

***Correspondence:**
Guang Ji
jiliver@vip.sina.com
Tao Wu
wutao001827@163.com

Endoplasmic reticulum stress (ERS) plays a key role in alcohol liver injury (ALI). Lysophosphatidylcholine acyltransferase 3 (LPCAT3) is a potential modifier of ERS. It was examined whether the protective effect of Qinggan Huoxue Recipe (QGHXR) against ALI was associated with LPCAT3 by suppressing ERS from *in vivo* and *in vitro* experiment. Male C57BL/6 mice were randomly divided into five groups (n = 10, each) and treated for 8 weeks as follows: the control diet-fed group (pair-fed), ethanol diet-fed group (EtOH-fed), QGHXR group (EtOH-fed + QGHXR), Qinggan recipe group (EtOH-fed + QGR), and Huoxue recipe group (EtOH-fed + HXR). QGHXR, QGR, and HXR groups attenuated liver injury mainly manifested in reducing serum ALT, AST, and liver TG and reducing the severity of liver cell necrosis and steatosis in ALI mouse models. QGHXR mainly inhibited the mRNA levels of *Lxrα*, *Perk*, *Eif2α*, and *Atf4* and activated the mRNA levels of *Lpcat3* and *Ire1α*, while inhibiting the protein levels of LPCAT3, eIF2α, IRE1α, and XBP1u and activating the protein levels of GRP78 to improve ALI. QGR was more inclined to improve ALI by inhibiting the mRNA levels of *Lxrα*, *Perk*, *Eif2α*, *Atif4*, and *Chop* and activating the mRNA levels of *Lpcat3* and *Ire1α* while inhibiting the protein levels of LPCAT3, PERK, eIF2α, IRE1α, and XBP1u. HXR was more inclined to improve ALI by inhibiting the mRNA levels of *Perk*, *Eif2α*, *Atf4*, and *Chop* mRNA while inhibiting the protein levels of LPCAT3, PERK, eIF2α, IRE1α, and XBP1u and activating the protein levels of GRP78. Ethanol (100 mM) was used to intervene HepG2 and AML12 to establish an ALI cell model and treated by QGHXR-, QGR-, and HXR-medicated serum (100 mg/L). QGHXR, QGR, and HXR groups mainly reduced the serum TG level and the expression of inflammatory factors such as IL-6 and TNF-α in the liver induced by ethanol. In AML12 cells, QGHXR and its disassembly

Abbreviations: AC, alcoholic cirrhosis; AFL, alcoholic fatty liver; AH, alcohol hepatitis; AHF, alcoholic hepatic fibrosis; ALI, alcohol liver injury; ALT, alanine transaminase; AST, aspartate transaminase; ATF4, activating transcription factor 4; ATF6, activating transcription factor 6; CHOP, C/EBP homologous protein 10; eIF2α, eukaryotic translation factor 2; ERS, endoplasmic reticulum stress; GRP78, glucose-regulated protein 78; HXR, Huoxue Recipe; IRE1α, inositol-requiring enzyme 1α; LPCAT3, lysophosphatidylcholine acyltransferase 3; LXRα, liver X receptor alpha; MAI, mild alcoholic injury; PERK, PKR-like endoplasmic reticulum kinase; QGHXR, Qinggan Huoxue Recipe; QGR, Qinggan Recipe; RT-qPCR, real-time-quantitative polymerase chain reaction; TG, triglyceride; TC, total cholesterol; and XBP1, X-box-binding protein 1.

mainly activated *Grp78* mRNA expression together with inhibiting *Lxrα*, *Lpcat3*, *Eif2α*, *Atf4*, and *Xbp1* mRNA expression. The protein expression of eIF2α and XBP1u was inhibited, and the expression of PERK and GRP78 was activated to alleviate ALI. In HepG2 cells, QGHXR mainly alleviated ALI by inhibiting the mRNA expression of *LPCAT3*, *CHOP*, *IRE1α*, *XBP1*, eIF2α, CHOP, and IRE1α protein. QGR was more inclined to inhibit the protein expression of PERK, and HXR was more likely to inhibit the protein expression of ATF4.

Keywords: LXRα, LPCAT3, QGHXR, QGR, HXR, endoplasmic reticulum stress, alcohol liver injury

INTRODUCTION

With the development of modern world, long-term and excessive drinking has become a global security problem, and it is closely related to many diseases, especially liver diseases (Menon et al., 2001; Im et al., 2021). They are all collectively referred to alcohol liver injury (ALI). The spectrum of development pathologically included mild alcoholic injury (MAI), alcoholic fatty liver (AFL), alcohol hepatitis (AH), alcoholic hepatic fibrosis (AHF), and alcoholic cirrhosis (AC). Epidemiology showed that 47.9% of all cirrhosis-related sclerosis patients died of AC (Rehm and Shield, 2013). The prevalence of ALI in China increased to 8.74% (Mathurin and Bataller, 2015; Chalasani et al., 2018; Wang et al., 2019) from 2000 to 2015 and showed a gradually increasing trend. In total, 90% of alcoholics develop AFL, while a small number of steatosis patients develop AH, and 10–20% eventually develops AC or even liver cancer (Mathurin and Bataller, 2015; Chalasani et al., 2018). ALI is one of the important processes in the development of liver diseases, mainly including the toxic effects of alcohol, acetaldehyde, lipid peroxidation, endotoxin, oxidative stress, and endoplasmic reticulum stress (ERS) (Suk et al., 2016), which straightly lead to the direct damage of the structure and function of the endoplasmic reticulum (ER) in hepatocytes (Howarth et al., 2012). When too many misfolded proteins accumulate in the ER, they stimulate downstream signaling pathways, mainly through the PKR-like ER kinase (*p*-PERK)/eucaryotic initiation factor 2α (eIF2α) pathway, inositol-requiring enzyme (IRE1)/X-box-binding protein 1 (XBP1) pathway, and activating the transcription factor 6 (ATF6) pathway. Early ERS is a cell self-protection mechanism, which can maintain cell homeostasis (Sugimoto et al., 2002; Singal and Shah, 2019), and long-term decompensated ERS can lead to steatosis, apoptosis, and inflammation (Longato et al., 2012). Our previous results confirmed the phosphorylation of eIF2α, and the expression of ERS molecular chaperone glucose-regulated protein 78 (GRP78) and apoptosis-related factor, caspase-3, was significantly downregulated in Qinggan Huoxue Recipe (QGHXR) (Han et al., 2011). Therefore, QGHXR is likely to alleviate ALI by regulating ERS; however, its mechanism needs to be further studied.

Lysophosphatidylcholine (lysoPCs), as the main component of cell membrane phospholipids (PLs), not only determines the biophysical properties of membrane but also affects the biological processes (Holzer et al., 2011), along with regulating immune cells, removing bacteria, and reducing neutrophils, tumor necrosis factor α (TNF α), and interleukin-1 β(IL-1β) (Drobnik et al., 2003; Yang et al., 2006). Stefanescu et al. (2016) found that serum lysoPC 16:1 and lysoPC 20:4 were specific biomarkers to predict the development of liver-related complications by observing 30 patients with ALD for 30 days. At the same time, our previous result showed that nine serum phospholipids decreased gradually with the progress of the disease from hepatitis, cirrhosis to liver cancer, especially lysoPCa C18:0, lysoPCa C18:2, lysoPCa C20:3, lysoPCa C20:4, lysoPCa C24:0, and PC ae C42:1 through targeted metabolomics (Wu et al., 2017). Our previous study first confirmed that LPCAT3 played a decisive role in the pathological changes of NASH (Xiang et al., 2021). All these results suggest that lysoPCs may be the key substance for predicting the occurrence and development of ALI. As another prevalent metabolic liver diseases globally, AFL also has shared and molecular regulatory mechanisms such as the SIRT1/AMPK (Berger et al., 2005; Chen et al., 2012) and PI3K/AKT signaling pathways (Zhang et al., 2021). Although the internal mechanism has not been fully clarified (Tarantino et al., 2019), further studies are required.

At present, clear and effective drugs for ALI are still lacking (Chalasani et al., 2018). Glucocorticoids, pentoxifylline, colchicine, insulin, and glucagon have been proved to have good curative effects in animals, but the clinical effect is not ideal (Singh et al., 2017). Traditional Chinese medicine (TCM) has stable efficacy in the treatment of ALI with fewer side effects such as gastrointestinal reactions and allergic reactions.

QGHXR includes five Chinese medicine including bupleurum, scutellaria, red sage, carapax trionycis, and radix puerariae. The main active ingredient of *Bupleurum* saikosaponin D has anti-inflammatory (Ma et al., 2016) and anticancer roles (Li et al., 2017). *Scutellaria baicalensis* flavonoids, the main active ingredient of scutellaria, can reduce liver injury caused by oxidative stress (Jia et al., 2021). Salvianolic acid A, the main active ingredient of red sage, can reduce the liver injury induced by concanavalin by activating SIRT1 and downregulating the p66shc pathway (Xu et al., 2013). Puerarin, the active ingredient of radix puerariae, can prevent the activation of pro-inflammatory factors and reduce lipopolysaccharide (LPS)/D-galactose (D-Gal)-induced liver injury by enhancing the ZEB2 expression level (Yang et al., 2021).

Our previous results had already confirmed that QGHXR not only significantly improved the clinical symptoms of ALI patients with total effective rate 95% but also reversed pathologic manifestations of hepatic steatosis and fibrosis (Gao and Shi, 2015). Animal experiments had also confirmed that QGHXR can inhibit liver lipid peroxidation damage caused by ethanol with anti-inflammatory and anti-hepatic fibrosis effects (Fu et al., 2005). *In vitro*, our previous result confirmed that QGHXR may inhibit CD14 and TLR4 by acting on the expression of nuclear factors NF-κB and AP-1 to protect hepatocytes (Wu et al., 2014), and QGHXR may inhibit epithelial–mesenchymal transition (EMT) by regulating the TGF-β1/Smads/Snail signaling pathway to alleviate AHF (Wu et al., 2016).

In order to study the effective parts of QGHXR for alleviating ALI, this study also analyzed the Qinggan Recipe (QGR) and Huoxue Recipe (HXR) according to their different roles. The present study is aimed to find the possible mechanism that QGHXR ameliorates ALI by inhibiting ERS through the LXRα-LPCAT3 signaling pathway both *in vivo* and *in vitro*.

MATERIALS AND METHODS

Reagents

QGHXR consists of bupleurum (Jiangyin Tianjiang Pharmaceutical Co., Ltd., No. 19102524), scutellaria (Jiangyin Tianjiang Pharmaceutical Co., Ltd., No. 19070598), red sage (Jiangyin Tianjiang Pharmaceutical Co., Ltd., No. 19101349), carapax trionycis (Jiangyin Tianjiang Pharmaceutical Co., Ltd., No. 19090910), and radix puerariae (Jiangyin Tianjiang Pharmaceutical Co., Ltd., No. 19091622). QGR consists of bupleurum (Jiangyin Tianjiang Pharmaceutical Co., Ltd., No. 19102524) and scutellaria (Jiangyin Tianjiang Pharmaceutical Co., Ltd., No. 19070598), and HXR consists of red sage (Jiangyin Tianjiang Pharmaceutical Co., Ltd., No. 19101349), carapax trionycis (Jiangyin Tianjiang Pharmaceutical Co., Ltd., No. 19090910), and radix puerariae (Jiangyin Tianjiang Pharmaceutical Co., Ltd., No. 19091622). They were concentrated and dissolved to 7.41, 2.34, and 5.07 g/kg by using double distilled water, respectively. The contents of puerarin, baicalin, baicalein, and wogonin were processed though high-performance liquid chromatography to ensure the quality control of herbal medicine based on our previous reported study (Lu et al., 2010).

Mice

Specific-pathogen-free 8-week-old male C57BL/6 J mice were provided by Shanghai SLAC Experimental Animal Co., Ltd. China and kept in the Animal Center of Shanghai University of Traditional Chinese Medicine at constant humidity (60 ± 5%), temperature (24 ± 1°C), and a 12 h light/dark cycle (6AM to 6PM light). The experiments were approved by the Guidelines for Animal Experiment of Shanghai University of Traditional Chinese Medicine, and the protocol was approved by the Institutional Animal Ethics Committee (PZSHUTCM200110003).

Experimental Design

According to the formulation of the Gao–Binge–Lieber–Decarli liquid diet (Bertola et al., 2013a), after adaptation to isocaloric liquid diet (Bio-Serv, product no. F1259SP) for a period of 5 days, all mice were randomly divided into two groups as follows: 1) pair-fed mice ($n = 10$) that received only the isocaloric liquid diet; 2) EtOH-fed mice ($n = 40$) that received isocaloric and ethanol-containing liquid diet (Bio-Serv, product no. F1258SP) from Day 6 to Day 61. From Day 6 to Day 61, the EtOH-fed mice were divided into four groups: EtOH-fed + QGHXR ($n = 10$), EtOH-fed + QGR ($n = 10$), EtOH-fed + HXR ($n = 10$), and the EtOH-fed mice group ($n = 10$). The pair-fed group and EtOH-fed mice group were administered with 10 ml/kg saline per day; the QGHXR group received 7.41 g/kg, the QGR group received 2.34 g/kg, and the HXR group received 5.07 g/kg, respectively. EtOH-fed mice were gavage 31.5% (vol/vol) ethanol solution (5 g ethanol per kg of body weight) on Day 62 in the morning just before administration between 7:00 am and 9:00 am and 45% (wt/vol) maltose dextrin solution (9 g of maltose dextrin per kg of body weight) to the pair-fed group. All mice were anesthetized with 1% pentobarbital sodium at the dosage of 50 mg/kg and sacrificed 9 h later. The blood samples were then centrifuged at 4°C at 3,000×g, and the supernatant were collected for further analysis. In addition, 1 × 1 cm liver tissue was fixed for the histopathology analysis; some liver tissue was used for the quantitative real-time polymerase chain reaction (qRT-PCR) and western blot analysis (WB), and the remaining liver tissue was stored at −80°C.

Biochemical Analysis

The serum level of alanine transaminase (ALT), aspartate transaminase (AST), triglyceride (TG), total cholesterol (TC) level, and hepatic TG and TC were analyzed using an automatic biochemical analyzer (Toshiba Accute Biochemical Analyzer TBA 40FR, Toshiba Medical Instruments, Otawara-shi, Tochigi-ken, Japan).

Liver Histological Analysis

For analysis, 5-μm liver tissue section fixed in 4% paraformaldehyde was processed on slides for hematoxylin and eosin (HE) staining and observed under a light microscope (Olympus BX41TF, Olympus Corporation, Tokyo, Japan). Frozen tissue sections were analyzed by oil red O staining (CRYOSTAR NX50, Thermo Fisher Scientific, United States).

Cell Culture and Treatment Including Collection and Production of Medicated Serum

HepG2 and AML12 cells were cultured in Dulbecco's modified Eagle's medium (DMEM) (Solarbio company, Beijing, China) (containing 10% fetal bovine serum, 100 U/ml penicillin, 100 μg/ml streptomycin, and 1‰ amphotericin B) and was maintained at 37°C, 95% air humidity, and 5% CO_2, taken from Cell Bank of Typical Culture Preservation Committee of Chinese Academy of Sciences. The cells were treated with 100 mM ethanol or control for 24 h together with medicated serum of QGHXR, QGR, and HXR (100 mg/L). The description of specific ALI cell model methods and dose selection of medicated serum is shown in **Supplementary Material**. Then, the cells were harvested and collected for RNA and total protein extraction.

Triglyceride Detection

Cell supernatant was extracted (2×10^4 cells per well) after 24 h incubation and detected according to the instructions in the intracellular TG kit (A110-1, Jiancheng, Nanjing, China).

qRT-PCR

Total RNA was extracted from both *in vivo* and *in vitro* using the Total RNA Extraction kit (19211ES60, YEASEN, Shanghai, China). The reverse transcript (cDNA) was transcribed from total RNA according to the Fast King-RT Super Mix kit (Tiangen, Beijing, China). qRT-PCR was performed with the SYBR Green PCR Master Mix (11201E03, YEASEN, Shanghai, China). Results were quantified by the $2^{-\Delta\Delta Ct}$ method relative to the housekeeping gene actin. Primer pairs are listed in **Supplementary Table S1**.

Western Blotting

The protein samples of liver tissue and cells are carried out with phenylmethylsulfonylfluoride (PMSF) (WB0122, Weiao, Shanghai, China) containing the radioimmunoprecipitation assay (RIPA) buffer (WB0102, Weiao, Shanghai, China). Then, the protein concentration was determined by a bicinchoninic acid (BCA) protein assay kit (B48110, YEASEN, Shanghai, China). Equal protein concentrations from liver tissue or cell homogenates at 30 ug of total protein were separated by sodium dodecyl sulfate–polyacrylamide (SDS-PAGE) gel electrophoresis (8–12%) and transferred onto a 0.22-um polyvinylidene fluoride membrane. Detailed information of antibodies and dilution ratio are listed in **Supplementary Table S2**. Then, membranes were incubated with the secondary horseradish peroxidase-conjugated antibody (1:5,000, peroxidase-conjugated affinity goat anti-mouse IgG, HA1001, HUABIO, China) for 2 h at room temperature. Washing steps were performed between all the steps, three times each for 10 min with 1X Tris-buffered saline (TBS) (ST665, Beyotime biotechnology, Shanghai, China) containing Tween 20 buffer (ST825, Beyotime biotechnology, Shanghai, China). The bands were visualized with electrochemiluminescence (ECL) detection reagents (SB-WB012, Share bio, Shanghai, China). ImageJ software (National Institutes of Health, Bethesda, MD) was used to analyze the expression of related protein.

Statistical Analysis

Categorical data were described using descriptive statistics (proportions and percentages). Continuous data were described using means ± SEM. A statistical analysis of data with more than two groups was evaluated by one-way analysis of variance. Data from two groups were analyzed by two-tailed Student's t-test. p value <0.05 was considered as statistical significance. All data analysis was performed using SPSS version 22 (SPSS, Chicago, United States). GraphPad Prism 6.0 (GraphPad Software Inc., United States) was used to perform histograms among groups.

RESULTS

The Protective Effect of QGHXR Against Alcohol-Induced Liver Injury in C57BL/6 Mice Involved Modulation of LXRα and LPCAT3

First, the establishment of a stable and ideal ALI model is the basis for studying the pathogenesis of ALI. This model is given 8-weeks *ad libitum* oral feeding with the Lieber–Decarli ethanol liquid diet plus a single binge ethanol feeding (31.5%) according to the Bertola et al. (2013b) (**Figure 1A**). HE staining showed that compared with the pair-fed group, EtOH-fed mice showed steatosis dominated by vesicle fat, increased necrosis of hepatocytes, and inflammatory cell infiltration in the liver sinusoids, and each medication group had different degrees of improvement. The oil red O staining showed that a large number of lipid droplets were formed in the liver tissue of mice in the EtOH-fed group with hepatocyte swelling. In addition, the significantly upregulated cytochromes P450 2E1 (CYP2E1) protein expression from immunohistochemical staining and increased Il-6 and monocyte chemoattractant protein-1 (*Mcp-1*) mRNA expression from qRT-PCR in the EtOH-fed group than those in the pair-fed group indicated that alcohol caused severe liver damage (**Supplementary Figures S1A,B**). However, although the expression of CYP2E1 in the medication group was lower than that in the EtOH-fed group, there was no statistical difference (**Supplementary Figure S1C**). The mRNA expression of *Il-6* and *Mcp-1* was decreased in the medication group compared to the EtOH-fed group (**Supplementary Figure S1B**). Compared with the EtOH-fed group, inflammatory cell infiltration was not significantly decreased by QGHXR through HE staining, but fat deposition was significantly improved after treatment with QGHXR through oil red O staining (**Figure 1B**). Our results first confirmed that QGHXR improved liver injury in EtOH-fed mice including decreased liver weight ($p < 0.05$, **Figure 1C**), liver/body weight ratio ($p < 0.05$, **Figure 1D**), serum ALT ($p < 0.01$, **Figure 1E**), AST ($p < 0.01$, **Figure 1F**), and liver TG ($p < 0.01$, **Figure 1I**), while QGR improved liver injury by decreasing serum ALT ($p < 0.001$), AST ($p < 0.01$), liver TG ($p<0.05$), and HXR by decreasing serum ALT ($p < 0.01$), serum AST ($p < 0.001$), and liver TG ($p < 0.05$). Both serum and liver TC showed no obvious downward trend after 8-week intervention by QGHXR (**Figures 1H,J**). From the mRNA level and protein level, it was shown with significant changes in LXRα and LPCAT3 at the transcriptional level, suggesting that ethanol stimulation broke the steady-state of ER and the recovery of related factors of QGHXR may be the potential mechanism of its improvement of ALI. Compared with the pair-fed group, mRNA expression of *Lxrα* was significantly increased in the EtOH-fed group ($p < 0.05$). QGHXR ($p < 0.05$) and QGR ($p < 0.01$) can significantly inhibit mRNA expression of *Lxrα*, except HXR (**Figure 1K**). *Lpcat3* mRNA expression decreased significantly in the EtOH-fed group ($p < 0.001$) compared with the control group. Only QGHXR significantly promoted its expression ($p < 0.05$) (**Figure 1L**). There was no significant difference in the protein level of LXRα among the groups either from WB (**Figure 1M**) or IHC (**Supplementary Figures S2A,C**). The protein expression of LPCAT3 was drastically increased in the EtOH-fed group ($p < 0.01$), and each medication group could significantly inhibit its protein expression ($p < 0.05$) (**Figure 1M**). Furthermore, QGHXR, QGR, and HXR improved ALI by regulating the mRNA expression of fatty acid oxidation related factors such as peroxisome proliferator-activated receptor-α (PPAR-α) and carnitine palmitoyltransferase 1 (CPT1) ($p < 0.05$); less relationship with sterol regulatory element binding transcription factor 1(SREBP1) was observed (**Supplementary Figure S2B**).

Protective Effect of QGHXR Against Alcohol-Induced Liver Injury in C57BL/6 Mice Involved Modulation of Factors Related to ERS

Second, in order to further verify whether the mechanism of QGHXR on improving ALI was related to ERS, we detected the

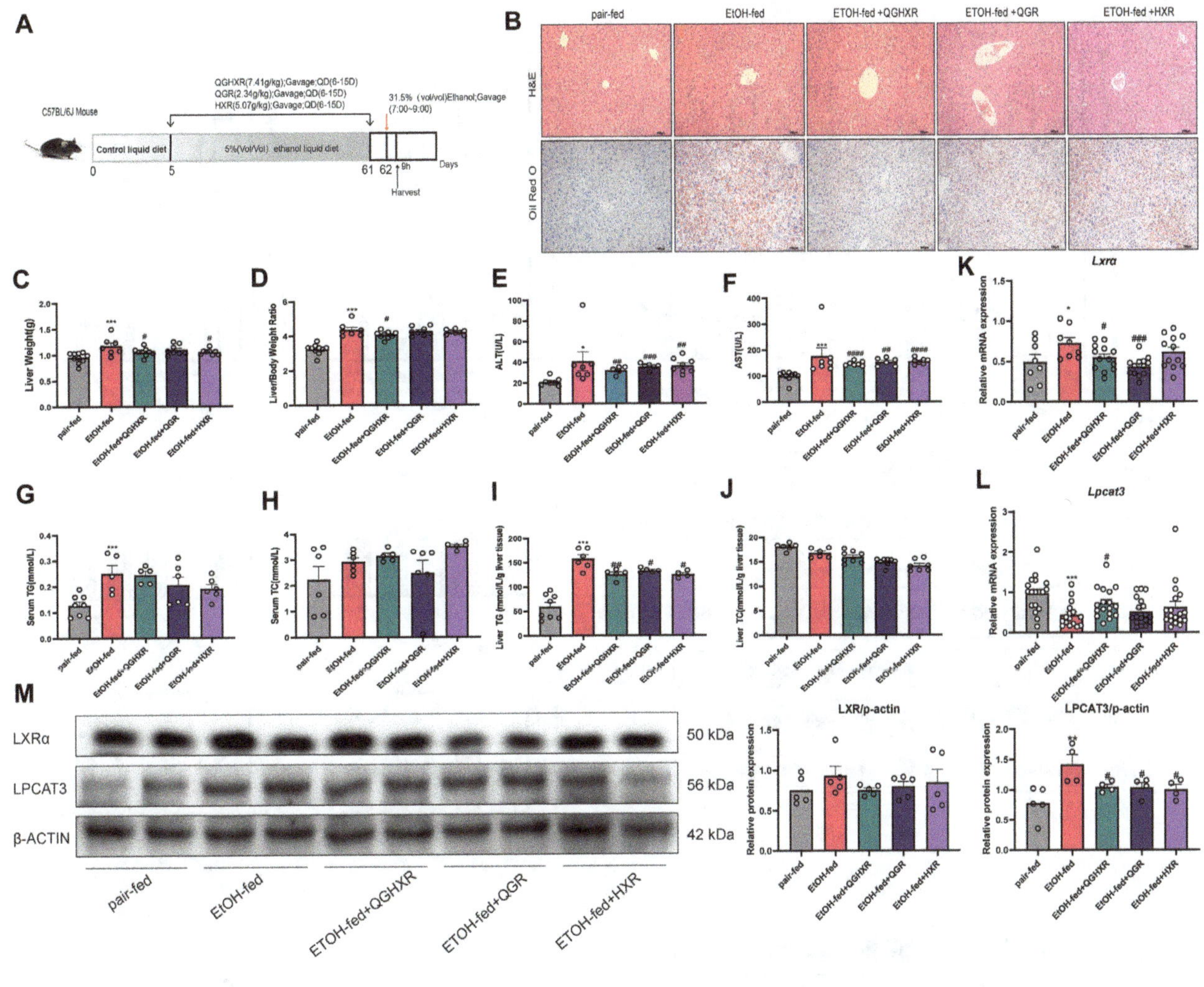

FIGURE 1 | Protective effect of QGHXR against alcohol-induced liver injury in C57BL/6 mice involved modulation of LXRα and LPCAT3. **(A)** Overview of the alcohol-induced liver injury mouse model procedure. **(B)** Representative photomicrographs of liver tissue with H&E and oil red O staining (×400, 100 μm). **(C)** Liver weight (g). **(D)** Liver/body weight ratio. **(E)** Serum level of alanine transaminase (ALT) (U/L). **(F)** Serum level of aspartate transaminase (AST) (U/L). **(G)** Serum level of cytoplasmic triglyceride (TG) (mmol/L). **(H)** Serum level of total cholesterol (TC) (mmol/L). **(I)** Liver level of cytoplasmic TG (mmol/L/g liver tissue). **(J)** Liver level of TC (mmol/L/g liver tissue). **(K)** mRNA expression of *Lxr* in liver tissues. **(L)** mRNA expression of *Lpcat3* in liver tissues. **(M)** The protein expression of LXR and LPCAT3 in liver tissues. Data were presented as means ± SEM. The pair-fed group; EtOH-fed: ethanol-fed group; EtOH-fed + QGHXR: Qinggan Huoxue Recipe group with ethanol-fed; EtOH-fed + QGR: Qinggan Recipe group with ethanol-fed; EtOH-fed + HXR: Huoxue Recipe group with ethanol-fed. Quantification of mRNA and protein level expression was normalized to β-actin levels. Compared with the control group, $^{*}p < 0.05$, $^{**}p < 0.01$, $^{***}p < 0.001$; Compared with the EtOH-fed group, $^{\#}p < 0.05$, $^{\#\#}p < 0.01$, $^{\#\#\#}p < 0.001$.

expression of mRNA and protein of ERS-related factors. Compared with the pair-fed group, mRNA expression of *Ire1α* were significantly decreased in the EtOH-fed group ($p < 0.05$), while mRNA expression of *Perk* was significantly increased ($p < 0.01$) (**Figure 2A**). Compared with the pair-fed group, protein expression of PERK ($p < 0.001$), eIF2α ($p < 0.001$), ATF4 ($p < 0.05$), IRE1α ($p < 0.001$), and XBP1u ($p < 0.05$) were significantly increased in the EtOH-fed group, while GRP78 ($p < 0.01$) protein expression was significantly decreased (**Figure 2B**). QGHXR mainly inhibited mRNA expression of *Perk* ($p < 0.05$), *Eif2α* ($p < 0.01$), and *Atf4* ($p < 0.01$) and activated the mRNA expression of *Ire1α* ($p < 0.05$) (**Figure 2A**), while it inhibited protein expression of eIF2α ($p < 0.001$), IRE1α ($p < 0.001$), and XBP1u ($p < 0.05$) and activates protein expression of GRP78 ($p < 0.05$) to improve ALI (**Figure 2B**). QGR was more inclined to improve chronic ALI by inhibiting mRNA expression of *Perk* ($p < 0.01$), *Eif2α* ($p < 0.05$), and *Atf4* ($p < 0.05$) (**Figure 2A**) and inhibiting protein expression of PERK ($p < 0.01$), eIF2α ($p < 0.001$), IRE1α ($p < 0.001$), and XBP1u ($p < 0.01$) (**Figure 2B**). HXR was more inclined to improve ALI by inhibiting mRNA expression of *Perk* ($p < 0.01$), *Eif2α* ($p < 0.01$), *Atf4* ($p < 0.05$), and *Chop* ($p < 0.05$) (**Figure 2A**), inhibiting protein expression of PERK ($p < 0.01$), eIF2α ($p < 0.01$), IRE1α ($p < 0.001$), XBP1u ($p < 0.05$), and activating protein expression of GRP78 ($p < 0.05$) (**Figure 2B**). The detailed modulation of QGHXR against ALI in C57BL/6 mice is summarized in **Table 1**.

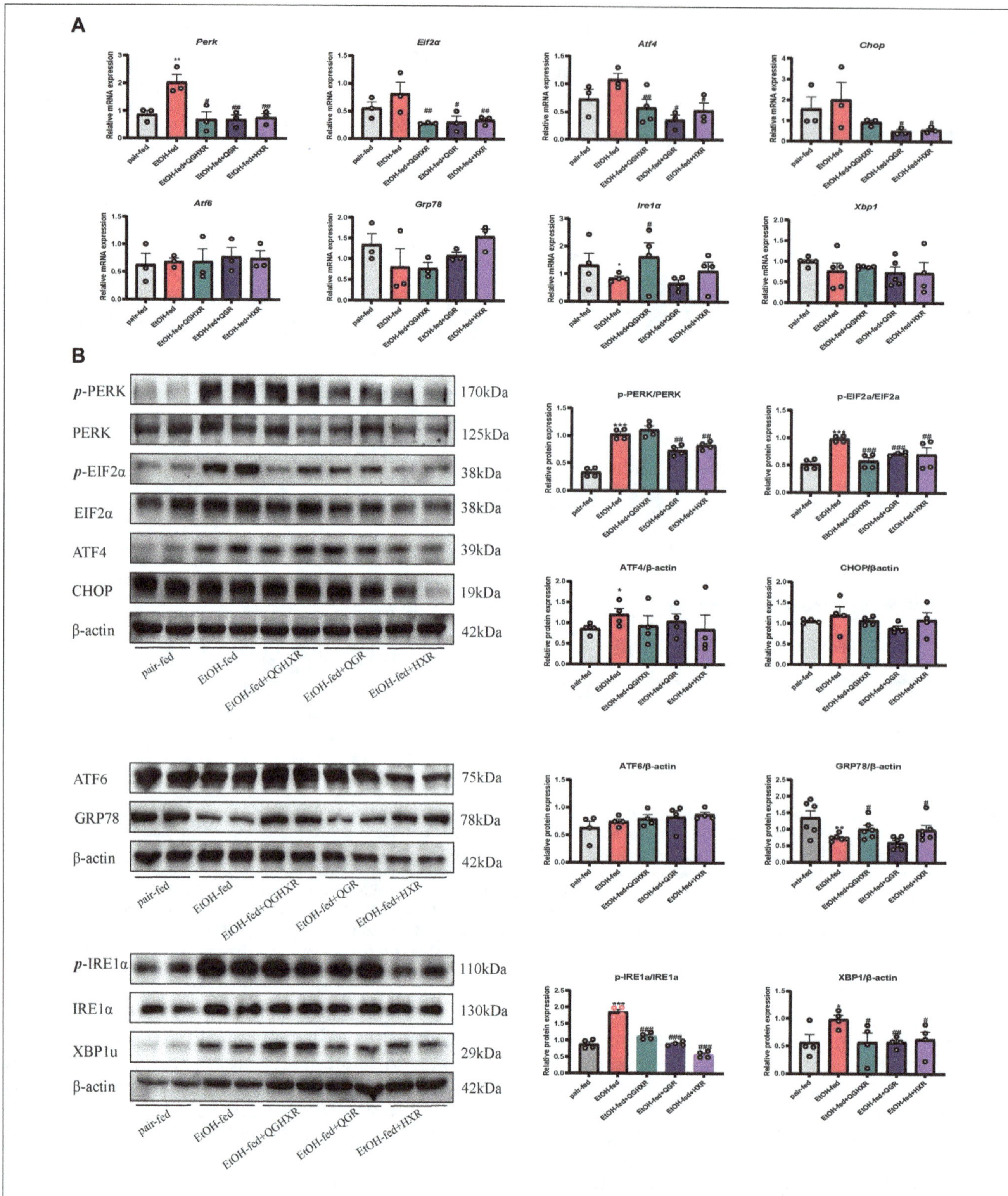

FIGURE 2 | Protective effect of QGHXR against alcohol-induced liver injury in C57BL/6 mice involved modulation of factors related to ERS. **(A)** mRNA expression in liver samples; **(B)** protein expression in liver samples. The pair-fed group; EtOH-fed: ethanol-fed group; EtOH-fed + QGHXR: Qinggan Huoxue Recipe group with ethanol-fed; EtOH-fed + QGR: Qinggan Recipe group with ethanol-fed; EtOH-fed + HXR: Huoxue Recipe group with ethanol-fed. For **(A,B)**, quantification of mRNA and protein level expression was normalized to β-actin levels, except protein phosphorylation level expression of PERK, eIF2α, and IRE1α was normalized to their prototypes. Data were presented as means ± SEM. Compared with the pair-fed group, $^{*}p < 0.05$, $^{**}p < 0.01$, $^{***}p < 0.001$; Compared with the EtOH-fed group, $^{\#}p < 0.05$, $^{\#\#}p < 0.01$, $^{\#\#\#}p < 0.001$.

TABLE 1 | Protective effect of QGHXR against alcohol-induced liver injury in C57BL/6 mice through the LXRα-LPCAT3-ERS pathway.

		ALI in C57BL/6 mice			
		M vs. C	**QGHXR vs. M**	**QGR vs. M**	**HXR vs. M**
PCR	*Lxrα*	↑	↓	↓	–
	Lpcat3	↓	↑	–	–
	Perk	↑	↓	↓	↓
	Eif2α	–	↓	↓	↓
	Atf4	–	↓	↓	↓
	Chop	–	–	↓	↓
	Atf6	–	–	–	–
	Grp78	–	–	–	–
	Ire1α	↓	↑	–	–
	Xbp1	–	–	–	–
WB	LXR/β-actin	–	–	–	–
	LPCAT3/β-actin	↑	↓	↓	↓
	p-PERK/PERK	↑	–	↓	↓
	p-EIF2α/EIF2α	↑	↓	↓	↓
	ATF4/β-actin	↑	–	–	–
	CHOP/β-actin	–	–	–	–
	ATF6/β-actin	–	–	–	–
	GRP78/β-actin	↓	↑	–	↑
	p-IRE1α/IRE1α	↑	↓	↓	↓
	XBP1u/β-actin	↑	↓	↓	↓

C, pair-fed group; M, EtOH-fed group; QGHXR, EtOH-fed + Qinggan Huoxue Recipe group; QGR, EtOH-fed + Qinggan Recipe group; HXR, EtOH-fed + Huoxue Recipe group.

QGHXR Regulates Lipid Accumulation and Inflammation in Ethanol-Induced Liver Injury Through Modulating of LXRα and LPCAT3

In order to further prove the efficacy of QGHXR on the ALI model, we further used the *in vitro* model. First, a liver injury cell model (100 mM ethanol) *in vitro* was established and best dosage of QGHXR-, QGR-, and HXR-medicated serum (100 mg/L) in cells were selected (**Supplementary Figure S3**). Compared with the control group, TG content in AML12 and HepG2 cells in the ethanol group was significantly increased ($p < 0.01$ and $p < 0.05$). The TG content of AML12 cells was significantly decreased after QGHXR, QGR, and HXR treatment ($p < 0.05$), and TG in HepG2 cell was significantly decreased after QGR and HXR treatment ($p < 0.01$) (**Figure 3A**). The mRNA levels of IL-6 and TNF-α were substantially upregulated in both HepG2 and AML12 cells induced by ethanol ($p < 0.05$, $p < 0.001$). After QGHXR, QGR, and HXR intervention, the mRNA transcription of IL-6 and TNF-α were significantly downregulated in both cells ($p < 0.05$, $p < 0.001$) (**Figure 3B**). In AML12 cells, *Lxrα* mRNA expression was significantly increased in the ethanol group compared with control group, while QGHXR ($p < 0.01$) and QGR ($p < 0.01$) can significantly inhibit its expression, but HXR has no obvious effect. In HepG2 cells, compared with the control group, mRNA expression of *LXRα* was substantially increased in the ethanol group, and there was no significant increase in each medication group (**Figure 3C**). Western blot results showed that in AML12 cells, the protein expression of LXRα in the ethanol group was significantly higher than that of the control group ($p < 0.01$), and there was no significant difference between other two groups. In HepG2 cells, compared with the control group, the protein expression of LXRα in the ethanol group was significantly increased, and QGR ($p < 0.05$) can significantly inhibit its expression. In AML12 cells, the protein expression of LPCAT3 in the ethanol group was significantly higher than that in the control group ($p < 0.001$), and there was no significant difference between other two groups. In HepG2 cells, QGR ($p < 0.001$) and HXR ($p < 0.01$) can significantly inhibit its protein expression (**Figure 3C**).

QGHXR Regulates Liver Injury Cells Induced by Ethanol Through Modulating of Factors Related to ERS

In AML12 cells, the mRNA expression of *Eif2α* ($p < 0.001$), *Atf4* ($p < 0.001$), and *Xbp1* ($p < 0.001$) in the ethanol group was increased significantly, and QGHXR, QGR, and HXR could significantly inhibit its expression ($p < 0.001$). However, this trend of *Eif2α* was not obvious and only HXR can significantly inhibit *ATF4* ($p < 0.001$) mRNA expression in HepG2 cell (**Figure 4A**). In HepG2 cells, compared with the control group, the mRNA expression of *CHOP* in the ethanol group was significantly increased ($p < 0.001$). QGHXR ($p < 0.05$), QGR ($p < 0.01$), and HXR ($p < 0.01$) were all able to inhibit its expression ($p < 0.001$). There was no significant difference in *Atf6* and *ATF6* mRNA levels among three groups of in both cells. In AML12 cells, compared with the ethanol group, QGHXR ($p < 0.05$) and HXR ($p < 0.05$) can significantly promote the mRNA expression of *Grp78* mRNA, while QGR can significantly promote it compared to the ethanol group in HepG2 cells ($p < 0.01$). In HepG2 cells, the mRNA expressions of *IRE1α* in the ethanol group were significantly higher than those in the control group, and QGHXR, QGR, and HXR could significantly inhibit their expression ($p < 0.001$) (**Figure 4A**).

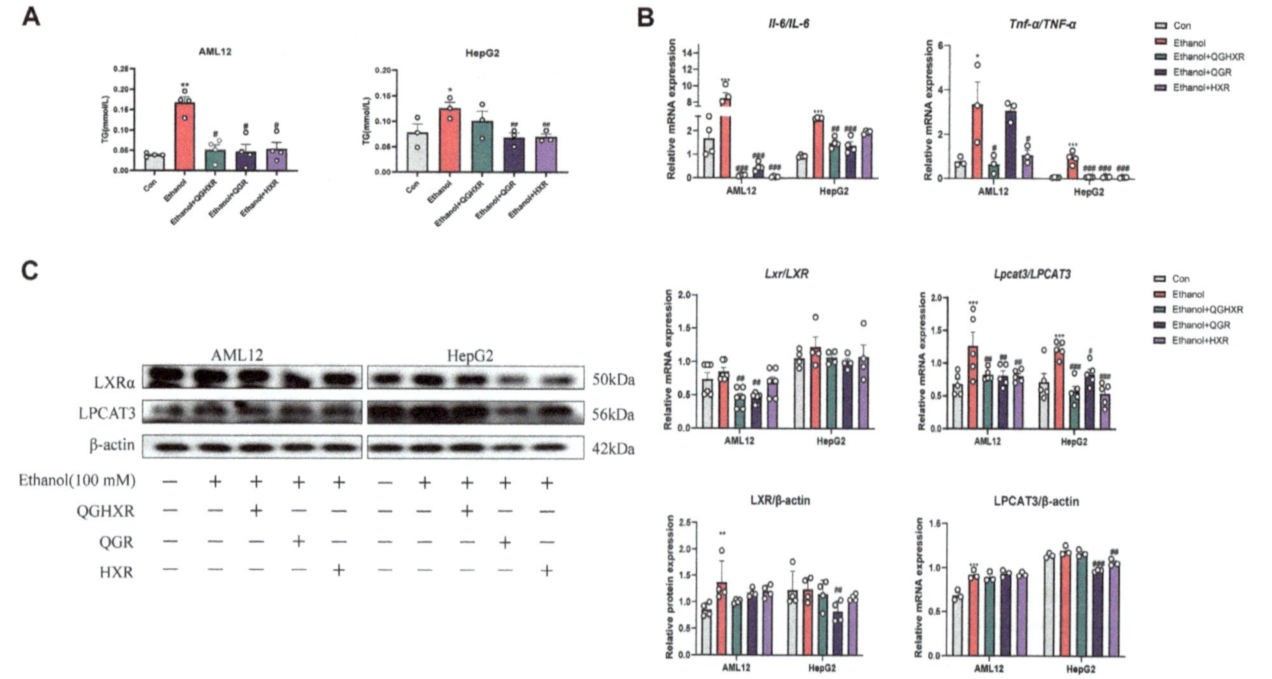

FIGURE 3 | Protective effect of QGHXR against alcohol-induced liver injury in AML12 and HepG2 cell involved modulation of LXRα and LPCAT3. **(A)** Level of TG (mmol/L) in AML12 and HepG2 cell. **(B)** mRNA expression of *Il-6* and *Tnf-α* in AML12 cell and HepG2 cell. **(C)** mRNA and protein expression of LXR and LPCAT3 in AML12 and HepG2 cell. Con: normal control group, ethanol: ethanol group (100 mM), ethanol + QGHXR: Qinggan Huoxue Recipe group induced by ethanol; ethanol + QGR: Qinggan Recipe group induced by ethanol; ethanol + HXR: Huoxue Recipe group induced by ethanol. Quantification of mRNA and protein level expression was normalized to β-actin levels. Data were presented as means ± SEM. Compared with the normal control group, $^{*}p < 0.05$, $^{**}p < 0.01$, $^{***}p < 0.001$; Compared with the ethanol group, $^{\#}p < 0.05$, $^{\#\#}p < 0.01$, $^{\#\#\#}p < 0.001$.

In terms of protein expression, in AML12 cells, the phosphorylation level of PERK and eIF2α in the ethanol group was significantly higher than that in the control group ($p < 0.001$), and the phosphorylation level of PERK in all three groups was significantly promoted, while QGHXR ($p < 0.05$), QGR ($p < 0.001$), and HXR ($p < 0.05$) can inhibit the phosphorylation level of eIF2α. In HepG2 cells, the phosphorylation level of PERK ($p < 0.001$) and the protein of CHOP ($p < 0.05$) in the ethanol group were significantly higher than that in the control group. Compared with the ethanol group, QGR ($p < 0.01$) and HXR ($p < 0.001$) can significantly inhibit the phosphorylation level of PERK, while QGHXR ($p < 0.001$), QGR ($p < 0.001$), and HXR ($p < 0.01$) can inhibit the phosphorylation level of eIF2α and the protein of CHOP ($p < 0.05$). In HepG2 cells, compared with the ethanol group, HXR could significantly inhibit the protein expression of ATF4 ($p < 0.05$). There was no significant difference in the protein level of ATF6 in both cells. In AML12 cells, compared with the ethanol group, QGHXR, QGR, and HXR could significantly promote the expression of GRP78 ($p < 0.001$). In HepG2 cells, compared with the control group, the protein expression of GRP78 in the ethanol group was significantly decreased ($p < 0.001$), and QGHXR ($p < 0.001$) and QGR ($p < 0.01$) could significantly promote its expression. In addition, the phosphorylation level of IRE1α in the ethanol group was higher than that in the control group both in AML12 cell ($p < 0.05$) and HepG2 cell ($p < 0.001$), and the expression of phosphorylation was significantly inhibited in all three treatment groups ($p < 0.001$) in HepG2 cell. In AML12 cells, the protein expression of XBP1u in the ethanol group was significantly higher than that in the control group ($p < 0.01$), and all three treatment groups could significantly inhibit its expression ($p < 0.01$). The protein expression of XBP1u in HXR was significantly promoted compared with that in the ethanol group ($p < 0.01$) (**Figure 4B**). The detailed modulation of QGHXR against ALI in AML12 and HepG2 is summarized in **Table 2**.

DISCUSSION

Liver is the most common target organ of alcohol toxicity (Arteel, 2003). It was shown that the prevalence of fatty liver caused by alcohol was as high as 4.7% in 2016 (Wong et al., 2019). Among them, more than 80% excessive drinking will produce fatty liver, of which 10–35% can develop into alcoholic hepatitis (Campollo et al., 2001). Therefore, it is important to timely prevent the development of ALI.

LXR is a nuclear cholesterol-sensing transcription factor that plays an important role in regulating fatty acid, cholesterol, and glucose metabolism (Gavini et al., 2018). Our previous study also found that downregulation of LXRα could improve liver lipid accumulation (Xiang et al., 2021). The similar mRNA results have been shown in our experiments, especially in animals, both *in vivo* and in AML12 cell. However there were no significant

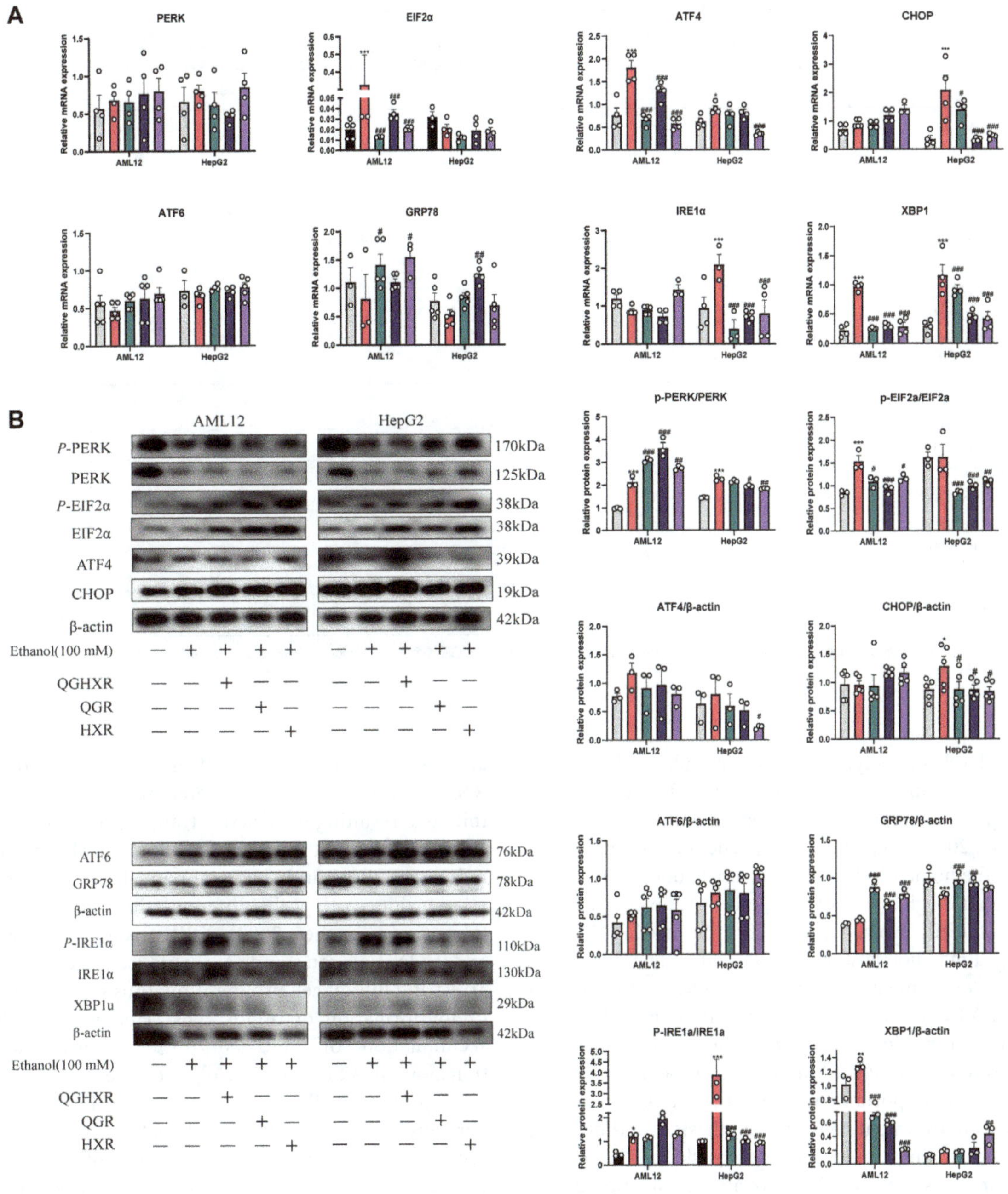

FIGURE 4 | Protective effect of QGHXR against alcohol-induced liver injury in AML12 and HepG2 cell involved modulation of factors related to ERS. **(A)** mRNA expression in both cell samples; **(B)** protein expression in both cell samples. Con: normal control group, ethanol: ethanol group (100 mM), ethanol + QGHXR: Qinggan Huoxue Recipe group induced by ethanol; ethanol + QGR: Qinggan Recipe group induced by ethanol; ethanol + HXR: Huoxue Recipe group induced by ethanol. For **(A,B)**, quantification of mRNA and protein level expression was normalized to β-actin levels, except protein phosphorylation level expression of PERK, eIF2α, and IRE1α was normalized to their prototypes. Data were presented as means ± SEM. Compared with the normal control group, $^{*}p < 0.05$, $^{**}p < 0.01$, $^{***}p < 0.001$; Compared with the ethanol group, $^{\#}p < 0.05$, $^{\#\#}p < 0.01$, $^{\#\#\#}p < 0.001$.

differences of the protein expression of LXRα among groups either WB or IHC detection.

LPCAT3 is a key molecule regulating intracellular PLs regulated by LXR, which regulates the formation of ERS and inflammation (Rong et al., 2013). As a direct target gene of LXR, LPCAT3 preferentially synthesized PC containing unsaturated fatty acids, such as arachidonic acid (20:4) and linoleic acid (18:2) at sn-2 position (Lands, 2000) of acylation of unsaturated fatty acids (Li et al., 2012). Some scholars believe that LPCAT3 can incorporate polyunsaturated fatty acids into phospholipids to promote the processing and lipogenesis of SREBP-1c (Liu et al., 2003). On the contrary, hepatocyte-deficient lpcat3 mice can

TABLE 2 | Protective effect of QGHXR against alcohol-induced liver injury in AML12 and HepG2 cell through the LXRα-LPCAT3-ERS pathway.

		AML12				HepG2			
		M vs. C	**QGHXR vs. M**	**QGR vs. M**	**HXR vs. M**	**M vs. C**	**QGHXR vs. M**	**QGR vs. M**	**HXR vs. M**
PCR	*Lxrα/LXRα*	–	↓	↓	–	–	–	–	–
	Lpcat3/ LPCAT3	↑	↓	↓	↓	↑	↓	↓	↓
	Perk/PERK	–	–	–	–	–	–	–	–
	Eif2α/EIF2α	↑	↓	↓	↓	–	–	–	–
	Atif4/ATF4	↑	↓	↓	↓	↑	–	–	↓
	Chop/CHOP	–	–	–	–	↑	↓	↓	↓
	Atf6/ATF6	–	–	–	–	–	–	–	–
	Grp78/GRP78	–	↑	–	↑	–	–	↑	–
	Ire1α/IRE1α	–	–	–	–	↑	↓	↓	↓
	Xbp1/XBP1	↑	↓	↓	↓	↑	↓	↓	↓
WB	LXR/β-actin	↑	–	–	–	–	–	↓	–
	LPCAT3/β-ctin	↑	–	–	–	–	–	↓	↓
	p-PERK/PERK	↑	↑	↑	↑	↑	–	↓	↓
	p-EIF2α/EIF2α	↑	↓	↓	↓	–	↓	↓	↓
	ATF4/β-actin	–	–	–	–	–	–	–	↓
	CHOP/β-actin	–	–	–	–	↑	↓	↓	↓
	ATF6/β-actin	–	–	–	–	–	–	–	–
	GRP78/β-actin	–	↑	↑	↑	↓	↑	↑	↑
	p-IRE1/IRE1α	↑	–	–	–	↑	↓	↓	↓
	XBP1u/β-actin	↑	↓	↓	↓	–	–	–	↑

C, normal control group; M, ethanol group; QGHXR, ethanol + Qinggan Huoxue Recipe group; QGR, ethanol + Qinggan Recipe group; HXR, ethanol + Huoxue Recipe group.

reduce the level of polyunsaturated phospholipids in ER membrane, reduce the level of SREBP-1c in nucleus, and slow down the lipogenic response when treated with LXR agonists (Walker et al., 2011; Rong et al., 2015). The role of LPCAT3 in maintaining the homeostasis of ER membrane under lipid stress in different physiological and pathological environments needs to be further studied. However, the key role of LPCAT3 in maintaining lipid homeostasis, ERS, and inflammation is obvious. Our experiment support that increasing the protein level of LPCAT3 in liver tissue of ALI mice may be more related to the promotion of fat production by LPCAT3, and the results were also confirmed *in vitro* experiments.

ER plays an important role in the stability of the intracellular environment and the synthesis, modification, secretion, and folding of proteins (Rutkowski and Kaufman, 2004). When excessive unfolded protein accumulates in the lumen and Ca+ is disturbed, a protective response called unfolded protein response (UPR) is triggered to respond to ERS. However, when too much UPR was coped with ERS, ERS can finally lead to a variety of pathological consequences, including liver fat accumulation, inflammation, and apoptosis (Ji and Kaplowitz, 2006) and activate PERK/elF2α, ATF6, and IRE1/XBP-1 signaling pathways along with dissociation of GRP78 from ER (Ye et al., 2000; Liu et al., 2003). The self-phosphorylation of PERK activates and phosphorylates eIF2α, thus protein synthesis is inhibited to reduce UPR overload and ERS (Hetz and Glimcher, 2009) along with the upregulated UPR target gene ATF4 and the downstream target gene CHOP (Malhi and Kaufman, 2011). After self-phosphorylation of IRE1α, the RNA enzyme activity is activated and XBP1 gene splicing is initiated, resulting in an active transcription factor XBP1s and a non-splicing body XBP1u. XBP1s controls protein folding, redox reaction, and UPR upregulation and has a great relationship with cell differentiation and DNA damage (Hetz and Glimcher, 2009). XBP1u is a precursor of XBP1s, and its deletion can significantly induce cell cycle g0-G1 phase arrest and inhibit cell proliferation, thus significantly reducing tumor formation of tumor cells (Huang et al., 2017). The accumulation of unfolded proteins also leads to the transport of ATF6 to the Golgi complex, where it is cut by site-1 protein (S1P) and site-2 protein (S2P). Free cytoplasmic domains as active transcription factors (Ye et al., 2000) are produced to activate the transcription of XBP1. Combined with the results of *in vivo* experiments, it is suggested that QGHXR can improve the imbalance of the LXRα-LPCAT3 pathway and prevent further development of ERS, which is mainly related to PERK-eIF2α and IRE1α, and a relatively small relationship with the ATF6 pathway (**Figure 5**).

The decreased expression of GRP78 also leads to the lack of sufficient GRP78 chaperone proteins in the downstream ERS to bind with them to form a stable and firm ER homeostatic state, resulting in more severe ERS and leading to severe liver injury (Ji et al., 2011). We found that the expression of GRP78 can be significantly increased through QGHXR, and the mechanism may be associated with the protective mechanism of ER by improving its expression (Maiers and Malhi, 2019). The detailed mechanism how GRP78 is expressed in the

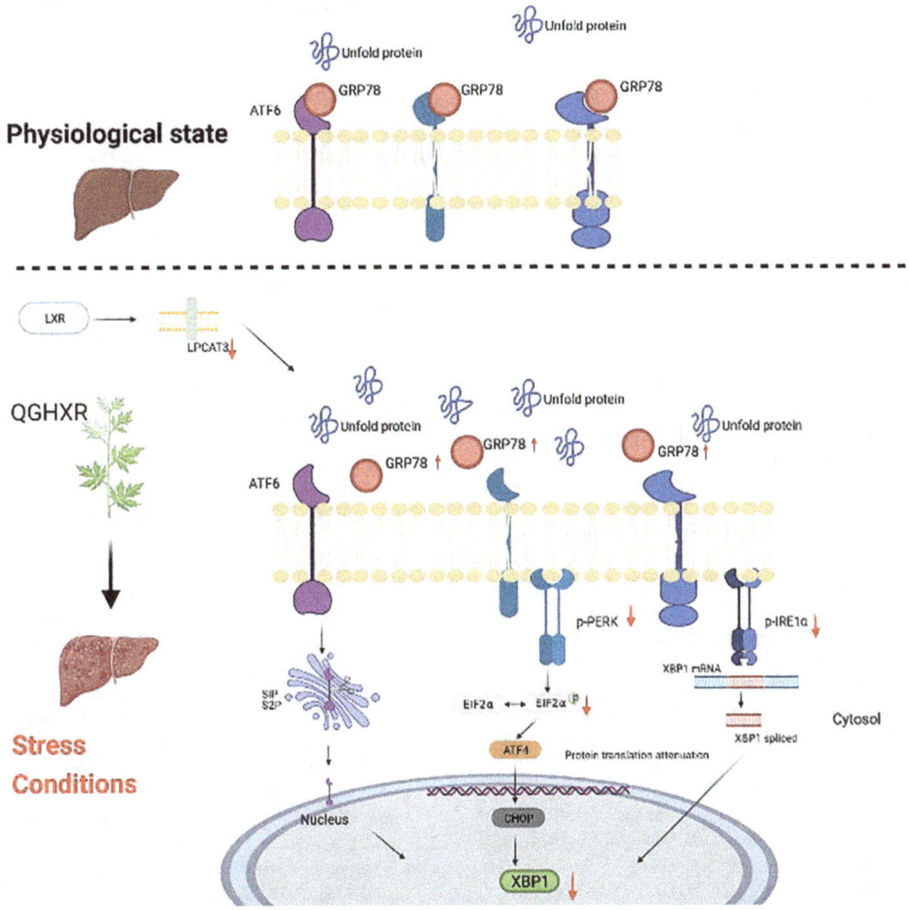

FIGURE 5 | Schematic diagram of the mechanism of QGHXR regulating the LXRα-LPCAT3 signaling pathway. It was created in the website QGHXR: Qinggan Huoxue Recipe group; LPCAT3: lysophosphatidylcholine acyltransferase 3; LXR α: liver X receptor alpha; PERK: protein kinase R-like ER kinase; eIF2α: eukaryotic translation initiation factor 2α; ATF6: activating transcription factor 6; IRE1: inositol-requiring enzyme 1; XBP1: X-box-binding protein 1; ATF4: activating transcription factor 4; CHOP: C/EBP homologous protein.

occurrence and development of ERS may be the focus of future research.

At the cellular level, PCR and western blot results showed that the mRNA and protein levels of LXRα and Lpcat3 were significantly increased in the ethanol-induced ALI model cells compared with the control group, suggesting that the stimulation of alcohol can result in imbalance of the LXRα-LPCAT3 pathway. QGHXR can significantly inhibit the expression of LPCAT3 mRNA to alleviate the ethanol-induced ALI. The mRNA and protein expression of ERS-related molecules eIF2α and PERK were significantly increased in ALI model cells compared with the control group. In the ALI model of AML12 cells, the mRNA and protein expressions of eIF2α and XBP1 were significantly increased, and the expression of PERK protein and ATF4 mRNA were significantly increased. In the ALI model of HepG2 cells, the expression of CHOP and IRE1α protein and mRNA was mainly increased, and the expression of PERK protein and ATF4 and XBP1 mRNA was increased. After the treatment with drug-containing serum of QGHXR, the mRNA and protein expressions of ERS-related factors tended to return to normal levels, and the pathways regulated by QGHXR were also different in different cell lines. QGHXR can effectively alleviate ALI by inhibiting the further development of ERS.

Limitation of the Study

There are still several limitations in the present study. First, the dynamic model *in vivo* animal experiment with different alcohol concentration and intervention time can be used to select a more appropriate and accurate animal model. Second, whole body-knockout or liver-specific knockout mice by CRISPR/CAS9 can used to further verify the key role of LPCAT3 and the exact mechanism of how QGHXR regulates ERS through the LXRα-LPCAT3 pathway to improve ALI. Finally, it should be noted that the animal model used in this research could not fully reflect the react human diseases. Therefore, our further experiments will further focus on the improvement effect and mechanism of the QGHXR on ALI patients.

CONCLUSION

In conclusion, this study confirmed that QGHXR can improve alcohol liver injury *in vivo* and alleviate the damage of ethanol on liver cells *in vitro*, mainly by regulating LXRα and LPCAT3 expression levels to improve ERS, and then alleviate liver steatosis inflammation and liver damage caused by alcohol.

AUTHOR CONTRIBUTIONS

GJ and TW: research design; YL and MS: animal feeding and sample collection; YL, MS and HX: performing the experiment; YL and JW: data analysis; YL: drafting the manuscript; and GJ and TW: supervising the study and revising the manuscript. All authors read and approved the final manuscript.

REFERENCES

Arteel, G. E. (2003). Oxidants and Antioxidants in Alcohol-Induced Liver Disease. *Gastroenterology* 124, 778–790. doi:10.1053/gast.2003.50087

Berger, J. P., Akiyama, T. E., and Meinke, P. T. (2005). PPARs: Therapeutic Targets for Metabolic Disease. *Trends Pharmacol. Sci.* 26, 244–251. doi:10.1016/j.tips.2005.03.003

Bertola, A., Mathews, S., Ki, S. H., Wang, H., and Gao, B. (2013). Mouse Model of Chronic and Binge Ethanol Feeding (The NIAAA Model). *Nat. Protoc.* 8, 627–637. doi:10.1038/nprot.2013.032

Bertola, A., Park, O., and Gao, B. (2013). Chronic Plus Binge Ethanol Feeding Synergistically Induces Neutrophil Infiltration and Liver Injury in Mice: A Critical Role for E-Selectin. *Hepatology* 58, 1814–1823. doi:10.1002/hep.26419

Campollo, O., Martínez, M. D., Valencia, J. J., and Segura-Ortega, J. (2001). Drinking Patterns and Beverage Preferences of Liver Cirrhosis Patients in Mexico. *Subst. Use Misuse* 36, 387–398. doi:10.1081/ja-100102632

Chalasani, N., Younossi, Z., Lavine, J. E., Charlton, M., Cusi, K., Rinella, M., et al. (2018). The Diagnosis and Management of Nonalcoholic Fatty Liver Disease: Practice Guidance from the American Association for the Study of Liver Diseases. *Hepatology* 67, 328–357. doi:10.1002/hep.29367

Chen, W. L., Kang, C. H., Wang, S. G., and Lee, H. M. (2012). α-Lipoic Acid Regulates Lipid Metabolism through Induction of Sirtuin 1 (SIRT1) and Activation of AMP-Activated Protein Kinase. *Diabetologia* 55, 1824–1835. doi:10.1007/s00125-012-2530-4

Drobnik, W., Liebisch, G., Audebert, F. X., Frohlich, D., Gluck, T., Vogel, P., et al. (2003). Plasma Ceramide and Lysophosphatidylcholine Inversely Correlate with Mortality in Sepsis Patients. *J. Lipid Res.* 44, 754–761. doi:10.1194/jlr.M200401-JLR200

Fu, Y. S., Zheng, P. Y., and Ji, G. (2005). Effect of QingganHuoxue Prescription on Hepatic Lipid Peroxidation in Rats with Alcoholic Liver Disease. *Hepatol. integrated Chin. West. Med.* 04, 218–220. CNKI:SUN:ZXGB.0.2005-04-010.

Gao, Q. F., and Shi, G. X. (2015). Clinical Study of Qinggan Huoxue Prescription in Treatment of Alcoholic Liver Disease. *Shenzhen J. Integrated Chin. West. Med.* 04, 1. doi:10.16458/j.cnki.1007-0893.2015.04.039

Gavini, C. K., Bookout, A. L., Bonomo, R., Gautron, L., Lee, S., and Mansuy-Aubert, V. (2018). Liver X Receptors Protect Dorsal Root Ganglia from Obesity-Induced Endoplasmic Reticulum Stress and Mechanical Allodynia. *Cell Rep* 25, 271–e4. doi:10.1016/j.celrep.2018.09.046

Han, X. H., Wang, J. Y., and Zheng, P. (2011). Effect and Mechanism of QingganHuoxue Prescription and its Disjunctive Prescription on Stress Induced Apoptosis of Endoplasmic Reticulum of Hepatocytes in Rats with Alcoholic Liver Injury. *Chin. J. Integrated Traditional West. Med.* 05, 78–83. doi:10.3969/j.issn.1009-3079.2009.13.002

Hetz, C., and Glimcher, L. H. (2009). Fine-tuning of the Unfolded Protein Response: Assembling the IRE1alpha Interactome. *Mol. Cel* 35, 551–561. doi:10.1016/j.molcel.2009.08.021

Holzer, R. G., Park, E. J., Li, N., Tran, H., Chen, M., Choi, C., et al. (2011). Saturated Fatty Acids Induce C-Src Clustering within Membrane Subdomains, Leading to JNK Activation. *Cell* 147, 173–184. doi:10.1016/j.cell.2011.08.034

Howarth, D. L., Vacaru, A. M., Tsedensodnom, O., Mormone, E., Nieto, N., Costantini, L. M., et al. (2012). Alcohol Disrupts Endoplasmic Reticulum Function and Protein Secretion in Hepatocytes. *Alcohol. Clin. Exp. Res.* 36, 14–23. doi:10.1111/j.1530-0277.2011.01602.x

Huang, C., Wu, S., Ji, H., Yan, X., Xie, Y., Murai, S., et al. (2017). Identification of XBP1-U as a Novel Regulator of the MDM2/p53 axis Using an shRNA Library. *Sci. Adv.* 3, e1701383. doi:10.1126/sciadv.1701383

Im, P. K., Millwood, I. Y., Kartsonaki, C., Chen, Y., Guo, Y., Du, H., et al. (2021). Alcohol Drinking and Risks of Total and Site-specific Cancers in China: A 10-year Prospective Study of 0.5 Million Adults. *Int. J. Cancer* 149, 522–534. doi:10.1002/ijc.33538

Ji, C., and Kaplowitz, N. (2006). ER Stress: Can the Liver Cope? *J. Hepatol.* 45, 321–333. doi:10.1016/j.jhep.2006.06.004

Ji, C., Kaplowitz, N., Lau, M. Y., Kao, E., Petrovic, L. M., and Lee, A. S. (2011). Liver-specific Loss of Glucose-Regulated Protein 78 Perturbs the Unfolded Protein Response and Exacerbates a Spectrum of Liver Diseases in Mice. *Hepatology* 54, 229–239. doi:10.1002/hep.24368

Jia, R., Du, J., Cao, L., Feng, W., Xu, P., and Yin, G. (2021). Effects of Dietary Baicalin Supplementation on Growth Performance, Antioxidative Status and protection against Oxidative Stress-Induced Liver Injury in GIFT tilapia (*Oreochromis niloticus*). *Comp. Biochem. Physiol. C Toxicol. Pharmacol.* 240, 108914. doi:10.1016/j.cbpc.2020.108914

Lands, W. E. (2000). Stories about Acyl Chains. *Biochim. Biophys. Acta* 1483, 1–14. doi:10.1016/s1388-1981(99)00177-8

Li, C., Xue, H. G., Feng, L. J., Wang, M. L., Wang, P., and Gai, X. D. (2017). The Effect of Saikosaponin D on Doxorubicin Pharmacokinetics and its MDR Reversal in MCF-7/adr Cell Xenografts. *Eur. Rev. Med. Pharmacol. Sci.* 21, 4437–4445. Available at: https://pubmed.ncbi.nlm.nih.gov/29077148/

Li, Z., Ding, T., Pan, X., Li, Y., Li, R., Sanders, P. E., et al. (2012). Lysophosphatidylcholine Acyltransferase 3 Knockdown-Mediated Liver Lysophosphatidylcholine Accumulation Promotes Very Low Density Lipoprotein Production by Enhancing Microsomal Triglyceride Transfer Protein Expression. *J. Biol. Chem.* 287, 20122–20131. doi:10.1074/jbc.M111.334664

Liu, C. Y., Xu, Z., and Kaufman, R. J. (2003). Structure and Intermolecular Interactions of the Luminal Dimerization Domain of Human IRE1alpha. *J. Biol. Chem.* 278, 17680–17687. doi:10.1074/jbc.M300418200

Longato, L., Ripp, K., Setshedi, M., Dostalek, M., Akhlaghi, F., Branda, M., et al. (2012). Insulin Resistance, Ceramide Accumulation, and Endoplasmic Reticulum Stress in Human Chronic Alcohol-Related Liver Disease. *Oxid Med. Cel Longev* 2012, 479348. doi:10.1155/2012/479348

Lu, Y. L., Wang, M., and Ji, G. (2010). Determination of Puerarin, Baicalin, Baicalein and Wogonin in Qinggan Huoxue Recipe by HPLC. *J. Chin. Pharm. Sci.* 45, 299–301. CNKI:SUN:ZGYX.0.2010-04-021.

Ma, Y., Bao, Y., Wang, S., Li, T., Chang, X., Yang, G., et al. (2016). Anti-Inflammation Effects and Potential Mechanism of Saikosaponins by Regulating Nicotinate and Nicotinamide Metabolism and Arachidonic Acid Metabolism. *Inflammation* 39, 1453–1461. doi:10.1007/s10753-016-0377-4

Maiers, J. L., and Malhi, H. (2019). Endoplasmic Reticulum Stress in Metabolic Liver Diseases and Hepatic Fibrosis. *Semin. Liver Dis.* 39, 235–248. doi:10.1055/s-0039-1681032

Malhi, H., and Kaufman, R. J. (2011). Endoplasmic Reticulum Stress in Liver Disease. *J. Hepatol.* 54, 795–809. doi:10.1016/j.jhep.2010.11.005

Mathurin, P., and Bataller, R. (2015). Trends in the Management and burden of Alcoholic Liver Disease. *J. Hepatol.* 62, S38–S46. doi:10.1016/j.jhep.2015.03.006

Menon, K. V., Gores, G. J., and Shah, V. H. (2001). Pathogenesis, Diagnosis, and Treatment of Alcoholic Liver Disease. *Mayo Clin. Proc.* 76, 1021–1029. doi:10.4065/76.10.1021

Rehm, J., and Shield, K. D. (2013). Global Alcohol-Attributable Deaths from Cancer, Liver Cirrhosis, and Injury in 2010. *Alcohol. Res.* 35, 174–183. Availabe at: https://pubmed.ncbi.nlm.nih.gov/24881325/.

Rong, X., Albert, C. J., Hong, C., Duerr, M. A., Chamberlain, B. T., Tarling, E. J., et al. (2013). LXRs Regulate ER Stress and Inflammation through Dynamic Modulation of Membrane Phospholipid Composition. *Cell Metab* 18, 685–697. doi:10.1016/j.cmet.2013.10.002

Rong, X., Wang, B., Dunham, M. M., Hedde, P. N., Wong, J. S., Gratton, E., et al. (2015). Lpcat3-dependent Production of Arachidonoyl Phospholipids Is a Key Determinant of Triglyceride Secretion. *Elife* 4. doi:10.7554/eLife.06557

Rutkowski, D. T., and Kaufman, R. J. (2004). A Trip to the ER: Coping with Stress. *Trends Cel Biol* 14, 20–28. doi:10.1016/j.tcb.2003.11.001

Singal, A. K., and Shah, V. H. (2019). Current Trials and Novel Therapeutic Targets for Alcoholic Hepatitis. *J. Hepatol.* 70, 305–313. doi:10.1016/j.jhep.2018.10.026

Singh, S., Osna, N. A., and Kharbanda, K. K. (2017). Treatment Options for Alcoholic and Non-alcoholic Fatty Liver Disease: A Review. *World J. Gastroenterol.* 23, 6549–6570. doi:10.3748/wjg.v23.i36.6549

Stefanescu, H., Suciu, A., Romanciuc, F., Crisan, D., Procopet, B., Radu, C., et al. (2016). Lyso-phosphatidylcholine: A Potential Metabolomic Biomarker for Alcoholic Liver Disease? *Hepatology* 64, 678–679. doi:10.1002/hep.28630

Sugimoto, T., Yamashita, S., Ishigami, M., Sakai, N., Hirano, K., Tahara, M., et al. (2002). Decreased Microsomal Triglyceride Transfer Protein Activity Contributes to Initiation of Alcoholic Liver Steatosis in Rats. *J. Hepatol.* 36, 157–162. doi:10.1016/s0168-8278(01)00263-x

Suk, K. T., Yoon, J. H., Kim, M. Y., Kim, C. W., Kim, J. K., Park, H., et al. (2016). Transplantation with Autologous Bone Marrow-Derived Mesenchymal Stem Cells for Alcoholic Cirrhosis: Phase 2 Trial. *Hepatology* 64, 2185–2197. doi:10.1002/hep.28693

Tarantino, G., Citro, V., and Capone, D. (2019). Nonalcoholic Fatty Liver Disease: A Challenge from Mechanisms to Therapy. *J. Clin. Med.* 9. doi:10.3390/jcm9010015

Walker, A. K., Jacobs, R. L., Watts, J. L., Rottiers, V., Jiang, K., Finnegan, D. M., et al. (2011). A Conserved SREBP-1/phosphatidylcholine Feedback Circuit Regulates Lipogenesis in Metazoans. *Cell* 147, 840–852. doi:10.1016/j.cell.2011.09.045

Wang, W. J., Xiao, P., Xu, H. Q., Niu, J. Q., and Gao, Y. H. (2019). Growing burden of Alcoholic Liver Disease in China: A Review. *World J. Gastroenterol.* 25, 1445–1456. doi:10.3748/wjg.v25.i12.1445

Wong, T., Dang, K., Ladhani, S., Singal, A. K., and Wong, R. J. (2019). Prevalence of Alcoholic Fatty Liver Disease Among Adults in the United States, 2001-2016. *Jama* 321, 1723–1725. doi:10.1001/jama.2019.2276

Wu, T., Chen, J. M., Xiao, T. G., Shu, X. B., Xu, H. C., Yang, L. L., et al. (2016). Qinggan Huoxue Recipe Suppresses Epithelial-To-Mesenchymal Transition in Alcoholic Liver Fibrosis through TGF-β1/Smad Signaling Pathway. *World J. Gastroenterol.* 22, 4695–4706. doi:10.3748/wjg.v22.i19.4695

Wu, T., Liu, T., Zhang, L., Xing, L. J., Zheng, P. Y., and Ji, G. (2014). Chinese Medicinal Formula, Qinggan Huoxue Recipe Protects Rats from Alcoholic Liver Disease via the Lipopolysaccharide-Kupffer Cell Signal Conduction Pathway. *Exp. Ther. Med.* 8, 363–370. doi:10.3892/etm.2014.1740

Wu, T., Zheng, X., Yang, M., Zhao, A., Li, M., Chen, T., et al. (2017). Serum Lipid Alterations Identified in Chronic Hepatitis B, Hepatitis B Virus-Associated Cirrhosis and Carcinoma Patients. *Sci. Rep.* 7, 42710. doi:10.1038/srep42710

Xiang, H., Shao, M., Lu, Y., Wang, J., Wu, T., and Ji, G. (2021). Kaempferol Alleviates Steatosis and Inflammation during Early Non-alcoholic Steatohepatitis Associated with Liver X Receptor α-Lysophosphatidylcholine Acyltransferase 3 Signaling Pathway. *Front. Pharmacol.* 12, 690736. doi:10.3389/fphar.2021.690736

Xu, X., Hu, Y., Zhai, X., Lin, M., Chen, Z., Tian, X., et al. (2013). Salvianolic Acid A Preconditioning Confers protection against Concanavalin A-Induced Liver Injury through SIRT1-Mediated Repression of P66shc in Mice. *Toxicol. Appl. Pharmacol.* 273, 68–76. doi:10.1016/j.taap.2013.08.021

Yang, J., Wu, M., Fang, H., Su, Y., Zhang, L., and Zhou, H. (2021). Puerarin Prevents Acute Liver Injury via Inhibiting Inflammatory Responses and ZEB2 Expression. *Front. Pharmacol.* 12, 727916. doi:10.3389/fphar.2021.727916

Yang, J., Zhao, X., Liu, X., Wang, C., Gao, P., Wang, J., et al. (2006). High Performance Liquid Chromatography-Mass Spectrometry for Metabonomics: Potential Biomarkers for Acute Deterioration of Liver Function in Chronic Hepatitis B. *J. Proteome Res.* 5, 554–561. doi:10.1021/pr050364w

Ye, J., Rawson, R. B., Komuro, R., Chen, X., Davé, U. P., Prywes, R., et al. (2000). ER Stress Induces Cleavage of Membrane-Bound ATF6 by the Same Proteases that Process SREBPs. *Mol. Cel* 6, 1355–1364. doi:10.1016/s1097-2765(00)00133-7

Zhang, P., Wang, W., Mao, M., Gao, R., Shi, W., Li, D., et al. (2021). Similarities and Differences: A Comparative Review of the Molecular Mechanisms and Effectors of NAFLD and AFLD. *Front. Physiol.* 12, 710285. doi:10.3389/fphys.2021.710285

14

Essential Role of IFN-γ in Regulating Gut Antimicrobial Peptides and Microbiota to Protect Against Alcohol-Induced Bacterial Translocation and Hepatic Inflammation in Mice

*Ruichao Yue[1], Xiaoyuan Wei[2], Jiangchao Zhao[2], Zhanxiang Zhou[1,3] and Wei Zhong[1,3]**

[1]Center for Translational Biomedical Research, University of North Carolina at Greensboro, North Carolina Research Campus, Kannapolis, NC, United States, [2]Division of Agriculture, Department of Animal Science, University of Arkansas, Fayetteville, AR, United States, [3]Department of Nutrition, University of North Carolina at Greensboro, North Carolina Research Campus, Kannapolis, NC, United States

***Correspondence:**
Wei Zhong
w_zhong@uncg.edu

The mechanisms by which alcohol provokes bacterial translocation in the development of alcoholic liver disease (ALD) remain incompletely defined. Our previous study demonstrates that impaired gut epithelial antimicrobial defense is critically involved in the pathogenesis of ALD. The study was set to determine the mechanisms of how alcohol inhibits the antimicrobial ability of intestinal epithelial cells (IECs) and to explore possible solutions to this issue. C57BL/6J mice were fed either alcohol or isocaloric dextrin liquid diet for 8 weeks, and intestinal IFN-γ-signal transducer and activator of transcription (STAT) signaling was analyzed. We found that chronic alcohol exposure led to a significant reduction in intestinal IFN-γ levels compared to a control; the protein levels of phosphorylated STAT1 (p-STAT1) and p-STAT3 were both declined by alcohol. We then tested the effects of IFN-γ-STAT signaling on regulating antimicrobial peptides (AMPs), gut microbiota, and disease progression of ALD in a mouse model of chronic alcohol feeding, time-course acute IFN-γ treatment, and *in vivo* and *in vitro* IEC-specific STAT1 or STAT3 knockout mouse models, respectively. Administration of IFN-γ activated intestinal STAT1 and STAT3, upregulated the expression of Reg3 and α-defensins, orchestrated gut microbiota, and reversed alcohol-induced intestinal ZO-1 disruption and systemic endotoxin elevation as well as hepatic inflammation. Meanwhile, acute IFN-γ treatment time-dependently induced AMP expression and α-defensin activation. We then dissected the roles of STAT1 and STAT3 in this progress. Lack of IEC-specific STAT3 inhibited IFN-γ-induced expression of Reg3 and α-defensins and hindered activation of α-defensins *via* inactivating matrix metallopeptidase 7 (MMP7), whereas lack of IEC-specific STAT1 impaired IFN-γ-stimulated expression of α-defensins and the IEC marker, sodium-hydrogen exchanger 3. Lastly, we found that interleukin (IL)-18, a known IFN-γ inducer, was also reduced by alcohol in mice. IL-18 treatment to alcohol-fed mice normalized gut IFN-γ levels and ameliorated organ damages in both the intestine and liver. Taken together, the study reveals that IFN-γ is critically involved in the regulation of AMPs through regulation of STAT1 and STAT3; impaired IFN-γ-STAT signaling provides an explanation for alcohol-induced gut antimicrobial dysfunction and microbial dysbiosis. Therefore, IFN-γ remains a promising host defense-enhancing cytokine with unexplored clinical potential in ALD therapy.

Keywords: alcohol, IFN-γ, STAT, antimicrobial peptide, microbiota, PAMP translocation

INTRODUCTION

Alcoholicliver disease (ALD) is one of the leading causes of chronic liver disease, which encompasses a spectrum of liver pathologies ranging from steatosis, hepatitis, fibrosis, cirrhosis, and hepatocellular carcinoma (Gao and Bataller, 2011; Bajaj, 2019). Among the various factors affecting the development of ALD, the role of a disrupted gut-liver axis is very crucial. In general, alcohol consumption leads to disrupted gut barrier as well as intestinal bacterial overgrowth and enteric dysbiosis. These factors contribute to the increased translocation of microbial products, namely pathogen associated molecular patterns (PAMPs), to the liver and subsequent alcohol-related damage (Yan et al., 2011; Bull-Otterson et al., 2013; Zhong et al., 2019). One well-known PAMP is lipopolysaccharide (LPS), levels of which have been shown to correlate with the severity of liver damage in patients with alcoholic hepatitis (Hanck et al., 1998; Parlesak et al., 2000). Mice deficient in LPS receptor Toll-like receptor 4 (TLR4), CD14, or downstream signaling molecule, MyD88, are resistant to ALD (Uesugi et al., 2001; Yin et al., 2001; Hritz et al., 2008).

There has been growing emphasis on the importance of functional antimicrobial peptides (AMPs) in protecting the gut and liver from alcohol-induced enteric dysbiosis and damage. AMPs are produced and secreted by intestinal epithelial cells and Paneth cells and serve as important innate immune regulators in maintaining gut microbial growth and composition (Bevins and Salzman, 2011; Muniz et al., 2012). Chronic alcohol feeding reduces intestinal AMPs, including C-type lectins (Reg3β and Reg3γ; Yan et al., 2011; Wang et al., 2016), α-defensins (Zhong et al., 2019), and cathelicidin-related antimicrobial peptide (CRAMP; He et al., 2019). Moreover, overexpression of Reg3γ in mice restricted bacterial colonization and ameliorated alcohol-induced steatohepatitis (Wang et al., 2016). We previously reported alcohol-induced Paneth cell antimicrobial dysfunction and protection from ALD by human α-defensin 5 administration in mice (Zhong et al., 2019). However, it remains unclear how alcohol intoxication impairs the host antimicrobial defense system and whether such mechanism could be manipulated to combat abnormal gut microflora and ALD progression.

IFN-γ is a type II IFN cytokine critical to both innate and adaptive immunity, and helps fight against viral and bacterial infections (Ma et al., 2011). Most of the studies that established the role of IFN-γ in bacterial infection are based on the regulation of the host's ability to respond to bacteria. Treatment of animal cells with IFN-γ leads to changes in target gene expression, including an AMP - cathelicidin (Shtrichman and Samuel, 2001; Fabri et al., 2011). IFN-γ also acts as a direct intestinal secretagogue for both Paneth and goblet cells to release AMP and mucus (Farin et al., 2014). Furthermore, IFN-γ plays an essential role in intestinal epithelial cell proliferation and apoptosis through regulating β-catenin pathway (Nava et al., 2010). The downstream signaling of IFN-γ involves signal transducer and activator of transcription (STAT) proteins, including STAT1, STAT3, and STAT5 (van Boxel-Dezaire and Stark, 2007; Ruiz et al., 2015). Intestinal STATs have an essential role in the host antimicrobial responses (Gavrilescu et al., 2004; Lieberman et al., 2004; Ching et al., 2018). Mice deficient in STAT1 are highly susceptible to infections caused by bacterial pathogens and viruses (Meraz et al., 1996). STAT3 transcriptionally regulates the expression of a variety of molecules with antimicrobial ability, including AMPs (Choi et al., 2013; Wittkopf et al., 2015).

Taken together, these studies indicate an important role for IFN-γ-STAT signaling in intestinal antimicrobial defense and integrity, which necessitates investigation in the context of ALD. Here, we investigated whether aberrant IFN-γ-STAT signaling would be a causal factor driving alcohol-induced AMP dysfunction, gut microbiome dysbiosis, PAMP translocation, and hepatic inflammation. Mice deficient in intestinal epithelial cell (IEC)-specific STAT1 or STAT3 were used to dissect the role of STATs in regulating AMPs. We also tested the therapeutic effects of an IFN-γ inducer, IL-18, to protect against alcohol-induced intestinal and hepatic damage in mice.

MATERIALS AND METHODS

Mice

C57BL/6J wild type (WT) mice, villin-Cre transgenic mice (stock no. 004586), Stat1 floxed mice ($Stat1^{flox/flox}$; stock no. 012901), and Stat3 floxed mice ($Stat3^{flox/flox}$; stock no. 016903), were purchased from the Jackson Laboratory (Bar Harbor, ME, United States). Conditional knockout mice with Stat1 or Stat3 deletion in IECs ($Stat1^{IEC-/-}$ or $Stat3^{IEC-/-}$) were created using villin promoter driving Cre recombinase in mouse with floxed P sites in the introns of Stat1 or Stat3 gene ($Stat1^{flox/flox}$ or $Stat3^{flox/flox}$ mouse). Mice were handled and all experiments were performed in accordance with the protocol approved by the North Carolina Research Campus Institutional Animal Care and Use Committee (project no. 19017).

Chronic Alcohol Feeding and Treatments

For chronic alcohol feeding experiments, male C57BL/6J WT mice at 12-week-old were administrated with ethanol-containing Lieber-DeCarli liquid diet [alcohol-fed (AF)] or an isocaloric control liquid diet [pair-fed (PF)] for 8 weeks as previously described (Zhong et al., 2015). Recombinant mouse IFN-γ (Biolegend, San Diego, CA, United States; 575,308) or mouse IL-18 (MBL International Corporation, Woburn, MA, United States; B004-5) was given to AF mice at 100 ng/mouse (IFN-γ) and 1 μg/mouse (IL-18), respectively, every other day through intraperitoneal injection for the last 2 weeks.

For the acute time course experiment, male WT mice were intraperitoneally treated with a single dose of either recombinant mouse IFN-γ at 100 ng/mouse or same volume of saline. The mice were sacrificed 1, 3, or 8 h after injection.

Mouse Small Intestinal Organoid Culture and Treatments

Small intestinal organoids were established from isolated crypts of the proximal small intestine of $Stat1^{flox/flox}$, $Stat1^{IEC-/-}$, $Stat3^{flox/flox}$, or $Stat3^{IEC-/-}$ mice as described (Sato et al., 2009) and grown with crypt niche factors and Matrigel (Corning, Corning, NY, United States). Organoids were cultured in mouse IntestiCult organoid growth medium (Stemcell Technologies, Cambridge, MA, United States) and passaged at a 1:5 ratio. Morphology of organoids, including budding and total area of the organoid cultures, was examined by light microscope during culture.

Organoid cells at 6 days after passage were treated with 1 ng/ml IFN-γ for 3 h and harvested for quantitative PCR (qPCR) using RNeasy Mini Kit (Qiagen) or immunofluorescence (IF) staining by fixing with 2% paraformaldehyde with 0.1% glutaraldehyde.

Cecal Microbial Community Analysis

Cecal content samples were collected after feeding experiment and were stored at −80°C until further processing. Microbial DNA was extracted with DNeasy PowerLyzer PowerSoil kit (Qiagen, Germantown, MD, United States) according to the manufacturer's instructions. The V4 region of the bacterial 16S rRNA gene was amplified and sequenced on Illumina MiSeq platform using the MiSeq Reagent kit v2 (Illumina, Inc., SanDiego, CA, United States). Mothur software package (v.1.39.5) was used to analyze the 16S rRNA MiSeq data (Schloss et al., 2009). After quality-filtering and alignment against SILVA v132 database (Quast et al., 2013), sequences were clustered into operational taxonomic units (OTU) with 97% similarity and were classified against the Ribosomal Database Project (Cole et al., 2009). The number of observed OTUs was calculated to measure alpha diversity. Bray-Curtis distance metrics were calculated to explore the dissimilarities in community structure. The analysis of similarity (ANOSIM) test was used to determine whether there is a significant difference between groups in beta diversity. Linear discriminant analysis effect size (LEfSe)[1] was performed on the complete sequence data (no OTU threshold) to detect differentially abundant taxa among groups (Segata et al., 2011). Phylogenetic investigation of communities by reconstruction of unobserved states (PICRUSt) was used to predict the functional gene content in the cecal microbiota based on taxonomy obtained from the Greengenes reference database 13.5 (Langille et al., 2013). LEfSe analysis was then applied to explore functional gene with significantly different abundances between groups.

Quantitative Reverse-Transcriptase PCR

Total RNA was extracted from ileal tissue using TRIzol™ reagent (Thermo Fisher Scientific) according to the manufacturer's direction. Complimentary DNA was generated using TaqMan Reverse Transcription Reagents (Thermo Fisher Scientific). Real-time PCR was performed with SYBR green PCR master mix (Qiagen, Germantown, MD, United States) using the QuantStudio 5 real time reverse-transcriptase PCR (RT-PCR) system. Primers were designed and synthesized by Integrated DNA Technologies (Coralville, CA, United States). Primers used for qPCR were listed in **Table 1**. All data were normalized to the expression of 18S rRNA gene and calculated using the $2^{-\Delta\Delta Ct}$ method (Livak and Schmittgen, 2001) setting the values of PF as 1.

Plasma ALT and AST Levels

The alanine aminotransferase (ALT) and aspartate aminotransferase (AST) levels were measured with Thermo Scientific ALT/GPT reagent and AST/GOP reagent, respectively.

Endotoxin Levels

Endotoxin levels in mouse blood and livers were tested using an ELISA-based method (EndoLISA Endotoxin Detection Kit; Biovendor, Asheville, NC, United States) as per the manufacturer's instructions. The concentrations of endotoxin were expressed in endotoxin units (EU) per milliliter for plasma and EU per milligram liver tissue.

Hepatic Lipids

Quantification assay of lipids was conducted by measuring the concentrations of triglyceride (TG) and free fatty acid (FFA) in liver tissues using BioVision (Milpitas, CA, United States) assay kits.

ELISA

The levels of IFN-γ, IL-18, and IL-22 in the ileum were determined by ELASA kit purchased from R&D Systems (Minneapolis, MN, United States) following the manufacturer's instructions.

[1]http://huttenhower.sph.harvard.edu/galaxy/

TABLE 1 | Primer sequences used for quantitative PCR (qPCR) analysis.

Gene	Genebank accession number	Forward primer (5'-3')/reverse primer (5'-3')	Amplicon size
Ifng	NM_008337	CTCTTCCTCATGGCTGTTTCT TTCTTCCACATCTATGCCACTT	105 bp
Defa2	NM_001195634	AGACACTTGTCCTCCTCTCT CTGCCTGCTCCTCAGTATTAG	102 bp
Defa4	NM_010039	CCAGGGGAAGATGACCAGGCTG TGCAGCGACGATTTCTACAAAGGC	110 bp
Defa5	NM_007851	CAGGCTGATCCTATCCACAAA CTTGGCCTCCAAAGGAGATAG	97 bp
Defa20	NM_183268	AGACACTTGTCCTCCTCTCT GCTGCTCCTCAGTATTAGTCTC	99 bp
Reg3b	NM_011036	AATGGAGGTGGATGGGAATG CCACAGAAAGCACGGTCTAA	95 bp
Reg3g	NM_011260	TTCTCAGGTGCAAGGTGAAG GGCATAGCAATAGGAGCCATAG	97 bp
Lbp	NM_008489	CAGATCCGCAAGGACTTCTTAT CCACTGAGACCCATCTTTCTTC	85 bp
Cd14	NM_009841	CTGGCACAGAATGCCCTAAT TTCCTCCTAACAGCCCTACTC	110 bp
Ass1	NM_007494	GAAGAGCTGGTGAGCATGAA AGCCTGAGCGAGTTGATATTG	83 bp
Cxcl1	NM_030845	ACCCAAACCGAAGTCATAGCCAC ACTAGTGTTGTCAGAAGCCAGCGT	181 bp
Mcp1	NM_031530	TGCTGTCTCAGCCAGATGCAGTTA TACAGCTTCTTTGGGACACCTGCT	131 bp
Nhe3	NM_001081060	CTGGCTTCGTCTTTGTCATTTC GTTGGCCTTCACGTACTTCT	119 bp
Rn18s	NR_046237	ACGGACCAGAGCGAAAGCAT TGTCAATCCTGTCCGTGTCC	152 bp

Acid Urea Polyacrylamide Gel Electrophoresis (AU-PAGE)

Ileal peptides were isolated using a modified procedure described previously (Wilson et al., 2015). Briefly, 5 cm fresh ileum were excised from the mouse and homogenized in 30% (v/v) acetic acid, incubated at 4°C with constant rocking overnight, and then ultracentrifuge at 100,000 × *g* at 4°C for 90 min. Resulting supernatants were lyophilized, and solubilized in loading solution (3 M urea in 5% acetic acid). Fifteen percent AU-PAGE gel was pre-electrophoresis for 90 min at 150 V. Samples were loaded into the gel for an additional 85 min at 150 V until methyl green had run off the bottom of the gel. Human α-defensin-5 (HD5; Peptide International, Louisville, KY, United States) was used as a positive control. After electrophoresis, gels were washed with double distilled water, stained with blue safe protein stain (Thermo Fisher Scientific, Rockford, IL, United States), and de-stained by double distilled water for 2 h.

Immunohistochemistry

For the detection of phosphorated-STAT1 (Tyr701; Abcam, Cambridge, MA, United States; ab29045), phosphorated-STAT3 (Tyr705; 9145S) in the ileum and neutrophil infiltration (myeloperoxidase/MPO; Lifespan Biosciences, Seattle, WA, United States; LS-B6699) in the liver, immunohistochemistry was performed using the paraffin-embedded sections as described in our previous study (Zhong et al., 2013).

Immunofluorescence

Immunofluorescence was applied to determine the levels of ileal IFN-γ, tight junction protein, ZO-1, and IEC marker, sodium-hydrogen exchanger 3 (NHE3). Cryostat sections of mouse ileum were incubated with anti-IFN-γ (Thermo Scientific; MM700), anti-ZO-1 (Millipore, Burlington, MA, Unites States; MABT11), or anti-NHE3 (Novus Biologicals, Centennial, CO, United States; NBP1-82574) followed by Alexa Fluor 594-conjugated donkey anti-rat IgG (Jackson ImmunoResearch Laboratories, West Grove, PA, United States). The nuclei were counterstained by 4',6-diamidino-2-phenylindole (DAPI; Thermo Fisher Scientific).

Immunoblotting

Whole tissue protein was extracted using T-PER Tissue Protein Extraction Reagent (Fisher Scientific) containing a cocktail of protease inhibitors. Protein samples were separated by 10% SDS-PAGE, transblotted onto polyvinylidene difluoride membranes (Bio-Rad, Hercules, CA, United States), and then blocked with the following primary antibodies overnight, including anti-phosphorated-STAT1, anti-phosphorated-STAT3, anti-STAT1

(Cell Signaling Technology, Danvers, MA, United States; 9172S), anti-STAT3 (Cell Signaling Technology; 9139S), anti-matrix metallopeptidase 7 (MMP7; Cell Signaling Technology; 3801S), and anti-β-actin (Sigma-Aldrich; A5316). HRP-conjugated goat anti-rabbit IgG or goat anti-mouse IgG (Thermo Scientific) were used to amplify the signal. The immunoreactive bands were visualized by enhanced chemiluminescence (Thermo Scientific) and quantified by densitometry analysis.

Statistics

All data are expressed as mean ± SD. The data were analyzed using GraphPad Prism software (La Jolla, CA, United States). Statistical significance was carried out using unpaired two-tailed Student's t-test or one-way ANOVA followed by *post hoc* Newman-Keuls test where appropriate and considered significant at $p < 0.05$.

RESULTS

Chronic Alcohol Feeding Impairs Intestinal IFN-γ-STAT Signaling

Chronic alcohol feeding has been shown to reduce intestinal AMP levels, such as Reg3β and Reg3γ (Yan et al., 2011; Wang et al., 2016), α-defensins (Zhong et al., 2019), and CRAMP (He et al., 2019), in mice. We explored if IFN-γ is involved in alcohol-induced AMP reduction using a mouse model of ALD. Intestinal IFN-γ levels were significantly lower in AF group than in PF group as indicated at both mRNA and protein levels (**Figures 1A,B**). This observation was further confirmed by IF staining of IFN-γ; fair amount of positive staining was detected in intestinal lamina propria of PF mice where IFN-γ-producing immune cells reside, whereas fewer positive cells were apparent in AF group (**Figure 1C**). In accordance with lower IFN-γ levels, AF mice had a 50–60%

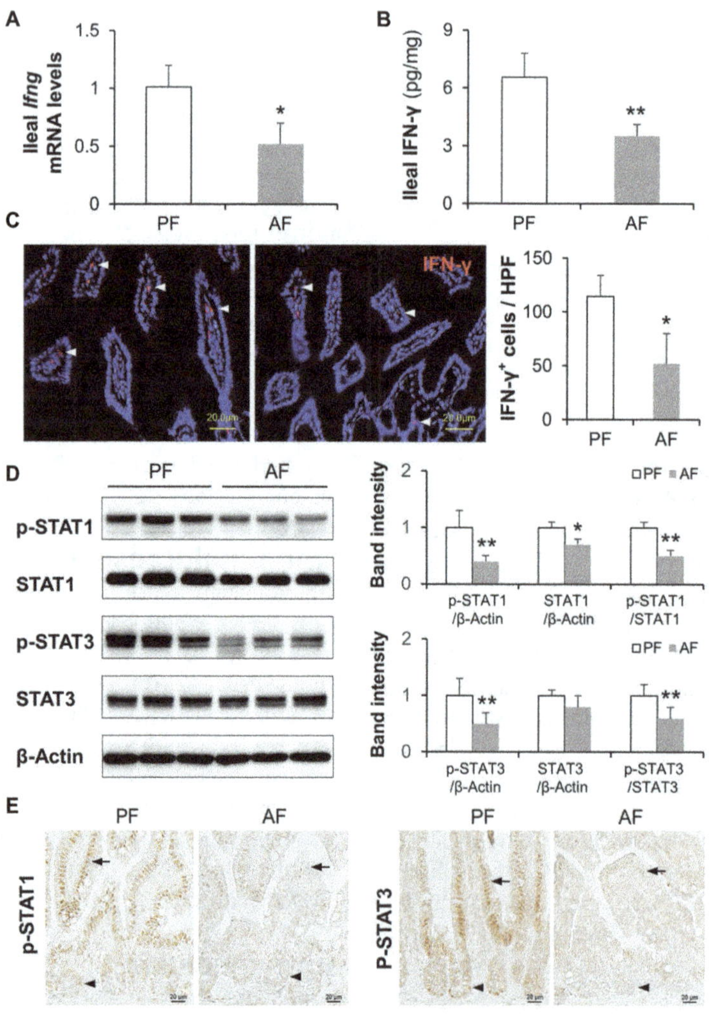

FIGURE 1 | Intestinal IFN-γ-signal transducer and activator of transcription (STAT) signaling is impaired in mice fed alcohol. **(A)** mRNA levels of ileal IFN-γ (n = 6 per group). **(B)** Protein levels of ileal IFN-γ measured by ELISA. **(C)** Representative immunofluorescence (IF) staining of ileal IFN-γ (red). Nuclei were counterstained by 4′,6-diamidino-2-phenylindole (DAPI; blue). Scale bar, 20 μm. IFN-γ positive stained cells were quantified and compared to high power field (HPF). **(D)** Western blot (WB) and quantification of ileal STAT1 and STAT3. **(E)** Representative immunohistochemistry (IHC) staining of phosphorylated STAT1 and STAT3 in the ileum of mice. $^{*}p < 0.05$ and $^{**}p < 0.01$. PF, pair-fed; AF, alcohol-fed.

reduction in ileal phosphorylated STAT1 and STAT3 compared with PF mice. Total STAT1 but not total STAT3 was also slightly decreased by alcohol (**Figure 1D**). Immunohistochemical staining showed that alcohol reduced positive staining of phosphorylated STAT1 (p-STAT1) and p-STAT3 in both IECs (**Figure 1E**; arrows) and crypt cells (**Figure 1E**; arrowheads). These findings indicate a defective IFN-γ-STAT signaling in the intestine after chronic alcohol exposure.

Restitution of IFN-γ Ameliorates Alcohol-Induced Hepatic Inflammation in Mice

To determine if the reduction of intestinal IFN-γ levels is linked to alcohol-induced hepatic inflammation possibly through PAMP translocation, we administrated AF mice with recombinant IFN-γ to restore IFN-γ levels and evaluated systemic LPS levels as well as hepatic inflammatory responses. As shown in **Figures 2A,B**, alcohol-elevated plasma and hepatic LPS levels were both blunted by IFN-γ treatment. Accumulation of infiltrated inflammatory cells was more frequently observed in AF group compared to that in PF or AF+IFN-γ group (**Figure 2C**; arrows). IFN-γ treatment did not alter the amount of lipids accumulated in the liver (**Figure 2C**; arrowheads). Staining of myeloperoxidase (MPO), a heme-containing peroxidase expressed mainly by neutrophils, showed that IFN-γ treatment resulted in a compelling reduction of alcohol-induced hepatic neutrophil infiltration (**Figure 2D**). We further analyzed expressions of hepatic LPS signaling molecules and cytokines. Alcohol exposure significantly increased the mRNA levels of LPS binding protein (*Lbp*), *Cd14*, and argininosuccinate synthase 1 (*Ass1*), which were all reversed by IFN-γ treatment (**Figure 2E**). Meanwhile, IFN-γ treatment also decreased the production of alcohol-induced chemokines, including *Cxcl1* and *Mcp1* (**Figure 2E**). IFN-γ treatment, however, did not improve plasma ALT and AST levels (ALT levels: PF 15.3 ± 4.2 U/L vs. AF 70.0 ± 8.9 U/L, $p < 0.01$, AF vs.

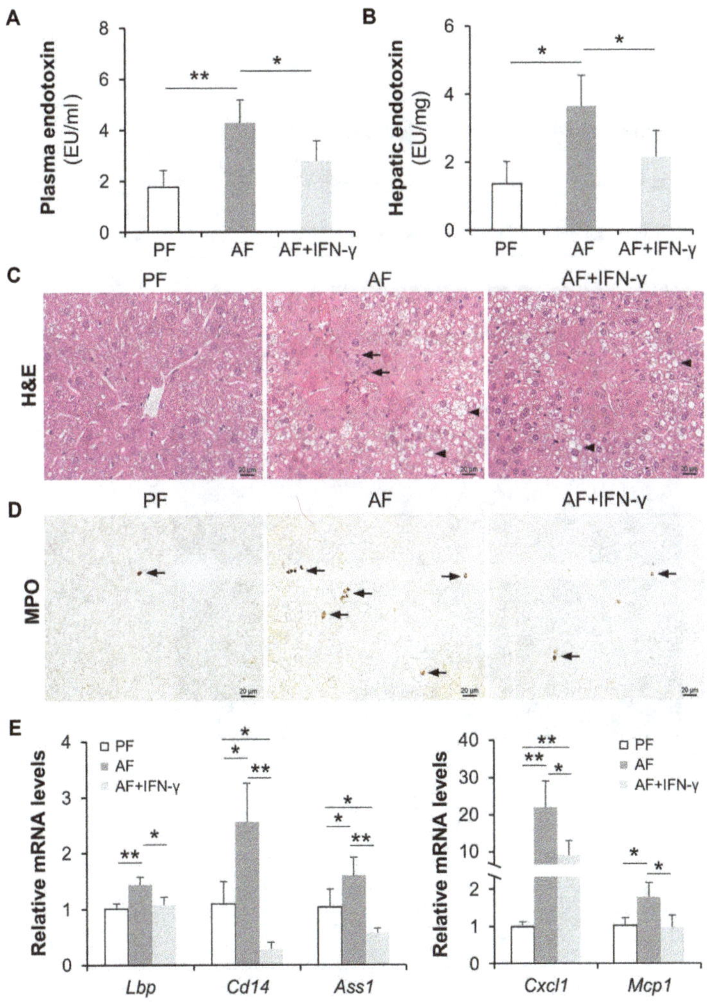

FIGURE 2 | IFN-γ treatment reduces alcohol-induced lipopolysaccharide (LPS) translocation and hepatic inflammation. **(A)** Plasma endotoxin levels (n = 8 per group). **(B)** Hepatic endotoxin levels. **(C)** Hematoxylin and eosin (H&E) staining of mouse liver sections. Arrowheads indicate lipid accumulation and arrows indicate inflammatory cells. Scale bar, 20 μm. **(D)** Representative IHC staining of neutrophil marker, MPO, in the liver of mice. Arrows indicate positive staining. Scale bar, 20 μm. **(E)** mRNA levels of hepatic LPS signaling molecules and inflammatory chemokines. $^*p < 0.05$ and $^{**}p < 0.01$. PF, pair-fed; AF, alcohol-fed.

AF+IFN-γ 62.9 ± 8.4 U/L, $p = 0.125$; AST levels: PF 19.7 ± 4.0 U/L vs. AF 57.1 ± 8.3 U/L, $p < 0.01$, AF vs. AF+IFN-γ 63.2 ± 9.1 U/L, $p = 0.538$). Alcohol feeding significantly increased hepatic triglyceride (PF 25.2 ± 4.1 nmol/mg vs. AF 40.1 ± 8.6 nmol/mg, $p < 0.01$) and free fatty acid (PF 5.3 ± 2.5 nmol/mg vs. 17.7 ± 6.9 nmol/mg, $p < 0.05$) levels, whereas IFN-γ treatment did not have an impact on lipid compositions in the liver (42.6 ± 6.8 nmol/mg TG, $p = 0.647$, and 19.6 ± 4.9 nmol/mg FFAs, $p = 0.329$). It suggests that short term IFN-γ treatment has beneficial effects in ameliorating alcohol-induced hepatic inflammation, but not lipid accumulation, through reducing PAMP translocation.

Restitution of IFN-γ Improves Alcohol-Impaired Gut Barrier and AMP Production

We further investigated gut barrier and AMP production to explore possible mechanisms of how IFN-γ treatment reduces alcohol-induced PAMP translocation. Alcohol-suppressed protein levels of p-STAT1, total STAT1, p-STAT3, and total STAT3 were reversed by IFN-γ treatment in mouse ileum to a level that were even higher than those in PF mice (**Figure 3A**). Disassembly of intestinal tight junction protein, ZO-1, was detected in AF mice compared to a continuous circumferential distribution of ZO-1 in PF mice, and IFN-γ treatment significantly improved ZO-1 distribution (**Figure 3B**). NHE3 is highly expressed at the apical part of differentiated IECs and used as a functional marker of IECs (Kozuka et al., 2017). We found that chronic alcohol feeding decreased the fluorescent intensity of ileal NHE3 compared to PF group and IFN-γ treatment dramatically reversed alcohol-reduced NHE3 (**Figure 3C**). In consistent with previous reports by our and others' laboratory (Yan et al., 2011; Wang et al., 2016; Zhong et al., 2019), expression of small intestinal AMPs, including Reg3β, Reg3γ produced by IECs and Paneth cells, and α-defensins produced exclusively by Paneth cells, were all decreased by alcohol and reversed by IFN-γ treatment (**Figure 3D**). Thus, IFN-γ treatment

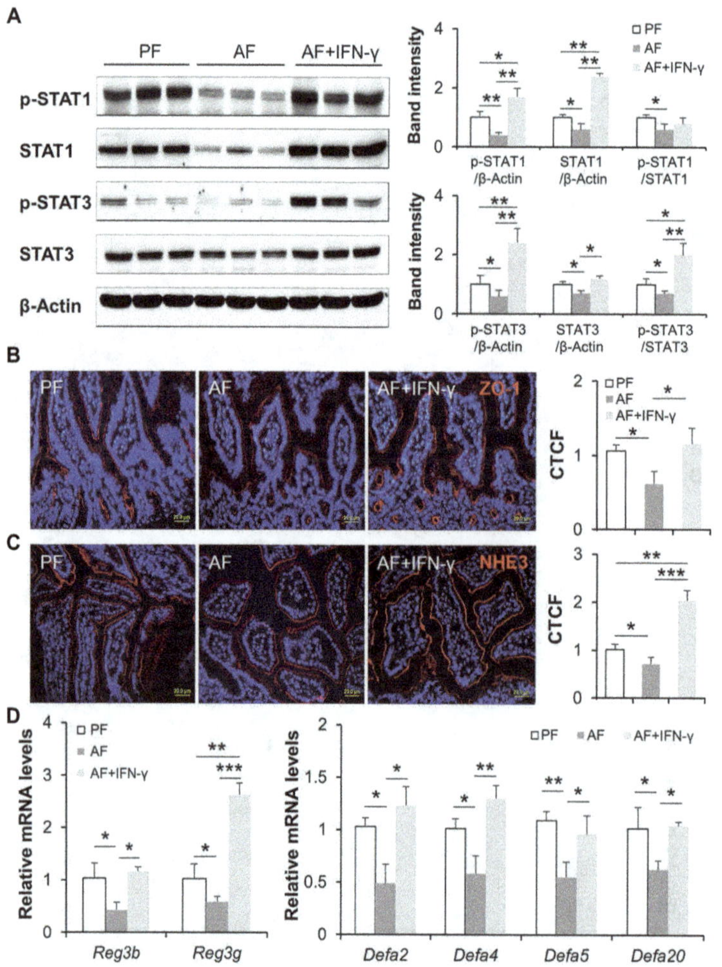

FIGURE 3 | IFN-γ treatment activates intestinal STATs, improves gut barrier, and reversed alcohol-reduced antimicrobial peptide (AMP) levels. **(A)** WB and quantification of ileal STAT1 and STAT3. **(B)** IF staining of ileal ZO-1 (red) and nuclei (blue). Scale bar, 20 μm. Corrected total cell fluorescence (CTCF) of ZO-1 was quantified. **(C)** IF staining and quantification of ileal sodium-hydrogen exchanger 3 (NHE3; red). Nuclei were counterstained by DAPI (blue). Scale bar, 20 μm. **(D)** mRNA levels of ileal AMPs ($n = 6$ per group). $^{*}p < 0.05$, $^{**}p < 0.01$, and $^{***}p < 0.001$. PF, pair-fed; AF, alcohol-fed.

restored intestinal STAT signaling, allowing repair of alcohol-damaged gut barrier and regulation of AMP production.

IFN-γ Orchestrates Gut Microbiota Composition and Microbial Functional Pathways

Due to the intimate relationship between AMPs and gut microbiota homeostasis, we hypothesized that IFN-γ treatment would improve alcohol-induced gut microbial dysbiosis in association with upregulated AMP expression. Cecal microbiome was analyzed by metagenomic sequencing of the 16S rRNA gene. Compared with PF group, the observed OTUs index, an α-diversity value showing overall microbial richness, was significantly higher in AF group and normalized in AF+IFN-γ group (**Figure 4A**). Bray-Curtis distance matrices, which evaluate phylogenetic similarities between microbial communities, were used to calculate β-diversity; the three groups were clearly separated into different clusters (ANOSIM, $p < 0.001$, $r = 0.926$),

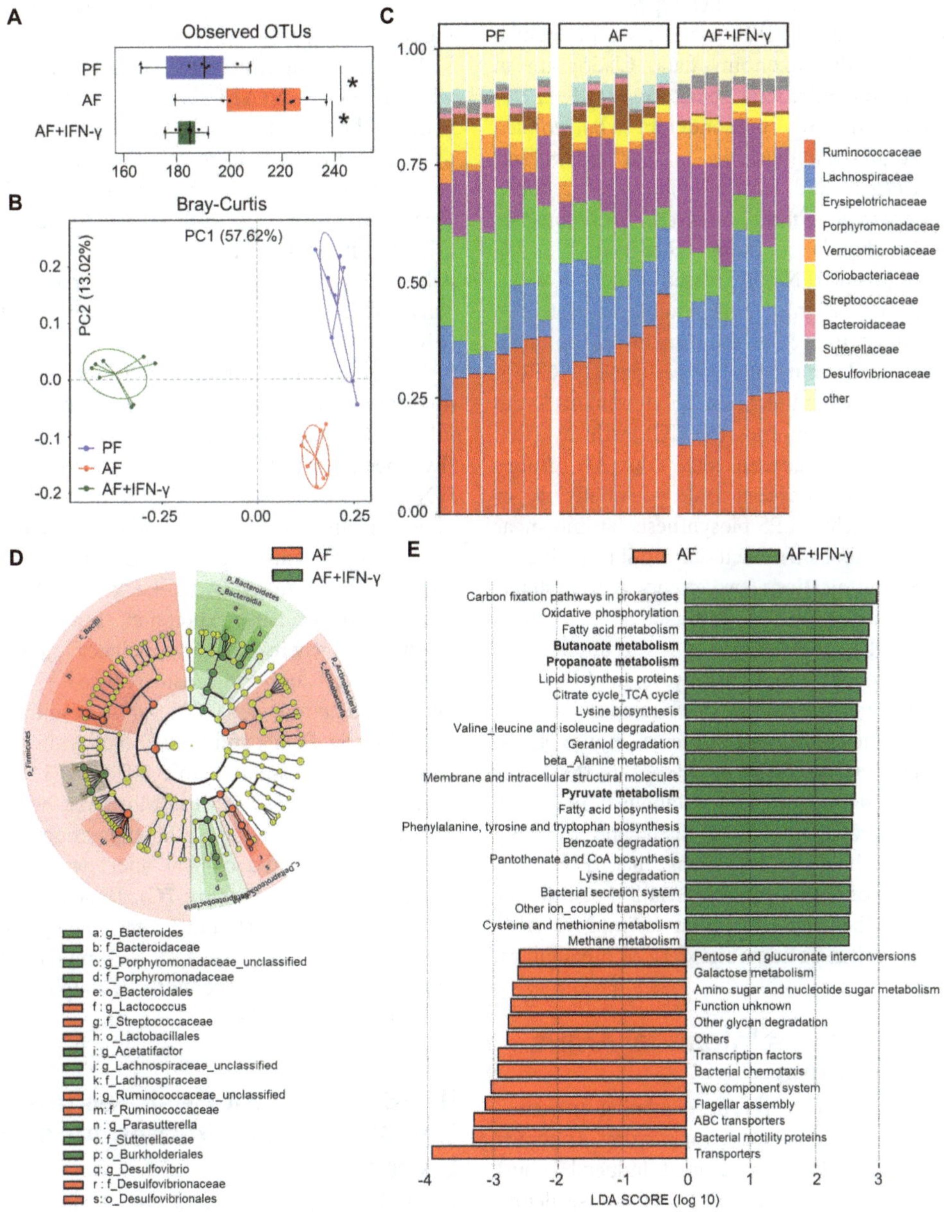

FIGURE 4 | IFN-γ treatment ameliorates chronic alcohol exposure-induced cecal microbial dysbiosis in mice. **(A)** Alpha-diversity measurement of observed number of operational taxonomic units (OTUs). **(B)** PCoA plot showing dissimilarity in bacterial community structures based on Bray-Curtis distances. **(C)** Barplot showing the bacterial composition at family level. **(D)** Cladogram taxonomic abundances of bacteria. Legend of prominent taxons is shown at bottom. **(E)** Bacterial gene functions predicted based on 16S rRNA gene sequences using the PICRUSt algorithm and annotated from KEGG databases ($n = 8$ per group). $^{*}p < 0.05$. PF, pair-fed; AF, alcohol-fed.

indicating distinct gut microbial community structures among these groups (**Figure 4B**). Despite different microbial richness and diverse communities, IFN-γ treatment clearly affected the gut microbial configuration. At the family level, the relative abundances of *Verrucomicrobiaceae* and *Sutterellaceae* were significantly lower in AF group than in PF group ($p = 0.019$ and $p = 0.008$, respectively), which were restored by IFN-γ treatment ($p = 0.036$ and $p < 0.001$, respectively). Meanwhile, the relative abundance of *Streptococcaceae* was significantly higher in AF group than in PF group ($p = 0.045$) and was diminished by IFN-γ treatment ($p = 0.002$; **Figure 4C**). To further identify the distinguishing phylotypes in the gut microbiota between AF and AF+IFN-γ mice, we performed LEfSe analysis based on the taxonomy data. Cladogram in **Figure 4D** shows that the microbial structure of AF+IFN-γ mice was characterized by preponderant *Bacteroides, Bacteroidaceae, Porphyromonadaceae, Lachnospiraceae, Parasutterella, Sutterellaceae*, and *Burkholderiales*, and reduced *Lactococcus, Streptococcaceae, Ruminococcaceae, Desulfovibrio*, and *Desulfovibrionales* abundance [LDA score ($\log_{10}$) > 4.0; red, IFN-γ-decreased; green, IFN-γ-increased].

Apart from phylogenic insights, metagenomic analysis also provided an opportunity to assess the functional potential associated with the microbial community. We performed PICRUSt analysis of the microbiome and defined 35 dominant Kyoto Encyclopedia of Genes and Genomes (KEGG) pathways that were significantly different between the two AF groups (**Figure 4E**). Many microbial genes that could potentially trigger inflammatory responses, such as LPS biosynthesis (amino sugar and nucleotide sugar metabolism), bacterial motility (bacterial motility proteins), communication (two component system), chemotaxis, and flagellar assembly, were predicted to be inhibited by IFN-γ compared to that of AF group. On the other hand, the relative abundance of 22 KEGG pathways in AF+IFN-γ group was higher than in AF group. This includes bacterial genes involved in the metabolism of proteins, amino acids, carbohydrates, and fatty acids. Of great interest is the genes involved in short chain fatty acid (SCFA) metabolism, including butanoate metabolism, propanoate metabolism, and pyruvate metabolism (**Figure 4E**; bolded), suggesting that IFN-γ not only inhibits overgrowth of pathogenic bacteria but also drives gut microbiota toward a beneficial direction to improve ALD with the possible involvement of microbial-derived metabolites, such as SCFAs.

IFN-γ Directly Regulates Intestinal AMPs Through STAT Signaling

We next tested the effects of IFN-γ in regulating intestinal AMPs in an acute time-course IFN-γ treatment study. As shown in **Figure 5A**, one dose of IFN-γ treatment induced robust phosphorylation of both STAT1 and STAT3 in mouse ileum; the induction lasted for up to 8 h with 1 h being the most significant time point. At 8 h, the expression of Reg3β and Reg3γ was upregulated in IFN-γ-treated mice compared to the control. IFN-γ treatment also led to increased mRNA levels of α-defensins, including *Defa2, Defa4, Defa5*, and *Defa20* (**Figure 5B**). The presence and activation state of α-defensins in the lumen of ileum was directly assessed by AU-PAGE. Extracts from freshly isolated ileal peptides contained α-defensin species with mobilities consistent with HD5. Compared with the controls, the levels of active α-defensins were gradually increased by IFN-γ in a time-dependent manner (**Figure 5C**). MMP7, which is responsible for the activation of pro-α-defensins (Wilson et al., 1999), was also induced by IFN-γ, with the most significant induction at 3 h (**Figure 5D**).

Mice with IEC-specific deletion of STAT1 or STAT3 were generated to dissect the role of STATs in mediating IFN-γ-regulated intestinal AMPs. Immunoblotting confirmed successful deletion of corresponding STAT proteins in the knockout (KO) models (**Figure 6A**). With STAT1 deletion, the levels of intestinal STAT3 were slightly increased compared to floxed controls, whereas KO of STAT3 did not affect STAT1 levels. We first compared the levels of active α-defensins in these mice. Deletion of STAT3 in IECs decreased the levels of active α-defensins compared to the control. Meanwhile, cleaved MMP7, the active form that cleaves pro-α-defensins to active α-defensins, was dramatically declined in $Stat3^{IEC-/-}$ mice (**Figure 6B**). IEC-specific deletion of STAT1, however, led to increased levels of intestinal active α-defensins and elevated levels of cleaved MMP7 (**Figure 6C**).

To exclude the possible interference of immune cells and microbiota in IFN-γ-STAT signaling, we established small intestinal organoid cultures isolated from floxed control and IEC-specific STAT KO mice and treated them with IFN-γ. IFN-γ triggered more than 20-fold elevation in mRNA levels of Reg3β and Reg3γ in organoids isolated from floxed mice; it also significantly upregulated expression of *Defa4, Defa5*, and *Defa20* (**Figures 7A,B**). Lack of STAT1 prevented IFN-γ-induced α-defensin expression but not Reg3 expression (**Figure 7A**), whereas STAT3 deficiency impaired the upregulation of both Reg3 and α-defensins caused by IFN-γ (**Figure 7B**). Of note, deletion of STAT3 *per se* resulted in lower levels of *Reg3b, Reg3g, Defa5*, and *Defa20* even without IFN-γ stimulation, indicating an essential role of STAT3 in maintaining the expression of these AMPs. Moreover, we found that IFN-γ was capable of inducing NHE3 expression in cultured organoids isolated from floxed control mice, which was diminished by KO of IEC STAT1 (**Figure 7C**). IF staining showed increment in NHE3 positive staining after IFN-γ treatment in floxed group, whereas the induction was much weaker in $Stat1^{IEC-/-}$ group (**Figure 7D**). Therefore, through *in vivo* and *in vitro* experiments, we identified an important role of IFN-γ in regulating intestinal AMPs *via* STAT signaling.

IL-18 Treatment Restores Intestinal IFN-γ Levels and Ameliorates Alcohol-Induced Liver Damage

It was not fully understood how alcohol intoxication leads to suppressed intestinal IFN-γ production, so we explored the levels of IFN-γ inducing factor (interleukin-18/IL-18; Nakamura et al., 1989) after chronic alcohol feeding and the effects of IL-18 in restoring intestinal IFN-γ levels as well as in reversing the pathogenesis of ALD. Compared with PF mice, AF mice had lower levels of IL-18 in the ileum (**Figure 8A**).

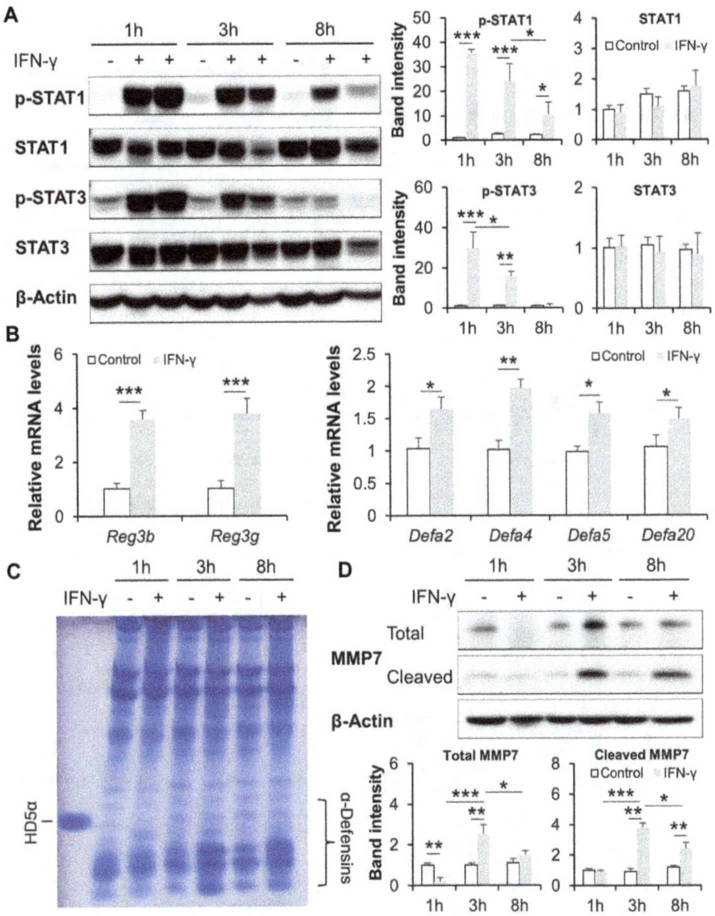

FIGURE 5 | IFN-γ time dependently activates intestinal STATs and stimulates AMPs in mice. **(A)** WB and quantification of ileal STAT1 and STAT3. **(B)** mRNA levels of ileal AMPs. **(C)** Acid urea polyacrylamide gel electrophoresis (AU-PAGE) of freshly isolated ileal peptides. Synthetic human α-defensin 5 (HD5) was included as a control. **(D)** WB and quantification of total and cleaved matrix metallopeptidase 7 (MMP7) in the ileum of mice (n = 3 per group). $^{*}p < 0.05$, $^{**}p < 0.01$, and $^{***}p < 0.001$.

Recombinant mouse IL-18 was then given to AF mice for the last 2 weeks in an 8-week feeding experiment. As expected, IL-18 treatment effectively restored alcohol-declined ileal IFN-γ levels (**Figure 8B**), without affecting the levels of IL-22 (AF 21.66 ± 11.66 pg/mg vs. AF+IL-18 10.13 ± 4.54 pg/mg, $p = 0.084$, compared to PF 59.47 ± 9.46 pg/mg, $p < 0.001$) which is known to be decreased by alcohol and could protect against ALD (Ki et al., 2010; Hendrikx et al., 2019). Intestinal barrier function was significantly improved by IL-18 as indicated by refined distribution of tight junction protein ZO-1 (**Figure 8C**) and enhanced expression of NHE3 (**Figure 8D**). In association with restored IFN-γ levels, IL-18-treated AF mice had higher levels of ileal *Reg3b* and *Reg3g* than AF mice. IL-18 treatment also reinstated alcohol-reduced expression of α-defensins (**Figure 8E**). In accordance with improved gut barrier and antimicrobial ability, AF mice received IL-18 exhibited lower plasma endotoxin levels than AF mice (**Figure 8F**). Alcoholic liver damage was compared between the two AF groups. IL-18 treatment reduced alcohol-elevated plasma ALT and AST levels (ALT levels: AF 78.9 ± 16.6 U/L vs. AF+IL-18 41.8 ± 15.4 U/L, $p < 0.05$; AST levels: AF 62.9 ± 14.3 U/L vs. AF+IL-18 35.4 ± 11.1 U/L, $p < 0.05$). IL-18 treatment ameliorated alcohol-induced hepatic inflammation as evidenced by reduced inflammatory cell infiltration (**Figure 8G**, arrows), less positive staining of neutrophil marker MPO (**Figure 8H**, arrows), and diminished expression of inflammatory chemokines *Cxcl1* and *Mcp1* (**Figure 8I**). Similar to IFN-γ treatment, IL-18 treatment did not further alter hepatic TG or FFA levels (TG levels: AF 46.1 ± 11.6 nmol/mg vs. AF+IL-18 40.6 ± 8.8 nmol/mg, $p = 0.531$; FFA levels: AF 15.1 ± 4.6 nmol/mg vs. AF+IL-18 16.6 ± 5.8 nmol/mg, $p = 0.255$). These results suggest that IL-18 treatment is potent in restoring intestinal IFN-γ levels and treating ALD.

DISCUSSION

Sustained gut microbial dysbiosis causes disequilibrium in energy homeostasis, disrupted gut barrier, as well as stress and inflammatory responses that ultimately leads to metabolic

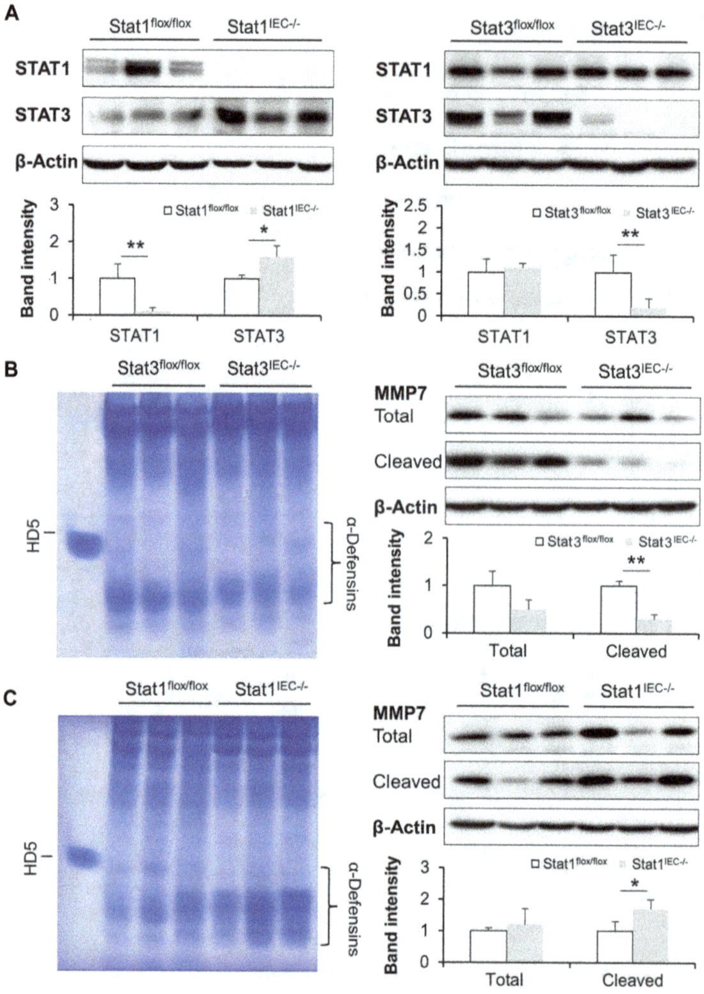

FIGURE 6 | Intestinal epithelial STAT1 and STAT3 regulate MMP7 and activation of α-defensins. **(A)** WB and quantification of STAT1 and STAT3 in the ileum of $Stat1^{IEC-/-}$ and $Stat3^{IEC-/-}$ mice. **(B)** AU-PAGE of freshly isolated ileal peptides, and WB and quantification of MMP7 in control and $Stat3^{IEC-/-}$ mice. **(C)** AU-PAGE of freshly isolated ileal peptides, and WB and quantification of MMP7 in control and $Stat1^{IEC-/-}$ mice (n = 3 per group). $^{*}p < 0.05$ and $^{**}p < 0.01$.

diseases, including ALD (Mutlu et al., 2012; Tilg et al., 2016). Human and animal studies show that modulation of gut microbiota seems to be a promising strategy to reduce alcohol-induced liver injury (Philips et al., 2017; Grander et al., 2018). Nevertheless, the precise mechanisms by which alcohol causes gut dysbiosis and the subsequent liver damage are still poorly understood. Our laboratory and others' have previously reported that alcohol intoxication hampers the antimicrobial ability of the host through reducing AMP production (Yan et al., 2011; Wang et al., 2016; He et al., 2019; Zhong et al., 2019). The present study revealed an essential role of intestinal IFN-γ-STAT signaling in regulating AMP levels, gut microbiota homeostasis, and alcohol-induced liver injury in mice (major findings summarized in **Figure 9**). We found that chronic alcohol feeding caused aberrant IFN-γ-STAT signaling in the intestine, which is responsible for maintaining AMP levels and gut microbiota symbiosis. We further demonstrate that IL-18 acts as an upstream regulator of IFN-γ and treatment of IL-18 restores intestinal IFN-γ levels and ameliorates liver injury induced by alcohol.

It is well-known that IFN-γ can enhance the innate immune response to epithelial cells and can boost the proinflammatory response of lymphocytes. It has been reported that IFN-γ strongly increased proliferation of intestinal epithelial T84 cells peaked at 24 h and substantially increased apoptosis from 24 to 72 h, which suggests that the effect of IFN-γ on epithelial proliferation is bidirectional and dose/time-dependent (Nava et al., 2010). There is mounting evidence, however, showing that IFN-γ also plays a protective role in a number of disease models (Ma et al., 2011). It has been reported that IFN-γ deficiency exacerbates inflammatory bowel disease in mice (Sheikh et al., 2010). Mechanically, IFN-γ can defend intestinal epithelium through upregulating cellular methylation pathways (Kominsky et al., 2011), inducing expression of indoleamine 2, 3-dioxygenase 1 (IDO1; Gurtner et al., 2003), and maintaining epithelial IL-10 signaling (Kominsky et al., 2014). This study

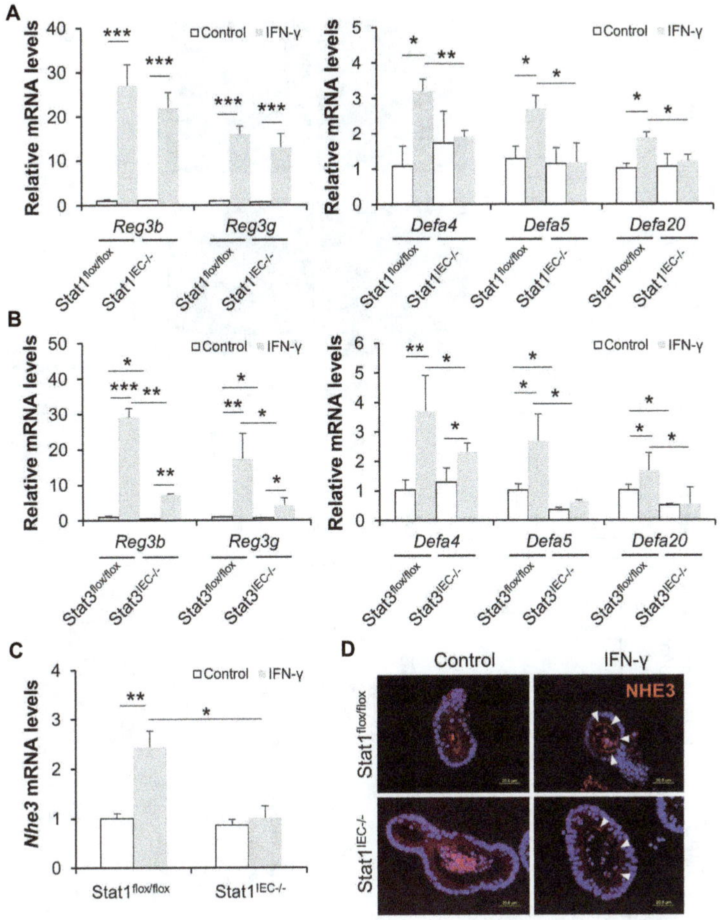

FIGURE 7 | IFN-γ directly stimulates AMP expression in cultured organoids through STAT pathway. **(A)** mRNA levels of AMPs in organoids isolated from control and Stat1$^{IEC-/-}$ mice after IFN-γ treatment. **(B)** mRNA levels of AMPs in organoids isolated from control and Stat3$^{IEC-/-}$ mice after IFN-γ treatment. **(C)** mRNA levels of *Nhe3* ($n = 3$ per group). **(D)** IF staining of NHE3 (red) in organoids. Nuclei were counterstained by DAPI (blue). Scale bar, 20 μm. $^{*}p < 0.05$, $^{**}p < 0.01$, and $^{***}p < 0.001$.

aimed to define the role of IFN-γ in mediating the antimicrobial ability of the host. We found that IFN-γ regulates a broad spectrum of AMPs at both transcriptional and post-translational levels. Through utilizing IEC-specific STAT1 or STAT3 KO mice models, we then elucidated that the effects of IFN-γ in regulating intestinal AMPs are through differential STAT1 and/or STAT3 signaling. We proved that restitution of IFN-γ levels by IFN-γ or IL-18 treatment ameliorated alcohol-induced gut and liver inflammation. This concept is not without precedence. IFN-γ has previously been reported to protect against bacterial and viral infections (Ma et al., 2011; Thiemann et al., 2017), regulate cathelicidin expression (Shtrichman and Samuel, 2001; Fabri et al., 2011), and directly stimulate AMP and mucus release (Farin et al., 2014). However, it remains unclear what is the turning point that directs IFN-γ toward protective or pathogenic directions. We presume that the intensity of IFN-γ signal, the condition of intestinal epithelium, and microenvironment cues inference with each other and all impact on the outcome. The goal of the present study was to restore intestinal IFN-γ to normal levels, and all data discussed are within this scope. It is noteworthy to mention that alcohol *per se* can directly disrupt the barrier of the intestine, such as colon (Zhong et al., 2010; Mutlu et al., 2012), and induce PAMP translocation. The present study, however, did not compare hepatic and systemic ethanol and acetaldehyde levels. Moreover, we found that neither IFN-γ nor IL-18 treatment altered major hepatic lipid compositions, including triglycerides and free fatty acids. Although inflammation and lipid metabolism are intertwined modulators of homeostasis and immunity, it is still obscure which specific lipid species would be impacted by inflammatory mediators given broad lipid categories, including triglycerides, free fatty acids, sterols, and phospholipids. Besides, we only treated the mice with IFN-γ or IL-18 for a short period during the 8-week alcohol feeding, and that may not be long enough to reverse lipid accumulation in the liver. One of the most interesting findings in this study is that IFN-γ orchestrates gut microbiota composition and possibly microbial-derived metabolites to an extend far beyond our current knowledge. First, IFN-γ treatment reduces overall gut microbial richness that is expanded by alcohol intoxication, which is in

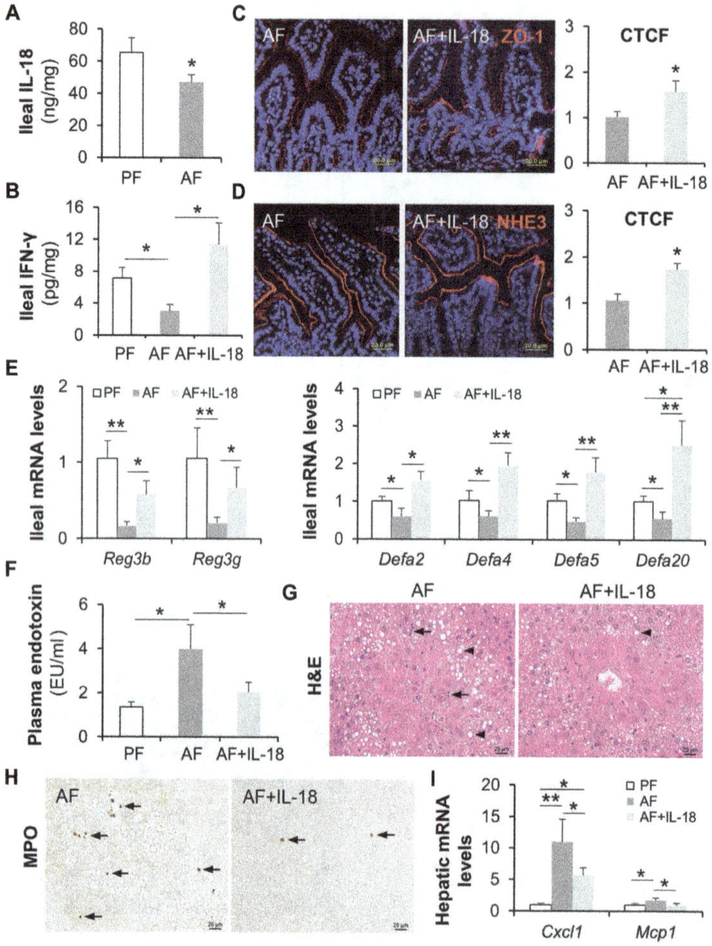

FIGURE 8 | IL-18 treatment restitutes intestinal IFN-γ levels and ameliorates alcohol-induced gut-liver damage in mice. **(A)** Ileal IL-18 levels measured by ELISA. **(B)** Ileal IFN-γ levels. **(C)** IF staining and quantification of ileal ZO-1 (red). Nuclei were counterstained by DAPI (blue). Scale bar, 20 μm. **(D)** IF staining and quantification of ileal NHE3 (red). Nuclei were counterstained by DAPI (blue). Scale bar, 20 μm. **(E)** mRNA levels of ileal AMPs. **(F)** Plasma endotoxin levels. **(G)** H&E staining of mouse liver sections. Arrowheads indicate lipid accumulation and arrows indicate inflammatory cells. Scale bar, 20 μm. **(H)** Representative IHC staining of neutrophil marker, MPO, in the liver of mice. Arrows indicate positive staining. Scale bar, 20 μm. **(I)** mRNA levels of hepatic inflammatory chemokines, *Cxcl1* and *Mcp1* ($n = 6$ per group). *$p < 0.05$ and **$p < 0.01$. PF, pair-fed; AF, alcohol-fed; CTCF, corrected total cell fluorescence.

line with stimulated AMP levels and the well-known antimicrobial function of AMPs. Second, it seems that IFN-γ specifically targets certain bacterial species rather than simple "correction" of a whole spectrum of microbiota. For example, IFN-γ treatment led to a proportional increase of *Verrucomicrobiaceae*. We previously reported that treatment of synthetic HD5 to AF mice resulted in a strikingly enriched *Verrucomicrobiaceae* population (Zhong et al., 2019). Similarly, another study also reported that HD5 increased *Akkermansia* sp. (the major genus of *Verrucomicrobiaceae*) without affecting microbial diversity in mice (Ehmann et al., 2019). Of note, *Akkermansia muciniphila* has been reported to be reduced upon alcohol intoxication, and treatment of *A. muciniphila* promotes gut barrier function and protects against ALD in mice (Grander et al., 2018). In addition, we also found that IFN-γ reversed alcohol-enriched *Streptococcaceae* and alcohol-diminished *Sutterellaceae*, which were not observed in HD5 treated mice, suggesting a HD5-independent regulatory mechanism of gut microbiota by IFN-γ. Third, functional pathway analysis of microbial genes revealed that IFN-γ also impacts on microbial metabolism, especially the production of SCFAs. SCFAs, especially butyric acid, are of great importance for their energy supply (Schonfeld and Wojtczak, 2016). They are also involved in intestinal epithelial AMP productions (Zhao et al., 2018; Pearce et al., 2020). This may partially explain the aforementioned beneficial effects of IFN-γ in regulating intestinal homeostasis and needs to be taken into consideration when interpreting data of the *in vivo* treatment experiments in the present study. We, therefore, used *in vitro* organoids and validated that IFN-γ can directly stimulate AMP expression in the absence of microbial-derived metabolites.

Although it has been established that IFN-γ-mediated signal transduction is mainly through Janus kinase (JAK)-STAT1 pathway, emerging evidence show that STAT1-independent

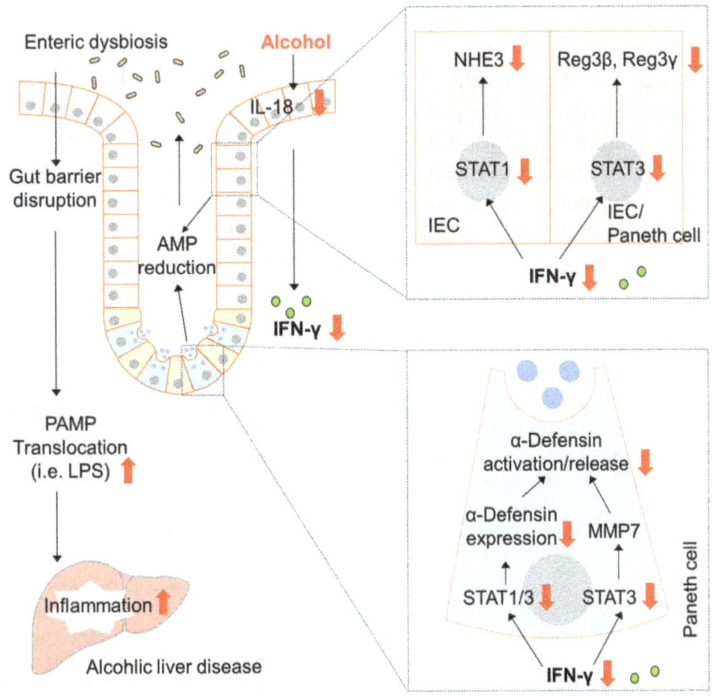

FIGURE 9 | Schematic diagram about the major findings of the present study. Red arrows indicate changes caused by alcohol. AMP, antimicrobial peptide; IFN-γ, interferon gamma; IEC, intestinal epithelial cells; IL-18, interleukin-18; LPS, lipopolysaccharide; MMP7, matrix metallopeptidase 7; NHE3, sodium-hydrogen exchanger 3; PAMP, pathogen-associated molecular pattern; STAT, signal transducer and activator of transcription.

pathways also play important roles in a wide range of biological responses of IFN-γ (Ramana et al., 2002; van Boxel-Dezaire and Stark, 2007). According to previous reports, STAT3 competes with STAT1 for activation at the same motif of IFN-γ receptor subunit 1 (IFNGR1; Qing and Stark, 2004). Moreover, IFN-γ-induced STAT3 activation was stronger and more prolonged in STAT1 deficient mouse embryo fibroblasts than in WT cells (Qing and Stark, 2004). The present study shows that both one and repeated administration of IFN-γ lead to substantial activation of intestinal STAT1 and STAT3. We further demonstrate that genetic deletion of IEC STAT1 causes STAT3 induction. This is not surprising as it has been reported that STAT1 may suppress STAT3 and compete it in many biological aspects, such as inflammation and tumorigenesis (Hu and Ivashkiv, 2009). We then dissected the roles of IEC STAT1 and STAT3 in mediating IFN-γ-regulated AMP levels and gut barrier. STAT3 is involved in the expression of Reg3 and α-defensins as well as the activation of α-defensins *via* activating MMP7, whereas STAT1 mediates the expression of α-defensins and NHE3. These synergistic interactions demonstrate that cross-regulation of STAT signaling processes can lead to a broad-spectrum of host response. These observations on the regulation of AMPs and gut microbiota by IFN-γ-STAT signaling indicate an essential role of IFN-γ-STAT signaling in intestinal homeostasis under normal and disease conditions.

IFN-γ is produced by a variety of immune cells, including CD4$^+$ T helper 1 (Th1) cells, natural killer (NK) cells, NK T cells, neutrophils, and macrophages (Beaurepaire et al., 2009). Alcohol abuse has been shown to be accompanied by suppressed immune response (Sibley et al., 2001). Alcohol abuse suppresses NK cell activity and decreases NK cell numbers (Meadows et al., 1989; Zhang et al., 2011). Moreover, in a mouse model of a combined insult of alcohol and burn injury, gut-associated lymphoid T cells are suppressed, intestinal IFN-γ is reduced, and bacterial translocation is elevated in association with exaggerated disease progression (Choudhry et al., 2002; Li et al., 2014). Here, we explored an epithelial-derived regulatory mechanism by IL-18 in regulating and maintaining physiological levels of IFN-γ. IL-18 was originally discovered as a cytokine that induces IFN-γ production by Th1 cells (Nakamura et al., 1989). Under homeostatic conditions, intestinal IL-18 is involved in epithelial cell repair, proliferation, and maturation (Wlodarska et al., 2014; Yasuda et al., 2019). The present study demonstrates that chronic alcohol feeding reduces IL-18 and administration of IL-18 restores intestinal IFN-γ levels (but not IL-22), reverses alcohol-reduced AMP expression, and alleviates alcoholic liver damage. In rats challenged with alcohol gavage and burn injury, however, a significant increase in IL-18 levels was observed, whereas alcohol gavage only did not change IL-18 levels (Li et al., 2006). This discrepancy may have resulted from different rodent species and disease models, administration routines, and the given dosages.

In summary, the present study demonstrates that constitutive expression of IFN-γ is instrumental in maintaining intestinal STAT signaling, innate immune responses of IECs, and gut microbial symbiosis to combat alcohol toxicity at the gut-liver axis, leading to a better control of the pathogenesis upon alcohol intoxication. Additionally, these findings provide new understanding of how the lack of adequate IFN-γ-STAT signaling may fail to elicit antimicrobial responses of IECs and thus provide an opportunity for progression of ALD. Therefore, IFN-γ-based interventions, such as IL-18 treatment, could be considered as a way of boosting intestinal epithelial innate immunity to halt systemic PAMP translocation and may also be one approach to preventing the development of ALD.

AUTHOR CONTRIBUTIONS

WZ conceived and designed research. RY, ZZ, and WZ performed experiments and analyzed data. XW and JZ analyzed gut microbiota and prepared figures. RY prepared figures and drafted manuscript. All authors contributed to the article and approved the submitted version.

REFERENCES

Bajaj, J. S. (2019). Alcohol, liver disease and the gut microbiota. *Nat. Rev. Gastroenterol. Hepatol.* 16, 235–246. doi: 10.1038/s41575-018-0099-1

Beaurepaire, C., Smyth, D., and McKay, D. M. (2009). Interferon-gamma regulation of intestinal epithelial permeability. *J. Interf. Cytokine Res.* 29, 133–144. doi: 10.1089/jir.2008.0057

Bevins, C. L., and Salzman, N. H. (2011). Paneth cells, antimicrobial peptides and maintenance of intestinal homeostasis. *Nat. Rev. Microbiol.* 9, 356–368. doi: 10.1038/nrmicro2546

Bull-Otterson, L., Feng, W., Kirpich, I., Wang, Y., Qin, X., Liu, Y., et al. (2013). Metagenomic analyses of alcohol induced pathogenic alterations in the intestinal microbiome and the effect of lactobacillus rhamnosus GG treatment. *PLoS One* 8:e53028. doi: 10.1371/journal.pone.0053028

Ching, C. B., Gupta, S., Li, B., Cortado, H., Mayne, N., Jackson, A. R., et al. (2018). Interleukin-6/Stat3 signaling has an essential role in the host antimicrobial response to urinary tract infection. *Kidney Int.* 93, 1320–1329. doi: 10.1016/j.kint.2017.12.006

Choi, S. M., McAleer, J. P., Zheng, M., Pociask, D. A., Kaplan, M. H., Qin, S., et al. (2013). Innate Stat3-mediated induction of the antimicrobial protein Reg3gamma is required for host defense against MRSA pneumonia. *J. Exp. Med.* 210, 551–561. doi: 10.1084/jem.20120260

Choudhry, M. A., Fazal, N., Goto, M., Gamelli, R. L., and Sayeed, M. M. (2002). Gut-associated lymphoid T cell suppression enhances bacterial translocation in alcohol and burn injury. *Am. J. Physiol. Gastrointest. Liver Physiol.* 282, G937–G947. doi: 10.1152/ajpgi.00235.2001

Cole, J. R., Wang, Q., Cardenas, E., Fish, J., Chai, B., Farris, R. J., et al. (2009). The Ribosomal Database Project: improved alignments and new tools for rRNA analysis. *Nucleic Acids Res.* 37, D141–D145. doi: 10.1093/nar/gkn879

Ehmann, D., Wendler, J., Koeninger, L., Larsen, I. S., Klag, T., Berger, J., et al. (2019). Paneth cell alpha-defensins HD-5 and HD-6 display differential degradation into active antimicrobial fragments. *Proc. Natl. Acad. Sci. U. S. A.* 116, 3746–3751. doi: 10.1073/pnas.1817376116

Fabri, M., Stenger, S., Shin, D. M., Yuk, J. M., Liu, P. T., Realegeno, S., et al. (2011). Vitamin D is required for IFN-gamma-mediated antimicrobial activity of human macrophages. *Sci. Transl. Med.* 3:104ra102. doi: 10.1126/scitranslmed.3003045

Farin, H. F., Karthaus, W. R., Kujala, P., Rakhshandehroo, M., Schwank, G., Vries, R. G., et al. (2014). Paneth cell extrusion and release of antimicrobial products is directly controlled by immune cell-derived IFN-gamma. *J. Exp. Med.* 211, 1393–1405. doi: 10.1084/jem.20130753

Gao, B., and Bataller, R. (2011). Alcoholic liver disease: pathogenesis and new therapeutic targets. *Gastroenterology* 141, 1572–1585. doi: 10.1053/j.gastro.2011.09.002

Gavrilescu, L. C., Butcher, B. A., Del Rio, L., Taylor, G. A., and Denkers, E. Y. (2004). STAT1 is essential for antimicrobial effector function but dispensable for gamma interferon production during toxoplasma gondii infection. *Infect. Immun.* 72, 1257–1264. doi: 10.1128/iai.72.3.1257-1264.2004

Grander, C., Adolph, T. E., Wieser, V., Lowe, P., Wrzosek, L., Gyongyosi, B., et al. (2018). Recovery of ethanol-induced *Akkermansia muciniphila* depletion ameliorates alcoholic liver disease. *Gut* 67, 891–901. doi: 10.1136/gutjnl-2016-313432

Gurtner, G. J., Newberry, R. D., Schloemann, S. R., McDonald, K. G., and Stenson, W. F. (2003). Inhibition of indoleamine 2,3-dioxygenase augments trinitrobenzene sulfonic acid colitis in mice. *Gastroenterology* 125, 1762–1773. doi: 10.1053/j.gastro.2003.08.031

Hanck, C., Rossol, S., Bocker, U., Tokus, M., and Singer, M. V. (1998). Presence of plasma endotoxin is correlated with tumour necrosis factor receptor levels and disease activity in alcoholic cirrhosis. *Alcohol Alcohol.* 33, 606–608. doi: 10.1093/alcalc/33.6.606

He, L., Li, F., Yin, X., Bohman, P., Kim, S., McClain, C. J., et al. (2019). Profiling of polar metabolites in mouse feces using four analytical platforms to study the effects of cathelicidin-related antimicrobial peptide in alcoholic liver disease. *J. Proteome Res.* 18, 2875–2884. doi: 10.1021/acs.jproteome.9b00181

Hendrikx, T., Duan, Y., Wang, Y., Oh, J. H., Alexander, L. M., Huang, W., et al. (2019). Bacteria engineered to produce IL-22 in intestine induce expression of REG3G to reduce ethanol-induced liver disease in mice. *Gut* 68, 1504–1515. doi: 10.1136/gutjnl-2018-317232

Hritz, I., Mandrekar, P., Velayudham, A., Catalano, D., Dolganiuc, A., Kodys, K., et al. (2008). The critical role of toll-like receptor (TLR) 4 in alcoholic liver disease is independent of the common TLR adapter MyD88. *Hepatology* 48, 1224–1231. doi: 10.1002/hep.22470

Hu, X., and Ivashkiv, L. B. (2009). Cross-regulation of signaling pathways by interferon-gamma: implications for immune responses and autoimmune diseases. *Immunity* 31, 539–550. doi: 10.1016/j.immuni.2009.09.002

Ki, S. H., Park, O., Zheng, M., Morales-Ibanez, O., Kolls, J. K., Bataller, R., et al. (2010). Interleukin-22 treatment ameliorates alcoholic liver injury in a murine model of chronic-binge ethanol feeding: role of signal transducer and activator of transcription 3. *Hepatology* 52, 1291–1300. doi: 10.1002/hep.23837

Kominsky, D. J., Campbell, E. L., Ehrentraut, S. F., Wilson, K. E., Kelly, C. J., Glover, L. E., et al. (2014). IFN-gamma-mediated induction of an apical IL-10 receptor on polarized intestinal epithelia. *J. Immunol.* 192, 1267–1276. doi: 10.4049/jimmunol.1301757

Kominsky, D. J., Keely, S., Macmanus, C. F., Glover, L. E., Scully, M., Collins, C. B., et al. (2011). An endogenously anti-inflammatory role for methylation in mucosal inflammation identified through metabolite profiling. *J. Immunol.* 186, 6505–6514. doi: 10.4049/jimmunol.1002805

Kozuka, K., He, Y., Koo-McCoy, S., Kumaraswamy, P., Nie, B., Shaw, K., et al. (2017). Development and characterization of a human and mouse intestinal epithelial cell monolayer platform. *Stem Cell Rep.* 9, 1976–1990. doi: 10.1016/j.stemcr.2017.10.013

Langille, M. G., Zaneveld, J., Caporaso, J. G., McDonald, D., Knights, D., Reyes, J. A., et al. (2013). Predictive functional profiling of microbial communities using 16S rRNA marker gene sequences. *Nat. Biotechnol.* 31, 814–821. doi: 10.1038/nbt.2676

Li, X., Rana, S. N., Schwacha, M. G., Chaudry, I. H., and Choudhry, M. A. (2006). A novel role for IL-18 in corticosterone-mediated intestinal damage in a two-hit rodent model of alcohol intoxication and injury. *J. Leukoc. Biol.* 80, 367–375. doi: 10.1189/jlb.1205745

Li, X., Rendon, J. L., and Choudhry, M. A. (2014). T cell IFN-gamma suppression following alcohol and burn injury is independent of miRNA155. *PLoS One* 9:e105314. doi: 10.1371/journal.pone.0105314

Lieberman, L. A., Banica, M., Reiner, S. L., and Hunter, C. A. (2004). STAT1 plays a critical role in the regulation of antimicrobial effector mechanisms, but not in the development of Th1-type responses during toxoplasmosis. *J. Immunol.* 172, 457–463. doi: 10.4049/jimmunol.172.1.457

Livak, K. J., and Schmittgen, T. D. (2001). Analysis of relative gene expression data using real-time quantitative PCR and the 2(-Delta Delta C(T)) method. *Methods* 25, 402–408. doi: 10.1006/meth.2001.1262

Ma, F., Xu, S., Liu, X., Zhang, Q., Xu, X., Liu, M., et al. (2011). The microRNA miR-29 controls innate and adaptive immune responses to intracellular bacterial infection by targeting interferon-gamma. *Nat. Immunol.* 12, 861–869. doi: 10.1038/ni.2073

Meadows, G. G., Blank, S. E., and Duncan, D. D. (1989). Influence of ethanol consumption on natural killer cell activity in mice. *Alcohol. Clin. Exp. Res.* 13, 476–479. doi: 10.1111/j.1530-0277.1989.tb00359.x

Meraz, M. A., White, J. M., Sheehan, K. C., Bach, E. A., Rodig, S. J., Dighe, A. S., et al. (1996). Targeted disruption of the Stat1 gene in mice reveals unexpected physiologic specificity in the JAK-STAT signaling pathway. *Cell* 84, 431–442. doi: 10.1016/s0092-8674(00)81288-x

Muniz, L. R., Knosp, C., and Yeretssian, G. (2012). Intestinal antimicrobial peptides during homeostasis, infection, and disease. *Front. Immunol.* 3:310. doi: 10.3389/fimmu.2012.00310

Mutlu, E. A., Gillevet, P. M., Rangwala, H., Sikaroodi, M., Naqvi, A., Engen, P. A., et al. (2012). Colonic microbiome is altered in alcoholism. *Am. J. Physiol. Gastrointest. Liver Physiol.* 302, G966–G978. doi: 10.1152/ajpgi.00380.2011

Nakamura, K., Okamura, H., Wada, M., Nagata, K., and Tamura, T. (1989). Endotoxin-induced serum factor that stimulates gamma interferon production. *Infect. Immun.* 57, 590–595. doi: 10.1128/IAI.57.2.590-595.1989

Nava, P., Koch, S., Laukoetter, M. G., Lee, W. Y., Kolegraff, K., Capaldo, C. T., et al. (2010). Interferon-gamma regulates intestinal epithelial homeostasis through converging beta-catenin signaling pathways. *Immunity* 32, 392–402. doi: 10.1016/j.immuni.2010.03.001

Parlesak, A., Schafer, C., Schutz, T., Bode, J. C., and Bode, C. (2000). Increased intestinal permeability to macromolecules and endotoxemia in patients with chronic alcohol abuse in different stages of alcohol-induced liver disease. *J. Hepatol.* 32, 742–747. doi: 10.1016/s0168-8278(00)80242-1

Pearce, S. C., Weber, G. J., van Sambeek, D. M., Soares, J. W., Racicot, K., and Breault, D. T. (2020). Intestinal enteroids recapitulate the effects of short-chain fatty acids on the intestinal epithelium. *PLoS One* 15:e0230231. doi: 10.1371/journal.pone.0230231

Philips, C. A., Pande, A., Shasthry, S. M., Jamwal, K. D., Khillan, V., Chandel, S. S., et al. (2017). Healthy donor fecal microbiota transplantation in steroid-ineligible severe alcoholic hepatitis: a pilot study. *Clin. Gastroenterol. Hepatol.* 15, 600–602. doi: 10.1016/j.cgh.2016.10.029

Qing, Y., and Stark, G. R. (2004). Alternative activation of STAT1 and STAT3 in response to interferon-gamma. *J. Biol. Chem.* 279, 41679–41685. doi: 10.1074/jbc.M406413200

Quast, C., Pruesse, E., Yilmaz, P., Gerken, J., Schweer, T., Yarza, P., et al. (2013). The SILVA ribosomal RNA gene database project: improved data processing and web-based tools. *Nucleic Acids Res.* 41, D590–D596. doi: 10.1093/nar/gks1219

Ramana, C. V., Gil, M. P., Schreiber, R. D., and Stark, G. R. (2002). Stat1-dependent and -independent pathways in IFN-gamma-dependent signaling. *Trends Immunol.* 23, 96–101. doi: 10.1016/s1471-4906(01)02118-4

Ruiz, J., Kanagavelu, S., Flores, C., Romero, L., Riveron, R., Shih, D. Q., et al. (2015). Systemic activation of TLR3-dependent TRIF signaling confers host defense against gram-negative bacteria in the intestine. *Front. Cell. Infect. Microbiol.* 5:105. doi: 10.3389/fcimb.2015.00105

Sato, T., Vries, R. G., Snippert, H. J., van De Wetering, M., Barker, N., Stange, D. E., et al. (2009). Single Lgr5 stem cells build crypt-villus structures in vitro without a mesenchymal niche. *Nature* 459, 262–265. doi: 10.1038/nature07935

Schloss, P. D., Westcott, S. L., Ryabin, T., Hall, J. R., Hartmann, M., Hollister, E. B., et al. (2009). Introducing mothur: open-source, platform-independent, community-supported software for describing and comparing microbial communities. *Appl. Environ. Microbiol.* 75, 7537–7541. doi: 10.1128/AEM.01541-09

Schonfeld, P., and Wojtczak, L. (2016). Short- and medium-chain fatty acids in energy metabolism: the cellular perspective. *J. Lipid Res.* 57, 943–954. doi: 10.1194/jlr.R067629

Segata, N., Izard, J., Waldron, L., Gevers, D., Miropolsky, L., Garrett, W. S., et al. (2011). Metagenomic biomarker discovery and explanation. *Genome Biol.* 12:R60. doi: 10.1186/gb-2011-12-6-r60

Sheikh, S. Z., Matsuoka, K., Kobayashi, T., Li, F., Rubinas, T., and Plevy, S. E. (2010). Cutting edge: IFN-gamma is a negative regulator of IL-23 in murine macrophages and experimental colitis. *J. Immunol.* 184, 4069–4073. doi: 10.4049/jimmunol.0903600

Shtrichman, R., and Samuel, C. E. (2001). The role of gamma interferon in antimicrobial immunity. *Curr. Opin. Microbiol.* 4, 251–259. doi: 10.1016/s1369-5274(00)00199-5

Sibley, D. A., Osna, N., Kusynski, C., Wilkie, L., and Jerrells, T. R. (2001). Alcohol consumption is associated with alterations in macrophage responses to interferon-gamma and infection by Salmonella typhimurium. *FEMS Immunol. Med. Microbiol.* 32, 73–83. doi: 10.1111/j.1574-695X.2001.tb00537.x

Thiemann, S., Smit, N., Roy, U., Lesker, T. R., Galvez, E. J. C., Helmecke, J., et al. (2017). Enhancement of IFNgamma production by distinct commensals ameliorates Salmonella-induced disease. *Cell Host Microbe* 21, 682.e685–694.e685. doi: 10.1016/j.chom.2017.05.005

Tilg, H., Cani, P. D., and Mayer, E. A. (2016). Gut microbiome and liver diseases. *Gut* 65, 2035–2044. doi: 10.1136/gutjnl-2016-312729

Uesugi, T., Froh, M., Arteel, G. E., Bradford, B. U., and Thurman, R. G. (2001). Toll-like receptor 4 is involved in the mechanism of early alcohol-induced liver injury in mice. *Hepatology* 34, 101–108. doi: 10.1053/jhep.2001.25350

van Boxel-Dezaire, A. H., and Stark, G. R. (2007). Cell type-specific signaling in response to interferon-gamma. *Curr. Top. Microbiol. Immunol.* 316, 119–154. doi: 10.1007/978-3-540-71329-6_7

Wang, L., Fouts, D. E., Starkel, P., Hartmann, P., Chen, P., Llorente, C., et al. (2016). Intestinal REG3 lectins protect against alcoholic steatohepatitis by reducing mucosa-associated microbiota and preventing bacterial translocation. *Cell Host Microbe* 19, 227–239. doi: 10.1016/j.chom.2016.01.003

Wilson, C. L., Ouellette, A. J., Satchell, D. P., Ayabe, T., Lopez-Boado, Y. S., Stratman, J. L., et al. (1999). Regulation of intestinal alpha-defensin activation by the metalloproteinase matrilysin in innate host defense. *Science* 286, 113–117. doi: 10.1126/science.286.5437.113

Wilson, S. S., Tocchi, A., Holly, M. K., Parks, W. C., and Smith, J. G. (2015). A small intestinal organoid model of non-invasive enteric pathogen-epithelial cell interactions. *Mucosal Immunol.* 8, 352–361. doi: 10.1038/mi.2014.72

Wittkopf, N., Pickert, G., Billmeier, U., Mahapatro, M., Wirtz, S., Martini, E., et al. (2015). Activation of intestinal epithelial Stat3 orchestrates tissue defense during gastrointestinal infection. *PLoS One* 10:e0118401. doi: 10.1371/journal.pone.0118401

Wlodarska, M., Thaiss, C. A., Nowarski, R., Henao-Mejia, J., Zhang, J. P., Brown, E. M., et al. (2014). NLRP6 inflammasome orchestrates the colonic host-microbial interface by regulating goblet cell mucus secretion. *Cell* 156, 1045–1059. doi: 10.1016/j.cell.2014.01.026

Yan, A. W., Fouts, D. E., Brandl, J., Starkel, P., Torralba, M., Schott, E., et al. (2011). Enteric dysbiosis associated with a mouse model of alcoholic liver disease. *Hepatology* 53, 96–105. doi: 10.1002/hep.24018

Yasuda, K., Nakanishi, K., and Tsutsui, H. (2019). Interleukin-18 in health and disease. *Int. J. Mol. Sci.* 20:649. doi: 10.3390/ijms20030649

Yin, M., Bradford, B. U., Wheeler, M. D., Uesugi, T., Froh, M., Goyert, S. M., et al. (2001). Reduced early alcohol-induced liver injury in CD14-deficient mice. *J. Immunol.* 166, 4737–4742. doi: 10.4049/jimmunol.166.7.4737

Zhang, H., Zhu, Z., and Meadows, G. G. (2011). Chronic alcohol consumption decreases the percentage and number of NK cells in the peripheral lymph nodes and exacerbates B16BL6 melanoma metastasis into the draining lymph nodes. *Cell. Immunol.* 266, 172–179. doi: 10.1016/j.cellimm.2010.10.001

Zhao, Y., Chen, F., Wu, W., Sun, M., Bilotta, A. J., Yao, S., et al. (2018). GPR43 mediates microbiota metabolite SCFA regulation of antimicrobial peptide expression in intestinal epithelial cells via activation of mTOR and STAT3. *Mucosal Immunol.* 11, 752–762. doi: 10.1038/mi.2017.118

Zhong, W., Li, Q., Xie, G., Sun, X., Tan, X., Sun, X., et al. (2013). Dietary fat sources differentially modulate intestinal barrier and hepatic inflammation in alcohol-induced liver injury in rats. *Am. J. Physiol. Gastrointest. Liver Physiol.* 305, G919–G932. doi: 10.1152/ajpgi.00226.2013

Zhong, W., McClain, C. J., Cave, M., Kang, Y. J., and Zhou, Z. (2010). The role of zinc deficiency in alcohol-induced intestinal barrier dysfunction. *Am. J. Physiol. Gastrointest. Liver Physiol.* 298, G625–G633. doi: 10.1152/ajpgi.00350.2009

Zhong, W., Wei, X., Hao, L., Lin, T. D., Yue, R., Sun, X., et al. (2019). Paneth cell dysfunction mediates alcohol-related steatohepatitis through promoting bacterial translocation in mice: role of zinc deficiency. *Hepatology* 71, 1575–1591. doi: 10.1002/hep.30945

Zhong, W., Zhang, W., Li, Q., Xie, G., Sun, Q., Sun, X., et al. (2015). Pharmacological activation of aldehyde dehydrogenase 2 by Alda-1 reverses alcohol-induced hepatic steatosis and cell death in mice. *J. Hepatol.* 62, 1375–1381. doi: 10.1016/j.jhep.2014.12.022

15

Higher Frequency of Hospital-Acquired Infections but Similar In-Hospital Mortality Among Admissions with Alcoholic Hepatitis at Academic vs. Non-Academic Centers

*Muhammad Waleed[1], Mohamed A. Abdallah[1], Yong-Fang Kuo[2], Juan P. Arab[3], Robert Wong[4] and Ashwani K. Singal[1,5]**

[1] Department of Medicine, University of South Dakota Sanford School of Medicine, Sioux Falls, SD, United States,
[2] Department of Biostatistics, University of Texas Medical Branch at Galveston, Galveston, TX, United States,
[3] Departamento de Gastroenterología, Escuela de Medicina, Pontificia Universidad Católica de Chile, Santiago, Chile,
[4] Division of Gastroenterology and Hepatology, Alameda Health System Highland Hospital, Oakland, CA, United States,
[5] Division of Transplant Hepatology, Avera Transplant Institute, Sioux Falls, SD, United States

***Correspondence:**
Ashwani K. Singal
ashwanisingal.com@gmail.com

Background: Alcoholic hepatitis (AH) is a unique syndrome characterized by high short-term mortality. The impact of the academic status of a hospital (urban and teaching) on outcomes in AH is unknown.

Methods: National Inpatient Sample dataset (2006–2014) on AH admissions stratified to academic center (AC) or non-academic center (NAC) and analyzed for in-hospital mortality (IHM), hospital resource use, length of stay in days (d), and total charges (TC) in United States dollars (USD). Admission year was stratified to 2006–2008 (TMI), 2009–2011 (TM2), and 2012–2014 (TM3).

Results: Of 62,136 AH admissions, the proportion at AC increased from 46% in TM1 to 57% in TM3, Armitage trend, $p < 0.001$. On logistic regression, TM3, younger age, black race, Medicaid and private insurance, and development of acute on chronic liver failure (ACLF) were associated with admission to an AC. Of 53,264 admissions propensity score matched for demographics, pay status, and disease severity, admissions to AC vs. NAC (26,622 each) were more likely to have liver disease complications (esophageal varices, ascites, and hepatic encephalopathy) and hospital-acquired infections (HAI), especially *Clostridioides difficile* and ventilator-associated pneumonia. Admissions to AC were more likely transfers from outside hospital (1.6% vs. 1.3%) and seen by palliative care (4.8% vs. 3.3%), $p < 0.001$. Use of endoscopy, dialysis, and mechanical ventilation were similar. With similar IHM comparing AC vs. NAC (7.7% vs. 7.8%, $p = 0.93$), average LOS and number of procedures were higher at AC (7.7 vs. 7.1 d and 2.3 vs. 1.9, respectively, $p < 0.001$) without difference on total charges ($52,821 vs. $52,067 USD, $p = 0.28$). On multivariable logistic regression model after controlling for demographics,

ACLF grade, and calendar year, IHM was similar irrespective of academic status of the hospital, HR (95% CI): 1.01 (0.93–1.08, $p = 0.70$). IHM decreased over time, with ACLF as strongest predictor. A total of 63 and 22% were discharged to home and skilled nursing facility, respectively, without differences on academic status of the hospital.

Conclusion: Admissions with AH to AC compared to NAC have higher frequency of liver disease complications and HAI, with longer duration of hospitalization. Prospective studies are needed to reduce HAI among hospitalized patients with AH.

Keywords: academic, outcomes, acute on chronic liver failure (ACLF), cirrhosis, organ failure

INTRODUCTION

Alcohol contributed to 48% of cirrhosis-related deaths in the United States in 2017, and alcohol-associated liver disease (ALD) accounts for 27% of these (GBD 2017 Cirrhosis Collaborators, 2020). Alcohol-associated liver disease presents as a spectrum of injuries to the liver, including isolated fatty liver disease, alcoholic hepatitis (AH), and cirrhosis (Chacko and Reinus, 2016).

With the recent advances in the treatment of hepatitis B and C, ALD has emerged as the leading indication for liver transplantation (LT; Williams, 2008; Cholankeril and Ahmed, 2018). There are also increasing trends on alcohol consumption especially drinking in younger individuals (Siegel et al., 2011a,b). Of approximately $250 billion spent by the United States annually on alcohol-related problems, a significant proportion is spent on taking care of patients with AH and alcohol-associated cirrhosis (Singal et al., 2020). Additionally, AH most often occurs in individuals aged 40–60 years, with the majority of these individuals contributing to the most productive contingent of the workforce (Thompson et al., 2018). Taken together, these trends in alcohol consumption contribute toward burden on social, economic, and health care systems (Jinjuvadia and Liangpunsakul, 2015).

AH is a distinct clinical entity among ALD patients and presents with jaundice and acute on chronic liver failure (ACLF; Altamirano et al., 2017). With limited therapeutic options for AH, it has a potential for high short-term mortality of 15–40% within 28 days of presentation (Altamirano et al., 2017). Given the very high prevalence of AH among hospitalized patients with decompensated ALD, patients with AH are treated by non-hepatology providers such as hospitalists, internists, and gastroenterologists at both academic (AC) and non-academic centers (NAC; Singal and Anand, 2013). Data on outcomes of AH patients comparing hospitalizations at AC with those hospitalized at NAC are scanty. In this study, we aim to compare characteristics and outcomes of AH patients hospitalized to AC vs. NAC using the National Inpatient Sample (NIS) Database.

PATIENTS AND METHODS

Study Design and Data Source

The Healthcare Cost and Utilization Project NIS database on hospitalizations between 2006 and 2014 in the US was used for this study. The largest inpatient database in the US representing 20% stratified sample of all hospital discharges from 46 states (approximately 97% of the United States population), NIS database is developed and maintained by the Agency for Healthcare Research and Quality. It contains data from over 7 million hospital discharges annually, yielding national estimates of hospital inpatient stays. The NIS includes up to 25 International Classification of Diseases (ICD) discharge diagnoses or procedures. The database also provides information on patient demographics, payer status, comorbidities, in-hospital mortality (IHM), hospital characteristics (region, urban, or rural location, and teaching status), length of stay (LOS) in days, and total hospital charges in the United States dollars (USD). Given that the NIS is completely de-identified and publicly available, institutional review board (IRB) approval was not required for this study.

Study Population

Our study population included hospitalizations with discharge diagnosis of AH identified using the ICD-09 diagnosis code 571.1 for AH (**Supplementary Table 1**). The study population was stratified to three time frames: 2006–2008 (TM1), 2009–2011 (TM2), and 2012–2014 (TM3).

Definitions

Academic vs. Non-Academic Centers

Hospitals in urban locations with teaching status were classified as AC and the remaining as NAC.

Acute on Chronic Liver Failure

Acute on chronic liver failure was defined per North American Consortium for the Study of End-Stage Liver Disease (NACSELD) Criteria, as the presence of two or more extrahepatic organ failures [cardiovascular (CV), respiratory, renal, and brain] in patients with cirrhosis (Bajaj et al., 2014; Allen et al., 2016; O'Leary et al., 2018; O'Leary et al., 2019). Organ failures were defined using the ICD-09 codes (**Supplementary Table 1**; Allen et al., 2016; Singal et al., 2020). Severity of ACLF was graded to ACLF-1, ACLF-2, and ACLF-3 in the presence of two, three, or four extrahepatic organ failures.

Organ Failures

International Classification of Diseases-09 procedure codes were used to define CV failure by (need for central venous pressure, pulmonary artery/wedge pressure, use of arterial line, the presence of septic shock, or severe sepsis); respiratory failure (using code for mechanical ventilation); renal failure (need for hemodialysis or diagnosis code of acute renal failure), and brain failure (diagnosis code for hepatic encephalopathy) (**Supplementary Table 1**).

Liver Disease Complications

Ascites, variceal bleeding, hepatic encephalopathy, community-acquired infections [CAI; urinary tract infection, spontaneous bacterial peritonitis (SBP), pneumonia, skin, and soft tissue infections], or hospital-acquired infections (HAI; *Clostridioides difficile*, ventilator-associated pneumonia, central line-associated bloodstream infection, catheter-associated urinary tract infection) were identified using discharge ICD-09 diagnoses codes (**Supplementary Tables 1, 2**).

Study Outcomes

Primary outcomes of the study were IHM, LOS, and total hospital charges. Secondary outcomes were (a) use of hospital resources (blood transfusion, hemodialysis, endoscopic intervention, ventilator support, liver transplant, and palliative care) as identified using the ICD-09 procedure codes and (b) discharge destination of survivors (home with or without home health care, short-term hospitals, and intermediate/long-term nursing care facility) as available from the dataset.

Statistical Analyses

Baseline characteristics were compared for AC vs. NAC using chi-square and Student *t* test for categorical and continuous variables, respectively. Hospitalization trends over period were analyzed using Cochran-Armitage trend test. Hospitalizations to AC or NAC were propensity score matched (1:1) on variables associated with admission to AC, as identified by logistic regression model. Baseline characteristics were also compared in the matched cohort. Admissions to AC were compared to NAC on primary and secondary outcomes. Logistic regression analysis model was built to determine predictors of IHM and reported as odds ratio (OR) with 95% confidence interval (CI). p values < 0.05 were considered significant. SAS version 9.4 (SAS Institute, Cary, NC) was used for statistical analyses.

RESULTS

Study Population

A total of 62,136 admissions with discharge diagnosis of AH were admitted during 2006–2014, with 31,321 (50.5%) admitted to an AC. Over the period, frequency of admissions to AC increased from 45.6% in TM1 to 45.8% in TM2 to 57.4% in TM3, $p < 0.001$ (**Figure 1**). The proportion of patients with ACLF over time for AH admissions was higher for TM1 but similar for TM2 and TM3 comparing AC vs. NAC: 6.8% vs. 5.8% ($p < 0.001$); 11.2% vs. 11.9% ($p = 0.79$); and 10.8% vs. 10.9% ($p = 0.79$), respectively.

Baseline Characteristics Admissions With AH: AC vs. NAC

Admissions to AC compared to NAC differed on demographics (younger age and more likely to be females and minorities in AC). Further, admissions to AC were less likely to be electively admitted and associated with Medicare pay source. About 72% admissions were associated with underlying alcohol-associated cirrhosis, without difference between admissions to AC or NAC (**Table 1**). Admissions to AC were associated with more severe disease with ACLF (12% vs. 9%, $p < 0.001$) and various organ failures (**Table 1**). On logistic regression analysis, time period, younger age, African American race, pay source other than Medicare, and the presence of ACLF were associated with admission to an AC (**Table 2**).

Matching for Admissions to AC or NAC

Baseline characteristics

Using propensity score analysis, admissions to AC were matched (1:1) with admissions to NAC for age, race, pay source, time period of admission, and the presence of ACLF. Matched cohort included 53,264 admissions (26,622 each to AC or NAC). Baseline characteristics comparing admissions to AC vs. NAC in this

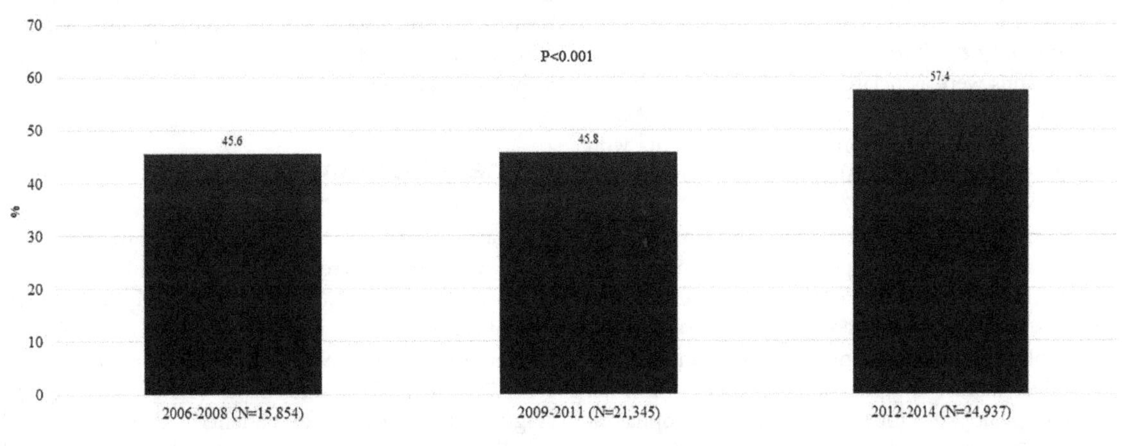

FIGURE 1 | Trends on the proportion of patients admitted with AH among admission to AC for the time periods 2006–2008 (TM1), 2009–2011 (TM2), and 2012–2014 (TM3). AC, academic centers; NAC, non-academic centers; AH, alcoholic hepatitis.

TABLE 1 | Comparison of baseline characteristics of admissions with diagnosis of alcoholic hepatitis (AH) to academic centers (AC) vs. non-academic centers (NAC).

Variables	Unmatched AH cohort			Matched AH cohort		
	AC (*N* = 31,321)	NAC (*N* = 30,815)	*p* value	AC (*N* = 26,622)	NAC (*N* = 26,622)	*p* value
Age in years (mean ± SD)	49 ± 10	50 ± 10	<0.001	49.7 ± 10.2	49.8 ± 10.2	0.34
Females (%)	34	33	<0.029	33	33	0.3
CA: AA: HI: OT (%)	67: 12: 15: 6	77: 7: 11: 5	<0.001	64:7: 12: 17	65: 7: 11: 17	0.2
Comorbidities, (mean ± SD)	7 ± 3.2	7.4 ± 3.3	<0.001	7.3 ± 3.3	7.3 ± 3.2	0.07
Obesity (%)	6.4	6.3	0.61	6.1	6.6	< 0.02
Alcoholic cirrhosis (%)	72	72	0.89	72	72	0.41
Elective admissions (%)	4.5	5.7	<0.001	4.9	4.6	0.12
Pay source (MC: MD: Self: Pvt. (%)	16: 30: 28: 26	20: 24: 29: 27	<0.001	17:27: 28: 28	18: 27: 29: 27	0.7
ACLF (%)	12.1	9.3	<0.001	9.9	10	0.64
Pulmonary failure (%)	10.1	8	<0.001	8.4	8.4	0.75
Cardiovascular failure (%)	6.2	4.5	<0.001	4.7	4.9	0.28
Brain failure (%)	29.2	29.3	0.81	29.6	28.3	< 0.002
Renal failure (%)	9.9	7.6	<0.001	8.2	8.2	0.79

CA, Caucasian; AA, African American; HI, Hispanic; OT, Other; MC, Medicare; MD, Medicaid; Pvt, private; ACLF, acute on chronic liver failure; HR, hazard ratio; CI, confidence interval; OR, odds ratio; NAC, non-academic center.

TABLE 2 | Factors associated with admission of patients with alcoholic hepatitis to academic centers.

Variable	Odds ratio	95% CI	*p* value
Age	0.99	0.989–0.993	<0.001
2009–2011 vs. 2006–2008	0.99	0.93–1.06	0.14
2012–2014 vs. 2006–2008	1.61	1.52–1.72	<0.001
AAvs. C	2.01	1.88–2.15	<0.001
H vs. C	1.40	1.32–1.48	0.76
Female vs. male	1.02	0.98–1.06	0.27
Medicaid vs. Medicare	1.31	1.24–1.40	<0.001
Pvt. insurance vs. Medicare	1.15	1.09–1.22	<0.001
ACLF	1.27	1.20–1.35	<0.001

AA, African American; C, Caucasian; H, Hispanic; ACLF, acute on chronic liver failure; CI, confidence interval.

matched cohort were similar except for obesity (6.1% vs. 6.6%, $p < 0.02$), **Table 1**. Admissions to AC were more often admitted as a transfer from another hospital (1.6% vs. 1.1%), $p < 0.001$.

Complications and organ failure

About 10% admissions were associated with ACLF at or during admission with no differences comparing admissions to AC or NAC (9.9% vs. 10%, $p = 0.64$). Among 5292 AH patients with ACLF (2630 at AC), distribution to ACLF grades to grades 1, 2, and 3 comparing NAC vs. AC were 70.5% vs. 71.1%, 24.3% vs. 23.3%, and 5.2% vs. 5.6%, respectively, $p = 0.89$. Similarly, all the organ failures were similar irrespective of academic status of the hospital, except brain failure which was more frequent among admissions to AC (30% vs. 28%, $p < 0.001$), **Table 1**. Of liver disease complications, admissions to AC were more often associated with liver disease complications on ascites (45% vs. 41%), hepatic encephalopathy (30% vs. 28%), and esophageal varices (14% vs. 12%), $p < 0.001$ for all analyses. However, there was no difference on variceal bleeding (7.3% vs. 7.5%, $p = 0.34$), **Figure 2**.

Infections

About 20% of admissions were associated with infection, without difference comparing admissions to AC vs. NAC (21% vs. 20%, $p = 0.13$), **Figure 3**. On analyzing the infection source whether acquired in the community or hospital, admissions to AC were more likely to develop HAI (4% vs. 3.1%, $p = 0.034$). However, there was no difference in CAI (18.2% vs. 18.4%, $p = 0.49$), **Figure 3**. Based on admission as transfer from outside hospital, the frequency of CAI was similar (18.7% vs. 18.4%, $p = 0.82$). However, transfers from outside hospital were associated with higher frequency of HAI (5.6% vs. 3.6%, $p = 0.002$), **Supplementary Figure 1**.

Of the HAI, *C. difficile* infection and ventilator-associated pneumonia were more frequent in AC vs. NAC, 2.6% vs. 1.8% and 0.18% vs. 0.08%, respectively, $p < 0.001$ for both analyses (**Supplementary Figure 2A**). Of CAI, urinary tract infection was most common in about 13% patients, without differences based on academic status of admitting hospital. Similarly, SBP and pneumonia were similar comparing admissions to AC with NAC. In contrast, skin and subcutaneous infections were more common among admissions to NAC (3.8% vs. 3.4%, $p < 0.001$), **Supplementary Figure 2B**.

Primary Outcomes

In-Hospital Mortality

A total of 4110 (7.7%) of admissions were associated with IHM, with no difference comparing admissions to AC vs. NAC (7.7% vs. 7.8%, $p = 0.93$) (**Figure 4**). In-hospital mortality comparing admissions to AC vs. NAC remained similar for TM1 (6.9% vs. 7.1%, $p = 0.72$), TM2 (8.5% vs. 8.7%, $p = 0.6$), and TM3 (7.5% vs. 7.3%, $p = 0.54$) (**Figure 4**). Moreover, for patients with concomitant AH and ACLF at the time of admission, IHM was found similar for AC vs. NAC (43.7% vs. 42.7%, $p = 0.47$). Patients who did not undergo LT had higher IHM than patients who

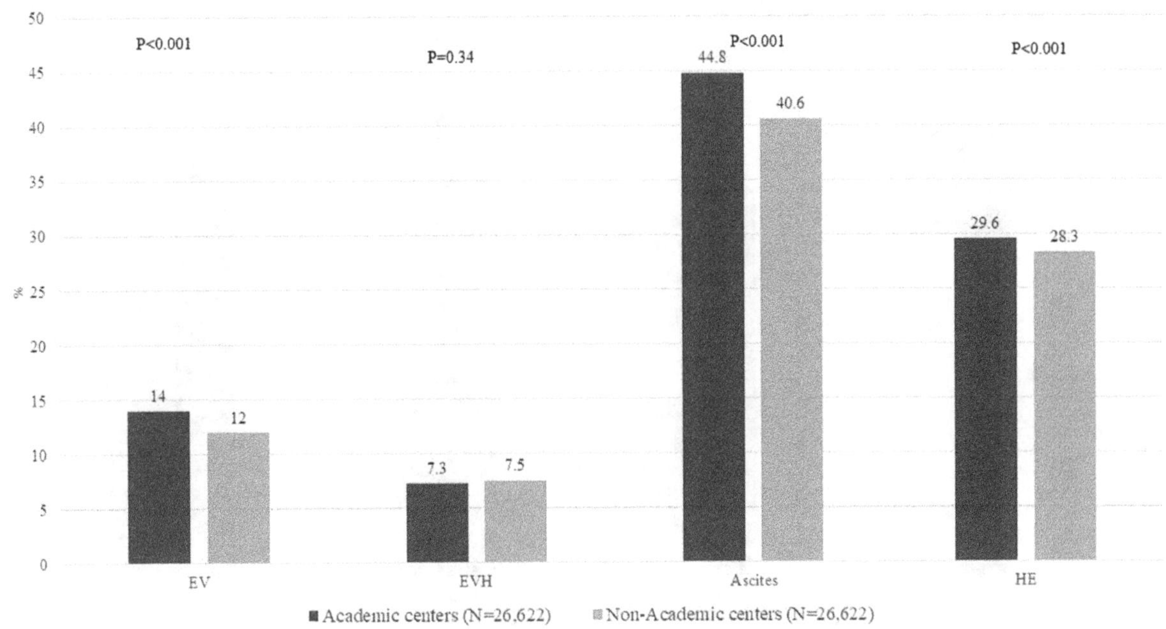

FIGURE 2 | Proportion of all admissions with AH on liver disease complications including EV, EVH, ascites, and HE, comparing admissions to AC vs. NAC. AH, alcoholic hepatitis; EV, esophageal varices; EVH, esophageal variceal hemorrhage; HE, hepatic encephalopathy; AC, academic centers; NAC, non-academic centers.

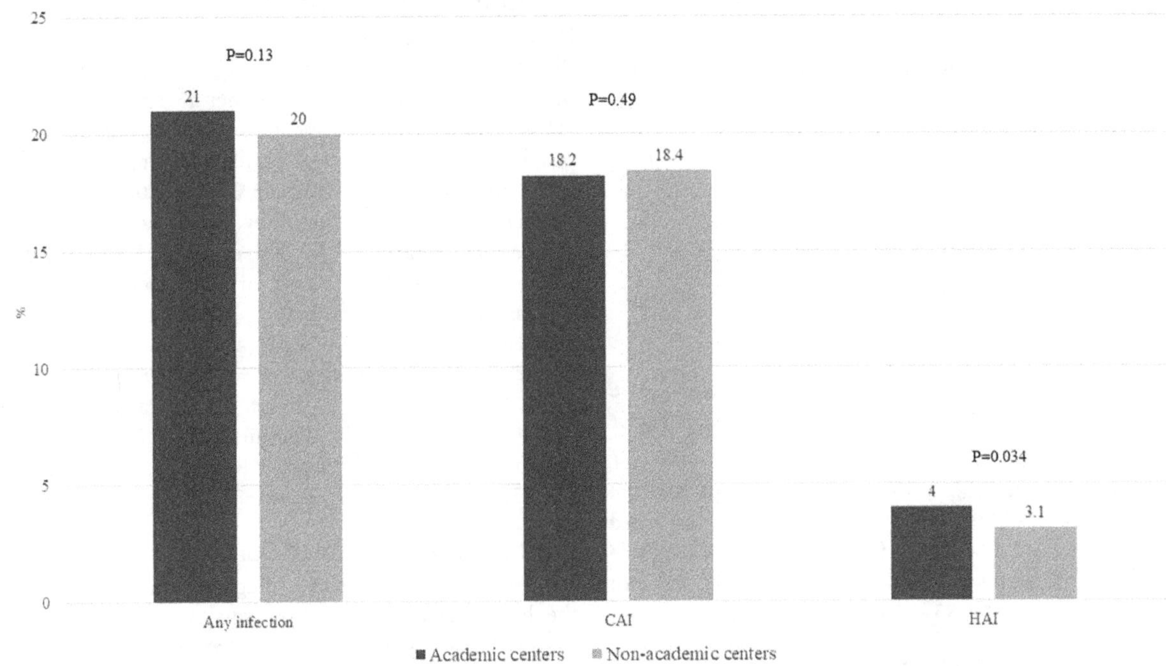

FIGURE 3 | Proportion of admissions with alcoholic hepatitis to academic or non-academic centers complicated by any infection, CAI, and HAI. CAI, community-acquired infections; HAI, hospital-acquired infections.

underwent LT, 8.2% vs. 4.5%, $p = 0.32$. IHM was higher among admissions from other hospitals compared to admissions from within the admitting center (13.4% vs. 8.2%, $p < 0.001$), **Supplementary Figure 3A**.

On multivariate logistic regression analysis, the presence of ACLF had strongest association with IHM with 20 folds higher IHM in the presence of ACLF. Other predictors were older age and transfer from outside hospital (**Table 3**). Conversely,

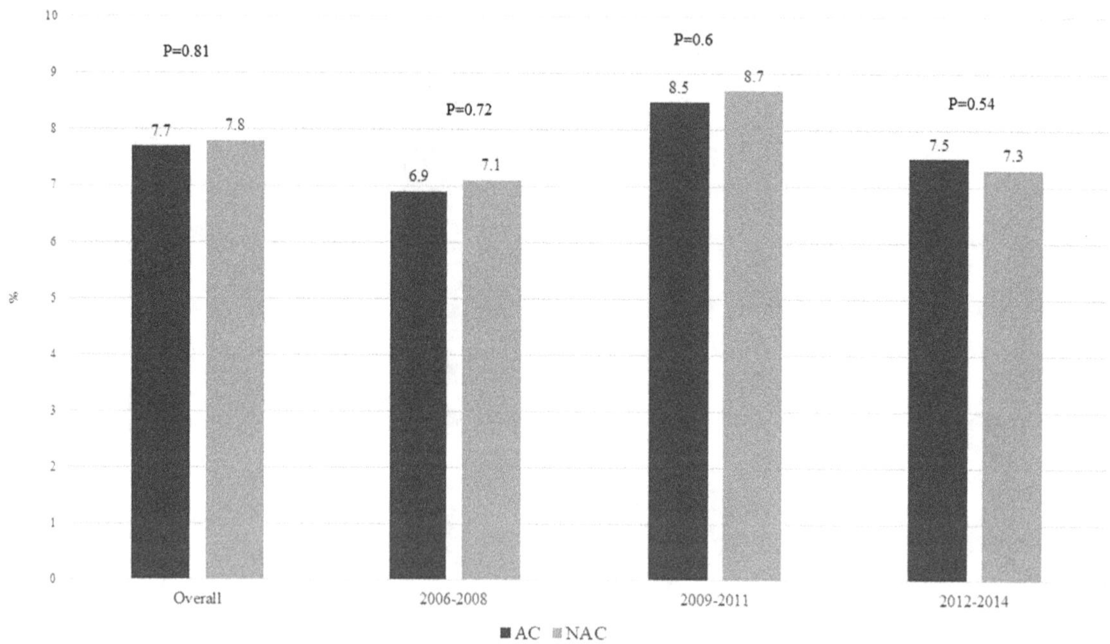

FIGURE 4 | In-hospital mortality comparing admissions with alcoholic hepatitis at academic vs. non-academic centers during 2006–2008, 2009–2011, and 2012–2014.

TABLE 3 | Predictors of in-hospital mortality among admissions with alcoholic hepatitis.

Effect	Hazard ratio	95% CI	*p* value
Age	1.03	1.026–1.035	<0.0001
2009–2011 vs. 2006–2008	0.95	0.83–1.09	0.16
2012–2014 vs. 2006–2008	0.81	0.71–0.92	<0.0001
Transfer from OSH	1.41	1.01–1.98	0.046
Females vs. males	1.00	0.92–1.09	0.25
AA vs. C	0.86	0.74–1.02	0.34
H vs. C	0.85	0.75–0.97	<0.0001
ACLF	20	18.5–21.7	<0.0001
ACvs. NAC	1.003	0.93–1.08	0.20

AA, African American; C, Caucasian; H, Hispanic; ACLF, acute on chronic liver failure; AC, academic centers; NAC, non-academic centers; OSH, outside hospital.

Hispanics were 15% less likely to die during hospitalization, and the IHM decreased by about 20% in 2012–2014 compared to admissions during 2006–2008. After controlling for all these variables, academic status of the admitting hospital was not associated with IHM, 1.00 (0.93–1.08, $p = 0.93$), **Table 3**.

Length of Stay and Total Hospital Charges

Mean (SD) LOS among admissions with discharge diagnosis of AH was 7.4 (7.8) days, longer among admissions to AC compared with admissions to NAC (7.7 vs. 7.1 days, $p < 0.001$), **Figure 5A**. Moreover, AH admissions to AC underwent higher number of procedures than NAC admissions, 2.3 vs. 1.9 $p < 0.001$. However, there was no difference on mean total hospital charges per hospitalization comparing admissions to AC vs. NAC, $52,067 vs. $52,821, $p = 0.28$ (**Figure 5B**).

Secondary Outcomes

Use of Hospital Resources

Blood transfusion was the most frequently used hospital resource in about 22% admissions, with higher use among NAC compared to admissions at AC (24% vs. 21%, $p < 0.001$). In contrast, palliative care consultation was more often obtained among admissions to AC (4.8% vs. 3.3%, $p < 0.001$). There were no differences on use of endoscopy, hemodialysis, or mechanical ventilation (**Figure 6**). A total of 63 AH-related admissions were associated with receipt of liver transplantation, 61 at AC and remaining 2 at NAC, $p < 0.001$. Receipt of LT was associated with reduced IHM (4.5% vs. 8.2%); however, this difference was not significant, $p = 0.32$, given small sample size of 63 liver transplants. Admissions as transfer from another hospital compared to those admitted directly underwent similar (mean ± SD) number of procedures (2.2 ± 2.5 vs. 2.1 ± 2.5, $p = 0.79$), **Supplementary Figure 3B**.

Discharge Disposition of Survivors

Admissions with discharge diagnosis of AH who survived the hospitalization were discharged to home in 63%, short-term rehabilitation in 3.5%, skilled nursing facility in 22%, and home with home health care in 3.5%. There were no differences on discharge disposition comparing admissions to AC vs. NAC (**Figure 7**).

DISCUSSION

The main findings of our study are that AH admissions in the United States (a) are increasing to AC compared to NAC, (b) have

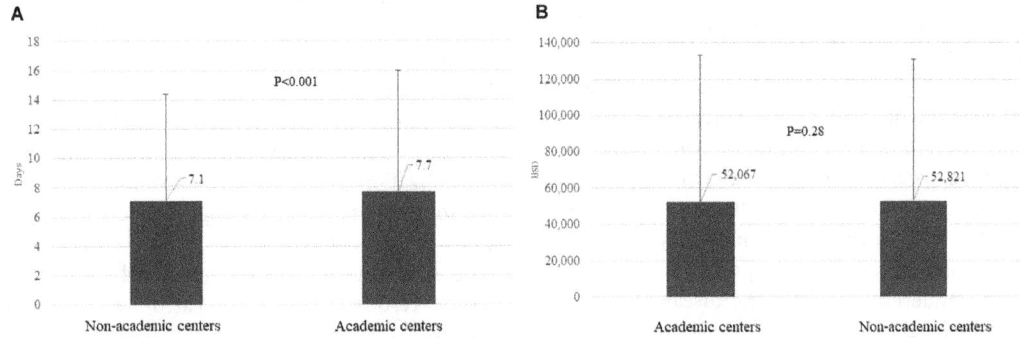

FIGURE 5 | LOS (mean and S.D.) in days **(A)** and total hospital charges in USD **(B)** per admission among AH admissions, comparing admissions to AC vs. NAC. LOS, length of stay; USD, US dollars; AH, alcoholic hepatitis; AC, academic centers; NAC, non-academic centers.

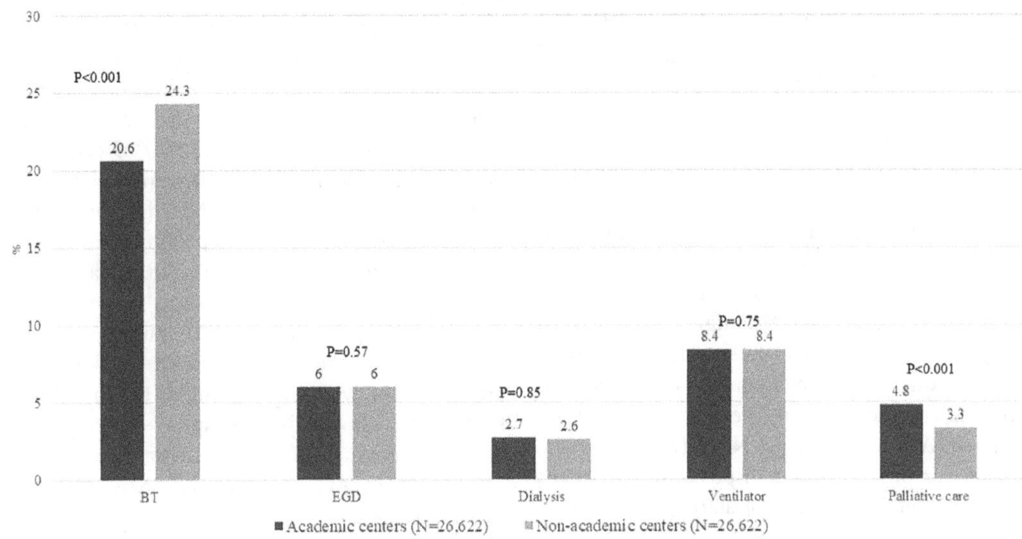

FIGURE 6 | Proportion of all admissions with AH on hospital resource utilization including BT, EGD, dialysis, ventilator use, and palliative care consult comparing admissions to AC vs. NAC. BT, blood transfusions; EGD, esophagogastroduodenoscopy; AH, alcoholic hepatitis; AC, academic centers; NAC, non-academic centers.

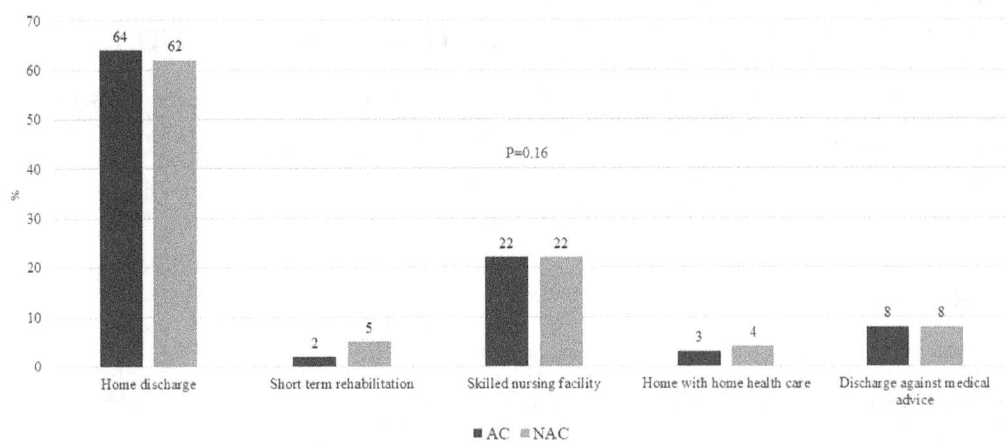

FIGURE 7 | Proportion of all admissions with AH on post-discharge disposition including home discharge, short-term rehabilitation, skilled nursing facility, home with home health care, discharge against medical advice, comparing admissions to AC vs. NAC. AH, alcoholic hepatitis; AC, academic centers; NAC, non-academic centers.

higher prevalence of liver disease and infectious complications, and (c) have longer length of hospital stay, in spite of similar IHM in AC compared to NAC.

Higher disease severity with liver disease complications, infections, and development of ACLF are potential reasons for this finding as also observed in this study. In an earlier study using the NIS database, we have also shown increasing frequency of admissions of patients with discharge diagnosis of cirrhosis who developed ACLF at or during hospitalization (Singal et al., 2020a). Another speculated reason may be potential coding error in AC vs. NAC and underestimation of the disease severity or comorbidities (Rangachari, 2007).

In an earlier study using the NIS database, infectious and other liver disease complications have been shown to be associated with higher mortality among patients with AH (Liangpunsakul, 2011; Jinjuvadia and Liangpunsakul, 2015). Studies have also shown higher mortality among hospitalizations with liver disease and complicated by HAI as compared to admissions with CAI (Bajaj et al., 2012; Arefian et al., 2016; Singal et al., 2020a). Patients with transfer from outside hospital should have low threshold for infection diagnosis and consider nosocomial or HAI, as they have implications on how we choose presumptive antibiotic coverage pending culture results.

Although in this study AH admissions to AC compared to those at NAC had higher frequency of liver disease complications and HAI, the IHM was similar irrespective of academic status of the hospital. Although exact reasons for these findings remain to be determined, it could be speculated to be due to more frequent availability of subspecialty expertise, multidisciplinary teams, and facilities with infrastructure at AC compared to NAC (Allison et al., 2000). Moreover, similar post-discharge disposition of patients from AC vs. NAC in spite of sicker population at AC may be due to the same reasons. Previous studies have also reported better outcomes for patients admitted to AC with complex surgical diseases and medical conditions, including myocardial infarction and pneumonia (Allison et al., 2000; Hayanga et al., 2010).

Health care resource utilization and estimated hospital costs with AH are on the rise (Thompson et al., 2018). We found similar use of hospital resources (other than less blood transfusions and more palliative care consults) between AC and NAC. A possible reason for less blood transfusions in AC could be the early availability of expert intervention from gastroenterology and interventional radiology for control of gastrointestinal bleeding in these patients. Further, longer LOS among admissions to AC for other medical and surgical conditions is likely due to sicker and complex cases at AC and is similar to other reports (Khuri et al., 2001; Dimick et al., 2004; Hayanga et al., 2010; Singal et al., 2020a). Interestingly, in spite of higher number of procedures and LOS at AC compared to NAC, there was no difference on hospitalization costs. Although overall palliative care use was low in these patients as reported in other studies, (Poonja et al., 2014; O'Leary et al., 2020; Singal et al., 2020a) its more frequent use at AC may likely explain similar use of hospital resources and total costs. Further, availability of trainee residents and fellows may have potentially reduced the cost of care and at the same time provided better care to sicker and complex patients.

The national database with large sample size and propensity-matched analysis for disease severity are potential strengths of our study. However, the authors suggest a cautious approach on interpreting these results given several limitations of the study. For example, there could be coding errors in adjudicating the discharge diagnoses given this is a database study with study population identified using the ICD-09 codes. Hence, it may be possible that patients with decompensated ALD and true AH may have been included. Further, NIS database stratifies admissions without linkage to a given patient, limiting identification of previous readmissions. Unavailability of laboratory values during the hospitalization and admissions to Veteran hospital systems are some other limitations of this study.

In summary, admissions with AH in the United States are increasingly being admitted to an AC and as transfer from other hospitals. In spite of longer hospitalizations, higher frequency of liver disease complications, and HAI, admissions to AC as compared to NAC are associated with similar IHM and hospitalization-related costs. These novel findings have epidemiological implications and suggest future large prospective studies overcoming limitations of database including NIS database to validate these findings and examine its mechanisms.

AUTHOR CONTRIBUTIONS

AS conceived the study idea and designed the study. MW and MA wrote the manuscript draft. Y-FK performed the statistical analyses. RW provided important intellectual input. All the authors reviewed the final version and approved it for submission.

REFERENCES

Allen, A. M., Kim, W. R., Moriarty, J. P., Shah, N. D., Larson, J. J., and Kamath, P. S. (2016). Time trends in the health care burden and mortality of acute on chronic liver failure in the United States. *Hepatology* 64, 2165–2172. doi: 10.1002/hep.28812

Allison, J. J., Kiefe, C. I., Weissman, N. W., Person, S. D., Rousculp, M., Canto, J. G., et al. (2000). Relationship of hospital teaching status with quality of care and mortality for Medicare patients with acute MI. *JAMA*. 284, 1256–1262. doi: 10.1001/jama.284.10.1256

Altamirano, J., López–Pelayo, H., Michelena, J., Jones, P. D., Ortega, L., Ginès, P., et al. (2017). Alcohol abstinence in patients surviving an episode of alcoholic hepatitis: Prediction and impact on long–term survival. *Hepatology* 66, 1842–1853. doi: 10.1002/hep.29338

Arefian, H., Hagel, S., Heublein, S., Rissner, F., Scherag, A., Brunkhorst, F. M., et al. (2016). Extra length of stay and costs because of health care-associated infections at a German university hospital. *Am. J. Infect. Control* 44, 160–166. doi: 10.1016/j.ajic.2015.09.005

Bajaj, J. S., O'Leary, J. G., Reddy, K. R., Wong, F., Biggins, S. W., Patton, H., et al. (2014). Survival in infection–related acute–on–chronic liver failure is defined by extrahepatic organ failures. *Hepatology* 60, 250–256. doi: 10.1002/hep.27077

Bajaj, J. S., O'Leary, J. G., Reddy, K. R., Wong, F., Olson, J. C., Subramanian, R. M., et al. (2012). Second infections independently increase mortality in hospitalized patients with cirrhosis: the North American consortium for the study of end–stage liver disease (NACSELD) experience. *Hepatology* 56, 2328–2335. doi: 10.1002/hep.25947

Chacko, K. R., and Reinus, J. (2016). Spectrum of alcoholic liver disease. *Clin.Liver Dis.* 20, 419–427. doi: 10.1016/j.cld.2016.02.002

Cholankeril, G., and Ahmed, A. (2018). Alcoholic liver disease replaces hepatitis C virus infection as the leading indication for liver transplantation in the United States. *Clin. Gastroenterol. Hepatol.* 16, 1356–1358. doi: 10.1016/j.cgh.2017.11.045

Dimick, J. B., Cowan, J. A. Jr., Colletti, L. M., Upchurch, G. R. Jr., (2004). Hospital teaching status and outcomes of complex surgical procedures in the United States. *Archives Sur.* 139, 137–141. doi: 10.1001/archsurg.139.2.137

GBD 2017 Cirrhosis Collaborators (2020). The global, regional, and national burden of cirrhosis by cause in 195 countries and territories, 1990–2017: a systematic analysis for the Global Burden of Disease Study 2017. *Lancet Gastroenterol. Hepatol.* 5, 245–266.

Hayanga, A. J., Mukherjee, D., Chang, D., Kaiser, H., Lee, T., Gearhart, S., et al. (2010). Teaching hospital status and operative mortality in the United States: tipping point in the volume-outcome relationship following colon resections? *Archives Surg.* 145, 346–350. doi: 10.1001/archsurg.2010.24

Jinjuvadia, R., and Liangpunsakul, S. (2015). Trends in alcoholic hepatitis related hospitalizations, financial burden, and mortality in the United States. *J. Clinic. Gastroenterol.* 49:506.

Khuri, S. F., Najjar, S. F., Daley, J., Krasnicka, B., Hossain, M., Henderson, W. G., et al. (2001). Comparison of surgical outcomes between teaching and nonteaching hospitals in the Department of Veterans Affairs. *Annal. Surg.* 234:370. doi: 10.1097/00000658-200109000-00011

Liangpunsakul, S. (2011). Clinical characteristics and mortality of hospitalized alcoholic hepatitis patients in the United States. *J. Clin. Gastroenterol.* 45:714. doi: 10.1097/mcg.0b013e3181fdef1d

O'Leary, J. G., Bajaj, J. S., Tandon, P., Biggins, S. W., Wong, F., Kamath, P. S., et al. (2019). Outcomes after listing for liver transplant in patients with Acute–on–Chronic liver failure: the multicenter North American Consortium for the study of End–Stage liver disease experience. *Liver Trans.* 25, 571–579. doi: 10.1002/lt.25426

O'Leary, J. G., Reddy, K. R., Garcia–Tsao, G., Biggins, S. W., Wong, F., Fallon, M. B., et al. (2018). NACSELD acute–on–chronic liver failure (NACSELD–ACLF) score predicts 30–day survival in hospitalized patients with cirrhosis. *Hepatology* 67, 2367–2374. doi: 10.1002/hep.29773

O'Leary, J. G., Tandon, P., Reddy, K. R., Biggins, S. W., Wong, F., Kamath, P. S., et al. (2020). Underutilization of Hospice in Inpatients with Cirrhosis: The NACSELD Experience. *Dig Dis Sci.* 65, 2571–2579. doi: 10.1007/s10620-020-06168-8

Poonja, Z., Brisebois, A., van Zanten, S. V., Tandon, P., Meeberg, G., and Karvellas, C. J. (2014). Patients with cirrhosis and denied liver transplants rarely receive adequate palliative care or appropriate management. *Clin Gastroenterol Hepatol.* 12, 692–698. doi: 10.1016/j.cgh.2013.08.027

Rangachari, P. (2007). Coding for quality measurement: the relationship between hospital structural characteristics and coding accuracy from the perspective of quality measurement. *Perspect. Health Inf. Manag.* 2007:4.

Siegel, M. B., DeJong, W., Naimi, T. S., Heeren, T., Rosenbloom, D. L., Ross, C., et al. (2011a). Alcohol brand preferences of underage youth: results from a pilot survey among a national sample. *Substance Abuse.* 32, 191–201. doi: 10.1080/08897077.2011.601250

Siegel, M. B., Naimi, T. S., Cremeens, J. L., and Nelson, D. E. (2011b). Alcoholic beverage preferences and associated drinking patterns and risk behaviors among high school youth. *Am. J. Prevent. Med.* 40, 419–426. doi: 10.1016/j.amepre.2010.12.011

Singal, A. K., Ahmed, Z., Axley, P., Arora, S., Arab, J. P., Haas, A., et al. (2020). Hospitalizations for Acute on Chronic Liver Failure at Academic Compared to Non-academic Centers Have Higher Mortality. *Dig Dis Sci.* 2020:32318884.

Singal, A. K., and Anand, B. S. (2013). Recent trends in the epidemiology of alcoholic liver disease. *Clinic. Liver Dis.* 2, 53–56. doi: 10.1002/cld.168

Singal, A. K., Arora, S., Wong, R. J., Satapathy, S. K., Shah, V. H., Kuo, Y.-F., et al. (2020a). Increasing burden of acute-on-chronic liver failure among alcohol-associated liver disease in the young population in the United States. *Am. J. Gastroenterol.* 115, 88–95. doi: 10.14309/ajg.0000000000000411

Thompson, J. A., Martinson, N., and Martinson, M. (2018). Mortality and costs associated with alcoholic hepatitis: A claims analysis of a commercially insured population. *Alcohol* 71, 57–63. doi: 10.1016/j.alcohol.2018.02.003

Williams, R. (2008). The pervading influence of alcoholic liver disease in hepatology. *Alcohol Alcoholism.* 43, 393–397. doi: 10.1093/alcalc/agn013

Comprehensive Analysis of the Expression Profiles of Hepatic lncRNAs in the Mouse Model of Alcoholic Liver Disease

Xiaobing Dou[1,2,3†], Wenwen Yang[1,2†], Qinchao Ding[2,4], Qiang Han[1,4], Qianyu Qian[2,3], Zhongyan Du[4], Yibin Fan[5], Cui Wang[2,3,4] and Songtao Li[1,3,4*]*

[1]School of Public Health, Zhejiang Chinese Medical University, Hangzhou, China, [2]School of Life Science, Zhejiang Chinese Medical University, Hangzhou, China, [3]Molecular Medicine Institute, Zhejiang Chinese Medical University, Hangzhou, China, [4]Academy of Chinese Medical Sciences, Zhejiang Chinese Medical University, Hangzhou, China, [5]Department of Dermatology, Zhejiang Provincial People's Hospital, People's Hospital of Hangzhou Medical College, Hangzhou, China

***Correspondence:**
Songtao Li
lisongtao@zcmu.edu.cn
Cui Wang
wangcui198506@163.com

†These authors have contributed equally to this paper

Background and Aim: The worldwide prevalence of alcoholic liver disease (ALD) due to escalating alcohol consumption has presented an unprecedented pressure on human health. A few studies have determined long non-coding RNAs (lncRNAs) involved in the pathogenesis of liver diseases. However, the roles of lncRNAs in ALD development is still poorly understood.

Methods: An ALD mouse model was established and confirmed. Expression profiles of lncRNAs were obtained by whole transcriptome sequencing. The altered lncRNAs in ALD mice were further verified by qRT-PCR. Gene Ontology (GO) and Kyoto Encyclopedia of Genes and Genomes (KEGG) enrichment analyses were used to enrich the functions of these lncRNAs. In combination with miRNA and mRNA profiles, we constructed concise endogenous RNA (ceRNA) networks. The function of the most up/downregulated lnRNA was further verified and investigated in both ALD model and AML-12 cells.

Results: Totally, five downregulated lncRNAs were obtained and verified in ALD mice. The GO term and KEGG pathway analyses revealed that the identified lncRNAs were associated with alcohol-induced hepatic oxidative damage, cellular inflammation, and lipid metabolism. Combination the differentially modulated miRNAs and mRNAs with ceRNA network analysis, we constructed five ceRNA networks and obtained 30 miRNAs and 25 mRNAs that may participate in ALD. Further, we verified and investigate the function of the most downregulated lnc_1700023H06Rik. Depletion lnc_1700023H06Rik reduced genes encoding for lipid metabolism, especially mRNA Acat2 (ENSMUST00000159697) and Pgrmc2 (ENSMUST00000058578) both *in vivo* and *in vitro*. Knocking down lnc_1700023H06Rik induced triglyceride accumulation and lactate dehydrogenase leakage in AML12 cells, consisting with that in alcohol-treated cells.

Conclusion: The five remarkably downregulated lncRNAs in ALD mouse model were identified as novel biomarkers, highlighting the key role of lncRNAs in the development of ALD. The effect of lnc_1700023H06Rik plays a pivotal role in lipid deposition and its pathological pathway in ALD needs further investigation.

Keywords: long non-coding RNA, alcoholic liver disease, messenger RNA, competitive endogenous RNA,, whole transcriptome sequencing

INTRODUCTION

Continued and excessive alcohol consumption is exacerbating the worldwide incidence of alcoholic liver disease (ALD) (Rehm et al., 2013), According to the Global Status Report on Alcohol and Health (2018), alcohol consumption caused approximately 3 million deaths and nearly half can be attributed to ALD (Lv et al., 2020; Shield et al., 2020). The pathological progression of ALD comprises a spectrum of diseases from liver steatosis and hepatitis to severe fibrosis or even cirrhosis (Liangpunsakul et al., 2016). Although ALD is well-characterized, it cannot be halted or reversed because the underlying mechanisms for ALD initiation or progression are still unclear.

In the past few decades, the proposed mechanisms for ALD have mainly focused on protein-coding genes of alcohol metabolism, reactive oxygen species, formation and inflammation responses (Beier and Arteel, 2010). Technologies such as RNA sequencing and microarray have revealed that non-coding RNAs (ncRNAs) compring up to 80% of the "transcriptional noise," and thus, also participated in ALD evelopment. However, the role of lncRNAs in ALD is still inconclusive as compared to that of the well-studied endogenous miRNA.

Long non-coding RNAs (lncRNAs, with lengths exceeding 200 nucleotides) are transcribed from various genomic regions, including introns and exons. The competitive endogenous RNA (ceRNA) regulates target gene expression through chromatin remodeling, transcription, and post-transcriptional processing (Zhang et al., 2016; Zhao et al., 2018). They play a critical role in various biological functions and disease processes (Peng et al., 2017). Recently, lncRNAs has been reported to involve in alcohol-related diseases. For instance, serum levels of AK054921 and AK128652 were downregulated in patients with alcohol-cirrhosis, and they were inversely correlated with the survival of these patients, indicating the pathological role in alcoholic cirrhosis (Yang et al., 2017). The lncRNAs NEAT1, Gm5091, and MEG3 participated in alcohol-induced hepatic steatosis and fibrosis in animal models (Wang et al., 2018; Zhou et al., 2018; Ye et al., 2020). Despite the definite role of lncRNAs in alcoholic diseases, the profiles of lncRNAs in ALD models have not been comprehensively investigated.

This study objective to screen the potential lncRNAs that may involved in the development of ALD in mice. We performed RNA sequencing to identify the differentially expressed lncRNAs in liver. The functions of lncRNAs were analyzed using Gene Ontology (GO) and Kyoto Encyclopedia of Genes and Genomes (KEGG) pathways. Several differentially expressed lncRNAs were further verified. A ceRNA network analysis was constructed to understand the lncRNA-miRNA-mRNA crosstalk. In addition to the miRNA sequencing assay, we proposed several key lncRNA pathways that may participate in the development of ALD. Our results may provide new insights into the underlying mechanisms of ALD.

MATERIALS AND METHODS

Animal Experiments

Male C57BL/6J mice weighing 25 ± 0.5 g (mean ± SD) were maintained at the Animal Center of Zhejiang Chinese Medical University. The ALD mouse model was established as previously described (Ding et al., 2017). Mice were divided into two groups of six animals each. The control groups, pair-fed (PF), were fed with an isocaloric control liquid diet (Bioserv, Frenchtown, NJ) and the treated groups, alcohol-fed (AF), were treated with Lieber-DeCarli diet (Bioserv, Frenchtown, NJ) for 5 weeks. In the first 3 days, mice were fed with Lieber-DeCarli diet without alcohol. At the following 2 days, the caloric content of alcohol in the diet was set at 5.5%, and increased to 11% on the 6th and 7th day, 22% at the 2nd week, 27% at the 3rd week, and maintained at 32% at the last 2 weeks. Animals were allowed ad libitum access to diet and water. Mice were euthanized using an intravenous injection of pentobarbital sodium (Merck, Darmstadt, Germany) without any pain after 12 h fasting.

Cell Culture and Treatment

The alpha mouse liver (AML)-12 hepatocyte cell line was obtained from the American Type Culture Collection (ATCC, Manassas, VA) and cultured in Dulbecco's Modified Eagle Medium/Ham's Nutrient Mixture F-12, 1:1 (Sigma, Aldrich, MO), containing 10% (v/v) fetal bovine serum (Life technologies), 5 mg/ml insulin (Sigma), 5 μg/ml transferrin (Sigma), 5 ng/ml selenium (Sigma), 40 ng/ml dexamethasone (Sigma), 100 U/mL penicillin, and 100 μg/ml streptomycin (Life technologies, 15,140–122) at 37°C in a humidified O_2/CO_2 (95:5) atmosphere (Li et al., 2014). Cells were plated into 12-well plates, and 200 μmol/L of ethanol was added when the cells volume reached about 80% confluence. After 12 h treatment, cells were collected for qRT-PCR.

RNA Interference

Based on the results of qRT-PCR, we selected the lncRNA with the most significant differential expression to investigate its function in AML12 cells. Cultured cells were transfected with small interfering RNA (siRNA) against mouse lnc_1700023H06Rik (Ribobio, Guangzhou, China) using Lipofectamine 2000 (Invitrogen, Carlsbad, CA) according to the manufacturer's instructions. In the control group (NC), cells were transfected with scrambled siRNA (Ribobio). Cells were collected after 24–48 h for qRT-PCR. Sequences of siRNA against mouse lnc_1700023H06Rik were listed in **Supplementary Table S1**, the sequences of scrambled siRNA were not disclosed.

To investigate the function of lnc_1700023H06Rik in the setting of alcohol treating. Cells were transfected with siRNAs as described aforementioned. Then, 200 μmol/L of ethanol was added into each well. After 12 h, the culture supernatants were for detection of Lactate dehydrogenase (LDH) and the cells were collected for triglyceride (TG) detection.

Histological and Biochemical Assays

Small pieces of liver were isolated and fixed immediately with 4% paraformaldehyde (Biosharp, Guangzhou, China). Samples were stained with hematoxylin (Sigma) and eosin (Sigma) to determine the histological change. Oil red O (Sigma) staining was performed on fresh liver samples to detect the lipid depostion according to our previous study (Ma et al., 2019). The amounts of liver cholesterol (TC), TG, plasma alanine aminotransferase (ALT), and aspartate aminotransferase (AST) were determined according to the manufacturer's instructions (Jiancheng, Nanjing, China).

Whole Transcriptome Sequencing

Total RNA was extracted, and quantified using Bioanalyzer 2100 (Agilent, CA, United States) with RNA Integrity Number (RIN) > 7.0. Subsequently, a small RNA library and a chain-specific library without ribosomal RNA were established and sequenced. The ribosome-deficient chain-specific library obtain the sequence information of lncRNA but also the sequence information of mRNA and circRNA. The small RNA library provided a miRNA sequence.

Transcripts that overlapped with known mRNAs and those that were shorter than 200 bp were discarded. The coding potential of transcripts was determined using Coding Potential Calculator (CPC) (Kong et al., 2007), Coding-Non-Coding Index (CNCI) (Sun et al., 2013), and Pfam (Punta et al., 2012). Transcripts with CPC scores <−1 and CNCI scores <0 was removed. StringTie and fragments per kilobase of transcript per million fragments (FPKM) (Pertea et al., 2015) were used to determine the levels of mRNAs and lncRNAs, respectively. LncRNAs were analyzed using the Ballgown R package. Those with $\log_2$ fold change (FC) > 1 or $\log_2$ FC <−1 and p value <0.05 were considered differentially expressed (Frazee et al., 2015).

Validation of Key lncRNAs and mRNA Using qRT-PCR

Total RNA was extracted using TRIzol (Invitrogen, Carlsbad, CA). The content and purity was determinated by, NanoDrop ND-1000 (NanoDrop, Wilmington, DE). The reaction systems containing cDNA templates, SYBR Green (Bimake, Houston, TX), ddH_2O (Bimake), and primers were mixed for qRT-PCR on ABI 7300 PCR instrument (Thermo Fisher Scientific, Waltha, MA). The gradient temperatures were set at 95°C for 5 min for Hot-Start DNA Polymer; 95°C for 15 s, 60°C for 1 min (40 cycles) for PCR; 95°C for 15 s, 60°C for 1 min, and 95°C for 15 s for melt curve. The relative gene expression was calculated using the $2^{-\Delta\Delta Ct}$ method, and it was normalized to the control group. All primer sequences were listed in **Supplementary Table S2-S3**.

Gene Ontology Enrichment Analysis

Gene Ontology functional enrichment analysis maps and calculates the numbers of all the differentially expressed genes to each term in the GO database, Then, the enrichment fractions and the number of differentially expressed genes (S gene number) enriched in each term were determined according to p values. Finally, the top 10 terms with $p < 0.05$ and largest numbers of S gene number were analyzed.

Kyoto Encyclopedia of Genes and Genomes Enrichment Analysis

Biological functions of differentially expressed lncRNAs were determined by KEGG (www.genome.jp/kegg), a public database for genome deciphering. The basic threshold for significant enrichment was set at $p < 0.05$. Subsequently, each pathway was sorted in a descending order according to S gene numbers, and the top ten pathways were displayed.

ceRNA Network Construction

After verification, lncRNAs with absolute values of $\log_2$ FC > 2 and $p < 0.05$ were selected. Combination with the differentially expressed miRNA and mRNA in sequence analysis we constructed the ceRNA networks. The RNAs which didn't obeyed the rule of negative regulation between lncRNA and miRNA, miRNA and mRNA, were removed. Finally, ceRNA network diagrams were prepared using Cytoscape (v3.8.2, http://www.cytoscape.org/) (Liu et al., 2019).

Detection of Triglyceride and Lactate Dehydrogenase Leakage

The supernatant of AML12 was collected and the activity of LDH leakage was detected according to the instructions of LDH assay kit (Beyotime, Shanghai, China). Cells were then washed with PBS and the triglyceride content in each group was measured according to the instructions of TG assay kit (Jiancheng, Nanjing, China).

Statistical Analysis

Statistical analyses were carried out using the Student's t-test and ANOVA-test accordingly via the SPSS 25.0 software (Chicago, IL, United States). Significant level was set at $p < 0.05$. The bar charts were prepared using GraphPad Prism 7.0 (GraphPad Software, California, United States).

RESULTS

Hepatic Lipid Accumulation and Hepatic Injury Under Alcohol Feeding

The successful establishment of ALD mouse model was verified by a sequence of well-characterized endpoints. As described, the amounts of TC (**Figure 1A**), TG (**Figure 1B**), ALT (**Figure 1C**), and AST (**Figure 1D**) remarkably increased in the AF group as compared to those in the PF group, indicating liver injury and hyperlipidemia. Additionally, a moderate amount of lipid droplets and obvious lipid vacuoles were observed in the liver (**Figure 1E**). The pathological morphology of the liver pointed toward hepatic steatosis and hepatitis, implicating a well-established ALD mouse model.

Differentially Expressed lncRNAs Identified in Alcoholic Liver Disease Mice

Totally, twenty-nine differentially expressed lncRNAs were identified by using RNA sequencing. We divided them into two groups: twelve upregulated and Seventeen downregulated, as separated and clustered by volcano graph and heat map (**Figure 2A,B**). In summary, eighteen lncRNAs with eleven

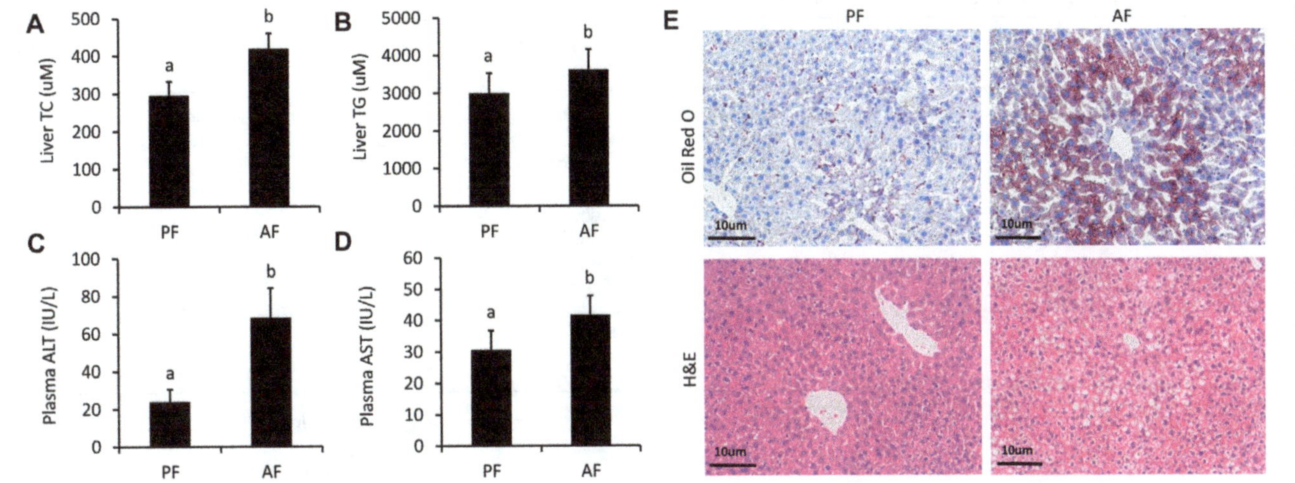

FIGURE 1 | Serum biochemical indices and liver morphologies of ALD mice. **(A)** Hepatic cholesterol (TC) contents. **(B)** Hepatic triglyceride (TG) contents. **(C)** Plasma alanine aminotransferase (ALT) levels. **(D)** Serum aspartate aminotransferase (AST) levels **(E)** Hematoxylin and eosin staining and Oil Red O staining of liver tissues. Bars represents 10 μm. Data are expressed as the mean ± SD (*n* = 6 mice per group).

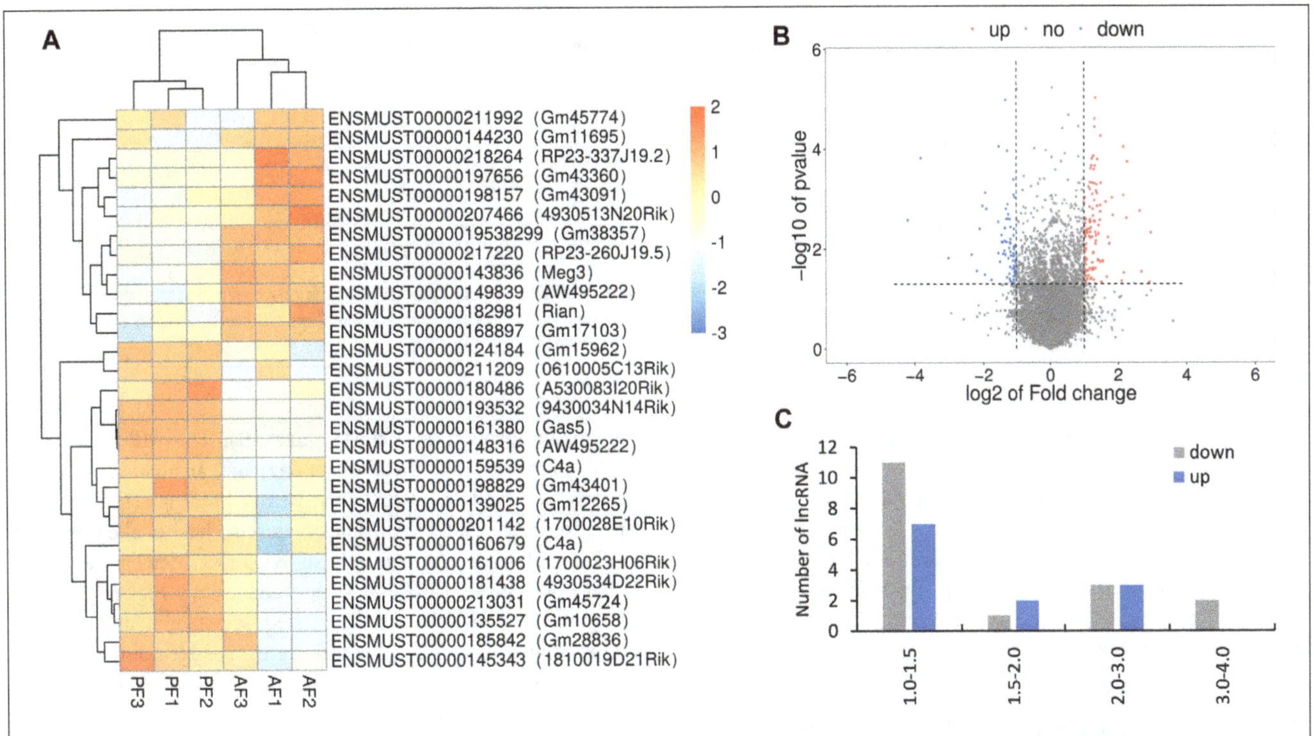

FIGURE 2 | Overview of the RNA sequencing signatures. **(A)** Volcanic map of differentially expressed lncRNAs. **(B)** Hierarchical clustering of the differentially expressed lncRNAs. **(C)** Categories of the 29 differentially expressed lncRNAs.

upregulated and seven downregulated genes changed nearly by 2 to 2.8 fold. Three lncRNAs (one upregulated and two downregulated) altered by 2.8 to 4-fold. Six lncRNAs, three upregulated and three downregulated, changed by 4 to 8-fold. The remaining two lncRNAs changed nearly by 8 to 16-fold (**Figure 2C**). Finally, eight lncRNAs with $\log_2$ FC change >2.0 (4-fold) and $p < 0.05$ were sent for PCR verification (**Table 1**).

Verification 5 Differentially Expressed lncRNAs via qRT-PCR

The differentially expressed lncRNAs were further verified by RT-PCR. Five of the selected lncRNAs in the AF group were maintained as the PF group. Among which, five (mmu_lnc_AW495222(39,807), mmu_lnc_1700023H06Rik, mmu_lnc_0610005C13Rik, mmu_lnc_Gm12265, and

TABLE 1 | Top 8 differently expressed lncRNAs in ALD mice model.

lncRNA	*p*-value	Log_2 of (FC)	Regulation	t_ID	chorm	Strand
mou_lnc_AW495222 (39807)	< 0.01	-3.8040	down	39807	Chr13	–
mou_lnc_AW495222 (39805)	< 0.01	2.6394	up	39805	Chr13	–
mou_lnc_1700023H06Rik	< 0.01	-2.1013	down	39407	chr13	–
mou_lnc_Gm38357	< 0.01	2.9613	up	84884	chr3	–
mou_lnc_0610005C13Rik	0.0276	-2.1850	down	128458	Chr7	–
mou_lnc_Gm12265	0.0131	-2.3356	down	23153	Chr11	–
mou_lnc_Gm45724	0.0153	-3.0207	down	143568	Chr8	–
mou_lnc_Rian	0.0442	2.1151	up	35221	Ch12	–

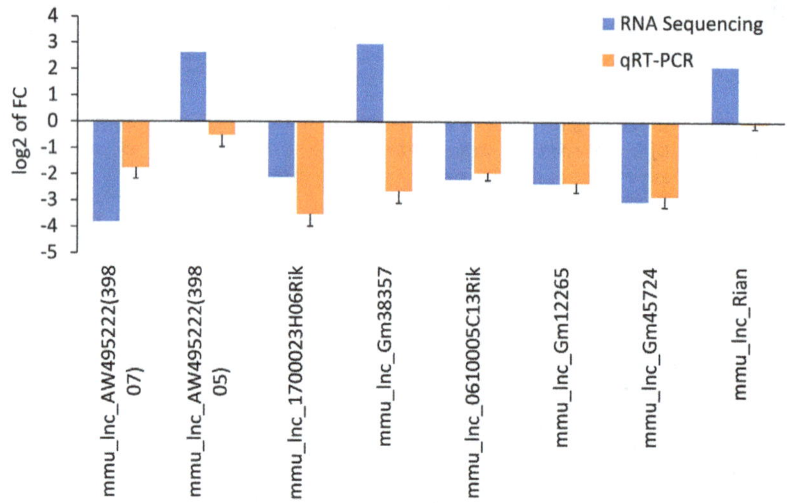

FIGURE 3 | Comparison of the expression levels of twelve lncRNAs between RNA sequencing and qRT-PCR. Data are displayed as log_2 transformed fold changes (log_2 FC), and the negative value indicates the downregulated lncRNAs in the AF group, the level of bar column indicates the differential expression multiple of target lncRNA in PF and AF groups ($p < 0.05$).

mmu_lnc_Gm45724) were consistent with the sequencing results, and two were reversed (mmu_lnc_Gm38357 and mmu_lnc_AW495222(39,805)) (**Figure 3**). Notably, mou_lnc_AW495222(39,807) and mou_lnc_Gm45724 demonstrated maximum inhibition both in RNA sequencing and PCR verification assays. The expression of mmu_lnc_Rian was not different in PF and AF groups. Altogether, about 5 lncRNAs were verified in RT-PCR.

Functional Enrichment of Differentially Expressed Genes

Functions of the differentially expressed lncRNAs were separately determined using GO and KEGG enrichment analyses. The first ten pathways enriched from BP, CC, and MF terms were selected using GO analysis. The enriched BP term (**Figure 4A**) included metabolic processes of lipids, fatty acids, steroid hormones, and oxidation-related pathways with rich factors higher than 0.1. The epoxygenase P450 pathway was ranked the first rich factor in the BP term. All the enriched CC terms had a high rich factor (>0.6) with the most significantly enriched pathway as intermediate density lipoprotein particle (**Figure 4B**). The MF terms were enriched in oxidative metabolism enzymes, aromatase, and lyase activity as well as iron and heme binding (**Figure 4C**). Specifically, the rich factor of aromatase activity peaked near 0.6.

The potential pathogenesis of ALD was determined using KEGG enrichment analysis with a rich factor higher than 0.1. In total, ten pathways were enriched, seven of which had rich factors higher than 0.2. They were ranked as retinol metabolism, arachidonic acid metabolism, steroid hormone biosynthesis, metabolism of xenobiotics by cytochrome P450 (CYP450), drug metabolism by CYP450, peroxisome proliferators activated receptor (PPAR) signaling pathway, and glutathione metabolism (**Figure 4D**).

The ceRNA interaction network of 5 differentially expressed lncRNAs.

The ceRNA network represents a novel regulatory mechanism among lncRNA, miRNA, and mRNA. We chose the top five significantly downregulated lncRNAs (mou_lnc_0610005C13Rik, mou_lnc_1700023H06Rik, mou _ lnc _ Gm12265, mou _ lnc _ AW495222(39,807), and mou_lnc_Gm45724) to construct the ceRNA network. The complex networks were further modified

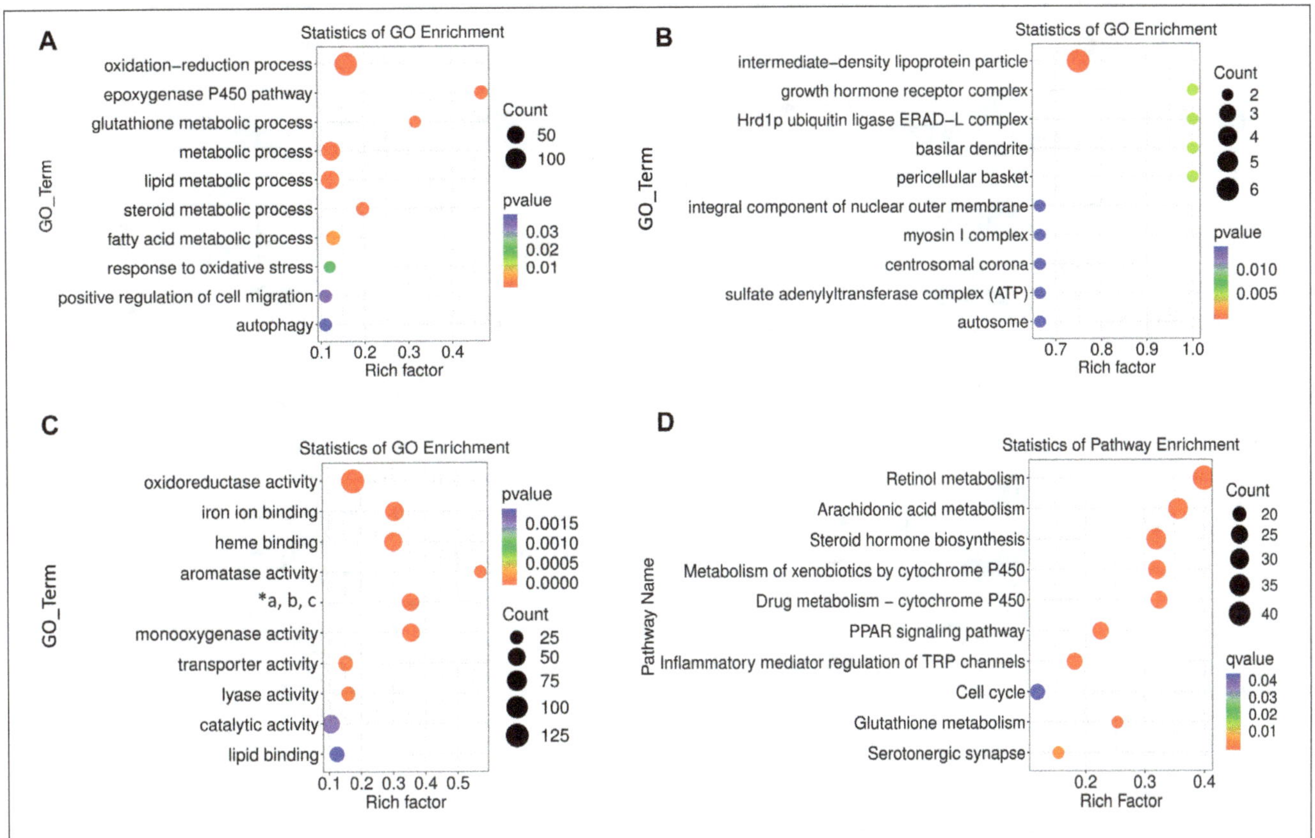

FIGURE 4 | GO and KEGG enrichment analysis of differentially expressed lncRNAs. BP **(A)**, CC **(B)**, and MF **(C)** terms for enrichment (rich factor) of differentially expressed lncRNAs in GO analysis ("*a, b, c" refers to "oxidoreductase activity, acting on paired donors, and molecular oxygen, respectively.") **(D)** KEGG pathways enriched by differentially expressed lncRNAs. The size of the circle represents S gene numbers. The color depth represents the statistical significance.

according to our whole transcriptome sequencing analysis data comprising thirty upregulated miRNAs and twenty-five downregulated mRNAs (**Supplementary Table S4**). Finally, the five aforementioned lncRNAs targeted eight miRNAs and eleven mRNAs (**Figure 5A**), ten miRNAs and eleven mRNAs (**Figure 5B**), five miRNAs and four mRNAs (**Figure 5C**), four miRNAs and seven mRNAs (**Figure 5D**), and five miRNAs and eight mRNAs (**Figure 5E**), respectively.

Verification on lnc_1700023H06Rik ceRNA network in both *in vivo* and *in vitro* model.

The mRNAs linked to the most downregulated lncRNA (lnc_1700023H06Rik) were verified in mouse liver and *in vitro* hepatocyte by RT-PCR. The expressions of Acat2 (ENSMUST00000159697), Pgrmc2 (ENSMUST00000058578), Acox1 (ENSMUST000000666587), Acox1 (ENSMUST00000072948), Mup3 (ENSMUST0000007488), Mup3 (ENSMUST 0000007472), Mup20 (ENSMUST00000074018), Slc22a28 (ENSMUST00000065651) and Slco1a1 (ENSMUST00000042119) were down-regulated in the AF group, which was consistent with the sequencing results (**Supplementary Table S4**). The mRNA level of Ptp4a2 (ENSMUST 00000165853) was upregulated and Prdx2 (ENSMUST00000164807) was not changed in AF groups (**Figure 6A**). The transcription level of Acat2 and Pgrmc2 was further corroborated in ethanol-treated AML-12 cells (**Figure 6B,C**). Knocking down lnc_1700023H06Rik (**Figure 6D**) revealed downregulation of both Acat2 and Pgrmc2 in AML-12 cells (**Figure 6E,F**), which was consistent with that in mice model.

Interference lnc_1700023H06Rik Resulted in Triglyceride Accumulation and Cell Damage

The biological function of lnc_170023H06Rik was further investigated in AML-12 cells. In line with the PCR and RNA-seq analysis, lnc_170023H06Rik was down-regulated in AML-12 cells after exposure to alcohol (**Figure 7A**). Depletion lnc_170023H06Rik was accompanied with apparent TG accumulation and LDH leakage in AML12 cells, which was consistent with that of ethanol treatment (**Figure 7B,C**).

DISCUSSION

In recent decades, many studies have been conducted to determine the pathology of ALD. Recently, the cardinal role of lncRNAs in ALD has been recognized. A few lncRNAs have been identified as biomarkers for predicting survival in patients with alcoholic cirrhosis (Yang et al., 2017). For the first time, we

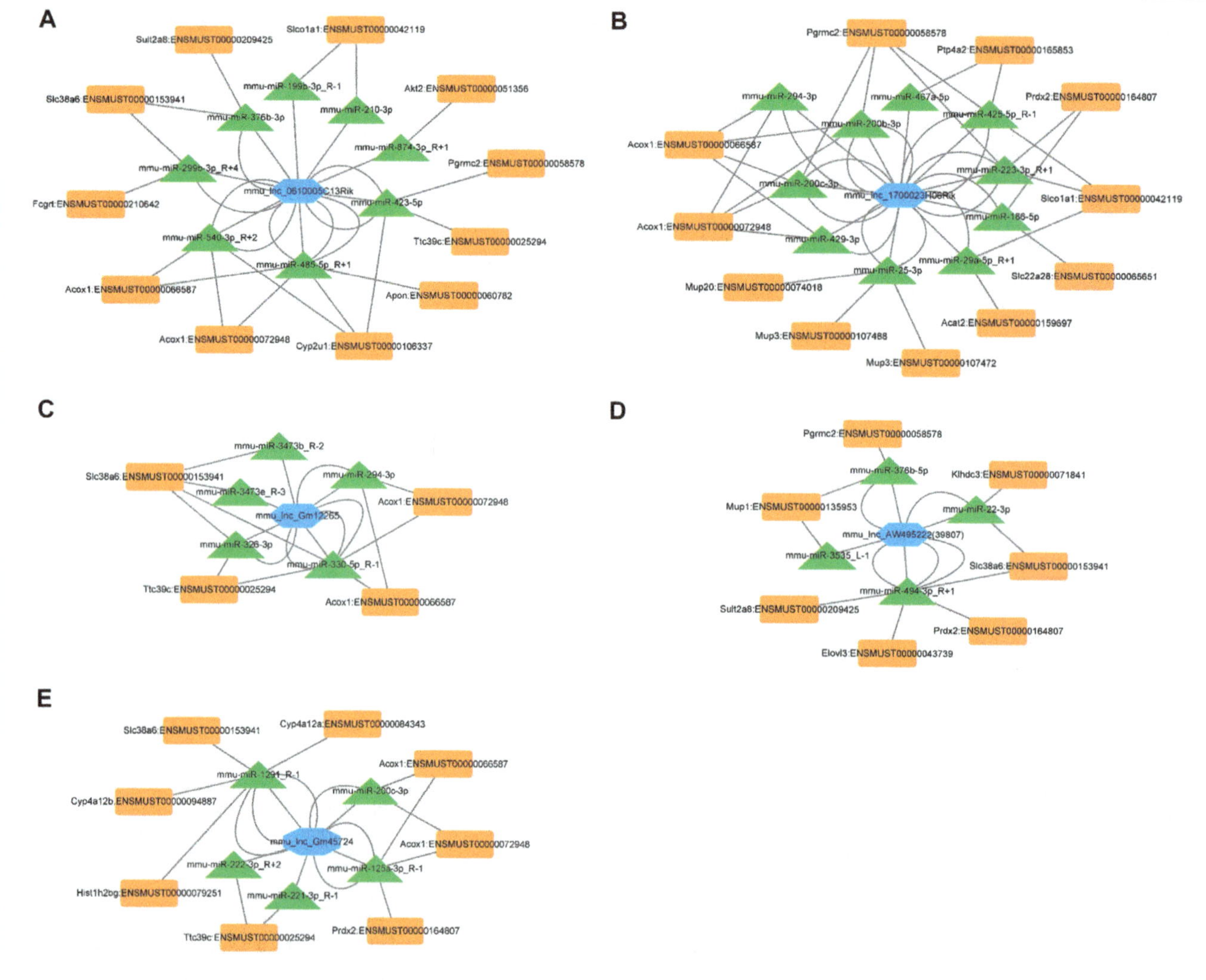

FIGURE 5 | ceRNA networks of mou_lnc_0610005C13Rik, mou_lnc_1700023H06Rik, mou _ lnc _ Gm12265, mou _ lnc _ AW495222(39,807), and mou_lnc_Gm45724. Blue hexagon represents the five lncRNAs. The green triangles and orange quadrilaterals represent differentially expressed miRNA and mRNA, respectively.

prioritized and confirmed eight new lncRNAs that may be involved in the pathological of ALD. Furthermore, we established the top five lncRNA-modulated networks based on the results of whole transcriptome sequencing.

Based on the co-expressed mRNAs functions of differentially expressed lncRNAs could be mainly ascribed to the following categories: oxidative stress, lipid metabolism and inflammatory reactions. According to the KEGG enrichment analysis, we determined the metabolism of xenobiotics by CYP450, drug metabolism by CYP450, retinol metabolism, and arachidonic acid metabolism as the most enriched pathways. Consistent with our present and previous findings, alcohol intake triggers RNAs involved in xenobiotic and drug biodegradation pathways (Dou et al., 2020). CYP450 is crucial for chemical metabolism. Alcohol-related hepatic oxidative stress is caused by ethanol oxidation by its superfamily CYP2E1, which ultimately promotes the development of ALD (Lu et al., 2018). Normally, the liver would exert anti-oxidative and anti-inflammatory processes by converting arachidonic acid into biologically active cyclic trienoic acid through arachidonic acid epoxygenase (Wells et al., 2016). However, CYP450 activation induces arachidonic acid hydroxylation and epoxidation, which partially lead to oxidative stress and liver peroxidation after alcohol intake (Seitz and Mueller, 2019). Additionally, alcohol can cause the decrease of retinol content in liver, and activation CYP2E1 is the main reason for this effect (Clugston et al., 2015). Results from the KEGG analysis were consistent with those of the GO analysis, as the most enriched CC, BF, and MF terms were occupied by lipid and alcoholic metabolism.

Although the functions of lncRNAs have not been fully recognized, the interacting with miRNAs and mRNAs from the ceRNA network enable the understanding of the pathological roles of lncRNAs in ALD. As mentioned above, the initial pathological feature of ALD is hepatic steatosis, that is,

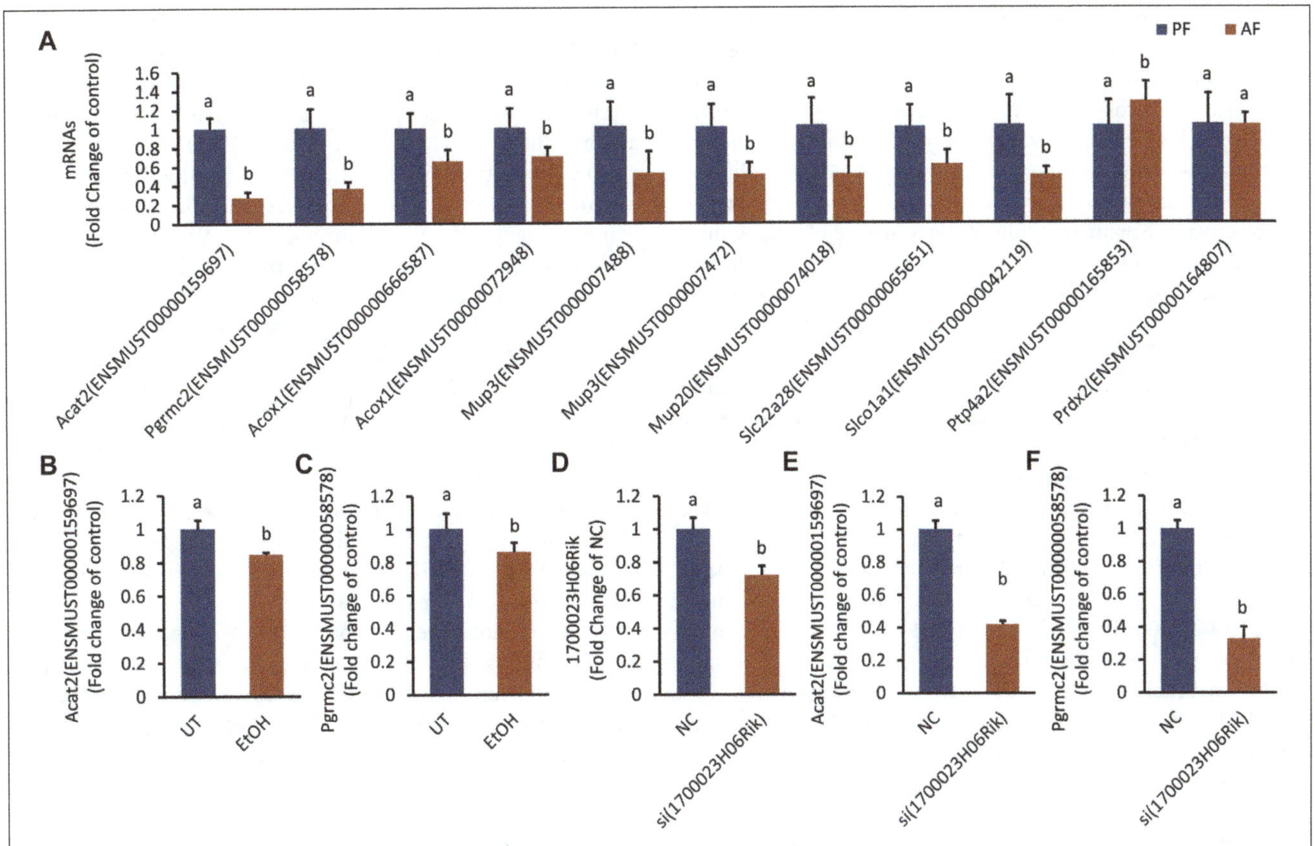

FIGURE 6 | The expression trend of mRNAs corresponding to lnc_1700023H06Rik. **(A)** The expression trends of 11 mRNAs in mouse liver tissues. **(B,C)** Expression of Acat2, Pgrmc2 in ethanol-treated AML-12 cells. **(D)** 1700023H06Rik expression in AML-12 cells by siRNA. **(E,F)** Expression of Acat2 and Pgrmc2 after knocking down lnc_1700023H06Rik.

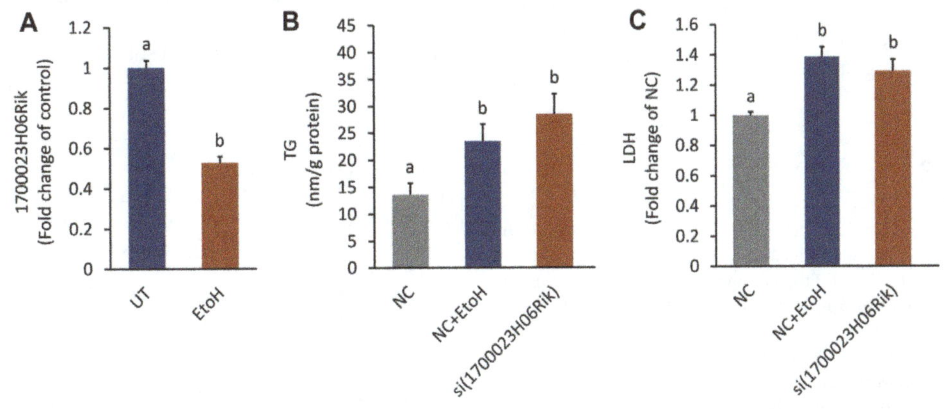

FIGURE 7 | Effect of lnc_1700023H06Rik on triglyceride accumulation and cell damage. **(A)** Expression of lnc_1700023H06Rik in ethanol-treated AML-12 cells. **(B)** TG accumulation in AML-12 cells after knocking down lnc_1700023H06Rik. **(C)** LDH leakage in AML-12 cells after knocking down lnc_1700023H06Rik.

ALD is closely related to lipid metabolism. This study found that lnc_0610005c13Rik-miR540, lnc_Gm45724-miR200c-3p, lnc_1700023H06Rik-miR294-3p, miR200c-3p, miR200b-3p, lnc_12,265-miR294-3p, and -miR 330-5p regulated the mRNA of Acox1, the first enzyme in fatty acid oxidation. Moreover, induction of miR540 inhibited the proteins involved in fatty acid oxidation, such as Acox1, PPARα, and cpt1α, in ALR-L-knockout mice (Kumar et al., 2019). And the expression of Acox1 was down-regulated in alcohol-treated mice with increased lipid accumulation in the mouse liver (Sun et al., 2016). Thus, mitigating these lncRNAs remarkably blocked the activities of enzymes involved in fatty acid oxidation, leading to lipid accumulation. These predictions were further verified in lnc_1700023H06Rik. Both lnc_1700023H06Rik and its related mRNAs, especially Acat2 and Pgrmc2 were downregulated in ALD mice and alcohol-treated cells. Genetic depletion of Acat2 and Pgrmc2 leads to excessive deposition of free fatty acid *in vivo*, and lipid metabolic dysfunction (Wang et al., 2017; Galmozzi et al., 2019). Ectopic Lipid accumulation and the consequence of lipotoxicity is the hallmark for liver injury in alcohol feeding mice (Alpini, 2019). Our study *in vitro* confirmed the blunted lnc_1700023H06Rik tightly contributed to lipid accumulation and cell injury when response to alcohol treatment.

Besides lipid deposition, oxidative stress and inflammation are two pathological factors in ALD. The mRNAs including Prdx2, slc38a6, and sult2a8, engaging in the network of lnc_1700023H06Rik-miR223-3p and lnc_AW49522-miR494-3p are responsible for the anti-oxidative and glutamate transportation pathways (Chan et al., 2016; Shimohira et al., 2018; Wang et al., 2020). Diminishing Prdx2 in hepatocyte of alcohol-treated mice endows lipid deposition (Han et al., 2020). Thus, attenuation of both lnc_1700023H06Rik and lnc_AW49522 in ALD mice indicated the deterioration of anti-oxidative system and lipid metabolism. Additionally, downregulation of lnc_Gm12265, lnc_Gm45724 and lnc_1700023H06Rik may involve in inflammation signaling. Activation of miR326 by inhibition the expression of lnc_Gm12265 may promoted hepatic inflammation as miR326 participates in the secretion of inflammation cytokines via TLR4/myD88/NFκB signaling (Liao et al., 2019). In contrast, miR223-3p, an emerging negative regulator of NLRP3 inflammation and inactivator of hematopoietic stem cells (Jimenez Calvente et al., 2020), was also triggered in the ALD mouse model through the downregulation of lnc_Gm45724 or lnc_1700023H06Rik. Thus, we posited that miR223-3p may participated in ALD given that NLRP3 is responsible for innate immunity during acute liver injury (Huang et al., 2013). The mRNA of Akt2, engaging in the network of lnc_0610005C13Rik, may also contribute to the inflammation status in ALD mice since inhibition on Akt2 attenuated the transcription of inflammation cytokine under alcohol challenge (Reyes-Gordillo et al., 2019).

The limitation of this study lies in the low sequence alignment between mice lncRNAs and the whole human genome via the sequence homological alignment. Most of lncRNAs that identified by our studies cannot be successfully paired in the sequences of humans. Only mmu _ lnc _ 170023H06Rik has a high homology between mice and human (ARRDC3-AS1, 89.58%, 600 bases, **Supplementary Table S5**). About 20 to 30 bases of mmu_lnc_Rian in mice has a full homology with human lncRNAs (LINC02315, LINC02307). Unexpectedly, none of the compared three human lncRNAs (ARRDC3-AS1, LINC02315, LINC02307) has been reported to be related to ALD. Despite this limitation, our study still sets the stage for further investigation on ALD development because the pathological mechanism of ALD in human is still in its infant stage.

In conclusion, the present study identified five lncRNAs functioning as anti-inflammation, anti-oxidation, and lipid metabolism in ALD mice model. Combination ceRNA network with miRNAs and mRNAs sequencing data, we got five ceRNA networks. Taken the most downregulated lncRNA as an example, we, for the first time, verified lnc_1700023H06Rik is tightly related to lipotoxicity in ALD mice model. However, the exact activities of the identified lncRNAs and the proposed pathways still need verification. Despite this limitation, our study highlights the identified lncRNAs as key factors responsible for ALD pathogenesis.

AUTHOR CONTRIBUTIONS

All authors listed have made a substantial, direct, and intellectual contribution to the work and approved it for publication.

REFERENCES

Alpini, G. (2019). Sphingosine Lipid Signaling in Alcoholic Liver Injury. *Dig. Liver Dis.* 51 (8), 1164–1165. doi:10.1016/j.dld.2019.04.002

Beier, J. I., and Arteel, G. E. (2010). Ethanol-Induced Hepatotoxicity. *Compr. toxicologe* 9, 421–435. doi:10.1016/B978-0-12-801238-3.95666-610.1016/b978-0-08-046884-6.01017-4

Chan, K., Busque, S. M., Sailer, M., Stoeger, C., Bröer, S., Daniel, H., et al. (2016). Loss of Function Mutation of the Slc38a3 Glutamine Transporter Reveals its Critical Role for Amino Acid Metabolism in the Liver, Brain, and Kidney. *Pflugers Arch.* 468 (2), 213–227. doi:10.1007/s00424-015-1742-0

Clugston, R. D., Huang, L. S., and Blaner, W. S. (2015). Chronic Alcohol Consumption Has a Biphasic Effect on Hepatic Retinoid Loss. *FASEB J.* 29 (9), 3654–3667. doi:10.1096/fj.14-266296

Ding, L., Wo, L., Du, Z., Tang, L., Song, Z., and Dou, X. (2017). Danshen Protects against Early-Stage Alcoholic Liver Disease in Mice via Inducing PPARα Activation and Subsequent 4-HNE Degradation. *PloS one* 12 (10), e0186357. doi:10.1371/journal.pone.0186357

Dou, X., Feng, L., Ying, N., Ding, Q., Song, Q., Jiang, F., et al. (2020). RNA Sequencing Reveals a Comprehensive Circular RNA Expression Profile in a Mouse Model of Alcoholic Liver Disease. *Alcohol. Clin. Exp. Res.* 44 (2), 415–422. doi:10.1111/acer.14265

Frazee, A. C., Pertea, G., Jaffe, A. E., Langmead, B., Salzberg, S. L., and Leek, J. T. (2015). Ballgown Bridges the gap between Transcriptome Assembly and Expression Analysis. *Nat. Biotechnol.* 33 (3), 243–246. doi:10.1038/nbt.3172

Galmozzi, A., Kok, B. P., Kim, A. S., Montenegro-Burke, J. R., Lee, J. Y., Spreafico, R., et al. (2019). PGRMC2 Is an Intracellular Haem Chaperone Critical for Adipocyte Function. *Nature* 576 (7785), 138–142. doi:10.1038/s41586-019-1774-2

Han, Y. H., Li, W. L., Jin, M. H., Jin, Y. H., Zhang, Y. Q., Kong, L. Z., et al. (2020). Peroxiredoxin II Inhibits Alcohol-Induced Apoptosis in L02 Hepatocytes through AKT/β-Catenin Signaling Pathway. *Anticancer Res.* 40 (8), 4491–4504. doi:10.21873/anticanres.14454

Huang, H., Chen, H. W., Evankovich, J., Yan, W., Rosborough, B. R., Nace, G. W., et al. (2013). Histones Activate the NLRP3 Inflammasome in Kupffer Cells during Sterile Inflammatory Liver Injury. *J. Immunol.* 191, 2665–2679. doi:10.4049/jimmunol.1202733

Jimenez Calvente, C., Del Pilar, H., Tameda, M., Johnson, C. D., and Feldstein, A. E. (2020). Del Pilar H.MicroRNA 223 3p Negatively Regulates the NLRP3 Inflammasome in Acute and Chronic Liver Injury. *Mol. Ther.* 28 (2), 653–663. doi:10.1016/j.ymthe.2019.09.013

Kong, L., Zhang, Y., Ye, Z.-Q., Liu, X.-Q., Zhao, S.-Q., Wei, L., et al. (2007). CPC:

Assess the Protein-Coding Potential of Transcripts Using Sequence Features and Support Vector Machine. *Nucleic Acids Res.* 35, W345–W349. doi:10.1093/nar/gkm391

Kumar, S., Rani, R., Karns, R., and Gandhi, C. R. (2019). Augmenter of Liver Regeneration Protein Deficiency Promotes Hepatic Steatosis by Inducing Oxidative Stress and microRNA-540 Expression. *FASEB J.* 33 (3), 3825–3840. doi:10.1096/fj.201802015R

Li, S., Li, J., Shen, C., Zhang, X., Sun, S., Cho, M., et al. (2014). tert-Butylhydroquinone (tBHQ) Protects Hepatocytes against Lipotoxicity via Inducing Autophagy Independently of Nrf2 Activation. *Biochim. Biophys. Acta* 1841 (1), 22–33. doi:10.1016/j.bbalip.2013.09.004

Liangpunsakul, S., Haber, P., and McCaughan, G. W. (2016). Alcoholic Liver Disease in Asia, Europe, and North America. *Gastroenterology* 150 (8), 1786–1797. doi:10.1053/j.gastro.2016.02.043

Liao, X., Zhan, W., Tian, T., Yu, L., Li, R., and Yang, Q. (2019). MicroRNA-326 Attenuates Hepatic Stellate Cell Activation and Liver Fibrosis by Inhibiting TLR4 Signaling. *J. Cell Biochem* 121, 3794–3803. doi:10.1002/jcb.29520

Liu, S., Xie, X., Lei, H., Zou, B., and Xie, L. (2019). Identification of Key circRNAs/lncRNAs/miRNAs/mRNAs and Pathways in Preeclampsia Using Bioinformatics Analysis. *Med. Sci. Monit.* 25, 1679–1693. doi:10.12659/MSM.912801

Lu, Y., and Cederbaum, A. I. (2018). Cytochrome P450s and Alcoholic Liver Disease. *Curr. Pharm. Des.* 24 (14), 1502–1517. doi:10.2174/1381612824666180410091511

Lv, Y., So, K. F., and Xiao, J. (2020). Liver Regeneration and Alcoholic Liver Disease. *Ann. Transl Med.* 8 (8), 567. doi:10.21037/atm.2020.02.168

Ma, Y., Chai, H., Ding, Q., Qian, Q., Yan, Z., Ding, B., et al. (2019). Hepatic SIRT3 Upregulation in Response to Chronic Alcohol Consumption Contributes to Alcoholic Liver Disease in Mice. *Front. Physiol.* 10, 1042. doi:10.3389/fphys.2019.01042

Peng, W. X., Koirala, P., and Mo, Y. Y. (2017). LncRNA-mediated Regulation of Cell Signaling in Cancer. *Oncogene* 36 (41), 5661–5667. doi:10.1038/onc.2017.184

Pertea, M., Pertea, G. M., Antonescu, C. M., Chang, T. C., Mendell, J. T., and Salzberg, S. L. (2015). StringTie Enables Improved Reconstruction of a Transcriptome from RNA-Seq Reads. *Nat. Biotechnol.* 33 (3), 290–295. doi:10.1038/nbt.3122

Punta, M., Coggill, P. C., Eberhardt, R. Y., Mistry, J., Tate, J., Boursnell, C., et al. (2012). The Pfam Protein Families Database. *Nucleic Acids Res.* 40, D290–D301. doi:10.1093/nar/gkr1065

Rehm, J., Samokhvalov, A. V., and Shield, K. D. (2013). Global burden of Alcoholic Liver Diseases. *J. Hepatol.* 59 (1), 160–168. doi:10.1016/j.jhep.2013.03.007

Reyes-Gordillo, K., Shah, R., Arellanes-Robledo, J., Cheng, Y., Ibrahim, J., and Tuma, P. L. (2019). Akt1 and Akt2 Isoforms Play Distinct Roles in Regulating the Development of Inflammation and Fibrosis Associated with Alcoholic Liver Disease. *Cells* 8 (11), 1337. doi:10.3390/cells8111337

Seitz, H. K., and Mueller, S. (2019). The Role of Cytochrom P4502E1 in Alcoholic Liver Disease and Alcohol Mediated Carcinogenesis. *Z. Gastroenterol.* 57 (1), 37–45. doi:10.1055/a-0784-8815

Shield, K., Manthey, J., Rylett, M., Probst, C., Wettlaufer, A., Parry, C. D. H., et al. (2020). National, Regional, and Global Burdens of Disease from 2000 to 2016 Attributable to Alcohol Use: a Comparative Risk Assessment Study. *Lancet Public Health* 5 (1), e51–e61. doi:10.1016/S2468-2667(19)30231-2

Shimohira, T., Kurogi, K., Liu, M. C., Suiko, M., and Sakakibara, Y. (2018). The Critical Role of His48 in Mouse Cytosolic Sulfotransferase SULT2A8 for the 7α-Hydroxyl Sulfation of Bile Acids. *Biosci. Biotechnol. Biochem.* 82 (8), 1359–1365. doi:10.1080/09168451.2018.1464897

Sun, L., Luo, H., Bu, D., Zhao, G., Yu, K., Zhang, C., et al. (2013). Utilizing Sequence Intrinsic Composition to Classify Protein-Coding and Long Non-coding Transcripts. *Nucleic Acids Res.* 41 (17), e166. doi:10.1093/nar/gkt646

Sun, Q., Zhang, W., Zhong, W., Sun, X., and Zhou, Z. (2016). Dietary Fisetin Supplementation Protects against Alcohol-Induced Liver Injury in Mice. *Alcohol. Clin. Exp. Res.* 40 (10), 2076–2084. doi:10.1111/acer.13172

Wang, Q., Li, M., Shen, Z., Bu, F., Yu, H., Pan, X., et al. (2018). The Long Non-coding RNA MEG3/miR-Let-7c-5p Axis Regulates Ethanol-Induced Hepatic Steatosis and Apoptosis by Targeting NLRC5. *Front. Pharmacol.* 9, 302. doi:10.3389/fphar.2018.00302

Wang, S., Chen, Z., Zhu, S., Lu, H., Peng, D., Soutto, M., et al. (2020). PRDX2 Protects against Oxidative Stress Induced by *H. pylori* and Promotes Resistance to Cisplatin in Gastric Cancer. *Redox Biol.* 28, 101319. doi:10.1016/j.redox.2019.101319

Wang, Y. J., Bian, Y., Luo, J., Lu, M., Xiong, Y., Guo, S. Y., et al. (2017). Cholesterol and Fatty Acids Regulate Cysteine Ubiquitylation of ACAT2 through Competitive Oxidation. *Nat. Cell Biol* 19 (7), 808–819. doi:10.1038/ncb3551

Wells, M. A., Vendrov, K. C., Edin, M. L., Ferslew, B. C., Zha, W., Nguyen, B. K., et al. (2016). Characterization of the Cytochrome P450 Epoxyeicosanoid Pathway in Non-alcoholic Steatohepatitis. *Prostaglandins Other Lipid Mediat* 125, 19–29. doi:10.1016/j.prostaglandins.2016.07.002

Yang, Z., Ross, R. A., Zhao, S., Tu, W., Liangpunsakul, S., and Wang, L. (2017). LncRNA AK054921 and AK128652 Are Potential Serum Biomarkers and Predictors of Patient Survival with Alcoholic Cirrhosis. *Hepatol. Commun.* 1 (6), 513–523. doi:10.1002/hep4.1061

Ye, J., Lin, Y., Yu, Y., and Sun, D. (2020). LncRNA NEAT1/microRNA-129-5p/SOCS2 axis Regulates Liver Fibrosis in Alcoholic Steatohepatitis. *J. Transl Med.* 18 (1), 445. doi:10.1186/s12967-020-02577-5

Zhang, Y., Xu, Y., Feng, L., Li, F., Sun, Z., Wu, T., et al. (2016). Comprehensive Characterization of lncRNA-mRNA Related ceRNA Network across 12 Major Cancers. *Oncotarget* 7 (39), 64148–64167. doi:10.18632/oncotarget.11637

Zhao, Y., Wang, H., Wu, C., Yan, M., Wu, H., Wang, J., et al. (2018). Construction and Investigation of lncRNA-Associated ceRNA Regulatory Network in Papillary Thyroid Cancer. *Oncol. Rep.* 39 (3), 1197–1206. doi:10.3892/or.2018.6207

Zhou, B., Yuan, W., and Li, X. (2018). LncRNA Gm5091 Alleviates Alcoholic Hepatic Fibrosis by Sponging miR-27b/23b/24 in Mice. *Cell Biol Int* 42 (10), 1330–1339. doi:10.1002/cbin.11021

17

Protective Effects of Ellagic Acid Against Alcoholic Liver Disease in Mice

Liang Zhao [1], Arshad Mehmood [1], Mohamed Mohamed Soliman [2], Asra Iftikhar [3], Maryam Iftikhar [1], Salama Mostafa Aboelenin [4] and Chengtao Wang [1]*

[1] Beijing Advance Innovation Center for Food Nutrition and Human Health, Beijing Engineering and Technology Research Center of Food Additives, Beijing Technology and Business University, Beijing, China, [2] Clinical Laboratory Sciences Department, Turabah University College, Taif University, Taif, Saudi Arabia, [3] Department of Pharmacy, Faculty of Pharmaceutical Sciences, The University of Faisalabad, Faisalabad, Pakistan, [4] Biology Department, Turabah University College, Taif University, Taif, Saudi Arabia

***Correspondence:**
Chengtao Wang
wangchengtao@th.btbu.edu.cn

Ellagic acid, a natural polyphenolic compound commonly present in vegetables, fruits, nuts, and other edible plants, exerts many pharmacological activities. The present project was designed to explore the hepatoprotective effect of ellagic acid against alcohol-induced liver disease (ALD) and the correlation among alcohol, oxidative stress, inflammation, and gut microbiota. Fifty percent (v/v) alcohol (10 mL/kg bw daily) was orally administrated for 4 weeks in mice along with ellagic acid (50 and 100 mg/kg bw). Alcohol administration significantly ($p < 0.05$) increased the activities of alanine aminotransferase and serum aspartate aminotransferase, levels of triglyceride, low density lipoprotein, free fatty acid, and total cholesterol, and decreased contents of the high-density lipoprotein in model group compared with the control group, which were further improved by ellagic acid (50 or 100 mg/kg bw). Furthermore, daily supplementation of ellagic acid alleviated hepatic antioxidant activities (glutathione peroxidase, catalase, malondialdehyde, superoxide dismutase, and glutathione), proinflammatory cytokines levels (IL-6, IL-1β, and TNF-α), genes expressions (*Tlr4*, *Myd88*, *Cd14*, *Cox2*, *Nos2*, and *Nfκb1*), and histopathological features in alcohol-induced liver injured mice. Additionally, results also revealed that ellagic acid supplementation improved alcohol-induced gut microbiota dysbiosis. In conclusion, ellagic acid mitigated oxidative stress, inflammatory response, steatosis, and gut microbiota dysbiosis in ALD mice. Our results suggested that ellagic acid could be applied as an ideal dietary therapy against ALD.

Keywords: alcoholic liver disease, polyphenolic compound, ellagic acid, inflammation, gut microbiota

INTRODUCTION

Alcohol-induced liver disease (ALD) is a leading source of morbidity and mortality in Europe, the United States, and China. ALD is a common liver disease and around 300 million people are affected by hepatitis B virus, non-alcoholic fatty liver disease, and ALD in China (1, 2). ALD is characterized by changes in hepatic morphological features such as alcoholic steatohepatitis (ASH), hepatitis, and even cirrhosis (3). The oxidative stress, steatosis, gut microbiota disorders, and inflammatory responses are currently proposed as the main causes of ALD (2, 4–6).

Emerging evidence suggests that consumption of alcohol caused the alternation of gut microbiota composition, known as gut dysbiosis, which plays a significant function in the progression of ASH (6–8). Briefly, chronic alcohol exposure leads to the overgrowth of intestinal bacterial, changes in gut microbiota composition, as well as the systemic elevation of inflammation, endotoxin [lipopolysaccharide (LPS)], and hepatic steatosis (9, 10). Particularly, dysbiosis of the gut microbiota is also found to be linked positively to alcohol-induced hepatic cirrhosis (11, 12). Moreover, results also revealed that relative abundance of *Actinobacteria* and *Firmicutes* markedly increased and *Bacteroidetes* decreased along with the inflammation and hepatic steatosis in alcohol-induced mice (13). Gut dysbiosis increases intestinal permeability, which in turn leads to LPS and gut-derived bacteria entering the liver (14, 15). The circulating endotoxin levels may initiate hepatic inflammation *via* multiple signaling pathways such as Toll-like receptor (TLR) 4, myeloid differentiation primary response gene 88 (MyD88), nuclear factor kappa-B (NF-κB), and others (16, 17). Therefore, gut dysbiosis has a significant impact on ALD, and treating ALD by focusing on the intestinal microbiota is an important clinical approach.

The available options for the treatment of ALD are limited, and most possess some adverse side effects. Therefore, there is an urgent need for alternative safe and inexpensive treatment strategies for coping with ALD. The use of natural products and nutritional agents attracts attention for the treatment of ALD due to their broad spectrum of antiinflammatory and antioxidant properties (5). Polyphenolic compounds have been reported to exert beneficial effects in the prevention and treatment of ALD (18–22). Ellagic acid is a natural polyphenol that belongs to the tannic acid group and is abundantly present in many medicinal plants, fruits, fruits peel of berries and nuts, possessing antiinflammatory, antiapoptotic and antioxidant effects (23–26). Previously studies confirmed that ellagic acid can protect the liver from aceclofenac (27), thioacetamide (28), valproic acid (29), D-galactosamine (30), carbon-tetrachloride (31), and ethanol (32). Previously, an *in vitro* study by Sohn et al. (32) also revealed that ellagic acid attenuated ethanol-induced liver toxicity in HepG2 cells *via* antioxidant and antiinflammatory mechanism. Notably, few studies were conducted before the protective effects of ellagic acid on ALD were understood. Therefore, the present study was designed to investigate the intervention effect of ellagic acid against ALD in mice induced by ethanol, and to further explore the possible mechanism.

MATERIALS AND METHODS

Chemicals and Reagents

Ellagic acid (98%) was purchased from Shanghai Yuanye Biotechnology Co., Ltd. (Nanjing, China). Formalin, sodium carboxymethyl cellulose (CMC-Na), and ethanol were procured from Shanghai Macklin Biochemical Co., Ltd (Shanghai, China). Alanine aminotransferase (ALT), aspartate aminotransferase (AST), total cholesterol (TC), triglycerides (TG), high-density lipoprotein (HDL), low-density lipoprotein (LDL), free fatty acid (FFA), and gamma glutamyl transferase (γGT) kits were procured from Nanjing Jiancheng Bioengineering Institute (Nanjing, China). The malondialdehyde (MDA), superoxide dismutase (SOD), catalase (CAT), glutathione (GSH) and glutathione peroxidase (GSH-Px) kits were procured from Nanjing Jiancheng Bioengineering Institute (Nanjing, China). The enzyme-linked immunosorbent assay (ELISA) kits (IL-6, IL-1β, and TNF-α) were purchased from Beijing Sinouk institute of biological technology (Beijing, China). TRIzol reagent and FastQuant RT kit were purchased from Tiangen Biotech Co., Ltd. (Beijing, China). All other chemicals used in the present study were analytical grade.

Animals

Forty male ICR mice, aged 7–9 weeks and weighing 22–24 g, were procured from Beijing Vital River Laboratory Animal Technology Co., Ltd. (Beijing, China) (Certificate SCXK (Beijing) 2012-0001). The mice were kept in a well-ventilated animal room for a 1-week acclimation period at 25°C, humidity (60–80%), under 12 h light/12 h dark cycle. The animal experiment project was approved by the Ethics Committee of the Beijing Key Laboratory of Functional Food from Plant Resources (Permit number: A330-19). All animal experimental procedures in this research also followed the National Institutes of Health's guidelines for the treatment and use of laboratory animals.

Design of Animal Experiment

After 1-week acclimation period, four groups of mice were formed ($n = 10$ in each group); control group (C), model group (M), low-dose of ellagic acid group (EL), and high-dose of ellagic acid group (EH); and were fed with normal pellet diet *ad libitum* and water. The C group was given CMC-Na (0.5%) *via* oral way whereas M group was administered with 50% (v/v) alcohol (10 mL/kg bw daily) after 1 h of 0.5% CMC-Na by oral route for 4 weeks. The mice in EL and EH were administered orally with low (50 mg/kg bw) or high (100 mg/kg bw) dose of ellagic acid (suspended in 0.5% CMC-Na) after 1 h of receiving 50% alcohol for 4 weeks. Every 3 days, the mice were weighted, and the amount of gastric infusion received was adjusted based on the weight. The total animal experiment lasted for 4 weeks. After 4 weeks, all mice were fasted for 12 h before being weighed and killed. Using a capillary tube, blood samples were taken from each mouse retroorbital venous plexus. Liver, kidney, and spleen tissues were dissected out, rinsed, washed with ice-cold PBS, and weighed to measured organ index according to the following formula:

$$\text{Organ index (\%)} = \text{organ weight/final body weight} \times 100\%$$

Following that, one section of the liver tissues was immersed in a 10% formaldehyde solution for histopathological examination whereas the remaining sections were kept for biochemical study, ELISA determination, and qPCR measurement.

Biochemical Analysis of Liver Tissues and Serum

The blood samples were clotted at 4°C for 6 h and then centrifugated at 4,000 g for 15 min to obtain the serum. After that, the serum was further subjected for the determination of various biochemical parameters such as ALT, AST, TC, TG, HDL, LDL,

FFA, and γGT by using commercially available kits according to the instruction manuals.

Liver tissue homogenates were prepared, and the lipids were separated according to the previously described method (13). Bicinchoninic acid protein assay kit was used to assess the total protein concentrations in the liver homogenate. The hepatic lipid profiles such as TG, TC, and FFA were measured by using the same protocol described for serum FFA, TC, and TG levels. The antioxidant activities such as MDA, SOD, CAT, GSH, and GSH-Px levels in liver tissue homogenates were examined by using commercially available kits following the protocol of the manufacturer.

Determination of Hepatic Proinflammatory Cytokines

The IL-6, IL-1β, and TNF-α (proinflammatory cytokines) concentrations in the liver were determined by using commercial ELISA kit, following the instruction manual.

Histological Investigation of Liver

Samples of liver were separated from each mouse and fixed in formalin solution (10%) for 24 h, and after that dehydrated using graded alcohol and xylene, and implanted in paraffin. Paraffin implanted segments were further cut into the thickness of 5 μm, stained with Masson's trichrome (MAS) and hematoxylin and eosin (H&E) for histological investigation. The degree of histological damage to the liver sections was further determined by using a light microscope (BA-9000L, Osaka, Japan).

Real-Time PCR Analysis

The total RNA was isolated from hepatic tissue by using TRIzol reagent according to the method reported by Mehmood et al. (33). RNA was reverse transcribed to cDNA using a FastQuant RT kit, and mRNA expression was quantified using real time polymerase chain reaction (qRT-PCR). The details of primers used in this study are presented in **Table 1**. To normalize mRNA expression, the expression of the housekeeping gene, glyceraldehyde-3-phosphate dehydrogenase (GAPDH), was measured.

Gut Microbiota Analysis

Colonic contents in mice were collected in individual sterile cryotube and stored in liquid nitrogen (34). The total DNA was extracted *via* the EZNA soil DNA extraction kit (Omega Bio-tek, Norcross, USA) according to instruction manuals. The V3–V4 region of the bacterial 16S ribosomal RNA gene was subjected to PCR amplification using primers 338F (5′-ACTCCTACGGGAGGCAGCAG-3′) and 806R (5′ - GGACTACHVGGGTWTCTAAT-3′).

The Illumina MiSeq sequencing technology along with multivariate statistical methods were conducted to detect the diversity of the V3-V4 region of the bacterial 16S rRNA gene. Related library construction and the Miseq high-throughput sequencing process were performed by Majorbio (Shanghai, China). Operational taxonomic units (OTUs) were clustered at 97% similarity, and Venn diagram, analyses of community composition, and Spearsman correlation analysis were performed.

TABLE 1 | List of primer sequences of genes used in this study.

Gene		Primer sequence (5′-3′)
Gapdh	Forward:	CCTTCATTGACCTCAACTACATGGT
	Reverse:	TCATTGTCATACCAGGAAATGAGCT
Cd14	Forward:	GGAAGCCAGAGAACACCATC
	Reverse:	CCAGAAGCAACAGCAACAAG
Myd88	Forward:	AGAACAGACAGACTATCGGCT
	Reverse:	CGGCGACACCTTTTCTCAAT
Nfkb1	Forward:	AGACAAGGAGCAGGACAT
	Reverse:	CCAGCAACATCTTCACATC
Cox2	Forward:	GGAGAGACTATCAAGATAGTGATC
	Reverse:	ATGGTCAGTAGACTTTTACAGCTC
Nos2	Forward:	GTGGTGACAAGCACATTTGG
	Reverse:	GGCTGGACTTTTCACTCTGC

Statistical Analysis

The data of the animal experiment was evaluated by using SPPSS version 22.0 (SPSS Inc., Chicago, IL, USA) and Graph Pad Prism version 8 (La Jolla, CA, USA). One-way analysis of variance (ANOVA) was used to compare variations between groups, followed by Duncan's multiple range test. Differences between groups were found statistically significant at $p < 0.01$ or $p < 0.05$ and the data was expressed as mean ± SD.

RESULTS

Effect of Ellagic Acid on Food Intake, Body Weight, and Organ Index in ALD Mice

The food intake by different groups of mice was measured in g/day. The normal group (C) utilized a healthy amount of food throughout the period of the experiment (**Table 2**). Compared with the normal group, food utilization in the model group (M) after alcohol administration was prominently decreased ($p < 0.05$), resulting in significant loss of body weight and activities ($p < 0.05$). However, the feed intake and weight loss were significantly improved in the two ellagic acid groups (EL and EH, $p < 0.05$), which was close to the C group. As shown in **Table 2**, the liver index of the M group was prominently raised compared with mice in the C group ($p < 0.05$). However, the administration of different doses of ellagic acid (EL and EH) attenuated the liver swelling compared with the M group. In addition, there were no significant changes in organ indices of kidney and spleen among mice in C, M, EL, and EH groups ($p > 0.05$).

Effect of Ellagic Acid on Serum Biomarkers and Lipids Profile in ALD Mice

As displayed in **Figures 1A–D**, a significant elevation ($p < 0.05$) in the serum AST (**Figure 1A**), ALT (**Figure 1B**), γGT (**Figure 1C**), and ALP (**Figure 1D**) activities occurred in

TABLE 2 | Effect of ellagic acid on food intake, body weight, and organ index in mice.

Variable	C	M	EL	EH
Food intake, g/day	4.65 ± 0.35^a	3.22 ± 0.52^b	4.18 ± 0.57^a	4.20 ± 0.55^a
Initial body weight, g	25.51 ± 0.97^a	25.39 ± 0.88^a	25.91 ± 0.81^a	25.82 ± 0.83^a
Final body weight, g	33.01 ± 2.84^a	26.63 ± 1.34^b	29.90 ± 2.11^a	30.13 ± 2.71^a
Liver index, %	3.85 ± 0.30^a	4.65 ± 0.34^b	4.00 ± 0.20^a	3.98 ± 0.31^a
Kidney index, %	1.45 ± 0.11^a	1.67 ± 0.30^a	1.60 ± 0.30^a	1.57 ± 0.30^a
Spleen index, %	0.23 ± 0.04^a	0.28 ± 0.02^a	0.25 ± 0.03^a	0.26 ± 0.05^a

Values represent the mean ± SD (n ≥ 6). Labeled means without a common letter difference. p < 0.05 by one-way ANOVA followed by Duncan's test. C, normal group; M, model group; EL, low dose of ellagic acid group; EH, high dose of ellagic acid.

the M group when compared with the C group. The treatment with ellagic acid (EL and EH) markedly ($p < 0.05$) downregulated the activities of the enzymes; AST, ALT, γGT, and ALP; when compared with the M group.

The results regarding serum lipid profiles such as TG, TC, HDL-C, LDL-C, and FFA are presented in **Figures 2A–E**. Compared with the C group, a significant rise in the serum TC, TG, LDL-C, and FFA levels and a downregulation of HDL-C level were observed in the M group ($p < 0.05$). Interestingly, the serum TG, TC, HDL-C, LDL-C, and FFA levels were significantly downregulated ($p < 0.05$), and HDL-C level was upregulated by ellagic acid treatment (EL and EH) compared with the M group.

Effect of Ellagic Acid on Hepatic Lipids Profile of Alcohol-Induced ALD Mice

As shown in the **Figures 3A–C**, hepatic lipid indicators such as TC (**Figure 3A**), TG (**Figure 3B**), and FFA (**Figure 3C**) were markedly upregulated in M group compared with the C group ($p < 0.05$). Ellagic acid treatment (EL and EH) induced a significant decline in the hepatic lipid indicators, e.g., TC, TG, and FFA ($p < 0.05$). However, EL failed to restore FFA level compared to the M group.

Effect of Ellagic Acid on Hepatic Oxidative Stress Parameters in ALD Mice

One of the major pathological events during the development of alcoholic fatty liver disease is oxidative stress since it connects lipid metabolism dysfunction to downstream inflammation and apoptosis (2, 4). Antioxidant enzymes, e.g., GSH-Px, CAT, MDA, SOD, and GSH, play significant roles in protecting alcohol-induced hepatic damage and oxidative stress. **Figures 4A–E** showed the effect of ellagic acid on hepatic antioxidant enzymes (GSH-Px, CAT, MDA, SOD, and GSH). Hepatic MDA level significantly elevated in the M group compared with C group ($p < 0.05$). The ellagic acid-treated groups (EL and EH) markedly decreased the MDA content compared with the M group ($p < 0.05$). In addition, hepatic GSH-Px, CAT, SOD, and GSH levels were significantly decreased in M group compared with C group ($p < 0.05$), which was restored by ellagic acid administration (EL and EH groups). The results clearly indicated that ellagic acid showed strong potential to alleviate hepatic damage in alcohol-induced mice *via* downregulating MDA content and increasing the antioxidant enzymes (GSH-Px, CAT, MDA, SOD, and GSH).

Effect of Ellagic Acid on the Hepatic Histopathological Features of Alcohol-Induced ALD Mice

To determine the protective effect of ellagic acid against ALD, we investigated the histopathological changes in the hepatic tissue by using H&E and MAS staining assay. As presented in the **Figure 5**, the structure of liver lobule was complete and clear with no evident inflammatory cell infiltration, and hepatocytes were in an ordered arrangement with centrally and round located nuclei in C group mice. However, after alcohol exposure (M group), a significant inflammatory cell infiltration, fibrosis, and enlargement of hepatocytes around the central vein was observed. The ellagic acid-treated groups (EL and EH) exhibited less edema, fibrosis, and inflammatory cell infiltration compared with M group.

Effect of Ellagic Acid on Hepatic Proinflammatory Cytokines Levels in ALD Mice

The results regarding proinflammatory cytokines such as IL-6, IL-1β, and TNF-α in the hepatic tissues are presented in the **Figures 6A–C**. A significant ($p < 0.05$) elevation in the hepatic IL-6, IL-1β, and TNF-α were observed in M group mice compared with C group. Interestingly, treatment of ellagic acid (EL and EH) was able to markedly decrease the levels of TNF-α, IL-1β, and IL-6 compared with the M group ($p < 0.05$). These results suggested that ellagic acid treatment was an effective approach to attenuate alcohol-induced hepatic inflammation.

Effect of Ellagic Acid on the Hepatic Inflammation Associated Genes Expression of ALD Mice

According to the results, hepatic mRNA expression of TLR4, a trigger of inflammation in ALD was significantly increased in M group mice ($p < 0.05$), which further caused the upregulation of MyD88 and downstream genes compared with the C group (**Figures 7A–F**). However, it has been observed that EL and EH significantly reduced the expression of TLR4 (*Tlr4*) and downstream MyD88 genes (*Myd88*) in a dose-dependent

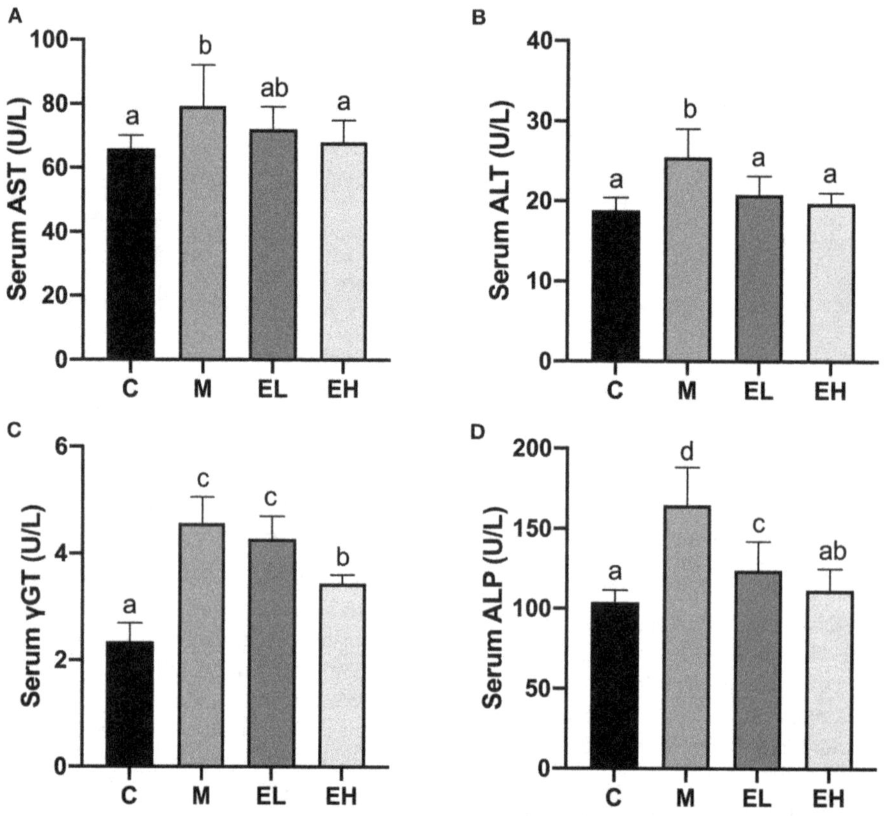

FIGURE 1 | Effect of ellagic acid on serum biochemical makers in mice. **(A)** AST; **(B)** ALT; **(C)** γGT; **(D)** ALP. Values represent the mean ± SD ($n \geq 6$). Labeled means without a common letter difference. $p < 0.05$ by one-way ANOVA followed by Duncan's test. C, normal group; M, model group; EL, low dose of ellagic acid group; EH, high dose of ellagic acid group.

manner resulting in reduced inflammatory changes ($p < 0.05$). Expression of inflammatory mediators (NF-κB and COX-2) and a cluster of differentiation (CD14) was significantly higher in the liver of M group of mice ($p < 0.05$). However, treatment with ellagic acid considerably reversed the inflammatory necrosis by downregulating the NF-κB (*Nfkb1*), COX-2 (*Cox2*), and CD14 (*Cd14*) genes expression ($p < 0.05$). Furthermore, a high dose of ellagic acid (100 mg/kg bw) was more effective in inhibiting the overexpression of TLR4, COX-2, CD14, and NF-κB genes than the low dose of ellagic acid (50 mg/kg bw, $p < 0.05$). It was also noticed that both doses of ellagic acid (EL and EH) reduced the hepatic inflammation by suppressing the expression of iNOS gene (*Nos2*) compared with the M group.

Effect of Ellagic Acid on the Intestinal Microbial Composition in ALD Mice

In the **Figure 8A**, Venn chart showed the number and overlap of sample OTUs in each and among the group. The results revealed that a total of 454 OTUs were shared by all the samples. At the phylum level (**Figure 8B**), ethanol administration elevated the relative abundance of *Firmicutes*, *Verrucomicrobia*, *Actinobacteria*, and decreased the relative abundance of *Bacteroidetes* and *Proteobacteria* compared with the C group. The administration of ellagic acid markedly modulated gut microbiota to some extent such as decreasing the relative abundance of *Actinobacteria* and *Verrucomicrobia* compared with the model group. At the genus level (**Figure 8C**), the *norank_f__Muribaculaceae*, *Lactobacillus*, *Kurthia*, *Akkermansia*, *Bacteroides*, and *Lachnospiraceae_NK4A136*_group were found to be the most prevalent six genera in colonic samples of tested mice. Alcohol administration decreased the relative abundance of *norank_f__Muribaculaceae* and *Bacteroides*, which were modulated to some extent by the treatment of EL and EH. In addition, the relative abundance of *Bacteroides* increased and *Lachnospiraceae_NK4A136*_group decreased in the EH group compared with the M group. The EL also improved the relative abundance of *Bifidobacterium* compared with the M group. Collectively, our results indicated that ellagic acid could significantly modulate gut microbiota composition.

Correlations between the microbiome and several biochemical indicators were tested by Spearman's correlation analysis. As shown in **Figure 8D**, the relative abundance of *Bifidobacterium* was significantly correlated with hepatic FFA, γGT, LDL, IL-6, and GSH. The relative abundance of *Lactobacillus* was significantly correlated with SOD. The relative abundance of *Akkermansia* was significantly correlated with IL-1β. The relative abundance

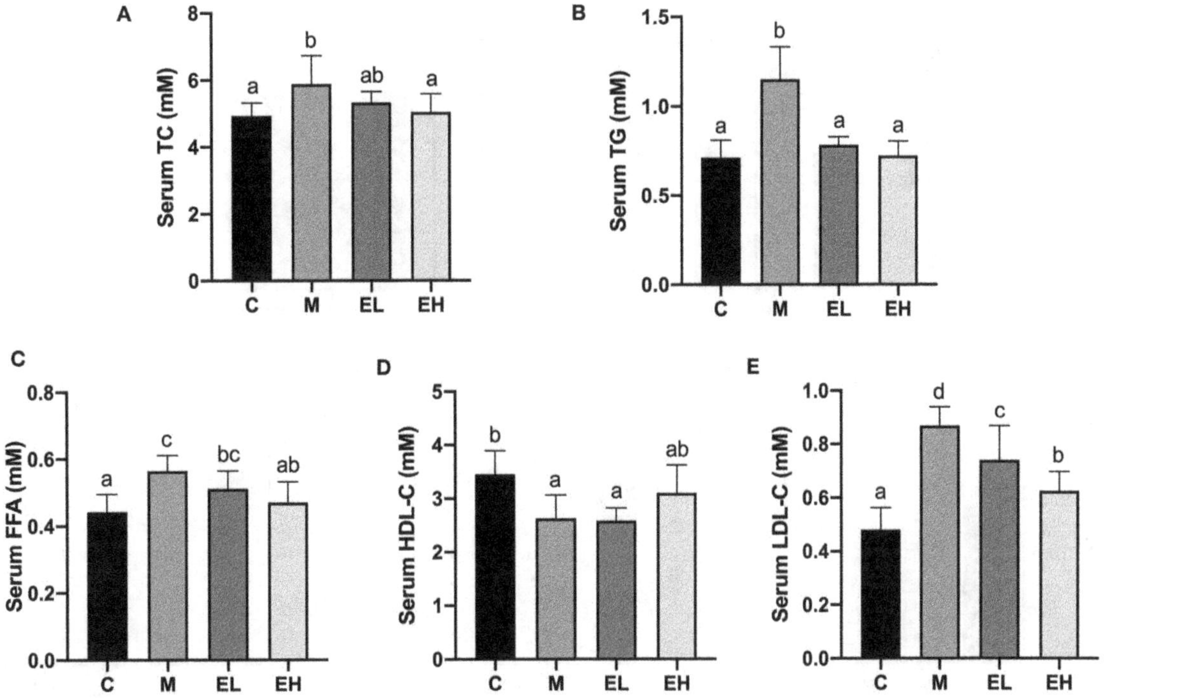

FIGURE 2 | Effect of ellagic acid on serum lipid profile in mice. **(A)** TC; **(B)** TG; **(C)** FFA; **(D)** HDL-C; **(E)** LDL-C. Values represent the mean ± SD ($n \geq 6$). Labeled means without a common letter difference. $p < 0.05$ by one-way ANOVA followed by Duncan's test. C, normal group; M, model group; EL, low dose of ellagic acid group; EH, high dose of ellagic acid group.

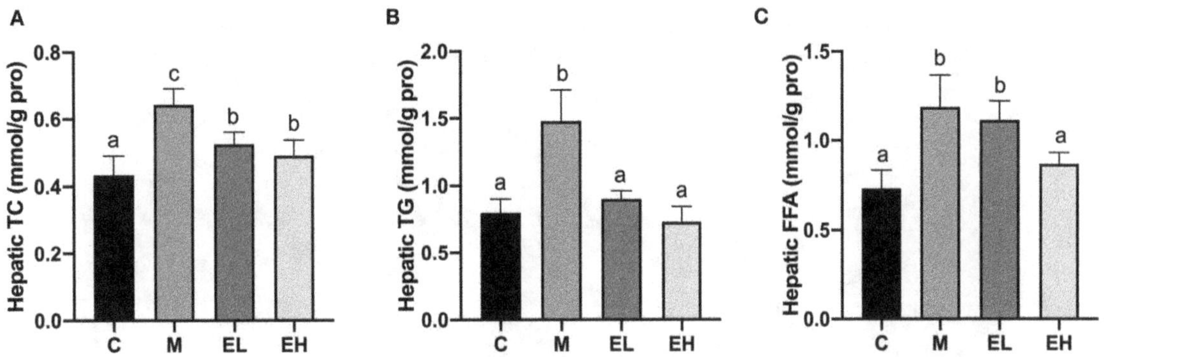

FIGURE 3 | Effect of ellagic acid on hepatic lipid profile in mice. **(A)** Hepatic TC; **(B)** Hepatic TG; **(C)** Hepatic FFA. Values represent the mean ± SD ($n \geq 6$). Labeled means without a common letter difference. $p < 0.05$ by one-way ANOVA followed by Duncan's test. C, normal group; M, model group; EL, low dose of ellagic acid group; EH, high dose of ellagic acid group.

of *Parasutterella* was significantly correlated with serum TG. The relative abundance of *Candidatus_Arthromitus* was significantly correlated with γGT and HDL. The relative abundance of *(Eubacterium)_coprostanoligenes*_group was significantly correlated with SOD. The relative abundance of *Alistipes* was significantly correlated with MDA.

DISCUSSION

Chronic alcohol intake could lead to ALD such as alcoholic fatty liver (AFL), steatohepatitis, and cirrhosis. The pathogenesis of ALD is very complex and may be associated with oxidative stress (OS) and inflammatory responses. Notably, despite years of ongoing research, the mechanisms of ALD remain obscure. Interestingly, recent studies confirmed that natural products (black rice, aged black garlic, Pinus thunbergii Parl, noni fruit, etc.) and bioactive compounds (apigenin, quercetin, naringenin, (-)-epigallocatechin gallate, genistein, and platycodin D, etc.) could attenuate ALD via multiple pathways (18–20, 22, 35–39). Based on the broad spectrum of antioxidant and antiinflammatory effects of ellagic acid, the present study was designed to evaluate the hepatoprotective effect of ellagic acid against ALD.

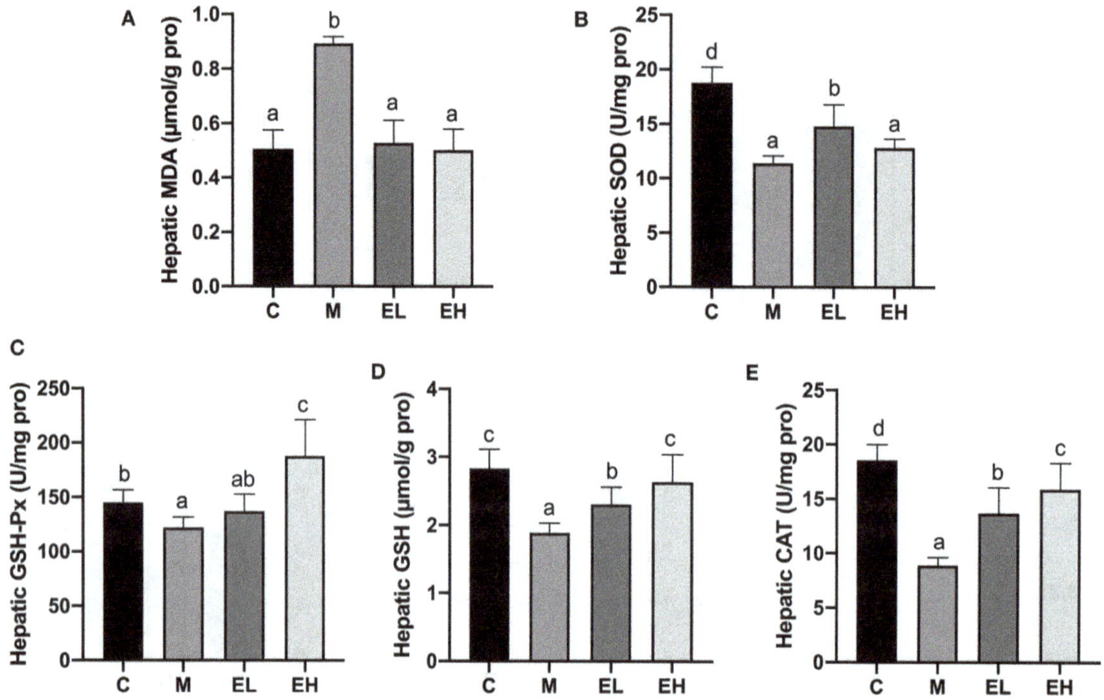

FIGURE 4 | Effect of ellagic acid on hepatic oxidative stress parameters in mice. **(A)** MDA; **(B)** SOD; **(C)** GSH-Px; **(D)** GSH; **(E)** CAT. Values represent the mean ± SD ($n \geq 6$). Labeled means without a common letter difference. $p < 0.05$ by one-way ANOVA followed by Duncan's test. C, normal group; M, model group; EL, low dose of ellagic acid group; EH, high dose of ellagic acid group.

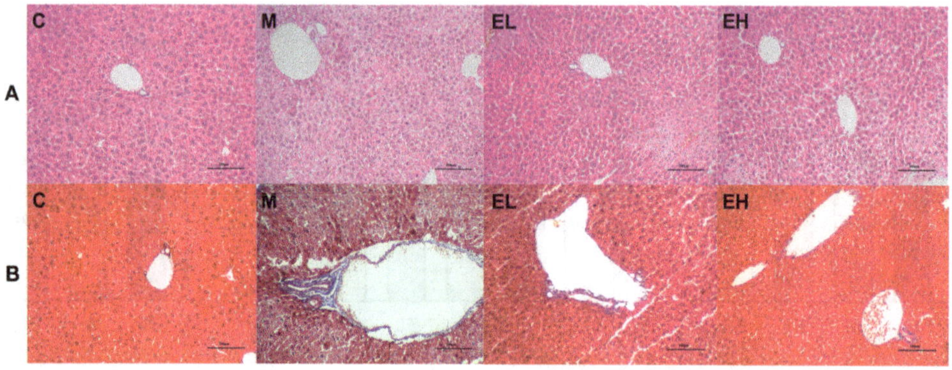

FIGURE 5 | Effect of ellagic acid on hepatic histopathology feature of alcohol induced ALD mice. **(A)** H&E staining; **(B)** MAS staining. C, normal group; M, model group; EL, low dose of ellagic acid group; EH, high dose of ellagic acid group.

Fatty liver is the earliest pathology of ALD, in which hepatocytes contain macrovesicular droplets of TG. It was reported that AFL is a result of fat metabolism imbalance, such as increased TG synthesis along with decreased mitochondrial lipid oxidation (40). Serum AST and ALT are also important biochemical indicators for hepatic cellular injury. Under the healthy condition, ALT and AST are present in hepatocytes. However, in the event of hepatic damage, these enzymes are released from hepatocytes into circulation (41). In the present study, we noticed that the consumption of alcohol markedly raised the serum TG level, and activities of ALT and AST, which clearly indicated the occurrence of hepatic injury caused by alcohol. However, the ellagic acid supplementation (at the dosage of 50 and 100 mg/kg bw) significantly alleviated lipid metabolism disorder and hepatocyte integrity in ALD mice, which is correlated with many previous reports in the same animal model (18, 37–39, 42–44).

Oxidative stress plays an important role in ALD. The consumption of alcohol aggravated OS *via* elevating reactive oxygen species (ROS). In the normal physiological environment, there are many antioxidants present in cells such as SOD,

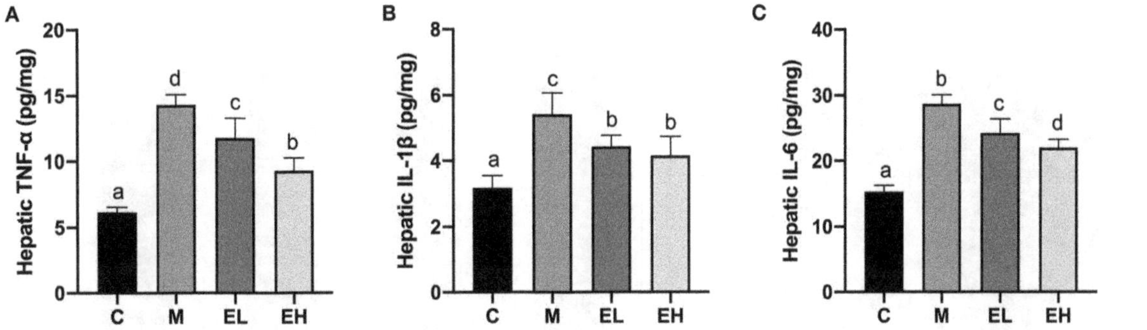

FIGURE 6 | Effect of ellagic acid on hepatic pro-inflammatory cytokines levels in mice. **(A)** TNF-α; **(B)** IL-1β; **(C)** IL-6. Values represent the mean ± SD ($n \geq 6$). Labeled means without a common letter difference. $p < 0.05$ by one-way ANOVA followed by Duncan's test. C, normal group; M, model group; EL, low dose of ellagic acid group; EH, high dose of ellagic acid group.

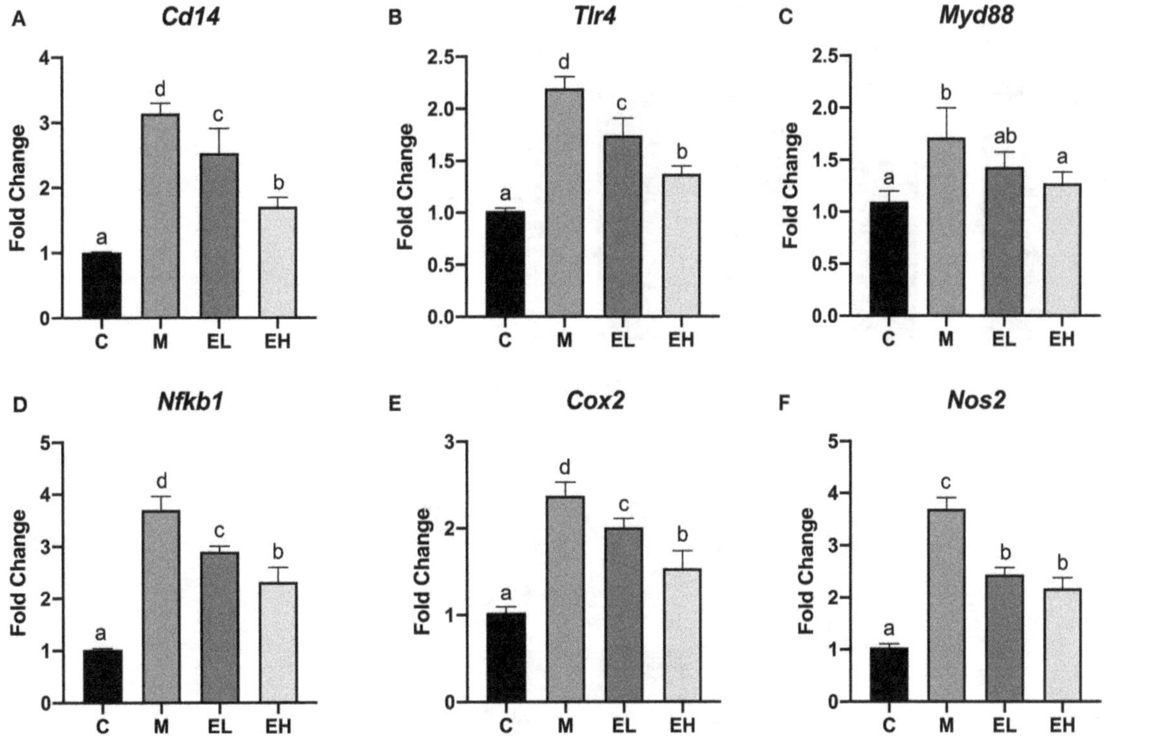

FIGURE 7 | Effect of ellagic acid on the hepatic inflammation associated genes expression in mice. **(A)** *Cd14*; **(B)** *Tlr4*; **(C)** *Myd88*; **(D)** *Nfkb1*; **(E)** *Cox2*; **(F)** *Nos2*. Values represent the mean ± SD ($n \geq 3$). Labeled means without a common letter difference. $p < 0.05$ by one-way ANOVA followed by Duncan's test. C, normal group; M, model group; EL, low dose of ellagic acid group; EH, high dose of ellagic acid group.

CAT, GSH, vitamin E, etc., which can eliminate harmful free radicals in the body. Therefore, the elimination and production of free radicals should be in dynamic equilibrium. However, excessive alcohol intake can lead to a loss of this dynamic equilibrium, and a higher generation of ROS surpasses the production of abundant antioxidants to remove ROS, causing OS and cell damage. Nrf2 (NF-E2-related factor 2) plays a key role in maintaining and regulating OS response mediated by alcohol, which can inhibit the OS-induced inflammation (3–5). In this study, protective effects of ellagic acid on the hepatic activities or levels of MDA, GSH, CAT, GSH-Px, and SOD were evaluated, and results revealed that ellagic acid markedly improved antioxidant defense status *via* increasing the hepatic GSH, CAT, GSH-Px, and SOD activities and decreasing the MDA content in ALD mice. Girish and Pradhan (31) documented that ellagic acid and curcumin treatment decreased hepatic MDA levels in CCl_4-induced liver toxicity in mice. In another study, Ding et al.

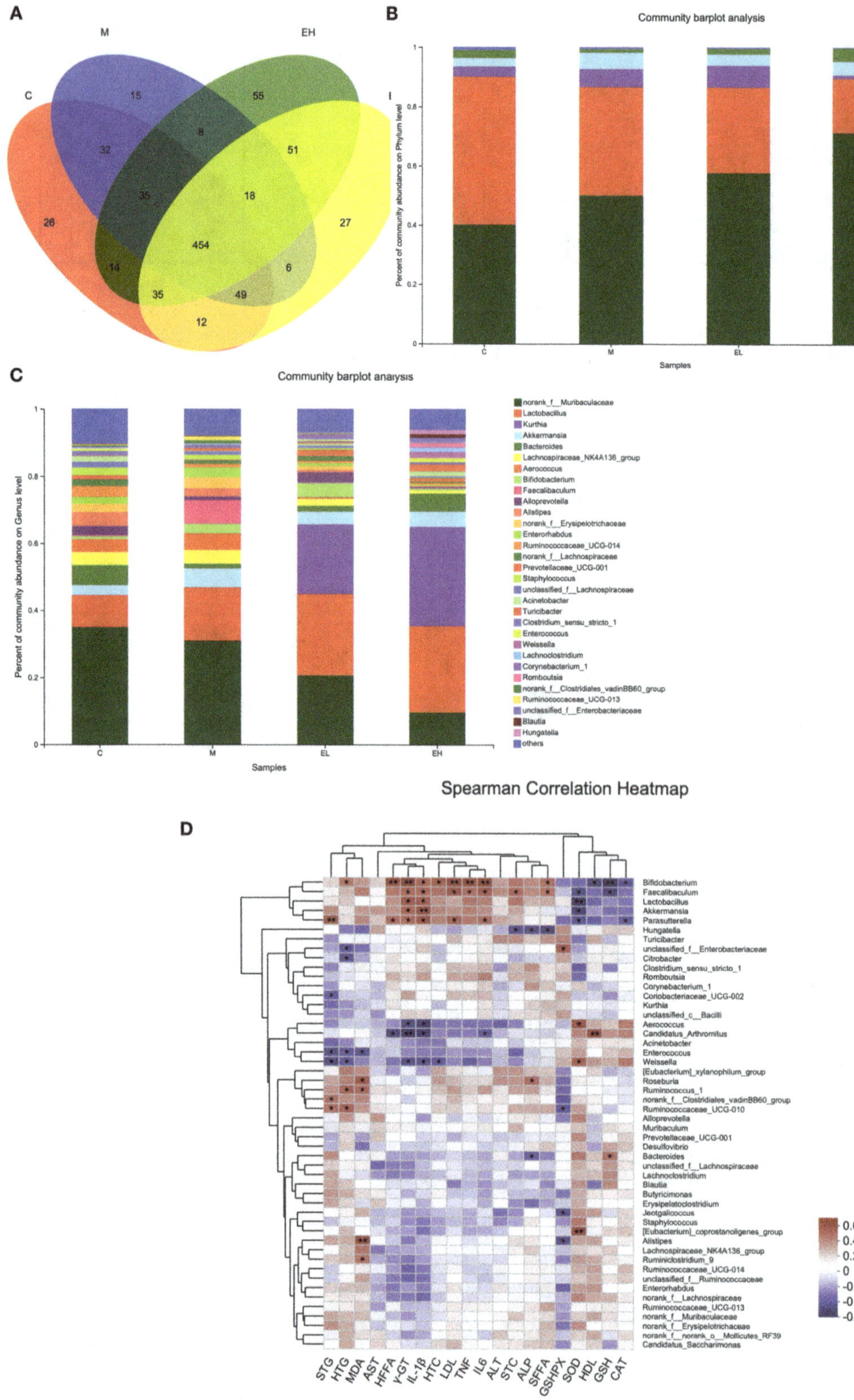

FIGURE 8 | Effect of ellagic acid on the intestinal microbial composition in ALD mice. **(A)** Venn plot; **(B)** Bacterial profile at phylum level; **(C)** Bacterial profile at genus level; **(D)** Heatmap of Spearman correlation analysis of physical parameters and microbiota based on species level. Values represent the mean ± SD ($n \geq 5$). C, normal group; M, model group; EL, low dose of ellagic acid group; EH, high dose of ellagic acid group.

(45) also reported that ellagic acid inhibited ROS release in CCl_4-induced cirrhotic mice. In addition, Girish et al. (46) observed that ellagic acid reduced the paracetamol-induced acute liver injury *via* enhancing antioxidant levels and inhibiting lipid peroxidation.

Proinflammatory cytokines (IL-6, IL-1β, and TNF-α) and their abnormal metabolism play a significant role in the pathogenesis of ALD (47). Earlier, Khan et al. (48) reported that ethanol administration led to the activation of NF-κB and elevated the TNF-α levels in the liver. With the consistence of Khan et al. (48), we also observed the elevation of hepatic proinflammatory cytokines levels (IL-6, IL-1β, and TNF-α) in the M group, clearly indicating that inflammatory factors play a major role in ALD. Interestingly, ellagic acid administration (EL and EH) could reduce the inflammatory factors in the hepatic tissues of ALD mice. Similarly, intervention with bioactive compounds and natural products could also reduce the inflammatory responses associated with acute alcoholic liver injury (18–20, 32, 35, 48).

In this study, histopathological findings showed a significant alteration in the liver architecture, edema, hepatocytes degeneration, and inflammatory cells infiltration in ALD mice. Interestingly, the administration of ellagic acid markedly improved histopathological features of ALD mice. These results were consistent with the previous reports of bioactive compounds protecting the liver from the toxic effects of alcohol (18–20, 43, 44, 49).

It has been reported that TLR4 plays a critical role in the development and pathogenesis of ALD *via* inducing inflammatory cytokine, TLR adapter, and the expression of MyD88 (50, 51). TLR4 has the potential to activate two different pathways, such as MyD88-independent/TRIF-dependent and MyD88-dependent pathways (52). Our results revealed that alcohol administration activated the TLR4 pathway *via* upregulating hepatic MyD88 and TLR4 genes expression. However, ellagic acid supplementation markedly decreased the hepatic genes expression of MyD88 and TLR4. Earlier, Lee et al. (53) demonstrated that ellagic acid could ameliorate concanavalin A-induced hepatitis through TLR4/MyD88/NF-κB signaling pathway. In another study, ellagic acid has also been reported to improve anxiety and sleep by inhibiting the TLR4 signaling pathway (54). Liu et al. (55) also reported that dioscin alleviated ALD in the hepatic stellate cell *via* the TLR4/MyD88/NF-κB signaling pathway. Similarly, many bioactive compounds were also reported to reduce the inflammatory responses *via* TLR4/NF-κB-mediated inflammatory pathway (56).

As stated in the introduction, alcohol consumption can elevate bacterial endotoxin levels, which disrupts intestinal integrity and barrier function, and significantly promotes the occurrence of ALD. In addition, alcohol consumption also changes the gut microbiota composition, leading to abnormalities in the gut–liver axis (6, 8, 57). Moreover, it has been documented that some intestinal microbiomes, such as *Bacteroides* and *Akkermansia*, have beneficial properties and can regulate inflammation (13, 58). Our results showed significant microbiota dysbiosis following ethanol exposure, which were consistent with previous studies (43, 44, 49, 59). As previously described in results sections, the relative abundance of microbiota such as *Firmicutes*, *Verrucomicrobia*, *Actinobacteria*, *Bacteroidetes*, and *Proteobacteria* at phylum level and *norank_f__Muribaculaceae*, *Lactobacillus*, *Kurthia*, *Akkermansia*, *Bacteroides*, and *Lachnospiraceae_NK4A136*_group at genus level were significantly altered after the intake of alcohol, which were further restored after ellagic acid treatment. Previously, it was reported that *Lactobacillus* species play an important role in the pathogenesis of ALD. The long-term alcohol intake decreases the *Lactobacillus* species abundance *via* altering the FFA level in serum circulation (49), which is relevant to our findings. Moreover, *Lactobacillus* species were also reported to exclude pathogens, stimulate mucin secretion, and regulate inflammatory responses (60). The ellagic acid supplementation increased the *Lactobacillus* species abundance. Okra seed oil supplementation could increase the *Lactobacillus* species population in ethanol-induced ALD mice (44). Similarly, lychee (*Litchi chinensis Sonn.)* pulp phenolic extract was also reported to modulate *Lactobacillus* species in ALD mice (43). The consumption of phenolic compounds (e.g., *p*-coumaric acid, caffeic acid, sinapic acid, rutin, hesperidin, and ferulic acid) and food rich with bioactive compounds (rhubarb, okra seed oil, and lychee) contributed to the increment of healthy gut microbiota in animal experiments (43, 44, 49, 59, 61–66). It is well-known that phenolic compounds are metabolized *via* microbiota in the colon but are not absorbed directly, thus contributing to the balance of gut microbiota (63, 64). Together, all these data suggest that ellagic acid could modulate the alcohol-induced gut microbiota dysbiosis.

In the present study, we demonstrated that ellagic acid (low and high doses) can attenuate alcohol-induced liver injury in mice. The ellagic acid supplementation exerted hepatoprotective effects *via* improving oxidative stress, decreasing inflammatory responses, and modulating gut microbiota composition. According to the above results, we can conclude that ellagic acid has strong potentials against ALD. Our results divulged that ellagic acid may be an ideal nutraceutical ingredient to prevent ALD. However, further mechanistic studies should be carried out prior to its clinical application.

AUTHOR CONTRIBUTIONS

LZ, AM, and CW had contributed to data collection and analysis, and manuscript preparation. AI, MI, SA, and MS supervised the whole study and revised the manuscript.

REFERENCES

Wang FS, Fan JG, Zhang Z, Gao B, Wang HY. The global burden of liver disease: the major impact of China. *Hepatology.* (2014) 60:2099– 108. doi: 10.1002/hep.27406

Osna NA, Donohue TM Jr, Kharbanda KK. Alcoholic liver disease: pathogenesis and current management. *Alcohol Res.* (2017) 38:147–61.

Smathers RL, Galligan JJ, Stewart BJ, Petersen DR. Overview of lipid peroxidation products and hepatic protein modification in alcoholic liver disease. *Chem Biol Interact.* (2011) 192:107–12. doi: 10.1016/j.cbi.2011.02.021

Zhao L, Zhang N, Yang D, Yang M, Guo X, He J, et al. Protective effects of five structurally diverse flavonoid subgroups against chronic alcohol- induced hepatic damage in a mouse model. *Nutrients.* (2018) 10:1754. doi: 10.3390/nu10111754

Gao B, Bataller R. Alcoholic liver disease: pathogenesis and new therapeutic targets. *Gastroenterology.* (2011) 141:1572– 85. doi: 10.1053/j.gastro.2011.09.002

Woodhouse CA, Patel VC, Singanayagam A, Shawcross DL. the gut microbiome as a therapeutic target in the pathogenesis and treatment of chronic liver disease. *Aliment Pharmacol Ther.* (2018) 47:192–202. doi: 10.1111/apt.14397

Engen PA, Green SJ, Voigt RM, Forsyth CB, Keshavarzian A. The gastrointestinal microbiome: alcohol effects on the composition of intestinal microbiota. *Alcohol Res.* (2015) 37:223–36.

Schnabl B, Brenner DA. Interactions between the intestinal microbiome and liver diseases. *Gastroenterology.* (2014) 146:1513– 24. doi:10.1053/j.gastro.2014.01.020

Bull-Otterson L, Feng W, Kirpich I, Wang Y, Qin X, Liu Y, et al. Metagenomic analyses of alcohol induced pathogenic alterations in the intestinal microbiome and the effect of *Lactobacillus rhamnosus* GG treatment. *PLoS ONE.* (2013) 8:e53028. doi: 10.1371/journal.pone.0053028

Yan AW, Fouts DE, Brandl J, Stärkel P, Torralba M, Schott E, et al. Enteric dysbiosis associated with a mouse model of alcoholic liver disease. *Hepatology.* (2011) 53:96–105. doi: 10.1002/hep.24018

Llopis M, Cassard AM, Wrzosek L, Boschat L, Bruneau A, Ferrere G, et al. Intestinal microbiota contributes to individual susceptibility to alcoholic liver disease. *Gut.* (2016) 65:830–9. doi: 10.1136/gutjnl-2015-310585

Leclercq S, Matamoros S, Cani PD, Neyrinck AM, Jamar F, Stärkel P, et al. Intestinal permeability, gut-bacterial dysbiosis, and behavioral markers of alcohol-dependence severity. *Proc Natl Acad Sci USA.* (2014) 111:E4485– 93. doi: 10.1073/pnas.1415174111

Ferrere G, Wrzosek L, Cailleux F, Turpin W, Puchois V, Spatz M, et al. Fecal microbiota manipulation prevents dysbiosis and alcohol-induced liver injury in mice. *J Hepatol.* (2017) 66:806–15. doi: 10.1016/j.jhep.2016.11.008

Tuomisto S, Pessi T, Collin P, Vuento R, Aittoniemi J, Karhunen PJ. Changes in gut bacterial populations and their translocation into liver and ascites in alcoholic liver cirrhotics. *BMC Gastroenterol.* (2014) 14:40. doi: 10.1186/1471-230X-14-40

Chen P, Stärkel P, Turner JR, Ho SB, Schnabl B. Dysbiosis-induced intestinal inflammation activates tumor necrosis factor receptor I and mediates alcoholic liver disease in mice. *Hepatology.* (2015) 61:883– 94. doi: 10.1002/hep.27489

Patel S, Behara R, Swanson GR, Forsyth CB, Voigt RM, Keshavarzian A. Alcohol and the intestine. *Biomolecules.* (2015) 5:2573–88. doi: 10.3390/biom5042573

Hao L, Sun Q, Zhong W, Zhang W, Sun X, Zhou Z. Mitochondria- targeted ubiquinone (MitoQ) enhances acetaldehyde clearance by reversing alcohol-induced posttranslational modification of aldehyde dehydrogenase 2: a molecular mechanism of protection against alcoholic liver disease. *Redox Bio.* (2018) 14:626–36. doi: 10.1016/j.redox.2017.11.005

Zhao L, Mehmood A, Yuan D, Usman M, Murtaza MA, Yaqoob S, et al. Protective mechanism of edible food plants against alcoholic liver disease with special mention to polyphenolic compounds. *Nutrients.* (2021) 13:1612. doi: 10.3390/nu13051612

Jeong MS, Park S, Han EJ, Park SY, Kim MJ, Jung K, et al. *Pinus thunbergii* PARL leaf protects against alcohol-induced liver disease by enhancing antioxidant defense mechanism in BALB/c mice. *J Funct Foods.* (2020) 73:104116. doi: 10.1016/j.jff.2020.104116

Guo M, Mao B, Sadiq FA, Hao Y, Cui S, Yi M, et al. Effects of noni fruit and fermented noni juice against acute alcohol induced liver injury in mice. *J Funct Foods.* (2020) 70:103995. doi: 10.1016/j.jff.2020.103995

Fiore M, Messina MP, Petrella C, D'Angelo A, Greco A, Ralli M, et al. Antioxidant properties of plant polyphenols in the counteraction of alcohol- abuse induced damage: impact on the Mediterranean diet. *J Funct Foods.* (2020) 71:104012. doi: 10.1016/j.jff.2020.104012

Li Y, Chen M, Wang J, Guo X, Xiao L, Liu P, et al. Quercetin ameliorates autophagy in alcohol liver disease associated with lysosome through mTOR-TFEB pathway. *J Funct Foods.* (2019) 52:177–85. doi: 10.1016/j.jff.2018.10. 033

Calixto JB, Beirith A, Ferreira J, Santos AR, Filho VC, Yunes RA. Naturally occurring antinociceptive substances from plants. *Phytother Res.* (2000) 14:401–18. doi: 10.1002/1099-1573(200009)14:6<401::AID-PTR762>3.0.CO;2-H

Firdaus F, Zafeer MF, Anis E, Ahmad M, Afzal M. Ellagic acid attenuates arsenic induced neuro-inflammation and mitochondrial dysfunction associated apoptosis. *Toxicol Rep.* (2018) 5:411– 7. doi: 10.1016/j.toxrep.2018.02.017

Ebrahimi R, Sepand MR, Seyednejad SA, Omidi A, Akbariani M, Gholami M, et al. Ellagic acid reduces methotrexate-induced apoptosis and mitochondrial dysfunction via up-regulating Nrf2 expression and inhibiting the IKBα/NFKB in rats. *J Pharm Sci.* (2019) 27:721–33. doi: 10.1007/s40199-019-0 0309-9

Lin Z, Lin C, Fu C, Lu H, Jin H, Chen Q, et al. The protective effect of Ellagic acid (EA) in osteoarthritis: an *in vitro* and *in vivo* study. *Biomed Pharmacother.* (2020) 125:109845. doi: 10.1016/j.biopha.2020.109845

Gupta A, Pandey AK. Aceclofenac-induced hepatotoxicity: an ameliorative effect of *Terminalia bellirica* fruit and ellagic acid. *World J Hepatol.* (2020) 12:949–64. doi: 10.4254/wjh.v12.i11.949

Afifi NA, Ibrahim MA, Galal MK. Hepatoprotective influence of quercetin and ellagic acid on thioacetamide-induced hepatotoxicity in rats. *Can J Physiol Pharmacol.* (2018) 96:624–9. doi: 10.1139/cjpp-2017-0651

Abdelkader NF, Elyamany M, Gad AM, Assaf N, Fawzy HM, Elesawy WH. Ellagic acid attenuates liver toxicity induced by valproic acid in rats. *J Pharmacol Sci.* (2020) 143:23–9. doi: 10.1016/j.jphs.2020.01.007

Cengiz M, Ali JH, Kutlu HM, Vejselova D, Ayhanci A. Potential recruiting and hepatoprotective effects of ellagic acid in D- galactosamine-induced liver damage in rats. *Pak J Zool.* (2017) 49:1251–9. doi: 10.17582/journal.pjz/2017.49.4.1251.1259

Girish C, Pradhan SC. Hepatoprotective activities of picroliv, curcumin, and ellagic acid compared to silymarin on carbon-tetrachloride- induced liver toxicity in mice. *J Pharmacol Pharmacother.* (2012) 3:149–55. doi: 10.4103/0976-500X.95515

Sohn EH, Koo HJ, Jang SA, Namkoong S, Lim JD, Kang SC. Protective effects of ellagic acid on ethanol-induced toxicity in hepatic HepG2 cells. *Mol Cell Toxicol.* (2013) 9:249–56. doi: 10.1007/s13273-013- 0032-1

Mehmood A, Zhao L, Ishaq M, Xin W, Zhao L, Wang C, et al. Anti-hyperuricemic potential of stevia (*Stevia rebaudiana Bertoni*) residue extract in hyperuricemic mice. *Food Func.* (2020) 11:6387–406. doi: 10.1039/C9FO02246E

Wang K, Yang Q, Ma Q, Wang B, Wan Z, Chen M, et al. Protective effects of salvianolic acid a against dextran sodium sulfate-induced acute colitis in rats. *Nutrients.* (2018) 10:791. doi: 10.3390/nu10060791

Zhao L, Wang Y, Liu J, Wang K, Guo X, Ji B, et al. Protective effects of genistein and puerarin against chronic alcohol-induced liver injury in mice via antioxidant, anti-inflammatory, and anti-apoptotic mechanisms. *J Agric Food Chem.* (2016) 64:7291–7. doi: 10.1021/acs.jafc.6b02907

Li W, Liu Y, Wang Z, Han Y, Tian YH, Zhang GS, et al. Platycodin D isolated from the aerial parts of Platycodon grandiflorum protects alcohol-induced liver injury in mice. *Food Funct.* (2015) 6:1418–27. doi: 10.1039/C5FO00094G

Kim MH, Kim MJ, Lee JH, Han JI, Kim JH, Sok DE, et al. Hepatoprotective effect of aged black garlic on chronic alcohol-induced liver injury in rats. *J Med Food.* (2011) 14:732–8. doi: 10.1089/jmf.2010.1454

Hou Z, Qin P, Ren G. Effect of anthocyanin-rich extract from black rice (*Oryza sativa L. Japonica)* on chronically alcohol-induced liver damage in rats. *J Agric Food Chem.* (2010) 58:3191–6. doi: 10.1021/jf904407x

Lu KH, Tseng HC, Liu CT, Huang CJ, Chyuan JH, Sheen LY. Wild bitter gourd protects against alcoholic fatty liver in mice by attenuating oxidative stress and inflammatory responses. *Food Funct.* (2014) 5:1027– 37. doi: 10.1039/C3FO60449G

You M, Considine RV, Leone TC, Kelly DP, Crabb DW. Role of adiponectin in the protective action of dietary saturated fat against a lcoholic fatty liver in mice. *Hepatology.* (2005) 42:568–77. doi: 10.1002/hep.20821

Limdi JK, Hyde GM. Evaluation of abnormal liver function tests. *Postgrad Med J.* (2003) 79:307–12. doi: 10.1136/pmj.79.932.307 Wang O, Cheng Q, Liu J, Wang Y, Zha o L, Zhou F, et al. Hepatoprotective effect of *Schisandra chinensis* (Turcz.) Baill. lignans and its formula with Rubus idaeus on chronic alcohol-induced liver injury in mice. *Food Funct.* (2014) 5:3018–25. doi: 10.1039/C4FO00550C

Xiao J, Zhang R, Zhou Q, Liu L, Huang F, Deng Y, et al. Lychee (*Litchi chinensis Sonn.*) pulp phenolic extract provides protection against alcoholic liver injury in mice by alleviating intestinal microbiota dysbiosis, intestinal barrier dysfunction, and liver inflammation. *J Agric Food Chem.* (2017) 65:9675–84. doi: 10.1021/acs.jafc.7b0379

Zhang J, Lu Y, Yang X, Zhao Y. Supplementation of okra seed oil ameliorates ethanol-induced liver injury and modulates gut microbiota dysbiosis in mice. *Food Func.* (2019) 10:6385–98. doi: 10.1039/C9FO00189A

Ding Y, Wang L, Song J, Zhou S. Protective effects of ellagic acid against tetrachloride-induced cirrhosis in mice through the inhibition of reactive oxygen species formation and angiogenesis. *Exp Ther Med.* (2017) 14:3375– 80. doi: 10.3892/etm.2017.4966

Girish C, Koner BC, Jayanthi S, Ramachandra Rao K, Rajesh B, Pradhan SC. Hepatoprotective activity of picroliv, curcumin and ellagic acid compared to silymarin on paracetamol induced liver toxicity in mice. *Fundam Clin Pharmacol.* (2009) 23:735–45. doi: 10.1111/j.1472-8206.2009.00722.x

Tilg H, Moschen AR, Szabo G. Interleukin-1 and inflammasomes in alcoholic liver disease/acute alcoholic hepatiti s and nonalcoholic fatty liver disease/ nonalcoholic steatohepatitis. *Hepatology.* (2016) 64:955–65. doi: 10.1002/ hep.28456

Khan AQ, Nafees S, Sultana S. Perillyl alcohol protects against ethanol induced acute liver injury in Wistar rats by inhibiting oxidative stress, NFκ- B activation and proinflammatory cytokine production. *Toxicology.* (2011) 279:108–14. doi: 10.1016/j.tox.2010.09.017

Chen P, Torralba M, Tan J, Embree M, Zengler K, Stärkel P, et al. Supplementation of saturated long-chain fatty acids maintains intestinal eubiosis and reduces ethanol-induced liver injury in mice. *Gastroenterology.* (2015) 148:203–14. doi: 10.1053/j.gastro.2014.09.014

Roh YS, Seki E. Toll-like receptors in alcoholic liver disease, non-alcoholic steatohepatitis and carcinogenesis. *J Gas troenterol Hepatol.* (2013) 28:38–42. doi: 10.1111/jgh.12019

Massey VL, Arteel GE. Acute alcohol-induced liver injury. *Front Physiol.* (2012) 3:193. doi: 10.3389/fphys.2012.00193

Takeda K, Akira S. Toll-like receptors. *Curr Protoc Immunol.* (2015) 109:11– 10. doi: 10.1002/0471142735.im1412s109

Lee JH, Won JH, Choi JM, Cha HH, Jang YJ, Park S, et al. Protective effect of ellagic acid on concanavalin A-induced hepatitis via toll-like receptor and mitogen-activated protein kinase/nuclear factor κB signaling pathways. *J Agric Food Chem.* (2014) 62:10110–17. doi: 10.1021/jf503188c

Wang W, Yang L, Liu T, Wang J, Wen A, Ding Y. Ellagic acid protects mice against sleep deprivation-induced memory impairment and anxiety by inhibiting TLR4 and activating Nr f2. *Aging.* (2020) 12:10457. doi: 10.18632/aging.103270

Liu M, Xu Y, Han X, Yin L, Xu L, Qi Y, et al. Dioscin alleviates alcoholic liver fibrosis by attenuating hepatic stellate cell activation via the TLR4/MyD88/NF-B signaling pathway. *Sci Rep.* (2015) 5:1– 13. doi: 10.1038/srep18038

Saleh HA,Yousef MH, Abdelnaser A. The anti-inflammatory properties of phytochemicals and their effects on epigenetic mechanisms involved in TLR4/ NF-κB-mediated inflammation. *Front Immunol.* (2021) 12:606069. doi:10.3389/ fimmu.2021.606069

Minemura M, Shimizu Y. Gut microbiota and liver diseases. *World J Gastroenterol.* (2015) 21:1691. doi: 10.3748/wjg.v21.i6.1691

Dao MC, Everard A, Aron-Wi snewsky J, Sokolovska N, Prifti E, Verger EO, et al. *Akkermansia muciniphila* and improved metabolic health during a dietary intervention in obesity: relationship with gut microbiome richness and ecology. *Gut.* (2016) 65:426–36. doi: 10.1136/gutjnl-2014-308778

Neyrinck AM, Etxeberria U, Taminiau B, Daube G, Van Hul M, Everard A, et al. Rhubarb extract prevents hepatic inflammation induced by acute alcohol intake, an effect related to the modulation of the gut microbiota. *Mol Nutr Food Res.* (2017) 61:1500899. doi: 10.1002/mnfr.201500899

Oelschlaeger TA. Mechanisms of probiotic actions'a review. *Int J Med Microbiol.* (2010) 300:57–62. doi: 10.1016/j.ijmm.2009.08.005

Hidalgo M, Oruna-Concha MJ, Kolida S, Walton GE, Kallithraka S, Spencer JP, et al. Metabolism of anthocyanins by human gut microflora and their influence on gut bacterial growth. *J Agric Food Chem.* (2012) 60:3882– 90. doi: 10.1021/ jf3002153

Celebioglu HU, Delsoglio M, Brix S, Pessione E, Svensson B. Plant polyphenols stimulate adhesion to intestinal mucosa and induce proteome changes in the probiotic *Lactobacillus acidophilus* N CFM. *Mol Nutr Food Res.* (2018) 62:1700638. doi: 10.1002/mnfr.201700638

Del Rio D, Rodriguez-Mateos A, S pencer JP, Tognolini M, Borges G, Crozier A. Dietary (poly) phenolics in human health: structures, bioavailability, and evidence of protective effects against chronic diseases. *Antioxid Redox Signal.* (2013) 18:1818–92. doi: 10.1089/ars.20 12.4581

Ozdal T, Sela DA, Xiao J, Boyacioglu D, Chen F, Capanoglu E. The reciprocal interactions between polyphenols and gut microbiota and effects on bioaccessibility. *Nutrients.* (2016) 8:78. doi: 10.3390/nu80 20078

Wang K, Jin X, Li Q, Sawaya AC, Le Leu RK, Conlon MA, et al. Propolis from different geographic origins decreases intestinal inflammation and Bacteroides spp. populations in a model of DSS-Induced colitis. *Mol Nutr Food Res.* (2018) 62:1800080. doi: 10.1002/mnfr.2018 00080

Wang K, Wan Z, Ou A, Liang X, Guo X, Zhang Z, et al. Monofloral honey from a medical plant, Prunella Vulgaris, protected against dextran sulfate sodium-induced ulcerative colitis via modulating gut microbial populations in rats. *Food Funct.* (2019) 10:3828–38. doi: 10.1039/C9FO00460B

18

Kinsenoside Alleviates Alcoholic Liver Injury by Reducing Oxidative Stress, Inhibiting Endoplasmic Reticulum Stress and Regulating AMPK-Dependent Autophagy

Limin Gao[1], *Xingyu Chen*[2], *Zeyu Fu*[3], *Jie Yin*[4], *Yafen Wang*[4], *Weiguang Sun*[4*], *Hong Ren*[1*] *and Yonghui Zhang*[4*]

[1]Biobank, Union Hospital, Tongji Medical College, Huazhong University of Science and Technology, Wuhan, China, [2]Department of Clinical Laboratory, the Central Hospital of Wuhan, Wuhan, China, [3]Department of Anesthesiology, Union Hospital, Tongji Medical College, Huazhong University of Science and Technology, Wuhan, China, [4]Hubei Key Laboratory of Natural Medicinal Chemistry and Resource Evaluation, School of Pharmacy, Tongji Medical College, Huazhong University of Science and Technology, Wuhan, China

Correspondence:
Weiguang Sun
weiguang_sun@hust.edu.cn
Hong Ren
renhong@hust.edu.cn
Yonghui Zhang
zhangyh@mails.tjmu.edu.cn

Background: *Anoectochilus roxburghii* (Orchidaceae) is a traditional Chinese medicinal herb with anti-inflammatory, antilipemic, liver protective, immunomodulatory, and other pharmacological activities. Kinsenoside (KD), which shows protective effects against a variety types of liver damage, is an active ingredient extracted from *A. roxburghii*. However, the liver protective effects and potential mechanisms of KD in alcoholic liver disease (ALD) remain unclear. This study aimed to investigate the liver protective activity and potential mechanisms of KD in ALD.

Methods: AML12 normal mouse hepatocyte cells were used to detect the protective effect of KD against ethanol-induced cell damage. An alcoholic liver injury model was induced by feeding male C57BL/6J mice with an ethanol-containing liquid diet, in combination with intraperitoneal administration of 5% carbon tetrachloride (CCl_4) in olive oil. Mice were divided into control, model, silymarin (positive control), and two KD groups, treated with different doses. After treatment, hematoxylin–eosin and Masson's trichrome staining of liver tissues was performed, and serum alanine aminotransferase (ALT) and aspartate transaminase (AST) levels were determined to assess the protective effect of KD against alcoholic liver injury. Moreover, proteomics techniques were used to explore the potential mechanism of KD action, and ELISA assay, immunohistochemistry, TUNEL assay, and western blotting were used to verify the mechanism.

Results: The results showed that KD concentration-dependently reduced ethanol-induced lipid accumulation in AML12 cells. In ALD mice model, the histological examination of liver tissues, combined with the determination of ALT and AST serum levels, demonstrated a protective effect of KD in the alcoholic liver injury mice. In addition, KD treatment markedly enhanced the antioxidant capacity and reduced the endoplasmic reticulum (ER) stress, inflammation, and apoptosis compared with those in the model group. Furthermore, KD increased the phosphorylation level of AMP-activated protein kinase (AMPK), inhibited the mechanistic target of rapamycin, promoted the phosphorylation of ULK1 (Ser555), increased the level of the autophagy marker LC3A/B, and restored ethanol-suppressed autophagic flux, thus activating AMPK-dependent autophagy.

Conclusion: This study indicates that KD alleviates alcoholic liver injury by reducing oxidative stress and ER stress, while activating AMPK-dependent autophagy. All results suggested that KD may be a potential therapeutic agent for ALD.

Keywords: Kinsenoside, alcoholic liver injury, oxidative stress, endoplasmic reticulum stress, AMP-activated protein kinase, autophagy

INTRODUCTION

According to the 2016 World Health Organization survey (World Health Organization, 2018), excessive alcohol consumption accounts for 3 million deaths annually (5.3% of all deaths). Alcoholic liver disease (ALD) is a chronic disease caused by long-term heavy drinking and includes steatosis, steatohepatitis, fibrosis, cirrhosis, and hepatocarcinoma (Kong et al., 2019). Among long-term (months or years) heavy (>40 g of alcohol per day) drinkers, 90–100% develop alcoholic fatty liver, and 10–35% of them develop alcoholic steatohepatitis. Furthermore, 8–20% of patients with alcoholic steatohepatitis develop liver cirrhosis, and 2% of patients with liver cirrhosis progress to hepatocarcinoma (Seitz et al., 2018). ALD seriously affects human's health and quality of life.

The early stage of ALD is alcoholic fatty liver, caused by abnormal lipid accumulation. Autophagy is the mechanism of self-protection of cells under stress, which can prevent lipid accumulation by degrading lipids (You et al., 2018) and can also prevent cell damage (Dikic and Elazar, 2018). However, chronic alcohol drinking inhibits autophagy, which is one of the causes of lipid metabolism disorders (Chao et al., 2018). AMP-activated protein kinase (AMPK) is an important regulator of various metabolic and signal transduction pathways, including autophagy (Xiang et al., 2020). Ethanol can inhibit AMPK, induce fatty acid synthesis, inhibit fatty acid oxidation, and cause abnormal fat accumulation in the liver (You et al., 2004). Continuous drinking of alcohol can aggravate liver damage in patients with fatty liver. The damage can result in the transformation of hepatic stellate cells, which are normally in a resting state, into activated myofibroblasts, lead to the upregulation of α-smooth muscle actin and the deposition of the extracellular matrix, and cause liver fibrosis, a severe form of liver injury (Seitz et al., 2018). In addition, acetaldehyde and reactive oxygen species (ROS), the metabolites of ethanol, can trigger oxidative stress and endoplasmic reticulum (ER) stress in hepatocytes, which in turn triggers inflammation and apoptosis, also leading to liver injury (Dara et al., 2011; Ceni et al., 2014). Fibrosis is a critical pathological process in ALD, but recent studies have shown that fibrosis can be reversed with a timely intervention (Parola and Pinzani, 2019).

The clinical treatment for ALD mainly consists of antioxidant and anti-inflammatory drugs, such as silymarin and glycyrrhizic acid preparations; however, these drugs have limited curative effects and a limited therapeutic scope (Flora et al., 1998; Levy et al., 2004; Meng et al., 2018; Li X. et al., 2019). Thus, it is essential to develop novel, safe, and pathophysiology-oriented therapies for ALD.

Anoectochilus roxburghii (Wall.) Lindl. (Orchidaceae), also known as Jinxianlan (Simplified Chinese: 金线兰) and Jinxianlian (Simplified Chinese: 金线莲), is a perennial herb that is mainly grown in China, Japan, India, Nepal, and Sri Lanka. In China, *A. roxburghii* is a protected species and is used as a traditional Chinese medicinal material for the treatment of liver disease, diabetes, hypertension, cancers, hand-foot-and-mouth disease, and osteoarthritis (Ye et al., 2017; Tang et al., 2018; Guo et al., 2019; Liu Y. et al., 2020). Kinsenoside (KD), 3-*O*-β-D-glucopyranosyl-(3*R*)-hydroxybutanolide (**Figure 1A**), a major active ingredient extracted from *A. roxburghii*, exhibits anti-inflammatory, antilipemic, liver protective, immunomodulatory, and other pharmacological activities (Qi et al., 2018; Wang et al., 2019; Zhou et al., 2019). Our previous reports have demonstrated that KD treatment could alleviate the complications of 17α-ethinylestradiol-induced cholestatic liver injury and concanavalin A-induced autoimmune liver injury by inhibiting inflammatory responses and regulating immune balance (Xiang et al., 2016; Ming et al., 2021). However, it is unclear whether KD has therapeutic activity against alcohol-induced liver injury. In this study, we aimed to investigate the protective effect and the underlying mechanism of KD against ALD.

MATERIALS AND METHODS

Materials

A whole herb of *A. roxburghii* was purchased from Yongan City Huangnijia Co., Ltd. (Sanming, China) and identified by Prof. Jianping Wang at the School of Pharmacy, Huazhong University of Science and Technology. A voucher specimen (No. TJ20180901) has been deposited at the Hubei Key Laboratory of Natural Medicinal Chemistry and Resource Evaluation. KD was prepared using a previously reported method (Ming et al., 2021). The purity of KD (>98%) was analyzed using a high-pressure liquid chromatograph equipped with an evaporative light scattering detector, and the identity was confirmed by comparing its nuclear magnetic resonance data with those from a previous study (Xiang et al., 2016). Silymarin was

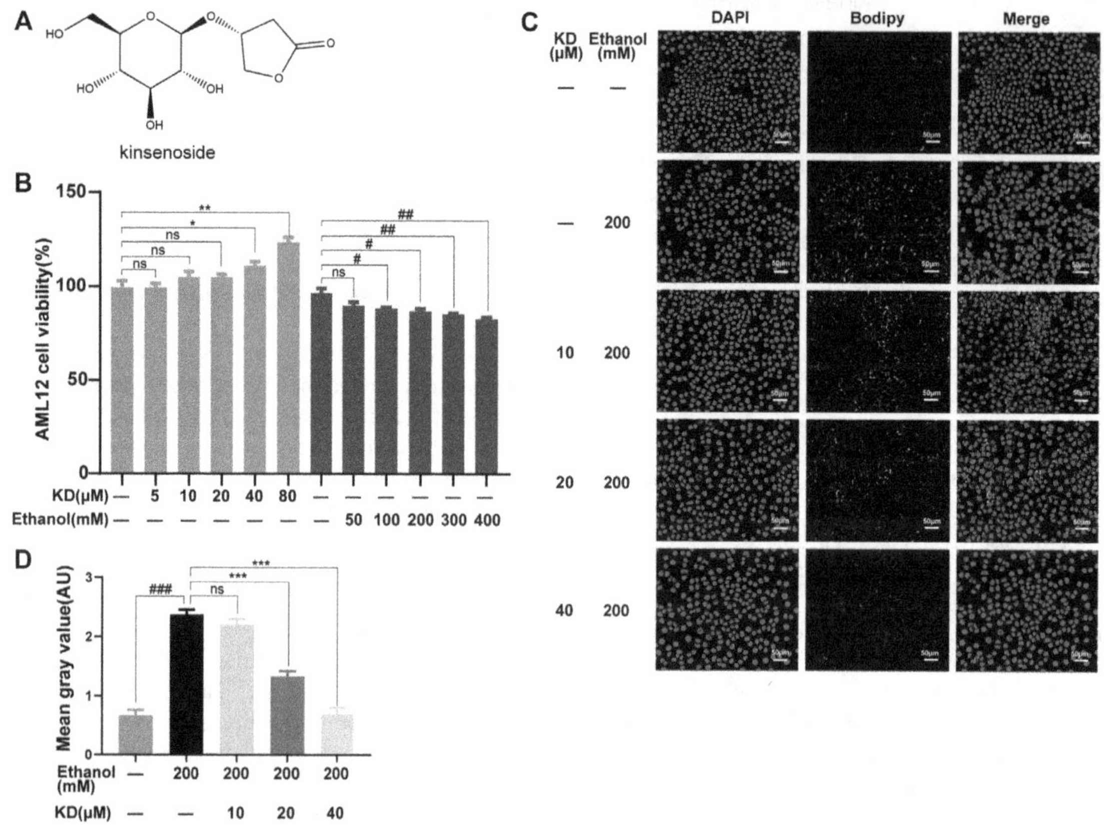

FIGURE 1 | Effects of KD on cellular ethanol-induced lipid accumulation. **(A)** The chemical structure of KD. **(B)** Effects of KD and ethanol on AML12 cell viability (n = 4). **(C)** Images of BODIPY-stained AML12 cells treated with KD and/or ethanol for 48 h. Scale bar: 50 μm. **(D)** Quantitative analysis of BODIPY staining (n = 3). Data represent the mean ± SEM. ns, not significant, $^{*}p < 0.05$, $^{**}p < 0.01$, $^{***}p < 0.001$, KD-treated vs. untreated cells. $^{\#}p < 0.05$, $^{\#\#}p < 0.01$, $^{\#\#\#}p < 0.001$, alcohol-treated vs. untreated cells.

purchased from Sigma Chemical Co. (St. Louis, MO, United States). The Lieber–DeCarli ethanol liquid diet was purchased from Trophic Animal Feed High-tech Co., Ltd. (Jiangsu, China). 3-Nitrotyrosine (3-NT; ab61392), 4-hydroxynonenal (4-HNE; ab46545), catalase (ab76110), aldehyde dehydrogenase 2 (ALDH2; ab108306), glyceraldehyde 3-phosphate dehydrogenase (GAPDH; ab181602), cluster of differentiation 3 (CD3; ab215212), Bcl-XL (ab32370), Bax (ab32503), STRAD (ab192879) and phospho (p)-mTOR (ab109268) antibodies were purchased from Abcam (Cambridge, United Kingdom). AMPKα (5832), p-AMPKα (2535), Beclin-1 (3495), p-Beclin-1 (84966S), BIP (3177), eIF2α (5324), p-eIF2α (3398), F4/80 (70076), JNK1 (3708), p-SAPK/JNK (4668), LC3A/B (12741), Raptor (2280), p-Raptor (2083), sequestosome-1 (SQSTM1)/p62 (5114), ULK1 (8054), p-ULK1 (5869), mTOR (2983), goat anti-rabbit (5151), and goat anti-mouse (5257) antibodies were purchased from Cell Signaling Technology (Beverly, MA, United States). Alcohol dehydrogenase 1B (ADH1B; 66939-1-Ig), LKB1 (10746-1-AP) and cytochrome P450 2E1 (CYP2E1; 19937-1-AP) antibodies were purchased from Proteintech (Rosemount, IL, United States). The CHOP (WL00880) antibody was purchased from Wanleibio (Liaoning, China). The mCherry-EGFP-LC3 adenovirus was purchased from Hanbio Co. Ltd. (Hanbio, Shanghai, China).

Cell Culture

The mouse hepatocyte cell line, AML12, was cultured in Dulbecco's modified Eagle's medium/F12 (Zhong Qiao Xin Zhou, China) supplemented with 10% fetal bovine serum, 1% penicillin–streptomycin, 10 μg/ml insulin, 5.5 μg/ml transferrin, 5 ng/ml selenium, and 40 ng/ml dexamethasone. Cells were cultured in a humidified atmosphere containing 5% CO_2 at 37°C.

Cell Viability

AML12 cells at the third passage were seeded into 96-well plates at a density of 1×10^4 cells per well. After 24 h of incubation, the cells were washed with phosphate-buffered saline (PBS) and then cultured with different concentrations of KD (0, 5, 10, 20, 40, and 80 μM) or ethanol (0, 50, 100, 200, 300, and 400 mM). After incubation for another 24 h, the culture media were replaced with a culture medium containing a 10% Cell Counting Kit-8 solution. After incubation for 2 h, the absorbance was measured at 450 nm (Varioskan LUX spectrophotometer; Thermo Fisher Scientific, Inc.).

BODIPY Staining

AML12 cells at the fifth passage were seeded at a density of 2×10^5 cell per well into a 6-well plate with slides. On the next day, the medium was changed, and the cells were incubated with KD (0, 10, 20, and 40 μM) for 1 h, followed by incubation with or without 200 mM ethanol for 24 h, after which medium containing KD or ethanol was replaced. After another 24 h, the cells were washed with PBS, fixed with paraformaldehyde, and then stained with the BODIPY staining solution (B&P Biotech, Hangzhou, China) according to the manufacturer's instructions. 4′,6-Diamidino-2-phenylindole (Servicebio, Wuhan, China) was used to counterstain the nuclei. Images were observed under a fluorescence microscope (Olympus, Tokyo, Japan). The ImageJ software was used for quantitative analysis of lipids.

Animal Experiments

The protocol of the animal study was reviewed and approved by the Institutional Animal Care and Use Committee of the Tongji Medical College, Huazhong University of Science and Technology. The Lieber–DeCarli ethanol liquid diet was used according to the manufacturer's instructions and was combined with carbon tetrachloride (CCl_4) to induce alcoholic liver injury in mice (Lamas-Paz et al., 2018). Eight-week-old male C57BL/6J mice (21–23 g) were purchased from SPF Biotechnology Co., Ltd. (Beijing, China) and were raised in a specific pathogen-free environment. Silymarin was chosen as the positive control (Federico et al., 2017; Gillessen and Schmidt, 2020). All mice were first fed a control (ethanol-free) liquid diet for 5 days. Subsequently, the mice were randomly divided into the following five groups: control, model, KD-20 mg/kg, KD-40 mg/kg, and silymarin-80 mg/kg. The control group was administered the control liquid feed, while the other groups were administered the ethanol liquid feed, and the ethanol concentration was gradually increased to 4% (w/v) in the first week and then maintained at the same level. On week 5, the mice in all groups, except the control group, were intraperitoneally injected with 5% CCl_4 in olive oil (2 ml/kg) twice a week and continued in subsequent weeks. The mice were sacrificed 5 weeks after the first injection of CCl_4 to obtain tissues and blood.

Tandem Mass Tag Quantitative Proteomics

Samples were lysed with a buffer containing 4% sodium dodecyl sulfate, 100 mM Tris-HCl, and 1 mM dithiothreitol (pH 7.6) to extract proteins, and the bicinchoninic acid method was used for protein quantification. An appropriate amount of protein from each sample was prepared using the filter-aided sample preparation method for trypsin digestion (Wisniewski et al., 2009). An Empore™ solid phase extraction cartridge (C18, standard density, bed internal diameter: 7 mm, volume: 3 ml; Sigma) was used to desalt the peptides. The peptides were concentrated by vacuum centrifugation and then reconstituted with 40 μL of 0.1% (v/v) formic acid. Peptides (100 μg) from each sample were labeled according to the manufacturer's instructions (Thermo Fisher Scientific) and then fractionated using a high pH reversed-phase peptide fractionation kit (Thermo Fisher Scientific). Liquid chromatography–tandem mass spectrometry was performed on a Q Exactive mass spectrometer (Thermo Fisher Scientific) coupled with an EASY-nLC liquid chromatograph (Thermo Fisher Scientific) to analyze the peptides. Protein identification and quantitative analyses were performed by searching the mass spectrometric raw data of each sample using the MASCOT search engine version 2.2 (Matrix Science, London, United Kingdom) integrated into the Proteome Discoverer 1.4 software. Finally, bioinformatics analysis was performed as previously described (Ashburner et al., 2000; Ross et al., 2004; Gotz et al., 2008).

Measurement of Serum and Liver Biochemical Parameters

Serum levels of tumor necrosis factor-alpha (TNF-α) and interleukin-6 (IL-6) were measured using an enzyme-linked immunosorbent assay kits (Neobioscience) according to the manufacturer's instructions. Serum levels of alanine aminotransferase (ALT) and aspartate transaminase (AST), as well as triglycerides (TG), reduced glutathione/oxidized glutathione (GSH/GSSG) and nicotinamide adenine dinucleotide (NAD^+)/reduced NAD^+ (NAD^+/NADH) ratios of liver homogenate, were determined according to the instructions of each kit obtained from Nanjing Jiancheng Bioengineering Institute. Activities of ADH, catalase, ALDH, and superoxide dismutase (SOD) in liver homogenates were also measured according to the instructions of each kit obtained from Nanjing Jiancheng Bioengineering Institute.

Histopathology

Liver tissue was fixed with 10% formalin and embedded in paraffin. The paraffinized tissue was cut into 5-μm sections and subjected to hematoxylin–eosin (H&E) and Masson's trichrome staining.

Immunohistochemistry

The levels of 3-NT, 4-HNE, F4/80, and CD3 in the liver were determined by immunohistochemical staining. Paraffin sections of the liver tissue were prepared using high temperature and pressure and then incubated with 3% hydrogen peroxide for 20 min to inactivate endogenous peroxidase. After incubation with 10% serum for 20 min to block nonspecific binding, the sections were separately incubated with the 3-NT, 4-HNE, F4/80, and CD3 primary antibodies in a working solution, followed by incubation with the corresponding secondary antibody to develop color. After the slides were rinsed with Tris-buffered saline, 3,3′-diaminobenzidine was added, and the sections were observed under a microscope. Subsequently, the slides were rinsed with tap water, counterstained with hematoxylin, dehydrated with gradient ethanol, and finally loaded with a neutral adhesive for microscopic examination.

Terminal Deoxynucleotidyl Transferase dUTP Nick-End Labeling Assay

A TUNEL kit (Roche, Shanghai, China) was used to detect apoptosis in liver tissue. Paraffin sections were deparaffinized and hydrated. A mixture of 3% bovine serum albumin and 20%

normal calf serum was used to block nonspecific reactions. The TUNEL working solution was added dropwise, and the sections were incubated in the dark for 60 min at 37°C. 4′,6-Diamidino-2-phenylindole was used to counterstain the nuclei, and images were observed under a fluorescence microscope.

Western Blotting

The liver tissue was removed from storage at −80°C and lysed in a buffer containing protease and phosphatase inhibitors. The lysate was then centrifuged at 12,000 × *g* for 10 min, and the protein concentration was quantified in the supernatant using the bicinchoninic acid method. After boiling with a sample loading buffer for 5 min, approximately 20–50 μg of total protein was separated by sodium dodecyl sulfate–polyacrylamide gel electrophoresis. The separated proteins were transferred onto nitrocellulose membranes, and the membranes were blocked with a fast blocking solution, followed by incubation with primary antibodies overnight at 4°C. After washing with Tris-buffered saline with 0.1% Tween 20, the membranes were incubated with secondary antibodies for 30–60 min at room temperature. A dual-color near-infrared fluorescence imaging system was used to detect protein bands. The ImageJ software was used for quantitative analysis of proteins.

Autophagy Progress in Ethanol Treated AML12 Cells

1×10^6 AML12 cells were seeded in a 6-well plate. The next day, the cells were treated with 100 mM ethanol for 0, 1, 4, 8, 12, and 24 h. After the cells were collected, western blotting was performed to detect the expression levels of LC3A/B-I, LC3A/B-II and SQSTM1.

The AML12 cells were seeded into 6-well plates at a density of 1×10^6 cells/well for 24 h. Then, 40 μM KD with or without 50 μM chloroquine (CQ) were added for 1 h according to the grouping, and cells were treated with 100 mM ethanol for another 8 h. The expression levels of LC3A/B-I, LC3A/B-II and SQSTM1 were further detected as described above.

Confocal Microscopy Assay

The AML12 cells were seeded in a confocal culture dish with a glass bottom (diameter of 15 mm; 1.5×10^5 cells/dish, and transfection was carried out on the next day. After 39 h of transfection, 40 μM KD or 50 μM CQ was added for 1 h, followed by addition of 100 mM ethanol for 8 h. After being washed with PBS, the cells were fixed with 4% paraformaldehyde for 10 min, and then washed with PBS again. The cells were immersed in PBS for observation by confocal fluorescence (Nikon, Tokyo, Japan).

Statistical Analysis

Data are presented as the mean ± standard error of the mean (SEM) and were analyzed with Dunnett's *t*-test or one-way analysis of variance using the GraphPad Prism software (GraphPad Software, Inc., San Diego, CA, United States). Statistical significance was set at $p < 0.05$.

RESULTS

Kinsenoside Reduces Ethanol-Induced Lipid Accumulation in Hepatocytes

AML12 normal hepatocytes were selected to analyze the effect of KD on ethanol-induced lipid accumulation. The cytotoxicity of KD and ethanol to AML12 cells was assayed to determine the optimal concentrations for subsequent experiments. As shown in **Figure 1B**, KD showed no cytotoxic effect on AML12 cells at 80 μM, while ethanol caused liver cell damage in a concentration-dependent manner in a range of 100–400 mM. Based on the above results, 200 mM ethanol was chosen for further treatment. BODIPY staining was used to localize lipids, which showed that 200 mM ethanol induced obvious lipid accumulation (green fluorescence intensity in **Figure 1C**). However, after pretreatment with different concentrations of KD, the lipid accumulation levels significantly decreased, and the lipid accumulation status was comparable to that of normal cells (**Figure 1C**). The BODIPY staining results showed that KD reduced ethanol-induced lipid accumulation in a concentration-dependent manner in a range from 20 to 40 μM (**Figure 1D**).

Kinsenoside Alleviates Alcoholic Liver Injury in Mice

A mouse model was established and pathologically analyzed to explore whether KD alleviates alcoholic liver injury. The detailed modeling method is illustrated in **Figure 2A**. The results of H&E staining showed ballooning degeneration and inflammatory cell infiltration in the model group. After KD treatment, ballooning degeneration was significantly reduced, and inflammation was alleviated (**Figure 2B**). Masson's trichrome staining showed that the number of blue collagen fibers dramatically increased in the model group and decreased after KD treatment, indicating the therapeutic effect of KD against liver tissue fibrosis (**Figure 2B**). The liver index of mice also changed after ethanol and KD treatment. KD reduced the increase in liver to body weight ratio caused by ethanol (**Figure 2C**) The essential indicators of hepatocellular damage were further assessed, including ALT, AST and TG. As shown in **Figures 2D–F**, the ALT, AST and TG levels were obviously elevated in the model group compared with those in the control group. KD at 20 and 40 mg/kg significantly ($p <$ 0.05) decreased the levels of these biomarkers. These findings demonstrated that KD alleviated alcoholic liver injury in mice, and its effects were comparable to those of silymarin.

Proteomic Analysis of the Mechanism of Action of Kinsenoside in Mice

To explore the mechanism of action of KD in alleviating alcoholic liver injury, proteomics was used for screening. The proteomic volcano plots and heatmap show that protein expression significantly differed between the model and control groups, with 836 proteins downregulated and 690 proteins upregulated in the model group. Compared with their expression in the model group, 165 proteins were downregulated and 75 proteins were upregulated in the KD

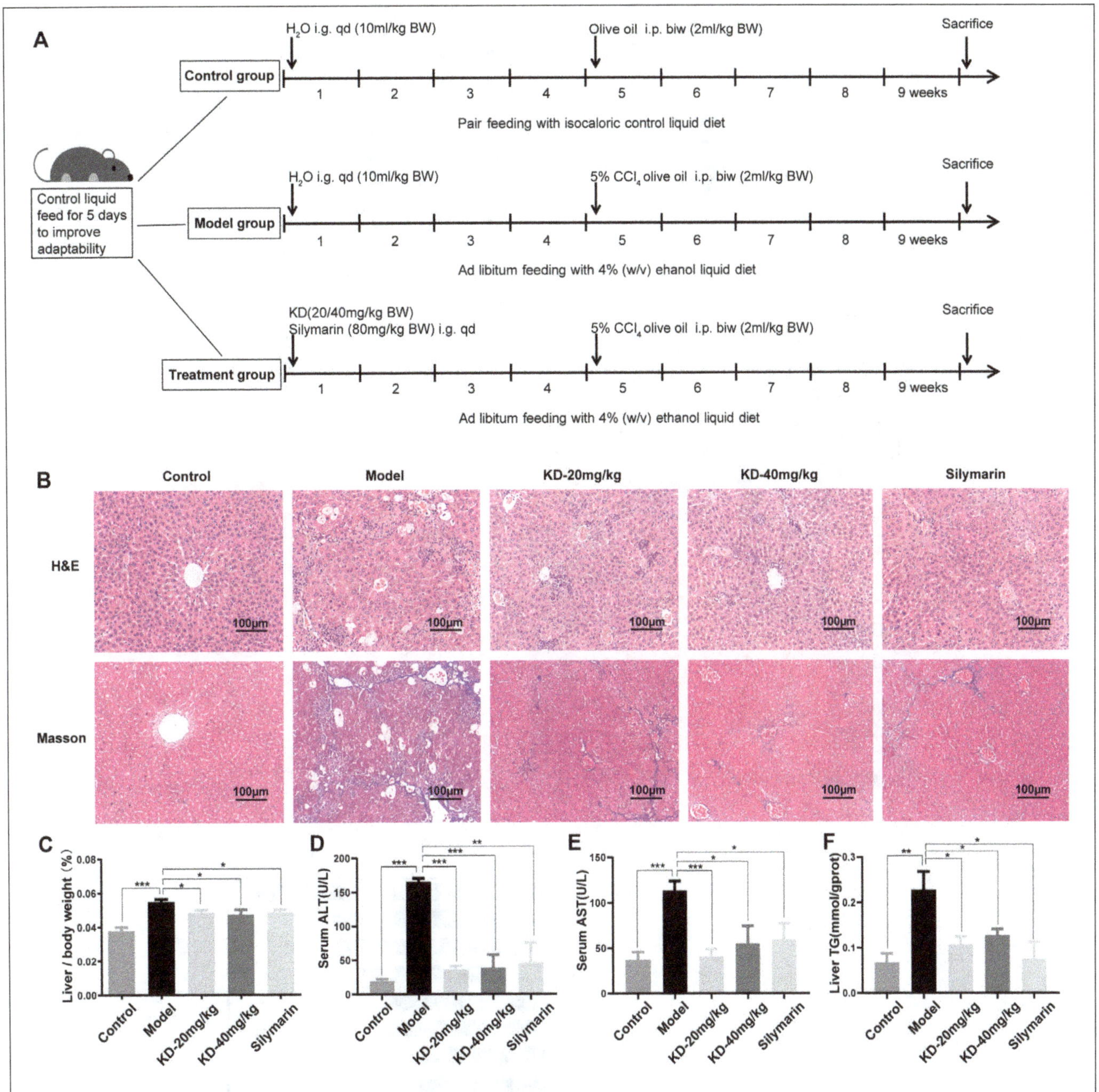

FIGURE 2 | Effects of KD on alcoholic liver injury in mice. **(A)** Schematic representation of the modeling of alcoholic liver injury in mice. **(B)** Images of H&E and Masson's trichrome-stained sections of the mice liver. Scale bar: 100 μm. **(C)** Liver to body weight ratio. **(D)** ALT levels in the mice serum. **(E)** AST levels in the mice serum. **(F)** TG content of mice liver homogenate. (n = 5–7). Data represent the mean ± SEM. $^{*}p < 0.05$, $^{**}p < 0.01$, $^{***}p < 0.001$ vs. the model group.

group (**Figure 3A**). Cluster analysis of differentially expressed proteins showed that the protein expression levels in the liver tissue after KD treatment were significantly different from that in model group (**Figure 3B**). Gene Ontology (GO) analysis of the differentially expressed proteins between the KD and model groups showed that the enriched biological process terms were mainly associated with acute inflammatory response, extracellular structure organization, acute-phase response and cell killing (**Figure 3C**). Kyoto Encyclopedia of Genes and Genomes (KEGG) pathway enrichment analysis showed that differentially expressed proteins between the KD and model groups (**Figure 3D**), in combination with the pathogenesis of ALD, were mainly involved in the ER, autophagy, and AMPK signaling pathways.

Kinsenoside Alleviates Oxidative Stress and ER Stress in Mice

The metabolism of ethanol *in vivo* is an important physiological and pathological process in ALD development. After entering the

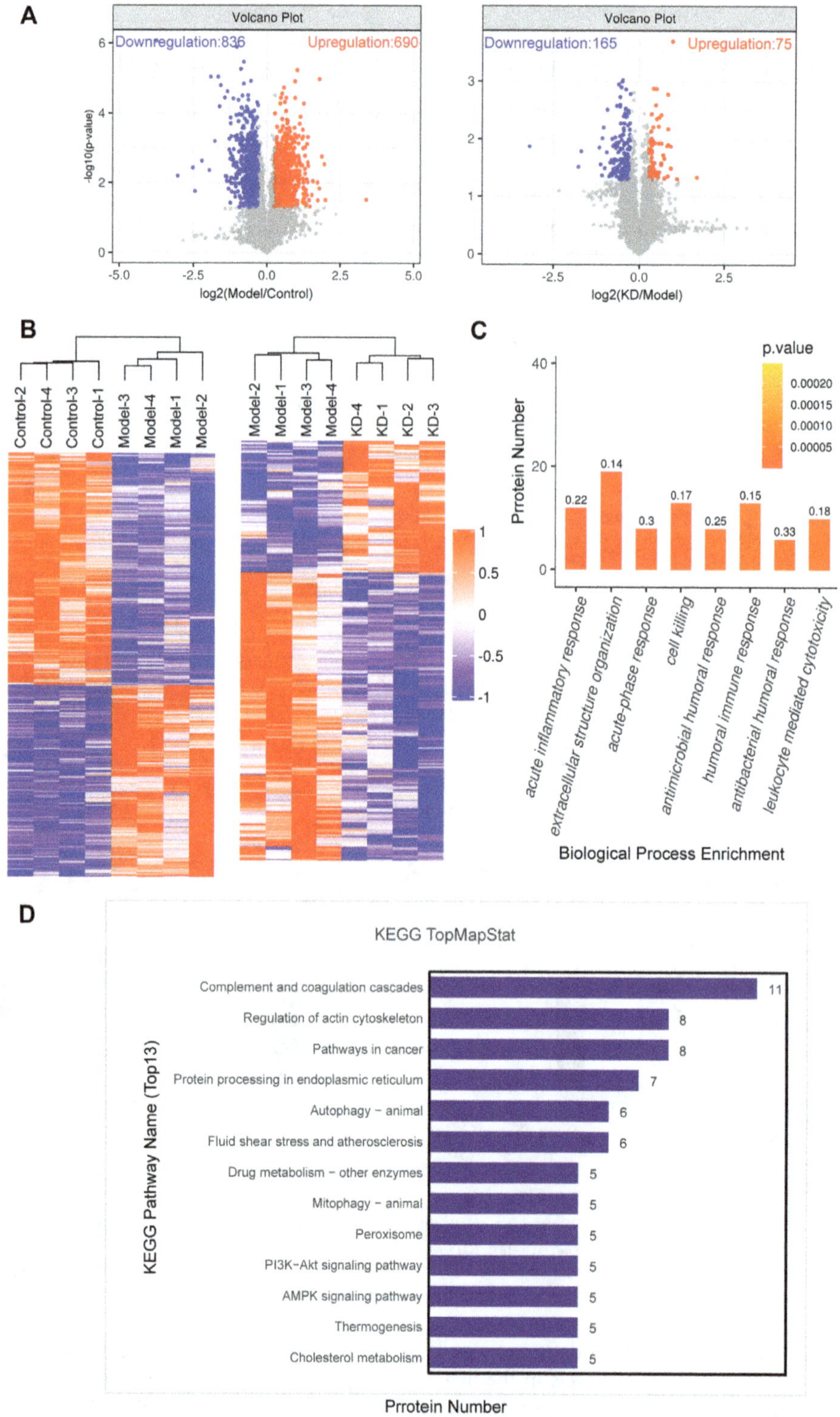

FIGURE 3 | Data from proteomic analysis of mice liver tissue. **(A)** Volcano plots of the number of differentially expressed proteins between the model and control groups and the KD and model groups. **(B)** Cluster analysis of the differentially expressed proteins in the control, model, and KD-treated groups of mice. **(C)** Biological process classification of GO functional enrichment histogram between the KD and model groups. The numbers on the histogram represent rich factor. The rich factor represents the ratio of the number of differentially expressed proteins annotated to a GO functional category to the number of all identified proteins annotated to the GO functional category. **(D)** KEGG pathway annotation of the top 13 differentially expressed proteins between the KD and model groups. (n = 4).

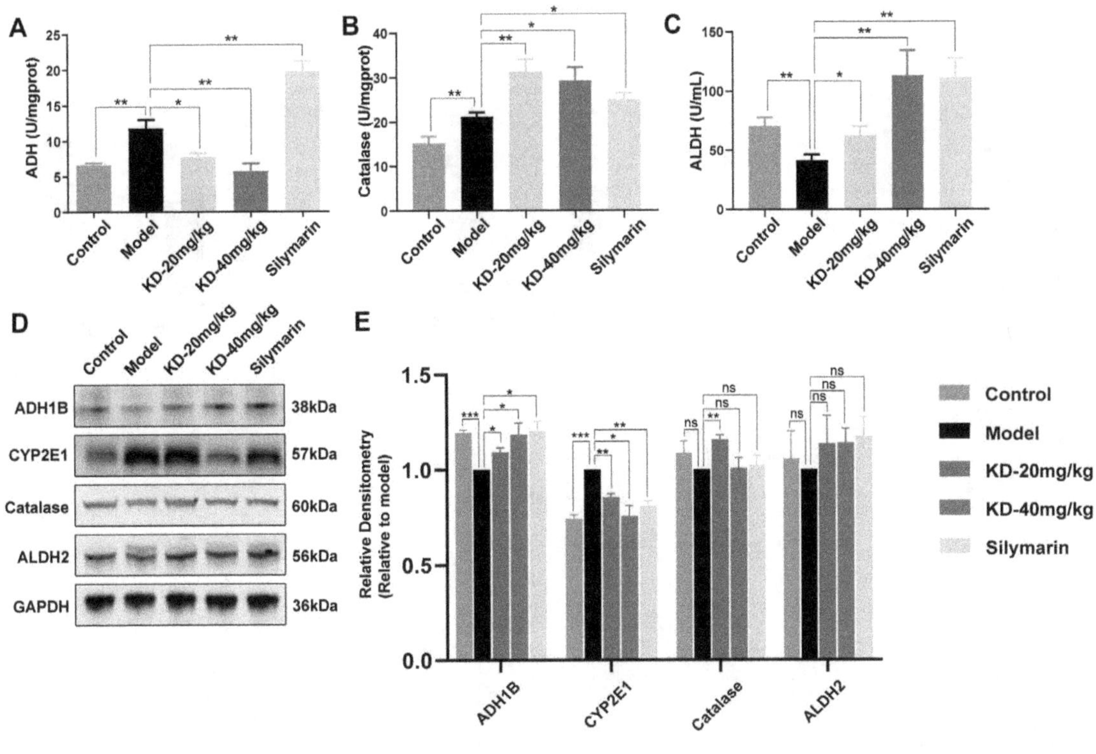

FIGURE 4 | Effects of KD on ethanol metabolism in mice. **(A)** ADH activity in mice liver homogenates. **(B)** Catalase activity in mice liver homogenates. **(C)** ALDH activity in mice liver homogenates. (n = 5–7). **(D)** Expression of the ADH1B, catalase, CYP2E1, and ALDH2 proteins in mice liver tissue. **(E)** Quantitative analysis of protein expression (n = 3). GAPDH was used as a loading control and for data normalization. Data represent the mean ± SEM. ns, not significant. *$p < 0.05$, **$p < 0.01$, ***$p < 0.001$ vs. the model group.

body, ethanol is converted into acetaldehyde by ADH, CYP2E1 and catalase. Acetaldehyde is then converted into nontoxic acetic acid by ALDH (Seitz et al., 2018). Analysis of enzymes of ethanol metabolism in the liver of mice showed that KD inhibited the ethanol-induced increase in ADH activity, enhanced the increase in catalase activity, and reversed the decrease in ALDH activity (**Figures 4A–C**). Western blotting revealed that KD reversed the ethanol-induced decrease in ADH1B (the main subunit of ADH) expression and the increase in CYP2E1 expression but had no effect on the expression of catalase and ALDH2 (the main subunit of ALDH) (**Figures 4D,E**).

ROS, another byproduct of ethanol metabolism, can cause oxidative stress, together with acetaldehyde (Farfan Labonne et al., 2009; Seitz et al., 2018). Analysis of the oxidative stress indicators SOD, GSH/GSSG, and NAD^+/NADH showed that KD improved the antioxidant status in mice (**Figures 5A–C**). In the presence of ROS, reactive nitrogen species are derived from NO and nitrify tyrosine or protein tyrosine residues to produce 3-NT. The 3-NT level in the diseased state is significantly higher than the normal 3-NT level (Li Y. et al., 2019). 4-HNE is an aldehyde product of lipid peroxidation and is considered a key mediator of oxidative stress-caused cell death (Ma et al., 2020; Hyatt et al., 2021). The ethanol-induced increases in the 3-NT and 4-HNE levels were reversed by KD treatment (**Figures 5D,E**). These results indicated that KD reduced the ethanol-induced oxidative stress.

ROS and acetaldehyde cause not only oxidative stress but also ER stress by damaging proteins and DNA (Ji, 2012; Ji, 2014; Ganne-Carrié and Nahon, 2019). KEGG analysis of proteomics data also showed the association of differentially expressed proteins with ER processes (**Figure 3D**). Western blotting showed that KD reduced the levels of the key ER stress protein BIP and the transcription factor CHOP, as well as the phosphorylation of eIF2α, thereby alleviating the translation block. JNK, a key kinase in ER stress, was also suppressed (**Figures 5F,G**). These results suggested that KD inhibited the persistent ER stress caused by long-term ethanol consumption.

Oxidative stress and ER stress can trigger inflammation and cell apoptosis. Our results showed that KD reversed the liver inflammation-associated increases in the levels of serum TNF-α and IL-6 (**Figures 6A,B**). Immunohistochemistry staining of liver tissue sections showed that the ethanol-induced increases in the F4/80 and CD3 levels were reversed by KD (**Figure 6C**). In addition, CHOP and JNK activation, which can trigger cell apoptosis, was inhibited, while the expression of the antiapoptotic factor Bcl-XL was increased and that of the proapoptotic factor Bax was decreased by KD treatment (**Figures 6D,E**). The TUNEL assay also confirmed that the ethanol-induced apoptosis of hepatocytes decreased after KD administration (**Figure 6F**). Thus, the results showed that KD inhibited the ethanol-induced liver inflammation and cell apoptosis. Together, KD alleviates oxidative stress and ER stress by affecting ethanol metabolism in the liver, thereby reducing

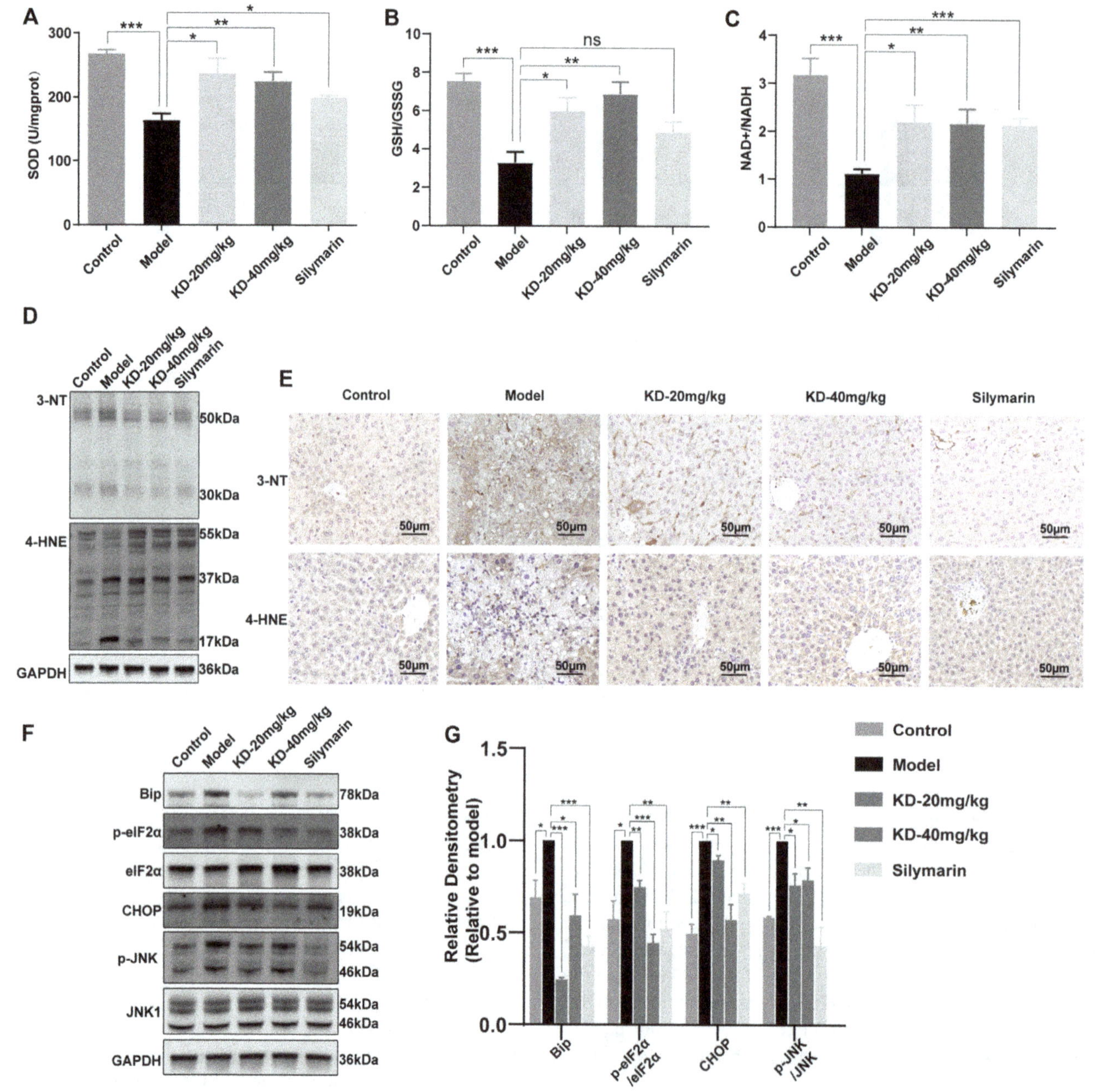

FIGURE 5 | Effects of KD on oxidative stress and ER stress in mice. **(A)** SOD activity in liver homogenates. **(B)** Liver GSH to GSSG ratios. **(C)** Liver NAD^+ to NADH ratios. ($n = 5–7$). **(D)** Liver 3-NT and 4-HNE expression determined by western blotting. **(E)** Immunohistochemistry staining of 3-NT and 4-HNE in the mice liver. Scale bar: 50 μm. **(F)** Expression of ER stress-related proteins determined by western blotting. **(G)** Quantitative analysis of protein expression ($n = 3$). GAPDH was used as a loading control. Data represent the mean ± SEM. ns, not significant. $^*p < 0.05$, $^{**}p < 0.01$, $^{***}p < 0.001$ vs. the model group.

inflammation and cell apoptosis, which in turn relieves alcoholic liver injury.

Kinsenoside Activates AMPK-Dependent Protective Autophagy in Mice With Alcoholic Liver Injury

AMPK, a central regulator of eukaryotic cell and organism metabolism, is a key protein involved in a variety of signaling pathways. Long-term drinking inhibits the activity of AMPK, thereby disrupting metabolic processes (Gao and Bataller, 2011; Seitz et al., 2018). Our results showed that KD increased the protein levels of STRAD and LKB1 (**Figures 7A,B**), which were the upstream of AMPK, thereby promoting the phosphorylation of AMPK.

Autophagy can remove damaged proteins, organelles, and lipids from cells and maintain intracellular balance. The increases in ROS and acetaldehyde levels caused by long-

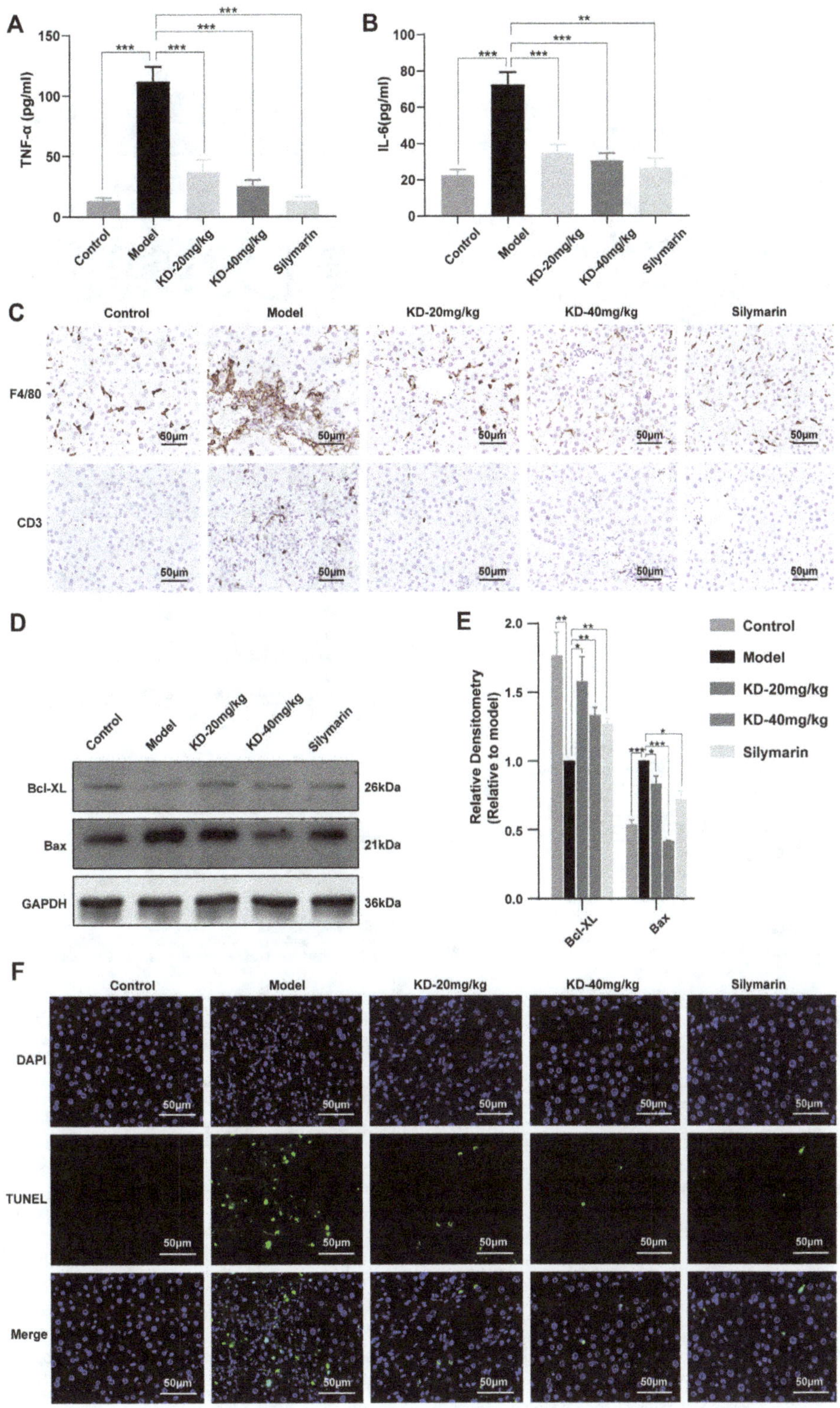

FIGURE 6 | Effects of KD on ethanol-induced liver inflammation and hepatocyte apoptosis in mice. **(A)** Serum TNF-α levels. **(B)** Serum IL-6 levels. (n = 5–7). **(C)** Immunohistochemistry staining for F4/80 and CD3 in the mice liver. **(D)** Expression of apoptosis-related proteins determined by western blotting. **(E)** Quantitative analysis of protein expression (n = 3). GAPDH was used as a loading control. **(F)** TUNEL-stained liver sections. Scale bar: 50 μm. Data represent the mean ± SEM. $^{*}p < 0.05$, $^{**}p < 0.01$, $^{***}p < 0.001$ vs. the model group.

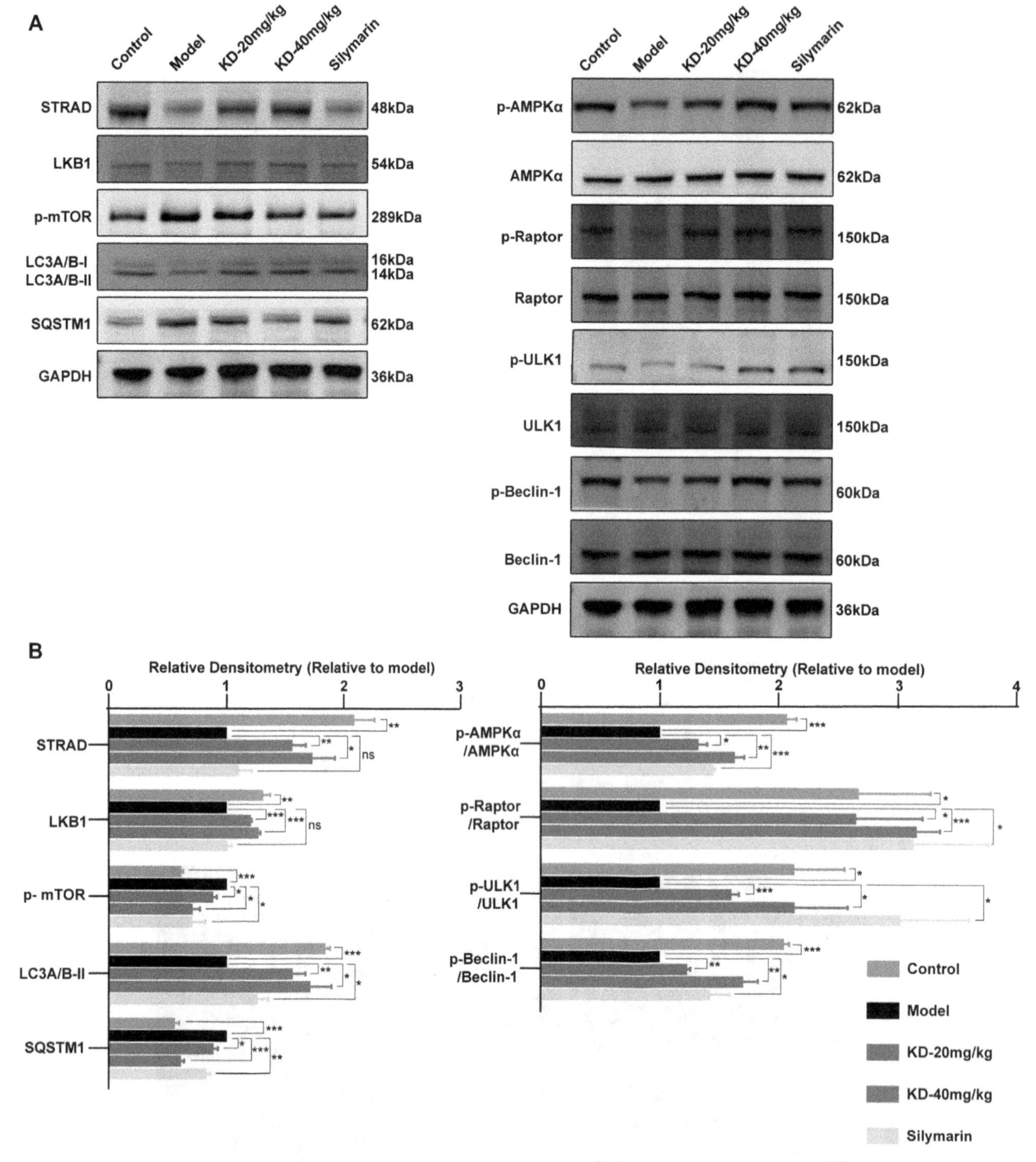

FIGURE 7 | Activation of AMPK-dependent protective autophagy in KD-treated mice with alcoholic liver injury. **(A)** Levels of AMPK and autophagy-related proteins determined by western blotting. **(B)** Quantitative analysis of protein expression ($n = 3$). Data represent the mean ± SEM. GAPDH was used as a loading control. ns, not significant. *$p < 0.05$, **$p < 0.01$, ***$p < 0.001$ vs. the model group.

term alcohol drinking can destroy proteins, cause lipid accumulation, and inhibit liver autophagy, thereby aggravating the alcohol-induced liver injury (Wang et al., 2015; Allaire et al., 2019). Our results showed that KD treatment led to the phosphorylation of Raptor by activated AMPK, thereby directly inhibiting the phosphorylation of mTOR (Total mTOR strip is shown in **Supplementary Figure S1**). MTOR is an autophagy inhibitory protein, and

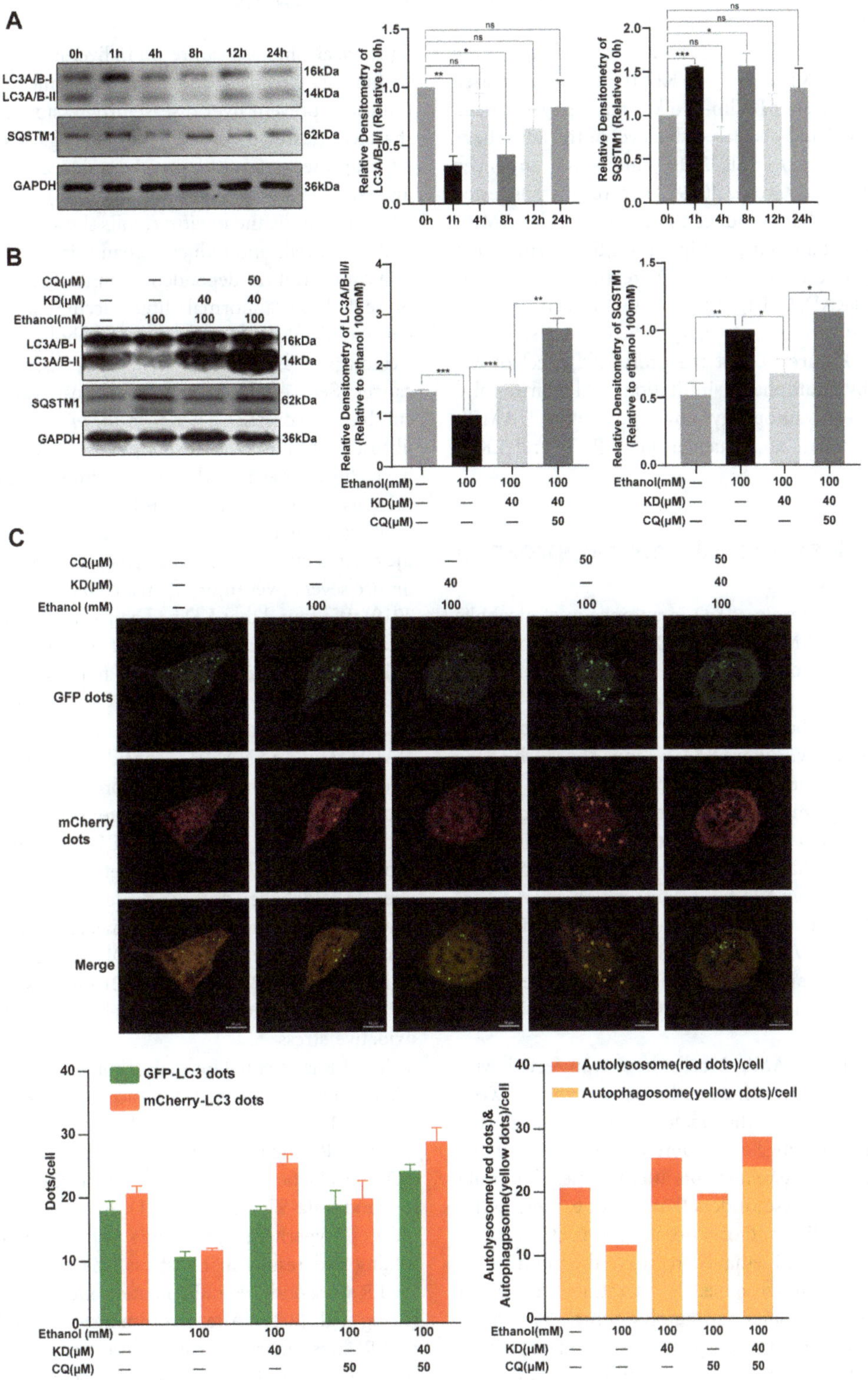

FIGURE 8 | KD restores ethanol-suppressed autophagic flux. **(A)** The effect of 100 mM ethanol for different time on autophagy. **(B)** KD affect the autophagy of ethanol in cells. **(C)** Confocal fluorescence image and analysis of KD promoting the recovery of autophagic flux. Red puncta represent autolysosomes, yellow puncta (merged by red and green) represent autophagosomes. (n = 3). Data represent the mean ± SEM. GAPDH was used as a loading control. ns, not significant. $^{*}p < 0.05$, $^{**}p < 0.01$, $^{***}p < 0.001$. Scale bar: 10 μm.

the inhibition of mTOR by AMPK can activate autophagy (Allaire et al., 2019). In addition, the activated AMPK in the KD group could directly activate autophagy *via* phosphorylation of ULK1 at Ser555. KD treatment increased the phosphorylation level of Beclin-1, a key autophagy protein, and that of LC3A/B-II and decreased the level of the autophagy substrate SQSTM1 (Turco et al., 2019), indicating enhanced autophagy (Galluzzi and Green, 2019). The results suggested that KD reversed the ethanol-induced inhibition of the AMPK signaling pathway and autophagy (**Figure 7A,B**). In summary, in mice with alcoholic liver injury, KD treatment led to the upregulation of STRAD/LKB1, resulting in the activation of AMPK-dependent protective autophagy; which was also shown in **Supplementary Figure S2** that the protective effect of KD was abrogated by autophagy inhibition. Silymarin also enhanced protective autophagy by promoting AMPK phosphorylation but had no influence on STRAD and LKB1 expression.

Kinsenoside Restores Ethanol-Suppressed Autophagic Flux

In order to determine the role of KD in autophagy of alcoholic liver injury, we exposed AML12 cells to 100 mM ethanol for 0, 1, 4, 8, 12, and 24 h. The results of multiple experiments demonstrated that the phenomenon of autophagy was a dynamic process and ethanol inhibited LC3A/B-II expression at 8 h with higher stability (**Figure 8A**), we thus chose 8 h as the end point to study the changes of autophagic flux.

Cells treat with 100 mM ethanol for 8 h showed reduced expression of LC3A/B-II and increased expression of SQSTM1, indicating that autophagy was inhibited. This change was reversed after KD treatment, which means that KD could activated the suppressed autophagy induced by 100 mM ethanol. LC3A/B-II and SQSTM1 both increased after adding KD and autophagy inhibitors CQ, revealing that KD had no effect on autophagy inhibited by CQ (**Figure 8B**).

For further proof, the AML12 cells were transfected with mCherry-EGFP-LC3 adenovirus. Because the EGFP fluorescence is quenched in the acidic environment of the lysosome, the EGFP and mCherry fluorescence express at the same time, which means the yellow dots after the merge indicate the autophagosomes. Fluorescent dots that do not express EGFP but express mCherry indicate autolysosomes (Liu B. et al., 2020). It was found that 100 mM ethanol reduced the number of autophagosomes and autolysosomes. KD treatment increased the number of autophagosomes and autolysosomes. Treatment with CQ inhibited the binding of autophagosomes and lysosomes, and further caused the accumulation of autophagosomes. After the cells treated with KD and CQ at the same time, the number of autophagosomes was increased, meanwhile the increase ratio of autolysosomes was less than that of KD alone. In summary, the data suggested that KD increases the production of autophagosomes, and could partially restore the autolysosome function inhibited by 100 mM ethanol, thereby enhancing autophagic flux (**Figure 8C**).

DISCUSSION

Chronic alcohol use can result in liver injury, which further leads to fibrosis, cirrhosis, and even liver cancer. Early treatment is critical to prevent liver disease progression. It has been reported that KD possesses broad pharmacological activities, including hepatoprotective, antihyperglycemic, anti-inflammatory, and antiosteoporosis effects (Qi et al., 2018).

In this study, the *in vitro* results showed that KD was nontoxic to AML12 cells and reduced ethanol-induced lipid accumulation in a concentration-dependent manner. The early stage of ALD is presented as abnormal lipid accumulation, and long-term chronic drinking can lead to alcoholic fatty liver, alcoholic steatohepatitis, alcoholic liver fibrosis, cirrhosis, and liver cancer (Seitz et al., 2018). Liver fibrosis is the most serious but curable form of ALD. Therefore, for *in vivo* studies, alcoholic liver fibrosis was chosen as the endpoint of liver injury. Many studies have shown that it is difficult to simulate severe liver injury in mice using ethanol alone, and the assistance of a second hit is required (Lamas-Paz et al., 2018; Brol et al., 2019). Therefore, in the current study, a combination of ethanol and CCl_4 was used to induce severe liver injury (Satishchandran et al., 2018; Brol et al., 2019). We found that KD had a protective effect in this model, as evidenced by the reduction of serum aminopherases, liver inflammation, and the degree of fibrosis.

Because of the reduction of NAD^+ to NADH by ADH and ALDH2, ethanol metabolism results in a decrease in the NAD^+/NADH ratio, and NADH is considered the main source of ROS in mitochondria (Ying, 2008). Moreover, previous studies have shown that long-term alcohol consumption induces CYP2E1 (Zhong et al., 2015). CYP2E1 metabolizes ethanol and produces ROS (Abdelmegeed et al., 2013), which, together with acetaldehyde, damage proteins and DNA. In this study, analysis of enzymes of ethanol metabolism in the liver showed that KD treatment increased ADH1B expression, enhanced the activity of ALDH2, reduced CYP2E1 expression, and reduced the accumulation of ROS and acetaldehyde *in vivo*, thereby inhibiting oxidative stress.

The ER is essential for maintaining hepatocyte metabolism and adapts to extracellular and intracellular stress signals (Lebeaupin et al., 2018). Upon prolonged ER stress, cells fail to maintain a normal ER function. Instead, pathways leading to an increase in ROS production induce cell death (Lebeaupin et al., 2018; Fernandes-da-Silva et al., 2021). Excessive alcohol consumption induces hyperhomocysteinemia, which interferes with protein folding and results in ER stress (Maiers and Malhi, 2019), and the ER stress-induced inflammation and apoptosis result in fibrosis (Liang et al., 2021). After the administration of KD, the expression of ER stress marker proteins was reduced, while the level of inflammation and the number of apoptotic cells also decreased.

Studies have indicated that the increase in AMPK phosphorylation alleviates liver injury (Hu et al., 2018; Wang et al., 2020). Hepatic autophagy alleviates liver injury by reducing cell apoptosis and inflammatory infiltration (Gilgenkrantz et al., 2021; Tong et al., 2021). These findings suggest that liver injury can be alleviated by activating AMPK and autophagy. Our results showed that KD treatment led to the activation of the AMPK

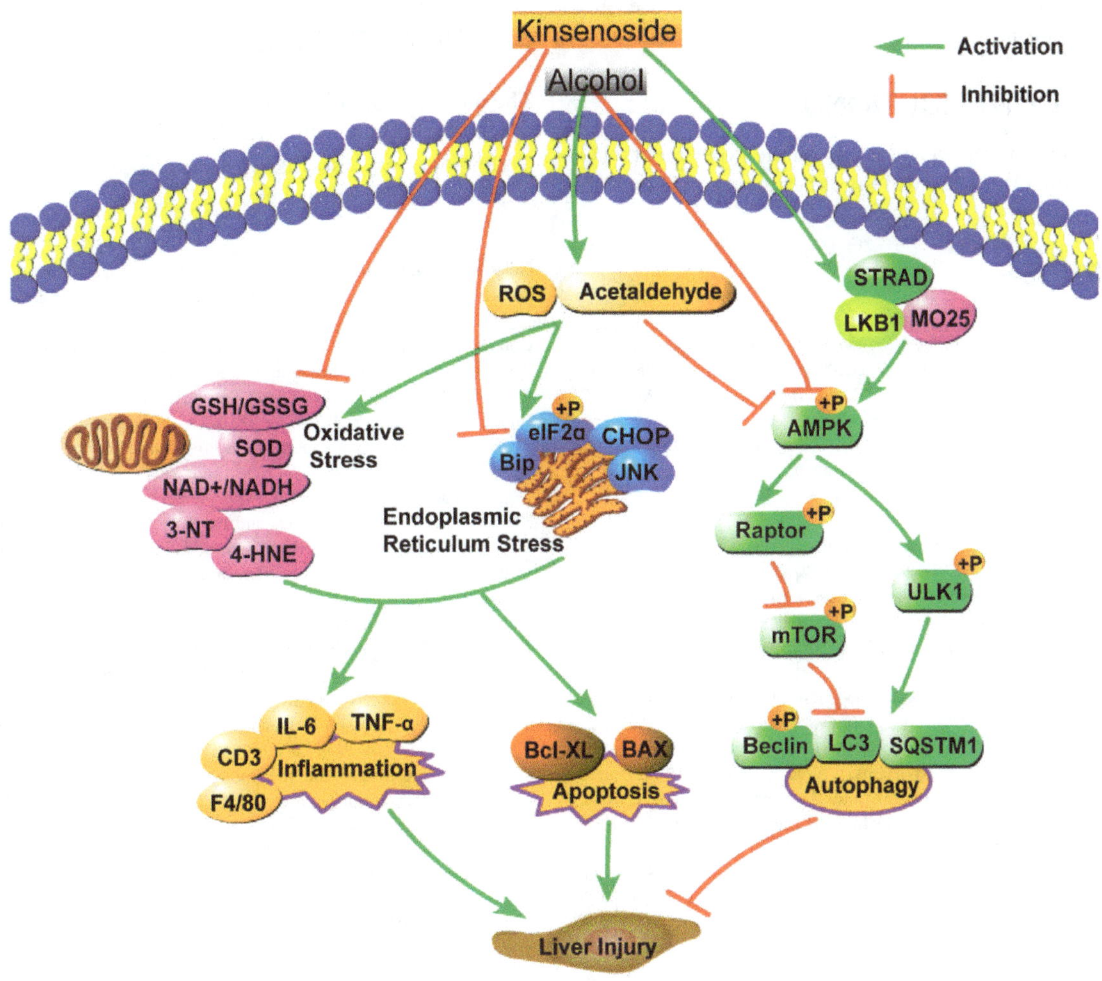

FIGURE 9 | A simplified diagram of the mechanism of KD on alcoholic liver injury.

signaling pathway by enhancing the expression of STRAD and LKB1, upstream of AMPK. Meanwhile, the activation of AMPK by silymarin did not involve LKB1, although both treatments reversed the inhibition of autophagy by ethanol.

Research shows that ALD is mainly caused by steatosis, oxidative stress, ER stress, and the toxic effects of acetaldehyde (Seitz et al., 2018; Maiers and Malhi, 2019). The diversity of the pathogenesis and the complexity of body functions allow drugs to play their roles *via* multiple mechanisms. Our research demonstrated that KD has a protective effect against alcoholic liver injury from oxidative stress, ER stress, and autophagy and has important preclinical value.

Although we found that KD alleviated alcoholic liver injury *via* multiple pathways, more studies are needed to clarify the specific target of KD. Subsequent studies should focus on ethanol metabolism, the AMPK signaling pathway, autophagy, oxidative stress, and ER stress to find the specific target of KD.

This study explored the pharmacological effects and mechanism of action of KD in alcoholic liver injury. A simplified diagram of the mechanism of KD action on alcoholic liver injury is shown in **Figure 9**. The results of this study suggested that KD can relieve inflammation and inhibit cell apoptosis by reducing oxidative stress and ER stress, while activating AMPK-dependent protective autophagy in mice with alcoholic liver injury. Currently, drugs for ALD treatment are limited and cannot meet the medication requirements of an increasing number of patients. Thus, together with the findings of previous studies, which have demonstrated the nontoxicity of KD *in vivo*, KD can be used as a supplement and candidate drug for the treatment of ALD.

the medication requirements of an increasing number of patients. Thus, together with the findings of previous studies, which have demonstrated the nontoxicity of KD *in vivo*, KD can be used as a supplement and candidate drug for the treatment of ALD.

AUTHOR CONTRIBUTIONS

YZ, HR, and LG conceived and designed the experiments; LG, XC, ZF, JY, and YW performed the experiments and analyzed the data; LG, HR, and WS wrote the manuscript. All authors have read and approved the manuscript.

ACKNOWLEDGMENTS

The authors would like to acknowledge the Tongji-Rongcheng Center for Biomedicine, Huazhong University of Science and Technology. We also thank Qianqian Xu, Jiaxiong Ming, and Yanfang Deng for their help.

REFERENCES

Abdelmegeed, M. A., Banerjee, A., Jang, S., Yoo, S. H., Yun, J. W., Gonzalez, F. J., et al. (2013). CYP2E1 Potentiates Binge Alcohol-Induced Gut Leakiness, Steatohepatitis, and Apoptosis. *Free Radic. Biol. Med.* 65, 1238–1245. doi:10.1016/j.freeradbiomed.2013.09.009

Allaire, M., Rautou, P. E., Codogno, P., and Lotersztajn, S. (2019). Autophagy in Liver Diseases: Time for Translation? *J. Hepatol.* 70, 985–998. doi:10.1016/j.jhep.2019.01.026

Ashburner, M., Ball, C. A., Blake, J. A., Botstein, D., Butler, H., Cherry, J. M., et al. (2000). Gene Ontology: Tool for the Unification of Biology. The Gene Ontology Consortium. *Nat. Genet.* 25, 25–29. doi:10.1038/75556

Brol, M. J., Rösch, F., Schierwagen, R., Magdaleno, F., Uschner, F. E., Manekeller, S., et al. (2019). Combination of CCl4 with Alcoholic and Metabolic Injuries Mimics Human Liver Fibrosis. *Am. J. Physiol. Gastrointest. Liver Physiol.* 317, G182–G194. doi:10.1152/ajpgi.00361.2018

Ceni, E., Mello, T., and Galli, A. (2014). Pathogenesis of Alcoholic Liver Disease: Role of Oxidative Metabolism. *World J. Gastroenterol.* 20, 17756–17772. doi:10.3748/wjg.v20.i47.17756

Chao, X., Wang, S., Zhao, K., Li, Y., Williams, J. A., Li, T., et al. (2018). Impaired TFEB-Mediated Lysosome Biogenesis and Autophagy Promote Chronic Ethanol-Induced Liver Injury and Steatosis in Mice. *Gastroenterology* 155, 865. doi:10.1053/j.gastro.2018.05.027

Dara, L., Ji, C., and Kaplowitz, N. (2011). The Contribution of Endoplasmic Reticulum Stress to Liver Diseases. *Hepatology* 53, 1752–1763. doi:10.1002/hep.24279

Dikic, I., and Elazar, Z. (2018). Mechanism and Medical Implications of Mammalian Autophagy. *Nat. Rev. Mol. Cel Biol* 19, 349–364. doi:10.1038/s41580-018-0003-4

Farfán Labonne, B. E., Gutiérrez, M., Gómez-Quiroz, L. E., Konigsberg Fainstein, M., Bucio, L., Souza, V., et al. (2009). Acetaldehyde-induced Mitochondrial Dysfunction Sensitizes Hepatocytes to Oxidative Damage. *Cell Biol Toxicol* 25, 599–609. doi:10.1007/s10565-008-9115-5

Federico, A., Dallio, M., and Loguercio, C. (2017). Silymarin/Silybin and Chronic Liver Disease: A Marriage of many Years. *Molecules* 22, 191. doi:10.3390/molecules22020191

Fernandes-da-Silva, A., Miranda, C. S., Santana-Oliveira, D. A., Oliveira-Cordeiro, B., Rangel-Azevedo, C., Silva-Veiga, F. M., et al. (2021). Endoplasmic Reticulum Stress as the Basis of Obesity and Metabolic Diseases: Focus on Adipose Tissue, Liver, and Pancreas. *Eur. J. Nutr.* 60, 2949–2960. doi:10.1007/s00394-021-02542-y

Flora, K., Hahn, M., Rosen, H., and Benner, K. (1998). Milk Thistle (Silybum marianum) for the Therapy of Liver Disease. *Am. J. Gastroenterol.* 93, 139–143. doi:10.1111/j.1572-0241.1998.00139.x

Galluzzi, L., and Green, D. R. (2019). Autophagy-independent Functions of the Autophagy Machinery. *Cell* 177, 1682–1699. doi:10.1016/j.cell.2019.05.026

Ganne-Carrié, N., and Nahon, P. (2019). Hepatocellular Carcinoma in the Setting of Alcohol-Related Liver Disease. *J. Hepatol.* 70, 284–293. doi:10.1016/j.jhep.2018.10.008

Gao, B., and Bataller, R. (2011). Alcoholic Liver Disease: Pathogenesis and New Therapeutic Targets. *Gastroenterology* 141, 1572–1585. doi:10.1053/j.gastro.2011.09.002

Gilgenkrantz, H., Mallat, A., Moreau, R., and Lotersztajn, S. (2021). Targeting Cell-Intrinsic Metabolism for Antifibrotic Therapy. *J. Hepatol.* 74, 1442–1454. doi:10.1016/j.jhep.2021.02.012

Gillessen, A., and Schmidt, H. H. (2020). Silymarin as Supportive Treatment in Liver Diseases: A Narrative Review. *Adv. Ther.* 37, 1279–1301. doi:10.1007/s12325-020-01251-y

Götz, S., García-Gómez, J. M., Terol, J., Williams, T. D., Nagaraj, S. H., Nueda, M. J., et al. (2008). High-throughput Functional Annotation and Data Mining with the Blast2GO Suite. *Nucleic Acids Res.* 36, 3420–3435. doi:10.1093/nar/gkn176

Guo, Y., Ye, Q., Yang, S., Wu, J., Ye, B., Wu, Y., et al. (2019). Therapeutic Effects of Polysaccharides from Anoectochilus Roxburghii on Type II Collagen-Induced Arthritis in Rats. *Int. J. Biol. Macromol* 122, 882–892. doi:10.1016/j.ijbiomac.2018.11.015

Hu, Y. B., Ye, X. T., Zhou, Q. Q., and Fu, R. Q. (2018). Sestrin 2 Attenuates Rat Hepatic Stellate Cell (HSC) Activation and Liver Fibrosis via an mTOR/AMPK-dependent Mechanism. *Cell Physiol Biochem* 51, 2111–2122. doi:10.1159/000495829

Hyatt, H. W., Ozdemir, M., Yoshihara, T., Nguyen, B. L., Deminice, R., and Powers, S. K. (2021). Calpains Play an Essential Role in Mechanical Ventilation-Induced Diaphragmatic Weakness and Mitochondrial Dysfunction. *Redox Biol.* 38, 101802. doi:10.1016/j.redox.2020.101802

Ji, C. (2012). Mechanisms of Alcohol-Induced Endoplasmic Reticulum Stress and Organ Injuries. *Biochem. Res. Int.* 2012, 216450. doi:10.1155/2012/216450

Ji, C. (2014). New Insights into the Pathogenesis of Alcohol-Induced ER Stress and Liver Diseases. *Int. J. Hepatol.* 2014, 513787. doi:10.1155/2014/513787

Kong, L. Z., Chandimali, N., Han, Y. H., Lee, D. H., Kim, J. S., Kim, S. U., et al. (2019). Pathogenesis, Early Diagnosis, and Therapeutic Management of Alcoholic Liver Disease. *Int. J. Mol. Sci.* 20, 2712. doi:10.3390/ijms20112712

Lamas-Paz, A., Hao, F., Nelson, L. J., Vázquez, M. T., Canals, S., Gómez Del Moral, M., et al. (2018). Alcoholic Liver Disease: Utility of Animal Models. *World J. Gastroenterol.* 24, 5063–5075. doi:10.3748/wjg.v24.i45.5063

Lebeaupin, C., Vallée, D., Hazari, Y., Hetz, C., Chevet, E., and Bailly-Maitre, B. (2018). Endoplasmic Reticulum Stress Signalling and the Pathogenesis of Non-alcoholic Fatty Liver Disease. *J. Hepatol.* 69, 927–947. doi:10.1016/j.jhep.2018.06.008

Levy, C., Seeff, L. D., and Lindor, K. D. (2004). Use of Herbal Supplements for Chronic Liver Disease. *Clin. Gastroenterol. Hepatol.* 2, 947–956. doi:10.1016/s1542-3565(04)00455-0

Li, X., Sun, R., and Liu, R. (2019). Natural Products in Licorice for the Therapy of Liver Diseases: Progress and Future Opportunities. *Pharmacol. Res.* 144, 210–226. doi:10.1016/j.phrs.2019.04.025

Li, Y., Cifuentes-Pagano, E., DeVallance, E. R., de Jesus, D. S., Sahoo, S., and Meijles, D. N. (2019), NADPH Oxidase 2 Inhibitors CPP11G and CPP11H Attenuate Endothelial Cell Inflammation & Vessel Dysfunction and Restore Mouse Hind-Limb Flow. *Redox Biol.* 22, 101143. doi:10.1016/j.redox.2019.101143

Liang, Y. J., Camacho, C. J., Ross, M., St Croix, C., Pagano, P. J., Huang, Y. H., et al. (2021). Clinical Implications on HBV preS/S Mutations and the Effects of preS2 Deletion on Mitochondria, Liver Fibrosis, and Cancer Development. *Hepatology* 74, 641. doi:10.1002/hep.31789

Liu, B., Deng, X., Jiang, Q., Li, G., Zhang, J., Zhang, N., et al. (2020). Scoparone Improves Hepatic Inflammation and Autophagy in Mice with Nonalcoholic Steatohepatitis by Regulating the ROS/P38/Nrf2 axis and PI3K/AKT/mTOR Pathway in Macrophages. *Biomed. Pharmacother.* 125, 109895. doi:10.1016/j.biopha.2020.109895

Liu, Y., Tang, T., Duan, S., Li, C., Lin, Q., Wu, H., et al. (2020). The Purification, Structural Characterization and Antidiabetic Activity of a Polysaccharide from Anoectochilus Roxburghii. *Food Funct.* 11, 3730–3740. doi:10.1039/c9fo00860h

Ma, Y. Y., Di, Z. M., Cao, Q., Xu, W. S., Bi, S. X., Yu, J. S., et al. (2020). Xanthatin Induces Glioma Cell Apoptosis and Inhibits Tumor Growth via Activating

Endoplasmic Reticulum Stress-dependent CHOP Pathway. *Acta Pharmacol. Sin* 41, 404–414. doi:10.1038/s41401-019-0318-5

Maiers, J. L., and Malhi, H. (2019). Endoplasmic Reticulum Stress in Metabolic Liver Diseases and Hepatic Fibrosis. *Semin. Liver Dis.* 39, 235–248. doi:10.1055/s-0039-1681032

Meng, X., Li, Y., Li, S., Gan, R. Y., and Li, H. B. (2018). Natural Products for Prevention and Treatment of Chemical-Induced Liver Injuries. *Compr. Rev. Food Sci. Food Saf.* 17, 472–495. doi:10.1111/1541-4337.12335

Ming, J., Xu, Q., Gao, L., Deng, Y., Yin, J., Zhou, Q., et al. (2021). Kinsenoside Alleviates 17α-Ethinylestradiol-Induced Cholestatic Liver Injury in Rats by Inhibiting Inflammatory Responses and Regulating FXR-Mediated Bile Acid Homeostasis. *Pharmaceuticals* 14, 452. doi:10.3390/ph14050452

Parola, M., and Pinzani, M. (2019). Liver Fibrosis: Pathophysiology, Pathogenetic Targets and Clinical Issues. *Mol. Aspects Med.* 65, 37–55. doi:10.1016/j.mam.2018.09.002

Qi, C. X., Zhou, Q., Yuan, Z., Luo, Z. W., Dai, C., Zhu, H. C., et al. (2018). Kinsenoside: A Promising Bioactive Compound from Anoectochilus Species. *Curr. Med. Sci.* 38, 11–18. doi:10.1007/s11596-018-1841-1

Ross, P. L., Huang, Y. N., Marchese, J. N., Williamson, B., Parker, K., Hattan, S., et al. (2004). Multiplexed Protein Quantitation in *Saccharomyces cerevisiae* Using Amine-Reactive Isobaric Tagging Reagents. *Mol. Cel Proteomics* 3, 1154–1169. doi:10.1074/mcp.M400129-MCP200

Satishchandran, A., Ambade, A., Rao, S., Hsueh, Y. C., Iracheta-Vellve, A., Tornai, D., et al. (2018). MicroRNA 122, Regulated by GRLH2, Protects Livers of Mice and Patients from Ethanol-Induced Liver Disease. *Gastroenterology* 154, 238. doi:10.1053/j.gastro.2017.09.022

Seitz, H. K., Bataller, R., Cortez-Pinto, H., Gao, B., Gual, A., Lackner, C., et al. (2018). Alcoholic Liver Disease. *Nat. Rev. Dis. Primers* 4, 16. doi:10.1038/s41572-018-0014-7

Tang, T., Duan, X., Ke, Y., Zhang, L., Shen, Y., Hu, B., et al. (2018). Antidiabetic Activities of Polysaccharides from Anoectochilus Roxburghii and Anoectochilus Formosanus in STZ-Induced Diabetic Mice. *Int. J. Biol. Macromol* 112, 882–888. doi:10.1016/j.ijbiomac.2018.02.042

Tong, M., Zheng, Q., Liu, M., Chen, L., Lin, Y.-H., Tang, S. G., et al. (2021). 5-methoxytryptophan Alleviates Liver Fibrosis by Modulating FOXO3a/miR-21/ATG5 Signaling Pathway Mediated Autophagy. *Cell cycle* 20, 676–688. doi:10.1080/15384101.2021.1897241

Turco, E., Witt, M., Abert, C., Bock-Bierbaum, T., Su, M. Y., Trapannone, R., et al. (2019). How RB1CC1/FIP200 Claws its Way to Autophagic Engulfment of SQSTM1/p62-Ubiquitin Condensates. *Autophagy* 15, 1475–1477. doi:10.1080/15548627.2019.1615306

Wang, L., Khambu, B., Zhang, H., and Yin, X. M. (2015). Autophagy in Alcoholic Liver Disease, Self-Eating Triggered by Drinking. *Clin. Res. Hepatol. Gastroenterol.* 39 (Suppl. 1), S2–S6. doi:10.1016/j.clinre.2015.05.023

Wang, Y., Li, C., Gu, J., Chen, C., Duanmu, J., Miao, J., et al. (2020). Celastrol Exerts Anti-inflammatory Effect in Liver Fibrosis via Activation of AMPK-SIRT3 Signalling. *J. Cel Mol Med* 24, 941–953. doi:10.1111/jcmm.14805

Wang, Y., Zuo, R., Wang, Z., Luo, L., Wu, J., Zhang, C., et al. (2019). Kinsenoside Ameliorates Intervertebral Disc Degeneration through the Activation of AKT-Erk1/2-Nrf2 Signaling Pathway. *Aging (Albany NY)* 11, 7961–7977. doi:10.18632/aging.102302

Wiśniewski, J. R., Zougman, A., Nagaraj, N., and Mann, M. (2009). Universal Sample Preparation Method for Proteome Analysis. *Nat. Methods* 6, 359–362. doi:10.1038/nmeth.1322

World Health Organization (2018). Global Status Report on Alcohol and Health 2018. Available at: https://apps.who.int/iris/handle/10665/274603 (Accessed July 12, 2021).

Xiang, H., Zhang, J., Lin, C., Zhang, L., Liu, B., and Ouyang, L. (2020). Targeting Autophagy-Related Protein Kinases for Potential Therapeutic Purpose. *Acta Pharm. Sin B* 10, 569–581. doi:10.1016/j.apsb.2019.10.003

Xiang, M., Liu, T., Tan, W., Ren, H., Li, H., Liu, J., et al. (2016). Effects of Kinsenoside, a Potential Immunosuppressive Drug for Autoimmune Hepatitis, on Dendritic cells/CD8+ T Cells Communication in Mice. *Hepatology* 64, 2135–2150. doi:10.1002/hep.28825

Ye, S., Shao, Q., and Zhang, A. (2017). Anoectochilus Roxburghii: A Review of its Phytochemistry, Pharmacology, and Clinical Applications. *J. Ethnopharmacol* 209, 184–202. doi:10.1016/j.jep.2017.07.032

Ying, W. (2008). NAD+/NADH and NADP+/NADPH in Cellular Functions and Cell Death: Regulation and Biological Consequences. *Antioxid. Redox Signal.* 10, 179–206. doi:10.1089/ars.2007.1672

You, M., Matsumoto, M., Pacold, C. M., Cho, W. K., and Crabb, D. W. (2004). The Role of AMP-Activated Protein Kinase in the Action of Ethanol in the Liver. *Gastroenterology* 127, 1798–1808. doi:10.1053/j.gastro.2004.09.049

You, Y., Li, W. Z., Zhang, S., Hu, B., Li, Y. X., Li, H. D., et al. (2018). SNX10 Mediates Alcohol-Induced Liver Injury and Steatosis by Regulating the Activation of Chaperone-Mediated Autophagy. *J. Hepatol.* 69, 129–141. doi:10.1016/j.jhep.2018.01.038

Zhong, W., Zhang, W., Li, Q., Xie, G., Sun, Q., Sun, X., et al. (2015). Pharmacological Activation of Aldehyde Dehydrogenase 2 by Alda-1 Reverses Alcohol-Induced Hepatic Steatosis and Cell Death in Mice. *J. Hepatol.* 62, 1375–1381. doi:10.1016/j.jhep.2014.12.022

Zhou, F., Mei, J., Han, X., Li, H., Yang, S., Wang, M., et al. (2019). Kinsenoside Attenuates Osteoarthritis by Repolarizing Macrophages through Inactivating NF-Kb/MAPK Signaling and Protecting Chondrocytes. *Acta Pharm. Sin B* 9, 973–985. doi:10.1016/j.apsb.2019.01.015

Permissions

All chapters in this book were first published Frontiers; hereby published with permission under the Creative Commons Attribution License or equivalent. Every chapter published in this book has been scrutinized by our experts. Their significance has been extensively debated. The topics covered herein carry significant findings which will fuel the growth of the discipline. They may even be implemented as practical applications or may be referred to as a beginning point for another development.

The contributors of this book come from diverse backgrounds, making this book a truly international effort. This book will bring forth new frontiers with its revolutionizing research information and detailed analysis of the nascent developments around the world.

We would like to thank all the contributing authors for lending their expertise to make the book truly unique. They have played a crucial role in the development of this book. Without their invaluable contributions this book wouldn't have been possible. They have made vital efforts to compile up to date information on the varied aspects of this subject to make this book a valuable addition to the collection of many professionals and students.

This book was conceptualized with the vision of imparting up-to-date information and advanced data in this field. To ensure the same, a matchless editorial board was set up. Every individual on the board went through rigorous rounds of assessment to prove their worth. After which they invested a large part of their time researching and compiling the most relevant data for our readers.

The editorial board has been involved in producing this book since its inception. They have spent rigorous hours researching and exploring the diverse topics which have resulted in the successful publishing of this book. They have passed on their knowledge of decades through this book. To expedite this challenging task, the publisher supported the team at every step. A small team of assistant editors was also appointed to further simplify the editing procedure and attain best results for the readers.

Apart from the editorial board, the designing team has also invested a significant amount of their time in understanding the subject and creating the most relevant covers. They scrutinized every image to scout for the most suitable representation of the subject and create an appropriate cover for the book.

The publishing team has been an ardent support to the editorial, designing and production team. Their endless efforts to recruit the best for this project, has resulted in the accomplishment of this book. They are a veteran in the field of academics and their pool of knowledge is as vast as their experience in printing. Their expertise and guidance has proved useful at every step. Their uncompromising quality standards have made this book an exceptional effort. Their encouragement from time to time has been an inspiration for everyone.

The publisher and the editorial board hope that this book will prove to be a valuable piece of knowledge for researchers, students, practitioners and scholars across the globe.

List of Contributors

Xiao-Han Tang, Marta Melis and Lorraine J. Gudas
Department of Pharmacology, Weill Cornell Medical College of Cornell University, New York, United States

Karen Mai
Nutrition Program, Hunter College, City University of New York, New York, United States

Steven E. Trasino
Department of Pharmacology, Weill Cornell Medical College of Cornell University, New York, United States
Nutrition Program, Hunter College, City University of New York, New York, United States

Manuela G. Neuman
In Vitro Drug Safety and Biotechnology, Department of Pharmacology and Toxicology, Temerity Faculty of Medicine, University of Toronto, Toronto, ON, Canada

Johannes Mueller
Center for Alcohol Research, University of Heidelberg, Heidelberg, Germany

Sebastian Mueller
Center for Alcohol Research, University of Heidelberg, Heidelberg, Germany
Department of Internal Medicine, Salem Medical Center, Heidelberg, Germany

Kalibixiati Aimulajiang
State Key Laboratory of Pathogenesis, Prevention, and Treatment of High Incidence Diseases in Central Asia, The First Affiliated Hospital of Xinjiang Medical University, Urumqi, China

Zongding Wang, Tiemin Jiang, Tuerganaili Aji and Hao Wen
State Key Laboratory of Pathogenesis, Prevention, and Treatment of High Incidence Diseases in Central Asia, The First Affiliated Hospital of Xinjiang Medical University, Urumqi, China
Hepatobiliary and Hydatid Disease Department, First Affiliated Hospital of Xinjiang Medical University, Urumqi, China

Xiaoyan Liang, Yanmei Lu, Huaxin Sun, Ling Zhang, Xianhui Zhou and Baopeng Tang
Department of Pacing and Electrophysiology, The First Affiliated Hospital of Xinjiang Medical University, Xinjiang, China
Xinjiang Key Laboratory of Cardiac Electrophysiology and Cardiac Remodeling, The First Affiliated Hospital of Xinjiang Medical University, Xinjiang, China

Antonio Riva, Elena Palma, Dhruti Devshi, Roger Williams and Shilpa Chokshi
Institute of Hepatology, Foundation for Liver Research, London, United Kingdom
Faculty of Life Sciences & Medicine, King's College London, London, United Kingdom

Debbie Shawcross
Faculty of Life Sciences & Medicine, King's College London, London, United Kingdom

Gavin Wright and Sarah Fairclough
Department of Gastroenterology, Basildon University Hospital, Basildon, United Kingdom

Douglas Corrigall
Institute of Hepatology, Foundation for Liver Research, London, United Kingdom
Faculty of Life Sciences & Medicine, King's College London, London, United Kingdom
Department of Gastroenterology, Basildon University Hospital, Basildon, United Kingdom

Alexander Evans
Department of Gastroenterology, Royal Berkshire Hospital, Reading, United Kingdom

Huyen Adams
Institute of Hepatology, Foundation for Liver Research, London, United Kingdom
Faculty of Life Sciences & Medicine, King's College London, London, United Kingdom
Department of Gastroenterology, Royal Berkshire Hospital, Reading, United Kingdom

Nigel Heaton, Krishna Menon, Melissa Preziosi and Ane Zamalloa
Institute of Liver Studies, King's College London, London, United Kingdom

Rosa Miquel
Liver Histopathology Laboratory, Institute of Liver Studies, King's College Hospital, London, United Kingdom

Jennifer M. Ryan
Gastrointestinal and Liver Services, Royal Free Hospital, London, United Kingdom

Robert Schierwagen, Sabine Klein and Frank E. Uschner
Translational Hepatology, Department of Internal Medicine I, University Hospital Frankfurt, Frankfurt, Germany

Michael Praktiknjo
Department of Internal Medicine I, University of Bonn, Bonn, Germany

Krum Katzarov, Tanya Hadzhiolova, Slava Pavlova and Marieta Simonova
Department of Gastroenterology, Hepatobiliary Surgery and Transplantology, Military Medical Academy, Sofia, Bulgaria

Jonel Trebicka
Translational Hepatology, Department of Internal Medicine I, University Hospital Frankfurt, Frankfurt, Germany
European Foundation for the Study of Chronic Liver Failure (EF-CLIF), Barcelona, Spain

Bei Gao, Atoosa Emami, Rongrong Zhou, Sonja Lang, Rohit Loomba and David A. Brenner
Department of Medicine, University of California, San Diego, San Diego, CA, United States

Yi Duan, Yanhan Wang, Lu Jiang and Bernd Schnabl
Department of Medicine, University of California, San Diego, San Diego, CA, United States
Department of Medicine, VA San Diego Healthcare System, San Diego, CA, United States

Peter Stärkel
St. Luc University Hospital, Université catholique de Louvain, Brussels, Belgium

Clayton W. Jordan, Elizabeth M. Staab and Sarah A. Sweeney
Department of Internal Medicine, University of Nebraska Medical Center, Omaha, NE, United States

Karuna Rasineni, Paul G. Thomes and Jacy L. Kubik
Department of Internal Medicine, University of Nebraska Medical Center, Omaha, NE, United States
Research Service, Veterans Affairs Nebraska-Western Iowa Health Care System, Omaha, NE, United States

Geoffrey A. Talmon
Department of Pathology and Microbiology, University of Nebraska Medical Center, Omaha, NE, United States

Terrence M. Donohue, Kusum K. Kharbanda and Carol A. Casey
Department of Internal Medicine, University of Nebraska Medical Center, Omaha, NE, United States
Research Service, Veterans Affairs Nebraska-Western Iowa Health Care System, Omaha, NE, United States
Department of Biochemistry and Molecular Biology, University of Nebraska Medical Center, Omaha, NE, United States

Mark A. McNiven
Department of Biochemistry and Molecular Biology and the Center for Digestive Diseases, Mayo Clinic, Rochester, MN, United States

Ran Yan and Ning Zhang
Department of Pharmacy, The Second Hospital of Dalian Medical University, Dalian, China

Xiaohui Kang, Yan Zhao, Zhecheng Wang, Ruimin Sun and Jihong Yao
College of Pharmacy, Dalian Medical University, Dalian, China

Junyi Chu, Sai Wang, Guoyang Li, Yan Hu and Musen Lin
Department of Pharmacy, The Second Hospital of Dalian Medical University, Dalian, China
College of Pharmacy, Dalian Medical University, Dalian, China

Wen Shan
Department of Pharmacy, The Second Hospital of Dalian Medical University, Dalian, China
Department of Pharmacy, The Third Hospital of Dalian Medical University, Dalian, China

Hongwei Lin, Qianjing Du, Tongtong Pan, Hanxiao Tu, Yuedong Xu, Teng Teng, Jingjing Tu, Ji Li, Zhuo Lin, Xiaodong Wang, Lanman Xu and Yong-Ping Chen
Department of Infectious Diseases, The First Affiliated Hospital of Wenzhou Medical University, Zhejiang Provincial Key Laboratory for Accurate Diagnosis and Treatment of Chronic Liver Diseases, Hepatology Institute of Wenzhou Medical University, Wenzhou, China

Dazhi Chen
Department of Gastroenterology, Peking University First Hospital, Beijing, China

Pengyi Zhang, Ruolin Gao, Wenting Shi, Bo Sui and Xuewen Tian
School of Sports and Health, Shandong Sport University, Jinan, China

Xiangjing Meng
Shandong Academy of Pharmaceutical Science, Jinan, China

Weiya Wang
School of Sports and Health, Shandong Sport University, Jinan, China
Shandong Academy of Pharmaceutical Science, Jinan, China

Min Mao
Department of Allied Health, University of North Carolina at Chapel Hill, Chapel Hill, NC, United States

Dongmei Li and Richard Calderone
Department of Microbiology and Immunology, Georgetown University Medical Center, Washington, DC, United States

Tian-xiang Zheng, Shi-lin Pu, Bao-lin Qian and Hao Chen
Department of Hepatobiliary Surgery, The Affiliated Hospital of Southwest Medical University, Luzhou, China

Peng Tan, Yi-chao Du and Mei-zhou Huang
Academician (Expert) Workstation of Sichuan Province, The Affiliated Hospital of Southwest Medical University, Luzhou, China

Wen-guang Fu
Department of Hepatobiliary Surgery, The Affiliated Hospital of Southwest Medical University, Luzhou, China
Academician (Expert) Workstation of Sichuan Province, The Affiliated Hospital of Southwest Medical University, Luzhou, China

Yuan-yuan Li, Yu-juan Zhong, Qi Cheng, Ying-zhao Wang, Yuan-yuan Fan, Cheng-fang Yang and Li Li
College of Pharmacy, Guilin Medical University, Guilin, China

Zuheng Ma
Department of Molecular Medicine and Surgery, Karolinska Institutet, Stockholm, Sweden

Yong-wen Li
College of Pharmacy, Guilin Medical University, Guilin, China
Center for Diabetic Systems Medicine, Guangxi Key Laboratory of Excellence, Guilin, China

Hongjiao Xiang and Junmin Wang
Institute of Interdisciplinary Integrative Medicine Research, Shanghai University of Traditional Chinese Medicine, Shanghai, China

Yifei Lu
Yueyang Hospital of Integrated Traditional Chinese and Western Medicine, Shanghai University of Traditional Chinese Medicine, Shanghai, China

Mingmei Shao
Teaching Department, Baoshan District Hospital of Intergrated Traditional Chinese and Western Medicine, Shanghai, China

Guang Ji
Institute of Digestive Disease, Longhua Hospital, Shanghai University of Traditional Chinese Medicine, Shanghai, China

Tao Wu
Institute of Interdisciplinary Integrative Medicine Research, Shanghai University of Traditional Chinese Medicine, Shanghai, China
Institute of Digestive Disease, Longhua Hospital, Shanghai University of Traditional Chinese Medicine, Shanghai, China

Ruichao Yue
Center for Translational Biomedical Research, University of North Carolina at Greensboro, North Carolina Research Campus, Kannapolis, NC, United States

Xiaoyuan Wei and Jiangchao Zhao
Division of Agriculture, Department of Animal Science, University of Arkansas, Fayetteville, AR, United States

Zhanxiang Zhou and Wei Zhong
Center for Translational Biomedical Research, University of North Carolina at Greensboro, North Carolina Research Campus, Kannapolis, NC, United States
Department of Nutrition, University of North Carolina at Greensboro, North Carolina Research Campus, Kannapolis, NC, United States

Muhammad Waleed and Mohamed A. Abdallah
Department of Medicine, University of South Dakota Sanford School of Medicine, Sioux Falls, SD, United States

Yong-Fang Kuo
Department of Biostatistics, University of Texas Medical Branch at Galveston, Galveston, TX, United States

Juan P. Arab
Departamento de Gastroenterología, Escuela de Medicina, Pontificia Universidad Católica de Chile, Santiago, Chile

Robert Wong
Division of Gastroenterology and Hepatology, Alameda Health System Highland Hospital, Oakland, CA, United States

Ashwani K. Singal
Department of Medicine, University of South Dakota Sanford School of Medicine, Sioux Falls, SD, United States
Division of Transplant Hepatology, Avera Transplant Institute, Sioux Falls, SD, United States

Wenwen Yang
School of Public Health, Zhejiang Chinese Medical University, Hangzhou, China
School of Life Science, Zhejiang Chinese Medical University, Hangzhou, China

Qiang Han
School of Public Health, Zhejiang Chinese Medical University, Hangzhou, China
Academy of Chinese Medical Sciences, Zhejiang Chinese Medical University, Hangzhou, China

Qianyu Qian
School of Life Science, Zhejiang Chinese Medical University, Hangzhou, China
Molecular Medicine Institute, Zhejiang Chinese Medical University, Hangzhou, China

Qinchao Ding
School of Life Science, Zhejiang Chinese Medical University, Hangzhou, China
Academy of Chinese Medical Sciences, Zhejiang Chinese Medical University, Hangzhou, China

Xiaobing Dou
School of Public Health, Zhejiang Chinese Medical University, Hangzhou, China
School of Life Science, Zhejiang Chinese Medical University, Hangzhou, China
Molecular Medicine Institute, Zhejiang Chinese Medical University, Hangzhou, China

Zhongyan Du
Academy of Chinese Medical Sciences, Zhejiang Chinese Medical University, Hangzhou, China

Songtao Li
School of Public Health, Zhejiang Chinese Medical University, Hangzhou, China
Molecular Medicine Institute, Zhejiang Chinese Medical University, Hangzhou, China
Academy of Chinese Medical Sciences, Zhejiang Chinese Medical University, Hangzhou, China

Cui Wang
School of Life Science, Zhejiang Chinese Medical University, Hangzhou, China
Molecular Medicine Institute, Zhejiang Chinese Medical University, Hangzhou, China
Academy of Chinese Medical Sciences, Zhejiang Chinese Medical University, Hangzhou, China

Yibin Fan
Department of Dermatology, Zhejiang Provincial People's Hospital, People's Hospital of Hangzhou Medical College, Hangzhou, China

Liang Zhao, Arshad Mehmood, Maryam Iftikhar and Chengtao Wang
Beijing Advance Innovation Center for Food Nutrition and Human Health, Beijing Engineering and Technology Research Center of Food Additives, Beijing Technology and Business University, Beijing, China

Mohamed Mohamed Soliman
Clinical Laboratory Sciences Department, Turabah University College, Taif University, Taif, Saudi Arabia

Asra Iftikhar
Department of Pharmacy, Faculty of Pharmaceutical Sciences, The University of Faisalabad, Faisalabad, Pakistan

Salama Mostafa Aboelenin
Biology Department, Turabah University College, Taif University, Taif, Saudi Arabia

Limin Gao and Hong Ren
Biobank, Union Hospital, Tongji Medical College, Huazhong University of Science and Technology, Wuhan, China

Xingyu Chen
Department of Clinical Laboratory, the Central Hospital of Wuhan, Wuhan, China

Zeyu Fu
Department of Anesthesiology, Union Hospital, Tongji Medical College, Huazhong University of Science and Technology, Wuhan, China

Jie Yin, Yafen Wang, Weiguang Sun and Yonghui Zhang
Hubei Key Laboratory of Natural Medicinal Chemistry and Resource Evaluation, School of Pharmacy, Tongji Medical College, Huazhong University of Science and Technology, Wuhan, China

Index

www.ingramcontent.com/pod-product-compliance
Lightning Source LLC
LaVergne TN
LVHW060516210926
848485LV00005B/1087
9781639278640